MOLECULAR IMAGING

Edited by **Bernhard Schaller**

Molecular Imaging
Edited by Bernhard Schaller

Published by InTech

Janeza Trdine 9, 51000 Rijeka, Croatia

Publishing Process Manager Martina Durovic

Technical Editor Teodora Smiljanic

Cover Designer InTech Design Team

Additional hard copies can be obtained from orders@intechopen.com

Molecular Imaging, Edited by Bernhard Schaller
p. cm.
ISBN 978-953-51-0359-2

For EU product safety concerns:
IN TECH d.o.o., Prolaz Marije Krucifikse Kozulić 3, 51000 Rijeka, Croatia,
info@intechopen.com or visit our website at intechopen.com.

Meet the editor

Bernhard Schaller (MD, PhD, DSC) studied Medicine in Switzerland and Biochemistry in Sweden and Great Britain. In later years, he developed an interest in Molecular Imaging and since than has been integrating this method into his other research activities. His principal contributions are in molecular imaging of stroke, brain and spinal tumors as well as stem cell therapy.

Contents

Preface

Molecular Imaging represents a unique project that was only possible by the exceptional InTech support. The authors of the book give therefore an overview of the relatively new topic of molecular imaging, with broad background to basic but also clinical sciences. The present book is best suited not only for the beginners in the area to gain some overview of the feature, but also for professionals to see trends of other groups from all over the world.

Molecular imaging has rapidly gained influence in medicine, not only for different research projects, but also in the view of personalized medicine. The door for personalized medicine is now widely open. Also in this direction, the present book gives more than only a little food for thought.

Even if *Molecular Imaging* covers a broad part of the whole topic, it was and it is not our goal to be comprehensive. Such a project can never be complete, and different authors from all over the world can only give some insights of their daily work. Ideas how molecular imaging will develop in the near future present a special delicacy.

We hope that readers will enjoy this book. I would like to thank all those who made the project possible, especially Ms Pantar and Mrs Durovic from InTech. They both were angels for the authors.

Prof. Bernhard Schaller, MD, PhD, DSC
Department of Neurosurgery,
University of Paris 7, Paris,
France

Part 1

Background, Theories and Methods of Molecular Imaging

1

Modern Quantitative Techniques for PET/CT/MR Hybrid Imaging

Babak Saboury*, Mateen Moghbel*, Sandip Basu and Abass Alavi
Radiology Department, School of Medicine, University of Pennsylvania, USA

1. Introduction

The relentless progress that is being made in tomographic imaging modalities is inexorably expanding the application of positron emission tomography (PET) in the clinical field. Some of the most noteworthy advances involve innovations in quantitative techniques for hybrid imaging modalities such as PET/Computed Tomography (CT) and PET/Magnetic Resonance Imaging (MRI), which have greatly improved the ability to segment and analyze functional images produced with radiotracers such as (^{18}F) Fluorodeoxyglucose (FDG). With continued technological progress, quantitative approaches can supplant the more subjective qualitative and semi-quantitative techniques that currently dominate the clinical use of PET.

Although it does not meet the rigorous standards for objectivity in medical research, the qualitative method of visual assessment continues to be very prevalent in the clinical field. The benefits of this technique's simplicity are offset by its immense subjectivity and the consequent lack of reproducibility and pervasiveness of inter-reader variability. These limitations are mitigated in the somewhat more consistent semi-quantitative technique of standardized uptake value (SUV), but concerns about reproducibility still linger. The manual delineation of the regions of interest (ROIs) within an image maintains a degree of subjectivity that hinders the reproducibility of the analysis. Therefore, while these methodologies may be less demanding, they open the door to the possibility of variability.

Using structural and functional imaging, namely PET/CT and PET/MRI, and combining structural information with functional data by various quantitative techniques provide a far more objective method of image analysis, but also carry their own set of inherent difficulties. This method of quantification is far more technically demanding and requires complex mathematical computations[1,2].

Despite its limitations, it appears likely that quantitative analysis of hybrid imaging will become the method of choice in the future. Recent developments in tomographic imaging have improved the ability of PET to accurately assess global function in addition to the more conventional ROI analysis. Global assessment, which combines data on the activity of a lesion measured by PET and its segmented volume defined by CT, has wide-reaching applications in a diverse range of medical fields. The viability of this alternative method

---

* Co-First Authors

depends on the accuracy of segmentation and quantification, as well as the alleviation of some of the inherent obstacles of hybrid imaging.

2. Classifications of PET data analysis

The techniques employed for the analysis of functional images can be subdivided into three categories: qualitative, semi-quantitative, and quantitative. The first of these three is by far the most subjective, and entails the visual interpretation of data by human observers. The second utilizes indices such as SUV and lesion-to-background ratio to measure activity in assigned regions of interest. Lastly, the third employs more complex mathematical and technical processes, such as non-linear regression and Patlak-Gjedde graphical analysis. Despite the superior reproducibility and objectivity it provides, this final technique is arguably rendered impractical for clinical use by its technical rigors. On the other hand, the other two techniques are far more susceptible to both inter-reader and intra-reader variability, but are widely employed due to their simplicity.

3. Models for quantifying absolute glucose metabolic rate

The metabolic rate of glucose is estimated with the aid of FDG, an analog of glucose that is currently the most widely used PET radiotracer[3,4,5]. The metabolism of FDG is in turn measured through kinetic modeling of the data[6]. This process reveals a series of rate constants that shed light not only on the absolute metabolic rate, but also the steps within glucose metabolism.

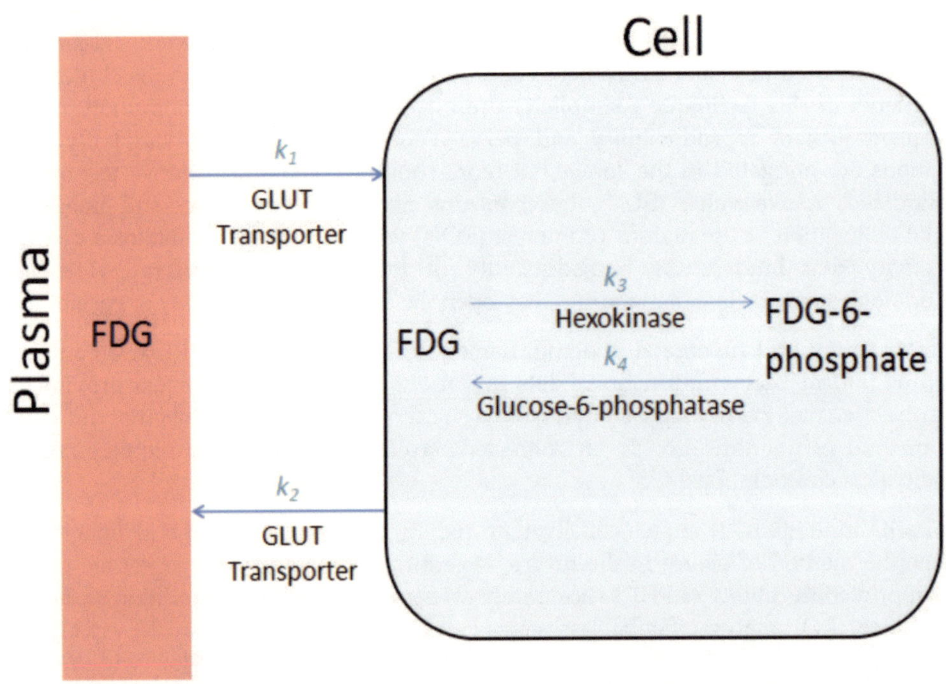

Fig. 1. The three-compartment model involves the transport of FDG from the plasma to the cell, as well as the phosphorylation and dephosphorylation of FDG within the cell. Simpler models ignore the dephosphorylation of FDG, thereby eliminating the k_4 rate constant.

When dealing with FDG, the tracer kinetic model comprises three compartments that encompass the processes of transportation and phosphorylation. More specifically, these compartments demarcate the FDG in the blood plasma, the FDG in the cell, and the FDG-6-phosphate in the cell (**Fig. 1**). The first compartment (C1) is assumed to be open, with free exchange with other tissues in the body. It is for this reason that the input function of this compartment (i.e., FDG levels in the plasma) cannot be calculated and must be measured by arterial sampling. The second compartment (C2) refers to FDG that is in the tissue and not in the vasculature. These pools of FDG in the cell are available for phosphorylation by hexokinase. Once FDG is in its phosphorylated form, it occupies the third compartment (C3).

If a kinetic model accounts for the dephosphorylation of FDG-6-phosphate by glucose-6-phosphatase in addition to transportation and phosphorylation, it is termed "reversible."[7] However, this three-compartment model is far from the only one in use; more simplified "irreversible" models often ignore the dephosphorylation of FDG on the assumption that the incorporation of fewer parameters will lower variance.[1] These methods include non-linear regression analysis, which estimates a single rate constant K_i in the place of k_1, k_2, and k_3, and Patlak-Gjedde graphical analysis, which calculates activity as a function of the concentration, distribution volume, and net rate of influx of FDG.[8]

By applying this simplified irreversible model to dynamic PET data, non-linear regression analysis can estimate the net rate of FDG influx. The advantages of this method of quantification include its lack of dependence on the length of time over which uptake occurs and its ability to provide insight into the rate constants behind glucose metabolism. But on the other hand, the technical complexity of the method makes it demanding and time-consuming, with the required arterial sampling only exacerbating these issues.

In comparison to non-linear regression, the method of Patlak-Gjedde graphical analysis is more robust due to a simpler scanning protocol that is less susceptible to noise. This technique, which also has the ability to produce parametric images, is modeled by the following equation:

$$c(t) = \lambda \cdot c_p(t) + K_i \int_0^t c_p(\tau)d\tau$$

where

$c(t)$ = activity in the tissue as measured by the PET scanner at time t,

$c_p(t)$ = concentration of FDG in the plasma,

λ = distribution volume of FDG,

K_i = net rate of FDG influx into the tissue, and

τ is a dummy integration variable

Unlike non-linear regression, Patlak-Gjedde graphical analysis cannot calculate individual rate constants for the metabolism of glucose. But similar to non-linear regression, it requires dynamic scanning, which carries with it a host of limitations.

Dynamic scanning, which is crucial to both non-linear regression and Patlak-Gjedde graphical analysis, entails an extended sequence of acquisitions that are subsequently reconstructed. The high availability of dynamic data, which is comparatively less dependent on imaging time, works to the advantage of these quantitative techniques. On the other hand, the rigors of the procedure make it technically demanding and time-consuming. Moreover, since only one bed position can be assumed per scan, each lesion may have to be acquired separately. The need to quantify FDG concentration in the plasma also necessitates arterial blood sampling at several points during the scan.

The arterial sampling performed during dynamic scans allows for the extrapolation of time-vs.-activity curves, which can yield rate constants through non-linear least squares approximation. This approach to quantifying FDG activity is certainly more objective than more popular alternatives such as SUV and visual assessment, but is far from immune to error. First and foremost, the assumption that FDG-6-phosphate is not dephosphorylated once it is inside the cell is overly simplistic and can lead to inaccurate estimates. Variance due to imaging noise and partial-volume effects further limit these methods of quantification.

In addition to non-linear regression and Patlak-Gjedde graphical analysis, there exist other, more simplified kinetic methods for quantifying the rate of glucose metabolism. This is done using only a single static scan, albeit with somewhat lower accuracy. An autoradiographic method developed by Sokoloff *et al.* is one such single-scan method, but is still limited by the need of arterial sampling to determine FDG concentration[9,10]. A similar technique devised by Hunter *et al.* is able to quantify metabolic rates with the aid of limited venous blood sampling[11].

4. Quantification of activity through SUV

Standardized uptake value (SUV)—also known as differential absorption ratio (DAR), differential uptake ratio (DUR), and standardized uptake ratio (SUR)—is currently the most common semi-quantitative index employed in the clinical field. It has the ability to measure FDG metabolism through tracer concentration in the tissue. It is calculated according to the following formula:

$$SUV = \frac{Mean\,ROI\,concentration(MBq\,/\,ml)}{Injected\,dose(MBq)/Body\,weight(g)} \times \frac{1}{decay\,factor\,of\,^{18}F}$$

The advantages of SUV lie in its ease of use; when compared to the aforementioned kinetic models, SUV is far less technically demanding and computationally complex. The fact that its values are automatically estimated by software makes the SUV method highly expedient for clinical use. The lack of dependency on arterial sampling and the comparatively short scanning time also work in its favor. In spite of these shortcuts, kinetic modeling reveals a strong correlation between SUV and glucose metabolic rate. However, that is not to say that SUV measurements are not just as—if not more—prone to error than kinetic modeling (**Table 1**).

Currently, PET scanners are most often normalized to the body weight of the patient. This causes the systematic overestimation of SUV in obese patients, since adipose tissue demonstrates comparatively low FDG uptake because of its dampened metabolic activity. Studies that employed the parameters of lean body mass and body surface area instead of body weight were found to be more accurate[12,13,14].

a. Patient-Related Factors

Factor	Effects	Corrective measures
Body size and habitus (3.3)	SUV in obese patients overestimates FDG uptake relative to normal patients	Use of lean body mass (SUV_{LBM}) or body surface area (SUV_{BSA})
Serum glucose levels (3.4)	Reduced FDG uptake in target tissues with increasing blood glucose levels	Control of blood glucose before administering FDG and applying correction factor for glucose level
Organ and lesion motion	Reduction of SUV	Respiratory gating or 4D reconstruction

b. Technical Factors

Factor	Effects	Corrective measures
Duration of uptake period (3.5)	Increase in SUV with increasing time in malignant lesions	Standardization of time of image acquisition
Attenuation correction and reconstruction methods (spatial filter kernel, image resolution, number of iterations)	Underestimation of SUV with highly smoothed reconstruction	Standardize acquisition and reconstruction algorithms
Partial-volume effects (4.1, 4.2)	Underestimation of SUV in lesions with diameters smaller than 2-3 × spatial resolution	Adopt an optimal partial volume correction factor
Size of the ROI and non-uniformity of tracer distribution in the lesion	Low SUV_{mean} for large ROIs and high random errors in smaller ROIs	Standard size ROIs placed reproducibly in the same location, SUV_{max} preferable to SUV_{mean}.
Organ and lesion motion	Mismatch between EM and CT data	Respiratory gating or 4D reconstruction

Table 1. Factors influencing standardized uptake value (SUV) determination for FDG at intended regions of interest, their undesirable effects, and associated required corrective measures. (Based on Basu *et al.* [95] with permission from Elsevier Inc.).

5. Effect of respiratory motion on SUV

The accuracy of quantification through PET/CT imaging is affected by several factors. Historically, one of the most problematic factors—especially in the scanning of thoracic lesions or non-small cell cancers—has been respiratory motion, which impacts diagnostic and staging accuracy. Misregistration due to respiratory motion in the thorax and abdomen between data acquired through PET and CT was reported soon after commercial introduction of PET/CT and has been one of the most challenging research topics in the field.

Fast gantry rotation of less than one second per revolution and sizeable detector coverage of over 2 cm enable CT systems to scan over 100 cm in the cranial-caudal direction in 20 seconds. By comparison, PET typically requires 2 to 5 minutes to scan 15 cm. The temporal resolutions of CT and PET are also disparate: less than 1 second for CT and about one respiratory cycle for PET. This discrepancy in temporal resolution may lead to a misalignment of the tumor position between the CT and PET data, and may compromise the quantification process.

These issues with misregistration due to motion can be remedied by respiratory gating. 4D-PET can also be performed on this PET/CT for RT, but its application has been limited due to the total acquisition time of approximately 40 minutes. Most patients cannot hold their arms over their heads for such a long period of time, and the inevitable motion that results compromises the PET data. Moreover, the splitting of coincident events into multiple bins or phases and the low spatial resolution of 5 to 10 mm further hinder the applicability of 4D-PET. When combined with respiratory gating, this technique of 4D-PET yields higher SUVs and more consistent tumor volumes between PET and CT.

6. Factors affecting SUV measurements

The SUVs of malignant lesion are heavily dependent on glycemic status. Hyperinsulinemia causes enhanced glycolysis in adipose tissue and muscles, leading to comparatively low SUVs elsewhere. For this reason, the glucose level of patients undergoing PET is normally capped at 150 to 200 mg/dl. Studies have shown the elevated blood glucose levels (up to 250 mg/dl) do not affect SUV in inflammatory or benign lesions.

Most centers measure SUV at a single time point by assigning ROIs. Variation in the time interval between tracer injection and image acquisition, which have a significant effect on SUV, is unavoidable to some extent. The confounding effect can be minimized by standardizing protocols outlining the time and direction of the scan. The SUV of tumors continues to rise for several hours after injection, whereas that of the surrounding non-malignant tissue can actually fall. As a result, delayed PET scans often demonstrate better contrast than early PET scans because of an increased lesion-to-background ratio.

The overlap between inflammatory and malignant lesions precludes SUV from being able to distinguish between them. Dual-time point imaging has been used instead to assess malignancies in the head, neck, lungs, breast, cervix, gallbladder, and CNS. The lack of glucose-6-phosphatase in the tumor cells relative to normal cells slows the dephosphorylation of FDG. This leads to increased contrast between tumor and normal cells over time. This also provides a means of differentiating between benign and malignant lesions.

In many studies of various malignancies, dual-time point imaging improved the sensitivity and specificity of PET. The higher specificity is due to the increasing difference in FDG uptake over time between malignant and benign lesions. On the other hand, the higher sensitivity is due to increased lesion-to-background ratio that results from increased uptake in malignancies and the clearance of FDG in other tissues.

7. Future Implications for SUV

It has been suggested that SUV is not optimal for classifying tumors. Dual-time point imaging and delayed PET imaging may be embraced as a more accurate method in the future. As structural and functional imaging become increasingly fused, it is likely that PET/CTs and PET/MRIs will be integral in the assessment of pathophysiological processes.

8. Correcting for Partial-Volume Effects

The partial-volume effect (PVE) affects objects that are less than 2 to 3 times the spatial resolution of the PET scanner. PVE causes the systematic underestimation of SUVs yielded from PET data. Physiological and patient motion also cause the degradation of spatial resolution and exacerbate PVE. These difficulties can be compensated for with 4D respiratory gated PET/CT. Studies have shown that using anatomic imaging (namely CT) to measure the true size of lesions also causes substantial increases in the accuracy of PET data.

The best resolution that can be achieved by modern clinical whole-body scanners is 4 mm. In the field, spatial resolution is normally worse by a significant margin. Structures that are less than 2 to 3 times the spatial resolution of the system, as measured by the full-width at half-maximum, are subject to PVE. Contrast between a lesion and the background decreases the smaller the region is. There are three broadly-defined approaches to minimizing PVE:

1. Correcting for the loss of resolution after reconstruction;
2. Incorporating PVE modeling into the reconstruction process;
3. Using the size of a lesion as determined by anatomic imaging to correct for PVE.

Correction of PVE was broached as early as the 1980s when CT and PET were used to examine patients with AD and other CNS disorders that cause cerebral atrophy. High resolution MR imaging has since led to accurate segmentation and measurement in the gray matter, white matter, and cerebrospinal fluid (CSF).

9. Factors affecting recovery coefficients

The recovery coefficient (RC) is the ratio of observed activity to true activity in PET. It is affected by lesion-to-background ratio, matrix size, etc. RC is usually measured in a static condition, but is subsequently applied in the field to scans with physiological and patient motion. A study carried out by Hickeson *et al.* reported an increase from 58% to 89% in the accuracy of metabolic activity measurements in lung nodues smaller than 2 cm when partial-volume effects were corrected for and a threshold SUV of 2.5 was used to differentiate between malignant and benign lesions[15].

10. Assessing global metabolic activity

Global metabolic activity is calculated by multiplying partial-volume corrected SUV and the volume of the organ of interest, as determined by CT or MRI. The ability to segment images into organs and even subcomponents of organs will no doubt have enormous value in the field of oncology. The therapeutic efficacy of treatment on multiple malignancies can be better measured in this manner.

The assessment of disease through global metabolic activity is particularly useful in neuropsychiatric disorders, where the measurement of glucose metabolism in the entire brain can be a more reliable indicator of disease than that of a single region of interest. Atrophy-corrected whole brain metabolism shows a high degree of sensitivity to and correlates well with cognitive function, as measured by mini-mental status examinations[16].

$$\text{Atrophy corrected average CMRGlc} = \frac{\text{Mean CMRGlc}}{\text{percentage of brain tissue in the intracranial volume}}$$

Global metabolic activity was first measured in studies of AD by Alavi *et al.*[1]. It was calculated by multiplying segmented brain volumes—as determined by MR—by the mean metabolic rate for glucose to yield metabolic volumetric product (MVP). Volume has to be measured accurately by algorithms on computers, while metabolic rate has to be corrected for partial-volume effects to be on target. Quantitative approaches that employ either structural or functional imaging are prone to more inaccuracy and variability than those utilizing both modalities.

The extent of athereosclerosis in the aorta can also be quantified by multiplying SUV in the aortic wall with volumetric data of the aortic wall, as determined by CT. The resulting MVP value is representative of the atheroscleoritc burden in each segment of the aorta[17]. The same principles can be applied to the diffuse hepatic steatosis; hepatic MVP can be calculated by multiplying the mean hepatic SUV by the liver volume measured by MRI[18].

Perhaps one of the most valuable applications of global metabolic activity is in the field of oncology. This technique of analysis can determine the metabolic burden of individual lesions. Metabolic burden (MB) is calculated by multiplying the partial-volume corrected SUV by the volume of the lesion measured by CT and dividing the product by the recovery coefficient.

$$MB = SUV_{meanCT}\left(V_{CT}\right)/RC$$

Metabolic burden is a promising method of assessing total body tumor burden, but there are other techniques that also draw from the concept of global metabolic activity. The measure of Total Lesion Glycolysis (TLG) multiplies SUV by lesion volume without accounting for the recovery coefficient.

11. Image segmentation in quantitative PET imaging

Segmentation, a crucial step in analyzing structural images, groups voxels into sets of distinct classes. Despite its technical complexity, the process of segmentation has breached the clinical field. Through segmentation, organ and tumor volume can be accurately measured, target treatment volumes can be defined, attenuation maps can be generated, and voxel-based anthropomorphic phantoms can be constructed from high resolution anatomical images. Approaches to segmentation are myriad, and include:

- Thresholding
- Region growing
- Classifiers
- Clustering
- Edge detection
- Markov random field models
- Artificial neutral networks
- Deformable models
- Atlas guidance

The process of segmenting CT images of regions such as the lungs is normally preceded by inhomogeneity correction and intensity standardization, and can be accomplished through thresholding and the construction of masks. Subtracting masks from one another allows for the segmentation of smaller structures. Lesion detectability is enhanced by similarity measures (e.g., cross-ψ_B-energy operator), while the reliability of the algorithms behind partial-volume correction is dependent on the accuracy of segmentation and coregistration. Errors in segmentation only affect the partial-volume correction of the mis-segmented region[19]. It is believed that errors in segmentation carry greater weight in measuring the true tracer concentration of a region in comparison to errors in coregistration.

12. Novel approaches to segmentation

Image segmentation is necessary for the quantification of tumor activity, assessment of tumor response to treatment, and definition of target volumes for treatment[20,21]. Demarcating target regions in noisy functional images is one of the most challenging aspects of the oncological applications of PET. Delineating target volumes is normally operator-dependent in the clinical setting. Since this methodology opens the door to high inter-reader variability, moving towards automated techniques would reduce subjectivity.

A method for automated segmentation involving Expectation Maximization-based mixture modeling using k-means clustering has been proposed. A multiscale Markov model can refine segmentation by modeling spatial correlations between neighboring image voxels[22]. Anthropomorphic phantom experiments evaluated the proposed segmentation algorithm. Segmentation using the Markov Random Field Model was shown to reduce relative error.

13. Conclusions

The incorporation of functional imaging such as MR and CT into PET analysis has expended and strengthened its applications in the medical field. Measures of global metabolic activity that can be made with PET/CT and PET/MRI may be superior to those of SUV_{max}, especially in oncology. Further refinements might prove invaluable for the optimal utilization of this powerful imaging technology.

14. View to the future

We believe that the future of imaging is going to shift rapidly from a single modality approach to hybrid imaging with heavy emphasis on PET-CT and possibly PET-MRI. Clearly, the impact of PET-CT has been substantial in many domains. In particular, this approach has revolutionized the practice of oncology and other disciplines with regard to monitoring the effects of various interventions. In particular, PET-CT has been critical in the preoperative assessment of the staging of disease and optimal characterization of the structural abnormalities noted before surgery. Similarly, the field of radiation oncology has rapidly adopted PET-CT imaging for effective control of a variety of cancers, in particular, those that originate in the lungs and the head/neck regions. The role of contrast enhanced CT can be expected to decline if PET data indicates that this extra step may be redundant and will not substantially alter the results generated from PET alone. The role of PET-MRI is unclear at this time. However, its applications in the brain will obviate the need for PET-CT for this anatomic site. This is mainly due to the fact that information provided by CT for central nervous disorders is suboptimal and therefore combined PET-MRI will provide superior data in the brain. It is possible that orthopedic applications of PET may substantially improve by combining PET and MRI, particularly in the structures of the feet and the knees. It is unclear whether PET-MRI will be as successful in assessing disease activity in the chest and abdomen. This is primarily due to the fact that attenuation correction in these anatomic sites is complex and may not be feasible with MR approaches alone. Efforts are on the way to estimate the degree of attenuation at these sites but we are uncertain that this will lead to overcoming the difficulties that exist in this particular domain. Finally, the use of hybrid imaging has substantially improved our ability to optimally quantify PET data. This will further enhance the role of functional imaging for accurate characterization of lesions and response to therapy.

15. Summary

The information provided in this chapter reveals a paradigm shift in medical imaging and has described in detail the need for hybrid imaging with an emphasis on PET-CT as major modality for the future in medicine. Therefore, practitioners of medicine must make every effort to amiliarize themselves with the capabilities of these modalities in order to optimize treatments and care for their patients.

16. References

[1] Alavi A, Reivich M, Greenberg J, Hand P, Rosenquist A, Rintelmann W, et al. Mapping of functional activity in brain with 18F-fluoro-deoxyglucose. Semin Nucl Med. 1981; 11:24-31.

[2] Reivich M, Alavi A, Wolf A, Greenberg JH, Fowler J, Christman D, et al. Use of 2-deoxy-D[1-11C]glucose for the determination of local cerebral glucose metabolism in humans: variation within and between subjects. J Cereb Blood Flow Metab. 1982; 2:307-19.

[3] Sokoloff L, Reivich M, Kennedy C, Des Rosiers MH, Patlak CS, Pettigrew KD, et al. The [^{14}C]deoxyglucose method for the measurement of local cerebral glucose utilization: theory, procedure, and normal values in the conscious and anesthetized albino rat. J Neurochem. 1977; 28:897-916.

[4] Reivich M, Kuhl D, Wolf A, Greenberg J, Phelps M, Ido T, et al. The [18F]fluorodeoxyglucose method for the measurement of local cerebral glucose utilization in man. Circ Res. 1979; 44:127-37

[5] Phelps ME, Huang SC, Hoffman EJ, Selin C, Sokoloff L, Kuhl DE. Tomographic measurement of local cerebral glucose metabolic rate in humans with (F-18)2-fluoro-2-deoxy-D-glucose: validation of method. Ann Neurol. 1979; 6:371-88.

[6] Carson R. Tracer kinetic modeling in PET. In: Valk PE, Bailey DL, Townsend DW, Maisey MN, editors. Positron Emission Tomography: Basic Science and Clinical Practice. Chapter 4 ed. London: Springer-Verlag; 2003. p. 147-79.

[7] Logan J. Graphical analysis of PET data applied to reversible and irreversible tracers. Nucl Med Biol. 2000 Oct;27(7):661-670.

[8] Zhou Y, Ye W, Brasic JR ,Wong DF. Multi-graphical analysis of dynamic PET. Neuroimage. 2010 Feb 15;49(4):2947-2957.

[9] Sokoloff L, Reivich M, Kennedy C, Des Rosiers MH, Patlak CS, Pettigrew KD, et al. The [^{14}C]deoxyglucose method for the measurement of local cerebral glucose utilization: theory, procedure, and normal values in the conscious and anesthetized albino rat. J Neurochem. 1977; 28:897-916.

[10] Schmidt KC, Lucignani G, Sokoloff L. Fluorine-18-fluorodeoxyclucose PET to determine regional cerebral glucose utilization: A reexamination. J Nucl Med 1996;37:394-39.

[11] Hunter G, Hamberg L, Alpert N, Choi N, Fischman A. Simplified measurement of deoxyglucose utilization rate. J Nucl Med. 1996; 37:950-5.

[12] Kim CK, Gupta N, Chandramouli B, Alavi A. Stardized uptake values of FDG: body ▯ surface area correction is preferable to body weight correction. J Nucl Med. 1994; 35:164-7.

[13] Kim CK, Gupta N. Dependency of standardized uptake values of fluorine-18 fluorodeoxyglucose on body size: Comparison of body surface area correction and lean body mass correction. Nucl Med Commun. 1996; 17:890-4.

[14] Gupta N, Frank A, Dewan N, et al. Solitary pulmonary nodules: detection of malignancy with PET with 2-[F-18]-fluoro-2-deoxy-D-glucose. Radiology. 1992; 184:441-4.

[15] Hickeson M, Yun M, Matthies A, Zhuang H, Adam LE, Lacorte L, et al. Use of a corrected standardized uptake value based on the lesion size on CT permits accurate characterization of lung nodules on FDG-PET. Eur J Nucl Med Mol Imaging. 2002; 29:1639-47.

[16] Basu S, Zaidi H, Houseni M, Udupa J, Acton P, Torigian D, et al. Novel quantitative techniques for assessing regional and global function and structure based on modern imaging modalities: Implications for normal variation, aging and diseased states. Sem Nucl Med. 2007; 37:223-39.

[17] Bural GG, Torigian DA, Chamroonrat W, Alkhawaldeh K, Houseni M, El-Haddad G, et al. Quantitative assessment of the atherosclerotic burden of the aorta by combined FDG-PET and CT image analysis: a new concept. Nucl Med Biol. 2006; 33:1037-43.

[18] Bural G, Torigian D, Burke A, Houseni M, Alkhawaldeh K, Cucchiara A, et al. Quantitative assessment of the hepatic metabolic volume product in patients with diffuse hepatic steatosis and normal controls through use of FDG-PET and MR imaging: A novel concept. Mol Imaging Biol. 2009.

[19] Zaidi H, Ruest T, Schoenahl F, Montandon M-L. Comparative evaluation of statistical brain MR image segmentation algorithms and their impact on partial volume effect correction in PET. Neuroimage. 2006; 32:1591-607.

[20] Zaidi H, Vees H, Wissmeyer M. Molecular PET/CT imaging-guided radiation therapy treatment planning. Acad Radiol. 2009: 16:1108-33.

[21] Paulino AC, Thorstad WL, Fox T. Role of fusion in radiotherapy treatment planning. Semin Nucl Med. 2003; 33:238-43.

[22] Montgomery D, Amira A, Zaidi H. Fully automated segmentation of oncological PET volumes using a combined multiscale and statistical model. Med Phys. 2007; 34:722-36.

2

Radiolabeled Nanoparticles for Molecular Imaging

Enrique Morales-Avila[1,2], Guillermina Ferro-Flores[1],
Blanca E. Ocampo-García[1,2] and Flor de María Ramírez[1]
[1]*Instituto Nacional de Investigaciones Nucleares,*
[2]*Universidad Autónoma del Estado de México,*
Mexico

1. Introduction

Molecular imaging (MI) comprises non-invasive monitoring of functional and spatiotemporal processes at molecular and cellular levels in humans and other living systems. In contrast to conventional diagnostic imaging, MI seeks to probe the molecular abnormalities that are the basis of disease rather than capture the images of the end effects of the molecular alterations. Imaging techniques such as magnetic resonance imaging (MRI), single photon emission computed tomography (SPECT), positron emission tomography (PET) and optical fluorescence imaging (OI) have been used to monitor such processes. Radionuclide-based imaging methods, such as SPECT and PET, use internal radiation that is administered through a target-specific molecule labeled with a radionuclide at doses free of pharmacologic side effects. Nuclear imaging is an established clinical MI modality that, compared to other modalities, offers better sensitivity and has no tissue penetration limits (Massoud & Gamghir, 2003; Ferro-Flores et. al., 2010a). Nuclear technologies have been evolving toward greater sensitivity due to enhanced hardware development, such as multi-pinhole acquisitions methods or pixelated semiconductor detectors. In parallel with the hardware advances, steady progress is being made in image-processing algorithms, and such algorithms may soon provide substantial reduction in SPECT acquisition times without sacrificing diagnostic quality (Madsen, 2007). The fusion of nuclear and anatomical images from computed tomography (CT) into a single imaging device (SPECT/CT and PET/CT) has been very useful for clinical oncology (Hong et al., 2009a).

According to the American Society for Testing and Materials (ASTM), the term nanoparticles describes a sub-classification of ultra-fine solids with dimensions from 1 nm to 100 nm and novel properties that distinguish them from the bulk material (ASTM, 2006). Nanoparticles produce multivalent effects due to multiple simultaneous interactions between the biomolecules conjugated to the nanoparticle surface and specific receptors for those biomolecules on the cell surface (Montet et al., 2006). Nanoparticles can be near infrared (NIR)-fluorescent (e.g. nanocrystals or quantum dots) or can have magnetic properties (e.g. iron oxide nanoparticles).

Therefore, the first aim during the development of radiolabeled nanoparticles is to maximize the binding affinity via multimeric receptor-specific biomolecules based on the multivalency principle. Large numbers of antibodies, peptides or any molecule with biological activity can be linked to the surface of a single radiolabeled nanocrystal (quantum dot), metal nanoparticle (iron oxide and gold) or single-walled carbon nanotube (SWNT) to improve imaging of tumors over-expressing those specific antigens or receptors.

In general, different imaging techniques are complementary rather than competitive. Consequently, the second aim of engineering radiolabeled nanoparticles is to develop dual-labeled imaging agents that target the same ligand. This allows for cross validation between nuclear and fluorescence optical images, MRI and nuclear images, or trimodal nuclear-MRI-fluorescence images.

The third aim is related to therapeutic properties. Gold nanoparticles and SWNT, which are designed to absorb in the NIR spectrum, cause irreversible thermal cellular destruction when they are irradiated using a laser (NIR light). It is important to remember that "the magic bullet does not exist" when it comes to cancer therapy; therefore, increasing the therapeutic response requires the application of combined modalities with multiple therapeutic agents. For example, gold nanoparticles or SWNT radiolabeled with beta-particle emitters could represent a unique, multifunctional and target-specific pharmaceutical that could be administered as a single drug. This pharmaceutical would be capable of functioning, simultaneously, as both a targeted radiotherapy system and a photothermal therapy system.

This chapter covers recent major advancements in design, synthesis, physicochemical characterization and molecular recognition assessment of radiolabeled synthetic nanoparticles for molecular imaging and highlights the therapeutic possibilities of these nanosystems.

2. General aspects of radiolabeled nanoparticles

Multivalent interactions regulate a wide variety of cellular processes, such as cell surface recognition events that involve inflammation and tumor metastasis. Multivalency is a design principle by which organized arrays amplify the strength of a binding process, e.g. the binding of multimeric peptides to specific receptors on a cell surface (Ocampo-Garcia et al., 2011a).

Nanoparticles can be design as multimeric systems to produce multivalent effects. The physical and chemical properties of nanoparticles play an important role in determining particle-cell interactions, cellular trafficking mechanisms, biodistribution, pharmacokinetics and optical properties. Important nanoparticle properties include chemical composition of the core, size, shape, surface charge and surface chemistry.

The synthesis of nanoparticles with a variety of physicochemical properties has led to important advances. Among these, gold nanoparticles are of particular importance to SPECT/CT or PET/CT molecular imaging due to the relative ease of surface modification and radiolabeling, their biocompatibility, resistance to oxidation and extraordinary optical properties (Giljohann et al., 2010).

Nanoparticles of semiconductors are densely packed inorganic fluorescent semiconductor crystals with excellent optical properties, and these can be radiolabeled for PET/NIR imaging (Erathodiyil & Ying, 2011).

Radiolabeled iron oxide nanoparticles have been designed for use in SPECT/MRI and PET/MRI dual techniques (Torres et al., 2011; Jarret et al., 2008). Other radiolabeled nanosystems have also been proposed for biomedical applications, and these include single wall carbon nanotubes (Hong et al., 2009b), fullerenes (Qingnuan et al., 2002), multiwall carbon nanotubes (Guo et al., 2007) and CuS nanoparticles (Zhou et al., 2010).

Radiolabeled nanoparticles conjugated to target specific molecules can be directly used as agents for diagnosis. The most common radionuclides for SPECT imaging include ^{99m}Tc ($t_{1/2}$= 6 h) and ^{111}In ($t_{1/2}$=2.8 days), and the most common for PET are ^{64}Cu ($t_{1/2}$ =12.7 h), ^{18}F ($t_{1/2}$=109.8 min) and ^{68}Ga ($t_{1/2}$= 68.1 min). Moreover, radiolabeling is used to study the biokinetics of new devices based on nanoparticles that comprise radiopharmaceuticals, drug/gene delivery systems or plasmonic photothermal therapy enhancers. Many types of radiolabeled nanoparticles have three main components: the core, the targeting biomolecule and the radiotracer group (Fig. 1). The targeting biomolecule includes a component with high affinity for target epitopes; radiolabeling can be performed with or without slight modifications of the original nanoparticle (NP) surface. For ligands to bind effectively, each radionuclide can be conjugated directly on the NP surface, with or without a spacer, or can be attached to the NP during chemical synthesis. The spacer groups between the NP surface and the radionuclide or the biomolecule can be a simple hydrocarbon chain, a peptide sequence or a poly-ethyleneglycol linker.

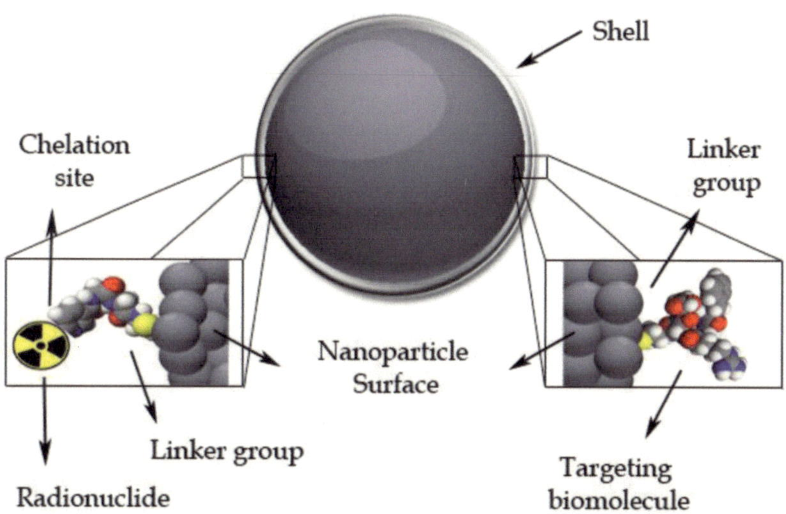

Fig. 1. Schematic structure of a radiolabeled nanoparticle design for molecular imaging

3. Radiolabeled nanoparticles for SPECT molecular imaging

Peptide receptors are proteins that are overexpressed in numerous human cancer cells. These receptors have been used as molecular targets, allowing radiolabeled peptides to identify tumors. The gastrin-releasing peptide receptor (GRP-r) is overexpressed in prostate and breast cancer, and ^{99m}Tc-Lys^{3}-bombesin has been reported as a radiopharmaceutical with specific binding to cells expressing GRP-r (Ferro-Flores et al., 2006; Santos-Cuevas et al., 2008). Integrin $\alpha_V\beta_3$ plays a critical role in tumor angiogenesis, and radiolabeled cyclic-Arg-Gly-Asp

(RGD) peptides have been used for noninvasive imaging of tumor $\alpha_V\beta_3$ expression (Liu, 2008, 2009). Mannosylated macromolecules labeled with ^{99m}Tc have displayed properties suitable for use in sentinel lymph node detection; these radiopharmaceuticals are considered target-specific because they exhibit specific binding to mannose receptors that are expressed on lymph node macrophages (Vera et al., 2001; Takagi et al., 2004).

Based on the observations above, ^{99m}Tc-labeled gold nanoparticles conjugated to Lys^3-bombesin, RGD peptides or thiol-mannose have been prepared as multimeric systems showing properties suitable for use as target-specific agents for molecular imaging of GRP receptor-positive tumors, tumor $\alpha_V\beta_3$ expression and sentinel lymph node detection, respectively. ^{99m}Tc- and ^{111}In-labeled carbon nanotubes, ^{125}I-labeled silver nanoparticles and ^{99m}Tc-labeled iron oxide nanoparticles have also been reported for SPECT imaging (Table 1). The strategies of synthesis and functionalization for these nanoparticles are discussed in the following sections.

3.1 Synthesis of NP cores

The most common nanomaterials reported for SPECT imaging are iron oxide NPs, gold NPs, silver NPs and carbon nanotubes. NPs usually have optical or magnetic properties that can be used for molecular imaging, whereas polymer- or liposome-based NPs do not produce imaging signals by themselves.

NP core synthesis generally follows standardized strategies; for example, the most popular method of synthesis for gold nanoparticles (AuNPs) is based on the use of $HAuCl_4$ (Au III) salt, which is reduced to metallic Au(0) in aqueous solution and stabilized with a chemical agent. The classical sodium citrate reduction is the oldest and most widely used method (Daniel & Astruc, 2004), but there are different techniques to produce AuNPs with different sizes and shapes using reduction agents stronger than citrate (such as $NaBH_4$), different organic solvents and/or different stabilizer surfactants. Most of the stabilizer surfactants are quaternary ammonium salts, such as cetyltrimethylammonium bromide (CTAB), didodecyldimethylammonium bromide (DDAB) and tetradodecylammonium bromide (TTAB). Anionic surfactant syntheses have also been reported (Zhang et al., 2006). Anisometric gold colloids (rods) can be prepared by adding gold nuclei to $HAuCl_4$ growth solutions (formed by reduction of $HAuCl_4$ with phosphorus), and the growth of the gold nanorods is initiate with the addition of H_2O_2 (Huang et al., 2009). Electrochemical and photochemical reduction, microwave, ultrasound and laser ablation have also been used for AuNP synthesis (Ferro-Flores et al., 2010b; Huang et al., 2009). The Au(0) core is essentially inert and non-toxic (Connor et al., 2005). AuNPs exhibit narrow and intense absorption and scattering bands due to the phenomenon of plasmon resonance. This occurs at the resonance condition of the collective oscillation that the conduction electrons experience in an electromagnetic field of the appropriate wavelength. The plasmon resonance band for ordinary 20 nm gold nanospheres is at 520 nm, in the middle of the visible spectrum, but this can be red-shifted into the NIR spectrum. Rod-shaped NPs exhibit two plasmon resonance bands due to oscillation of the conduction electrons along the short axis and the long axis of the particles. The former plasmon band is called the transverse resonance and the latter the longitudinal resonance. While the transverse plasmon band occurs in the neighborhood of 520 nm, the longitudinal band is red-shifted between 675–850 nm in the interest of optical imaging. This occupies the most important part of the "optical imaging window" where light penetration in tissue is high due to reduced scattering and absorption coefficients. Optical imaging techniques that rely on scattering and/or absorption contrast to detect pathological tissue could benefit from the use of gold nanoparticles with targeting capability (Huang et al., 2009).

Core	Surface molecule/ Target	Radionuclide and Chelator	Application (Reference)
Gold nanoparticles	RGD/ $\alpha_v\beta_3$ integrin	^{99m}Tc-HYNIC	SPECT/CT imaging of $\alpha_v\beta_3$ integrin expression, and multimodal probe for possible thermotherapy (Morales-Avila et al., 2011)
	Lys^3-Bombesin/ Gastrin releasing peptide receptors		SPECT/CT imaging of gastrin releasing peptide-receptor in breast and prostate cancer detection , and multimodal probe for possible thermotherapy (Mendoza-Sanchez et al., 2010)
	Mannose/ Mannose receptors		SPECT/CT imaging for mannose receptors in sentinel lymph node detection in breast cancer, and multimodal probe for possible thermotherapy (Ocampo-Garcia et al., 2011a, 2011b)
	--	^{99m}Tc-DTPA	PEG-coated AuNPs for drug delivery vehicles and diagnostic imaging agents (Zhang et al., 2009)
Carbon nanotubes	--	^{99m}Tc-$C_{60}(OH)_x$ ^{111}In-DTPA	SPECT/CT image and platform for delivery of biologic, radiologic and chemical cargo to target tissues. (Qingnuan et al., 2002; Guo et al., 2007; Chan et al., 2004; Singh et al., 2006; McDevitt et al., 2007)
	Rituximab (anti-CD20)/ CD20 epitope on human non Hodgkin lymphoma cells	^{111}In-DOTA	
Silver nanoparticles	Poly (N-vinyl-2-pyrrolidone)	^{125}I	*In vivo* imaging and biodistribution of radiolabeled NPs (Chrastina & Schnitzer, 2010)
Supermagnetic Iron oxide, SPIO	Alendronate/ osteoclastic surface	^{99m}Tc-DTPA	Platform for SPECT/MRI images (Torres et al., 2011)

Table 1. Radiolabeled nanoparticles for SPECT imaging

Iron oxide NPs can be synthesized via the coprecipitation of Fe^{2+} and Fe^{3+} aqueous salt solutions, which results in the addition of a base. The size, shape and composition of NPs depend on a number of factors, including: the type of salts used (e.g., chlorides, sulfates, nitrates or perchlorates), the Fe^{2+} and Fe^{3+} ratio, pH and ionic strength of the media. A variety of other methods, based on the principle of precipitation in highly constrained domains, have been developed and these include sol–gel preparation, polymer matrix-mediated synthesis and precipitation using microemulsions and vesicles (Kogan et al., 2007).

Silver nanoparticles can be synthesized in large quantities by reducing silver nitrate with ethylene glycol in the presence of poly(vinyl pyrrolidone) (PVP). The presence of PVP and its molar ratio relative to silver nitrate is important in determining the geometric shape and size of the product. The size, shape, and structure of metal nanoparticles are important because there is a strong correlation between these parameters and optical, electrical, and catalytic AgNP properties (Sun & Xia, 2002).

Carbon nanotubes (CNT) are essentially hexagonal networks of carbon atoms arranged like a layer of graphite rolled into a cylinder consisting of pure carbon units, the C_{60} fullerene. Methods such as electric arc discharge, laser vaporization and chemical vapor deposition techniques are well known to produce a wide variety of single- (SWNT) and multi-walled (MWNT) CNTs. Catalytic chemical vapor deposition is the most commonly used, whereas the water-assisted synthesis method for NTs produces highly organized intrinsic nanotube structures. The water-stimulated synthesis enhances catalytic activity resulting in massive growth of super-dense and vertically aligned nanotubes (Hata et al., 2004). SWNTs produce high optical absorbance in the NIR (Kam et al., 2005). It has been well documented that water-solubilized nanotubes with high hydrophilicity are non-toxic, even at high concentrations (Dumortier et al., 2006).

3.2 Preparation of radiolabeled NP-conjugates

To achieve recognition of the molecular target, specific biomolecules are used as ligands and these are conjugated to the AuNP surface. These ligands include sugars, antibodies, nucleic acids, proteins and peptides. All of these biomolecules must offer low nonspecific binding, high affinity to their binding sites, no immunogenicity, fast accumulation at the target, fast blood clearance, and preferably exhibit no peripheral metabolic activity or toxicity. The biomolecules are frequently attached to the surface of the nanoparticle via electrostatic interactions; however, a covalent bond is preferred to prevent release of the attached biomolecules *in vivo*. The chemical bond occurs between the AuNP surface and the peptide containing sulfhydryl (-SH) groups (usually from cysteine) with high affinity toward the gold atoms. The -SH group forms a 'staple motif' chemical model comprised of two thiol groups interacting with three gold atoms in a bridge conformation (Jadzinsky et al., 2009).

Two main strategies for binding peptides to AuNPs are commonly used. The first is the direct conjugation of the peptide by means of a terminal thiol (cysteine) or an *N*-terminal primary amine (Levy et al., 2004; Porta et al., 2007), and the second is an indirect conjugation with a linker that contains both a thiol group (that binds the nanoparticle) and a carbonyl terminal group, that is activated and conjugated to biological active peptides using the carbodiimide-coupling chemistry (Wang et al., 2005; Cheung et al., 2009). An advantage of the direct conjugation strategy is that it does not require the use of linkers with long chains as spacers between the NP and the conjugated peptides. This is important because the introduction of spacers and an increase in linker length has been proven to significantly alter the peptide-multivalency effect, which may correlate to a decrease in the effective peptide molarity (Kubas et al., 2010).

Current methodologies for SPECT molecular imaging require an additional ligand that is appended to the AuNP surface, and this ligand functions as a chelator of the radiometal. Two different kinds of molecules can be bound to the AuNP surface to produce hybrid radiolabeled AuNP-peptide systems. In our research, we have reported two different radionuclide chelators to generate radiolabeled gold nanoparticles. Mendoza-Sanchez et al., (2010), Ocampo-Garcia et al., (2011b) and Morales-Avila et al., (2011) demonstrated radiolabeling of AuNPs using 6-hydrazinopyridine-3-carboxylic(HYNIC)-GGC peptide. With this approach, HYNIC was added as a ^{99m}Tc chelator group, -Gly-Gly- as a spacer group and -Cys as the active group that interacted with the nanoparticle surface (Fig. 2). In the second approach, the HYNIC-Tyr^{3}-Octreotide (HYNIC-TOC) was used for AuNP radiolabeling, whereby the HYNIC group was the ^{99m}Tc chelator and the cysteine contained in the disulphide bridge or the ε-amine of lysine was the reactive group for AuNP conjugation (Ocampo-Garcia et al., 2011a) (Fig. 3).

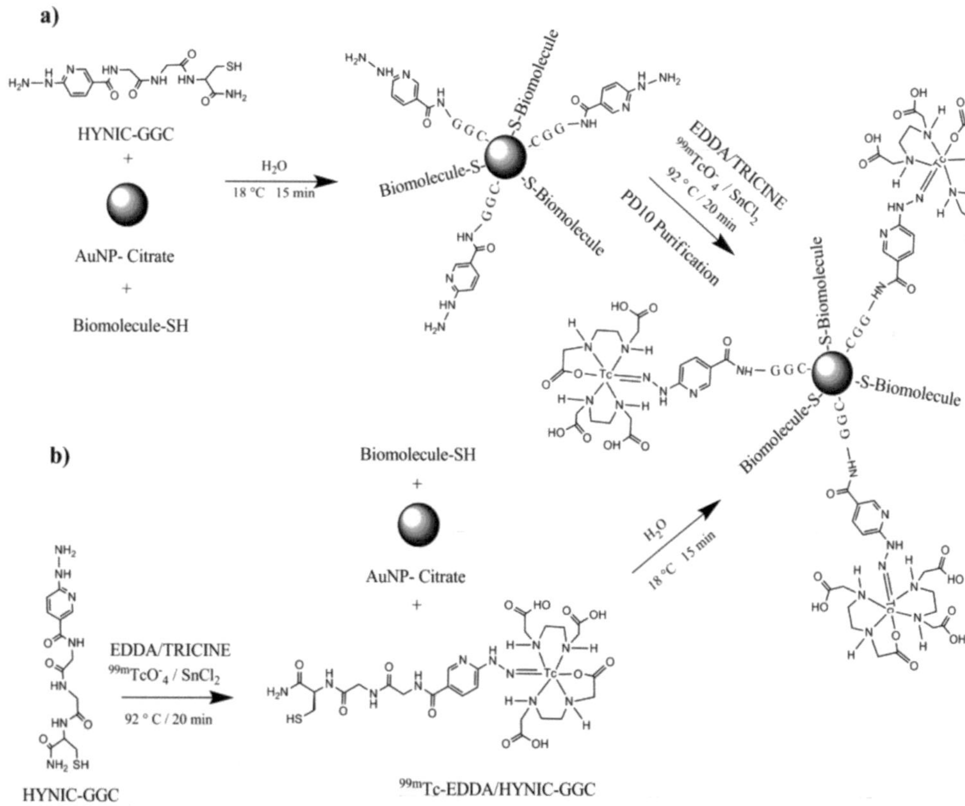

Fig. 2. Radiolabeling of gold nanoparticles conjugated to biomolecules using HYNIC-GGG as ^{99m}Tc chelator: a) radiolabeling after biomolecule conjugation to AuNP and b) conjugation and radiolabeling in a single step without further purification.

Mendoza-Sanchez et al., (2010) and Ocampo-Garcia et al., (2011b) conjugated peptides to the gold nanoparticle surface using a posterior radiolabeling process. This process was conducted by adding ethylenediaminediacetic acid (EDDA)/Tricine, $SnCl_2$ (as reducing agent) and ^{99m}Tc-pertechnetate to 1 mL of HYNIC-GGC-AuNP followed by incubation at 100 °C for 20 min. The mixture was purified by size-exclusion chromatography (PD-10 column, Sephadex G-25) using injectable grade water as the eluent by collecting 0.5 mL fractions. The first peak (3.0–4.0 mL) corresponded to the void volume of the column and contained ^{99m}Tc-EDDA/HYNIC-GGC-AuNP (a radioactive red color solution), while the second peak corresponded to ^{99m}Tc-EDDA (6.0–8.0 mL). Free $^{99m}TcO_4^-$ and ^{99m}Tc-colloid remained in the PD-10 column (Fig. 2a). In a second approach (Morales-Avila et al., 2011), the peptide conjugation to AuNPs and the radiolabeling were carried out in a single step without further purification (Fig. 2b).

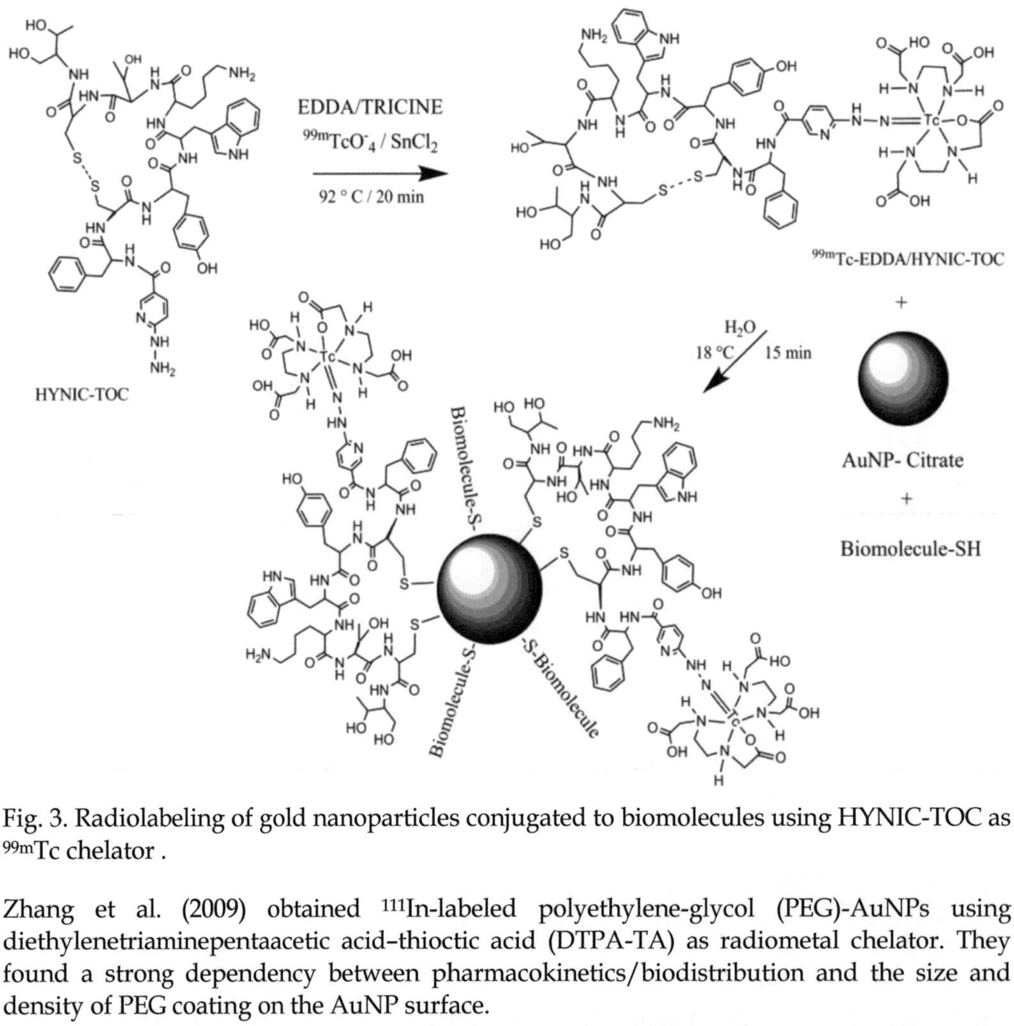

Fig. 3. Radiolabeling of gold nanoparticles conjugated to biomolecules using HYNIC-TOC as ^{99m}Tc chelator .

Zhang et al. (2009) obtained ^{111}In-labeled polyethylene-glycol (PEG)-AuNPs using diethylenetriaminepentaacetic acid–thioctic acid (DTPA-TA) as radiometal chelator. They found a strong dependency between pharmacokinetics/biodistribution and the size and density of PEG coating on the AuNP surface.

Chan et al. (2004) prepared carbon-encapsulated ^{99m}Tc nanoparticles. Fullerenes can be directly labeled with ^{99m}Tc using ascorbic acid/$SnCl_2$ as reducing agents to form

$^{99m}Tc-C_{60}(OH)_X$, however, biodistribution studies indicated that the radionanoparticles were distributed in all tissues (Qingnuan et al., 2002). The ^{99m}Tc-glucosamine-MWNT, also labeled by the direct method, is water-soluble, and further modification of this system may allow the development of a versatile delivery system for molecular targeting (Guo et al., 2007).

^{111}In-labeled carbon nanotubes were synthesized by Singh et al. (2006). The ammonium-functionalized CNTs (single- and multi-walled) were prepared following the 1,3-dipolar cycle addition method to be covalently bound to DTPA. Biodistribution studies showed a rapid blood clearance (half-life=3 h) with renal excretion. Radiolabeling of CNTs with ^{111}In has also been reported by McDevitt et al., 2007. In general, CNTs are functionalized with 2-(4-isothiocyanatobenzyl)-1,4,7,10-tetraazacyclododecane-1,4,7,10-tetraacetic (DOTA-NCS) via thiolurea bonding and radiolabeled by adding ^{111}In chloride to the DOTA-CNT conjugate.

Chrastina & Schnitzer (2010) reported the synthesis of silver nanoparticles labeled with iodine-125 to track *in vivo* tissue targeting with SPECT images. Poly(N-vinyl-2-pyrrolidone)-capped silver nanoparticles (average size 12 nm) were labeled by chemisorptions, whereby chloramine-T (N-chlorobenzenesulfonamide) was immobilized on a polystyrene backbone. The radio-solution was removed and added to a dispersion of unfunctionalized Ag nanoparticles. Unbound iodide-125 was removed by size exclusion chromatography on Sephadex G-25 columns. Radiochemical yields higher than 95% were obtained. Radiolabeled AgNPs were characterized by UV-Vis spectrometry (410 nm).

Torres et al., (2011) reported the development of a new class of dual-modality imaging agents based on the conjugation of radiolabeled bisphosphonates (BP) directly to the surface of superparamagnetic iron oxide (SPIO) nanoparticles (5 nm, Fe_3O_4 core). The SPIO labeling with ^{99m}Tc-DTPA-alendronate was performed in a single step at room temperature. The radiolabeled nanoparticles showed excellent stability, making the conjugate suitable for SPECT-CT/MRI imaging.

3.3 Structural, chemical and radiochemical characterization

Several methods have been used for the structural characterization of nanoparticles, including X-ray diffraction (XRD), small-angle X-ray scattering (SAXS), microscopic techniques such as scanning electron microscopy (SEM), high-resolution transmission microscopy (HRTEM) and scanning probe microscopy (SPM). For the chemical characterization of the biomolecule-nanoparticle conjugate, spectroscopic methods have been applied to confirm the chemical interaction and functionalization of NPs with the biomolecules. These methods include UV-Vis, infrared, Raman, fluorescence and XPS spectroscopy. For example, in the case of peptides conjugated to AuNPs, the vibrational spectroscopic techniques can be used to confirm that the biomolecule displaces the carboxylate groups of the citrate on the AuNP surface. The structured spectra can be used to confirm that AuNPs were functionalized with peptides, because several well defined bands with vibrational frequencies in the region of those associated with the main functional groups of the peptides can be observed in the AuNP-peptide conjugate, even though these will have characteristics of the AuNP-peptide because the bands shift to lower or higher energies and increase in intensities (Surujpaul et al., 2008; Morales-Avila et al., 2011). Additionally, the Au-S bond shows a characteristic band at 279 ± 1 cm^{-1} identified by far-infrared spectroscopy (Ocampo-Garcia et al., 2011a). In UV-Vis spectroscopy a red shift in the maximum absorbance of the AuNP is representative of the peptide conjugation process, while the small change in the surface plasmon resonance position occurs as the result of the peptide adsorption on the AuNP surface (Kogan et al., 2007; Ferro-Flores et al. 2010b). The orbital energies of Au-Au or AuNP (Au^0) and Au-S (Au^{+1}) bonds are related to changes in the oxidative states (Au^0 to Au^{+1}); therefore, in XPS analyses the shift of electron binding energies to higher values in the AuNP-peptide conjugates, with respect to AuNPs, is an intrinsic property of the interaction between gold core electrons and the peptide (Mendoza-Sanchez et al., 2010; Ocampo-Garcia et al., 2011b).

The methods frequently used to determine radiochemical purity and assess quality control of the radiolabelled nanoparticles include instant thin layer chromatography (ITLC), which has the advantage of being very quick and easy to use, and size-exclusion high performance liquid chromatography (SE-HPLC) that can be used as an accurate method depending on the NPs size. PD-10 columns and ultrafiltration can be used as easy purification methods and to determine radiochemical purity (Ocampo-Garcia et al., 2011a).

3.4 Biological recognition

It has been demonstrated that multimeric systems of ^{99m}Tc-AuNP-biomolecules exhibit properties that make them suitable for use as target-specific agents for molecular imaging of tumors and sentinel lymph node detection. For example, *in vitro* binding studies of ^{99m}Tc-AuNP-RGD conducted in $\alpha_V\beta_3$ receptor positive C6 glioma cancer cells showed specific recognition for those receptors (Morales-Avila et. al., 2011). Moreover, ^{99m}Tc-AuNP-Lys^3-bombesin showed specific recognitions for GRP receptors in PC3 cancer cells (Mendoza-Sanchez, et al., 2010) and ^{99m}Tc-AuNP-mannose demonstrated specificity for mannose receptors (Ocampo-Garcia et al., 2011a). Micro-SPECT/CT images of these radiopharmaceuticals have shown a clear tumor uptake or lymph node accumulation (Fig. 4).

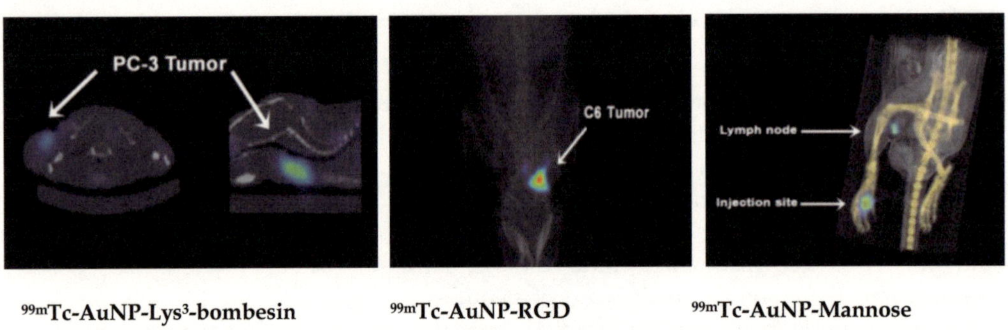

Fig. 4. Micro-SPECT/CT images of ^{99m}Tc-labeled gold nanoparticles in mice with induced tumors (conjugates of Lys^3-bombesin and RGD) and in Wistar rat (mannose conjugate).

The ^{111}In-DTPA-TA-AuNP-PEG system has shown a prolonged blood circulation and significant tumor uptake by the enhanced permeability and retention effect, making of the radiolabeled AuNPs a promising drug delivery vehicle and diagnostic imaging agent (Zhang et al., 2009).

The multifunctional system of carbon nanotubes, conjugated to both anti-CD20 (Rituximab) and ^{111}In-DOTA-NCS, demonstrated ability of this double conjugate to specifically target tumor cells *in vitro* (in CD20+ specific Daudi cells) and tumors *in vivo* using a murine model of disseminated Lymphoma (McDevitt et al. 2007).

4. Radiolabeled nanoparticles for PET molecular imaging

PET is a nuclear imaging technique used to map biological and physiological processes in living subjects following the administration of radiolabeled probes. In PET, the radionuclide decays and the resulting positrons subsequently interact with nearby electrons after travelling a short distance (~1 mm) within the body. Each positron-electron transmutation produces two 511-keV gamma photons in opposite trajectories, and these two gamma photons may be detected by the detectors surrounding the subject to precisely locate the source of the decay event. Subsequently, the "coincidence events" data can be processed by computers to reconstruct the spatial distribution of the radiotracer (Chen & Conti, 2011). Several positron-emitting radionuclides have been used in the development of radiolabeled nanoparticles. These radionuclides include ^{64}Cu (E_{max} 657 keV), ^{18}F (E_{max} 635 keV) and ^{68}Ga (E_{max} 1.90 MeV), which are described in the following sections.

4.1 ^{64}Cu-labeled nanoparticles

The ^{64}Cu radionuclide can be effectively produced using both reactor- and accelerator-based methods. Its use as a positron emitter has grown, and it has been reported to be suitable for the radiolabeling of proteins, antibodies and peptides. In addition, ^{64}Cu has been investigated as a promising radiotracer for real-time PET monitoring of regional drug concentration and for pharmacokinetics applications. Its integration as a structural component of nanoparticles produces multimeric systems suitable for therapy and PET imaging (Zhou et al., 2010).

To date, nanocrystals (quantum dot), iron oxide nanoparticles, SWNT and gold nanoparticles (nanoshells) have been functionalized with ^{64}Cu ligands for PET/MRI or PET/NIR fluorescence imaging and therapy. In these multiple combinations, the same molecular target can be evaluated with two different imaging modalities. These groupings allow the strengths of each to improve the overall diagnostic accuracy, and this approach provides a synergistic effect, increasing expectations for high sensitive and high-resolution imaging (Hong, 2009).

Quantum dots (QDs) or nanocrystals are fluorescent semiconductor nanoparticles (2-10 nm) with many unique optical properties including bright fluorescence, resistance to photobleaching, and a narrow emission bandwidth (Ferro-Flores et al., 2010a). Their fluorescence emission wavelength can be continuously tuned from 400 nm to 2000 nm by changing both the particle size and chemical composition. Their quantum yields are as high as 85 %. The particles are generally made from hundreds to thousands of atoms (~200-10,000 atoms) of IIB and VIA family elements (e.g. CdSe and CdTe) or IIIA and VA family elements (e.g. InP and InAs). Recent advances have allowed the precise control of particle size, shape and internal structure (core-shell, gradient alloy or homogenous alloy) (Yu et al., 2003). As cadmium is potentially toxic, Gao et al. (2004) developed a class of QD conjugates that contains an amphiphilic triblock copolymer for *in vivo* protection and multiple PEG molecules for improving biocompatibility and circulation. InAs/InP/ZnSe Core/Shell/Shell quantum dots without Cd have significantly lower intrinsic toxicity compared to QDs containing elements such as cadmium (Xie et al., 2008).

A dual-modality PET/NIR fluorescent peptide has been recently reported (Cai et al., 2007; Chen et al., 2010). A QD (QD705; emission maximum, 705 nm) with an amine-functionalized surface was modified with RGD (90 peptides per QD) or the vascular endothelial growth factor (VEGF) and 1,4,7,10-tetraazacyclodocecane-N,N',N'',N'''-tetraacetic acid (DOTA) chelator for integrin-$\alpha_v\beta_3$ or VEGF imaging. PET/NIR imaging, tissue homogenate fluorescence measurement, and immunofluorescence staining were performed with U87MG human glioblastoma tumor-bearing mice to quantify the ^{64}Cu-DOTA-QD-RGD and ^{64}Cu-DOTA-QD-VEGF uptake in tumor and major organs. Excellent linear correlation was obtained between the results measured by *in vivo* PET imaging and those measured by *ex vivo* NIR fluorescent imaging and tissue homogenate fluorescence. Histologic examination revealed that ^{64}Cu-DOTA-QD-RGD targets primarily the tumor vasculature through a RGD-integrin interaction, with little extravasation. The authors concluded that this dual-function probe has significantly reduced potential toxicity and overcomes the tissue penetration limitation of optical imaging, requisite for quantitative targeted imaging in deep tissue.

Iron oxide nanoparticles have magnetic properties and have been extensively investigated for biomedical applications due to their excellent biocompatibility and ease of synthesis. Jarrett et al. (2008) recently reported a dual-mode imaging probe for PET/MRI that was designed for vascular inflammation, and this probe was based on iron oxide nanoparticles coupled to ^{64}Cu. The labeling of SPIONs was made by coordination of ^{64}Cu to the chelating bifunctional ligand *S*-2-(4- isothiocyanatobenzyl)-1,4,7,10-tetraazacyclododecane-1,4,7,10-tetraacetic acid (*p*-SCNBz-DOTA) and followed by conjugation to the nanoparticle. For the dextran sulfate coated nanoparticles, the particle surface was modified to contain aldehyde groups that can be conjugated to the amine-reactive *p*-SCN-Bz-DOTA chelator. Xie et al. (2010) encapsulated iron oxide nanoparticles (IONPs) into human serum albumin (HSA) matrices. The HSA coated IONPs (HSA-IONPs) were dually labeled with ^{64}Cu-DOTA and Cy5.5, and tested in a subcutaneous U87MG xenograft mouse model. *In vivo* PET/NIR fluorescence/MRI tri-modality imaging showed massive accumulation in lesions, high extravasation rate, and low uptake of the particles by macrophages at the tumor area. Glaus et al. (2010) prepared ^{64}Cu-DOTA-PEG-SPIOs which demonstrated strong MR and PET signals and high stability in mouse serum for 24 h at 37 °C.

To image $\alpha_V\beta_3$ expression, multifunctional ^{64}Cu-labeled IONPs conjugated to RGD have been reported. Lee et al. (2008) developed the ^{64}Cu-DOTA-IO-RGD system (diameter: 45 ± 10 nm) containing 35 RGD peptide molecules and 30 DOTA chelating units per nanoparticle. The receptor-binding affinity studies for $\alpha_v\beta_3$ integrin in U87MG cells showed an IC50 value of 34 ± 5 nM. cRGDfC and the macrocyclic 1,4,7-triazacyclononane-N,N',N''-triacetic-thiol derivative (NOTA-SH) were conjugated onto the iron oxide nanoparticles. ^{64}Cu-labeled SPIONs conjugated to cRGDfC demonstrated a good U87MG tumor-targeting capability and tumor contrast by PET/MRI dual-modality imaging (Yang et al., 2011).

Liu et al. (2007) investigated the biodistribution of ^{64}Cu-labeled SWNTs conjugated to polyethylene-glycol-DOTA and RGD in mice with U87MG-induced tumors using PET, *ex vivo* biodistribution and Raman spectroscopy. The results showed a high ^{64}Cu-DOTA-PEG-

SWNT-RGD tumor accumulation (~7% at 1 h) that was attributed to the multivalent effect of the SWNTs.

Gold nanoshells (NSs) are core/shell particles comprised of a gold shell and a dielectric silica core with peak plasmon resonances tunable to desired wavelengths by adjusting the relative core and shell thicknesses. At NIR wavelengths, light penetrates up to several centimeters in tissue. NSs absorb in the NIR wavelength and efficiently convert incident light to heat (eg, a 120-nm core diameter and a 14-nm-thick shell result in an absorption peak between 780 nm and 800 nm). Xie et al. (2011) reported the preparation of ^{64}Cu-DOTA labeled NSs conjugated to cRGDfK and evaluated the *in vivo* biodistribution and tumor specificity of these in live nude rats bearing head and neck squamous cell carcinoma (HNSCC) xenografts. The potential therapeutic properties were also evaluated by subablative thermal therapy of tumors. PET/CT imaging showed a high tumor uptake even at ~20 h postinjection and the thermal therapy study showed a high degree of tumor necrosis.

Core	Surface molecule/Target	^{64}Cu Chelator	Imaging Modality	Reference
Quantum Dots	RGD/$\alpha_v\beta_3$ integrin or VEGF/VEGF-r	DOTA	PET/NIR fluorescence	Cai et al., 2007; Chen et al., 2010
Iron oxide nanoparticles	RGD/$\alpha_v\beta_3$ integrin	DOTA and *p*-SCN-Bz-DOTA	PET/MRI	Lee et al., 2008; Jarret et al., 2008
		NOTA-SH		Yang et al., 2011
	PEGylated phospholipids	DOTA	PET/MRI	Glaus et al., 2010
	Human serum albumin and Cy5.5	DOTA	PET/MRI/ NIR fluorescence	Xie et al., 2010
Carbon nanotubes	RGD/$\alpha_v\beta_3$ integrin	PEG-DOTA	PET/NIR fluorescence	Liu et al., 2007
Gold nanoshells	RGD/$\alpha_v\beta_3$ integrin	DOTA	PET/CT imaging and thermotherapy	Hie et al., 2011

Table 2. ^{64}Cu-labeled nanoparticles for PET imaging

4.2 ^{18}F labeled iron oxide nanoparticles for PET/MRI

The main requirement for MRI is the efficient capture of magnetic nanoparticles by the cell, and when a cell is sufficiently loaded with magnetic material, MRI can also be used for cell tracking. The synthesis and *in vivo* characterization of iron oxide nanoparticles labeled with ^{18}F was reported by Devaraj et al. (2009). This particle consists of cross-linked dextran molecules held together in core-shell formation by a superparamagnetic iron oxide core and functionalized with the radionuclide ^{18}F in high yield, via "click" chemistry. Such nanoparticles could accurately detect lymph nodes (LNs), which are critical for assessing cancer metastasis. *In vivo* PET/MRI images could clearly identify small (~1 mm) LNs along with precise anatomical information.

4.3 ^{68}Ga labeled nanoparticles

Stelter et al. (2009) covalently bound the transfection agent HIV-1 Tat (peptide derived from the transcription protein transactivator of the human immunodeficiency virus), the fluorescent dye fluorescein isothiocyanate and ^{68}Ga to the aminosilane-coated superparamagnetic nanoparticle. PET imaging and MRI revealed increasing hepatic and splenic accumulation of the particles over 24 h in Wistar rats. Hepatogenic HuH7 cells were labeled with the radionanoparticles and injected them intravenously into rats, followed by animal PET and MRI imaging. *In vitro* studies in hepatogenic HuH7 cells showed a rapid intracellular accumulation of the labeled nanoparticles and without any signs of toxicity. *In vivo* dissemination of the labeled cells was followed by dynamic biodistribution studies. This radionanoconjugate can be applicable to efficient cell labeling and subsequent multimodal molecular imaging. Moreover, their multiple free amino groups suggest the possibility of further modifications and might provide interesting opportunities for various research fields.

A quadruple imaging modality made using nanoparticles that is capable of concurrent fluorescence, bioluminescence, bioluminescence resonance energy transfer (BRET), PET and MRI has been reported (Hwang et al., 2009). A cobalt-ferrite nanoparticle surrounded by rhodamine (MF) was conjugated with luciferase (MFB) and p-SCNbnNOTA (2-(4-isothiocyanatobenzyl)-1,4,7-triazacyclonane-1,4,7-triacetic acid) followed by $^{68}GaCl_3$ (magnetic-fluorescent-bioluminescent-radioisotopic particle, MFBR). Confocal microscopy revealed good transfection efficiency of MFB into cells and BRET was also observed in MFB. A good correlation among rhodamine, luciferase, and $^{68}GaCl_3$ was found in MFBR, and the activities of each imaging modality increased dose-dependently with the amount of MFBR in the C6 cells. *In vivo* optical images were acquired from the thighs of mice after intramuscular and subcutaneous injections of MFBR-laden cells. MicroPET and MR images showed intense radioactivity and ferromagnetic intensities with MFBR-laden cells. The multimodal imaging strategy could be used as a potential imaging tool to improve the diagnostic accuracy.

5. Radiolabeled nanoparticle for therapy

Radiolabeled nanoparticles represent novel agents with huge potential for clinical radiotherapy applications. McDevitt et al. (2010) proposed the radiolabeling of carbon nanotubes (DOTA-NTs, diameter of 1.4 nm.) functionalized by the anti-CD20 monoclonal antibody (Rituximab), the α-particle emitter ^{225}Ac and the β-particle emitter ^{90}Y. Alpha-emitters can be efficient therapeutics against small-volume tumors and micrometastatic cancers due to the linear energy transfer that is 500 times greater than that of β particles; hence, damaged cells have inadequate capability to repair DNA injure, and cell death may result. Beta-particle emitters are the most widely used radionuclides among the cancer therapeutic agents because the localized decay in target cells generates DNA damaging free radicals, which can induce apoptosis (Fig. 4). Kucka et al. (2006) have also proposed the astatination of silver nanoparticles conjugated to poly(ethylene oxide) as possible carriers of the α-particle emitter ^{211}At.

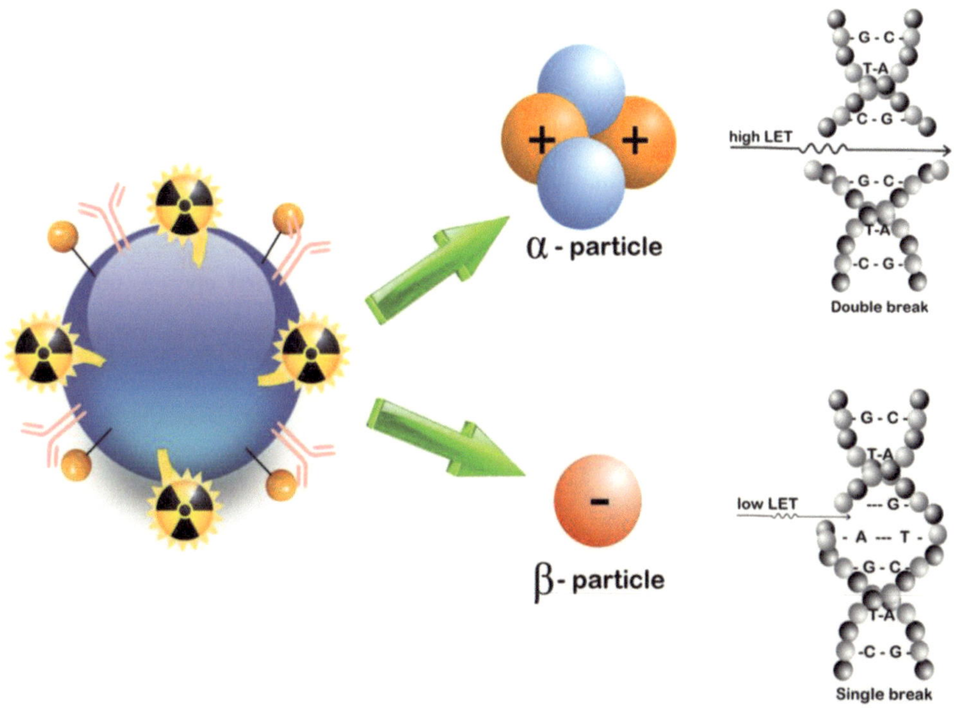

Fig. 4. Schematic representation of radiolabeled nanoparticles for therapeutic applications

The impermeable nature of the cell plasma membrane limits the therapeutic uses of many macromolecules. Several cell penetrating peptides, such as the HIV-1 Tat peptide, have been shown to traverse the cell membrane (where integral protein transduction domains (PTDs) are responsible for cellular uptake) and to reach the nucleus while retaining biological activity. PTDs can enable the cellular delivery of conjugated biomolecules and even nanoparticles, but nuclear delivery needs other strategies. Berry et al. (2007) developed biocompatible gold nanoparticles of differing sizes, functionalized with the HIV Tat-PTD, with the aim of producing nuclear targeting agents. The particles were subsequently tested *in vitro* on a human fibroblast cell line, and the results demonstrated successful nanoparticle transfer across the plasma membrane with 5 nm particles achieving nuclear entry while larger 30 nm particles were retained in the cytoplasm, suggesting entry was blocked via nuclear pores dimensions. ^{99m}Tc internalized in cancer cell nuclei acts as an effective system of targeted radiotherapy because of the Auger and internal conversion electron emissions near DNA. The HIV Tat(49-57) is a cell penetrating peptide that reaches DNA (Santos-Cuevas et al., 2011). Therefore, ^{99m}Tc-labeled gold nanoparticles (5nm) prepared by the methods previously described (Ocampo-Garcia et al., 2011b; Morales-Avila et al., 2011) and conjugated to the HIV Tat(49-57) peptide, could potentially be a multifunctional system with properties suitable for targeted radionuclide therapy.

The β-particle emitter ^{188}Re has been conjugated to NPs for radiotherapy purposes. In 2004, Cao et al. prepared silica-coated magnetite nanoparticles immobilized with histidine. ^{188}Re was linked on their surface by the complexation of $[^{188}Re(CO)_3(H_2O)_3]^+$ to the imidazolyl groups of histidine, obtaining a labeling yield of 91%. A direct labeling method has also been reported that radiolabels SPIONs with rhenium-188 (Liang et al., 2007). The radiolabeling efficiency was about 90%, with good *in vitro* stability. ^{188}Re labeled SPIONs demonstrated the ability to kill SMMC-7721 liver cancer cells.

Photothermal ablation (PTA) therapy is a minimally invasive alternative to conventional approaches for cancer treatment. NPs, primarily gold nanostructures such as gold nanoshells, nanorods, nanocages and hollow nanospheres but also carbon nanotubes, have been investigated as photothermal coupling agents to enhance the efficacy of PTA therapy. These plasmonic nanomaterials exhibit strong absorption in the NIR region (700-1100 nm) and offer the opportunity to convert optical energy into thermal energy, enabling the deposition of otherwise benign optical energy into tumors for thermal ablation of tumor cells, as recently demonstrated Xie et al. (2011). Furthermore, AuNPs can be labeled with α- or β-particle emitter radionuclides and linked to target specific biomolecules to produce both thermotherapy and radiotheraphy effects on cancer cells.

Zhou et al. (2010) synthesized and evaluated a novel class of chelator-free $[^{64}Cu]CuS$ nanoparticles (NPs) suitable both for PET imaging and as photothermal coupling agents for photothermal ablation. $[^{64}Cu]CuS$ NPs possess excellent stability, and allow robust noninvasive micro-PET imaging. The CuS NPs display strong absorption in the near-infrared (NIR) region (peak at 930 nm); passive targeting prefers the tumor site, and mediated ablation of U87MG tumor cells occurs upon exposure to NIR light both *in vitro* and *in vivo* after either intratumoral or intravenous injection. The combination of small diameter (11 nm), strong NIR absorption, and integration of ^{64}Cu as a structural component makes these $[^{64}Cu]CuS$ NPs suited for multifunctional molecular imaging and therapy.

6. View to the future

Looking into the future of the field of nuclear molecular imaging, we have to think about the development of the next generation of radiopharmaceuticals combining variety of properties and allowing for the simultaneous performance of multiple functions. The great diversity of nanoparticle cores and biomolecules that can be attached to the nanoparticle surface, offers the possibility of creating multifunctional devices to be used in hybrid imaging platforms.

In the field of molecular therapy, some nanoparticles offer novel proposals for the delivery of therapeutic and target-specific drugs. Multifunctional radiolabeled nanoparticles can combine imaging and therapeutic agents in one preparation and specifically target the site of the disease (accumulate there) via both non-specific and specific mechanisms, such as the enhanced permeability and retention (EPR) effect for macromolecules (Maeda et al., 2000) and the ligand-mediated recognition.

In all clinically relevant imaging modalities, contrast agents are used to absorb certain types of signal much stronger than do the surrounding tissues. To still further increase a local spatial concentration of a contrast agent for better imaging, it is a natural progression to use nanoparticles to carry multiple contrast moieties for an efficient enhancing of the signal from these areas (Torchilin, 2006).

A nanoparticle that has intrinsic imaging and therapeutic properties is advantageous. For gold and SWNT nanoparticles, the composition itself produces imaging contrast (optical imaging). Moreover, these nanoparticles have thermoablative properties. Local application of heat is a known concept in therapeutic medicine that has been extensively explored for cancer treatment and other conditions. Excitation sources, such as infrared lamps, ultrasound or lasers, can be used in the process, but there is always the problem of limiting the heat generated to just the area of the target tissue. This problem could be solved by using nanoparticles designed to absorb in the NIR region so that the resulting localized heating causes irreversible thermal cellular destruction. A laser irradiation (NIR light) of SWNT or gold nanoparticles leads to a rise in the temperature of the target regions from 40°C to 50°C, which selectively could destroy a carcinoma (Pissuwan et al., 2006).

An important benefit of receptor-specific radiopharmaceuticals is their use for targeted radiotherapy. Multiple specific biomolecules to target breast cancer cells, appended to one gold nanoparticle and labeled with an imaging radionuclide such as ^{99m}Tc as well as a β-particle-emitting radionuclide such as ^{90}Y, ^{177}Lu or ^{188}Re, could be a multifunctional system useful for the identification of malignant tumors (SPECT/NIR fluorescence imaging) and metastatic sites (avoiding immunohistochemistry studies), for targeted radiotherapy (high β-particle-energy delivered per unit of targeted mass) and for photothermal therapy (localized heating). Furthermore, ^{99m}Tc internalized in cancer cell nuclei acts as an effective system of targeted radiotherapy because of the Auger and internal conversion electron emissions near DNA. ^{99m}Tc-labeled gold nanoparticles described above and also conjugated to the HIV Tat(49-57) peptide to reach DNA, could potentially be a radiotherapeutic system at cellular level. However, for therapeutic purposes NPs should be administered by intratumoral injection or into a selective artery to avoid a high uptake by organs of the reticuloendothelial system because of the NPs' colloidal nature.

The traditional concept of separating diagnosis and treatment could conclude. The use of multifunctional radiolabeled nanoparticles that can simultaneously detect, image, and treat diseases may one day become the first alternative instead of the exception.

7. Conclusions

In our research we have demonstrated that it is possible to prepare stable hybrid radiolabeled gold nanoparticles. Multimeric systems of ^{99m}Tc-labeled gold nanoparticles conjugated to peptides or mannose can be prepared from kit formulations with high radiochemical purities (>94%). ^{99m}Tc-AuNP-Lys^{3}-bombesin, ^{99m}Tc-AuNP-c[RDGfK(C)] and ^{99m}Tc-AuNP-mannose show properties suitable for use as target-specific agents for molecular imaging of GRP receptor-positive tumors, tumor $\alpha_v\beta_3$ expression and sentinel lymph node detection, respectively, with the possibility to be used as photothermal therapeutic systems.

Multifunctional nanoparticles can combine diagnostic and therapeutic capabilities for targeted-specific diagnosis and the treatment of disease. Medical imaging modalities such as SPECT, PET and MRI can identify tumors non-invasively, but radiolabeled nanoparticle probes with multivalent properties can provide multimodal images with enhanced signal and sensitivity. Developments of radioactive QD-, AuNP-, SWNT-, CuS- or IO-target-specific biomolecules can be further developed to provide a visual guide during surgery. Radiolabeled SWNT and gold nanoparticles have a variety of real or potential applications in medical diagnosis and therapeutic treatments, due to their particularly combination of optical and photothermal properties. However, the work in this field is still in its infancy, and the achievement of more *in vivo* preclinical and clinical trials is required.

8. Acknowledgment

The authors are grateful for the support of the Mexican National Council of Science and Technology (CONACYT-SEP-CB-2010-01-150942).

9. References

ASTM E 2456-06: *Standard Terminology related to Nanotechnology.* ASTM International, 100 Barr Harbor Drive, PO Box C700, West Conshohocken, PA, 19428-2959 USA (2006). http://www.astm.org/Standards/E2456.htm

Berry, C.C.; de la Fuente, J.M.; Mullin, M.; Chu, S.W. & Curtis A.S. (2007). Nuclear Localization of HIV-1 Tat Functionalized Gold Nanoparticles. *IEEE Trans Nanobioscience*, Vol.6, No.4, (December 2007), pp. 262-269, ISSN 1536-1241

Cai, W.; Chen, K.; Li, Z.B.; Gambhir, S.S. & Chen, X. (2007). Dual-Function Probe for PET and Near-Infrared Fluorescence Imaging of Tumor Vasculature. *Journal of Nuclear Medicine*, Vol.48, No.11, (November 2007), pp. 1862-1870, ISSN 0161-5505

Cao, J.; Wang, Y.; Yu J.; Xia J.; Zhang C.; Yin D. & Häfeli U.O. (2004). Preparation and Radiolabeling of Surface-Modified Magnetic Nanoparticles with Rhenium-188 for Magnetic Targeted Radiotherapy. *Journal of Magnetism and Magnetic Materials*, Vol.277, No.1-2, (February 2004), pp. 165-174, ISSN 0304-8853

Chan, H.B.S.; Ellis, B.L.; Sharma, H.L.; Frost, W.; Caps, V.; Shields, R.A. & Tsang, S.C. (2004). Carbon-Encapsulated Radioactive ^{99m}Tc Nanoparticles. *Advanced Materials*, Vol.16, No.2, (January 2004), pp. 144-149, ISSN 0935-9648

Chen, K. & Conti, P.S. (2010). Target-Specific Delivery of Peptide-Based Probes for PET Imaging. *Advanced Drug Delivery Reviews*, Vol.62, No.11, (August 2010), pp. 1005–1022, ISSN 0169-409X

Chen, K.; Li, Z-B.; Wang, H.; Cai, W. & Chen, X. (2010). Dual-modality Optical and Positron Emission Tomography Imaging of Vascular Endothelial Growth Factor Receptor on Tumor Vasculature Using Quantum Dots. *European Journal of Nuclear Medicine and Molecular Imaging*, Vol.35, No.12, (December 2010), pp. 2235-2244, ISSN 1619-7089

Cheung, W.H.; Chan, V.S.; Pang, H.W.; Wong, M.K.; Guo, Z.H.; Tam, P.K.; Che, C.M.; Lin, C.L.; & Yu, W.Y. (2009). Conjugation of Latent Membrane Protein (LMP)-2 Epitope to Gold Nanoparticles as Highly Immunogenic Multiple Antigenic Peptides for Induction of Epstein-Barr Virus-Specific Cytotoxic T-lymphocyte Responses in Vitro. *Bioconjugate Chemistry*, Vol.20, No.1, (January 2009), pp. 24-31, ISSN 1520-4812

Chrastina, A. & Schnitzer, J.E. (2010). Iodine-125 Radiolabeling of Silver Nanoparticles for in Vivo SPECT Imaging. *International Journal of Nanomedicine*, Vol.5, (September 2010), pp. 653-659, ISSN 1176-9114

Connor, E.E.; Mwamuka, J.; Gole, A.; Murphy, C.J. & Wyatt, M.D. (2005). Gold Nanoparticles Are Taken Up by Human Cells But Do Not Cause Acute Cytotoxicity. *Small*, Vol.1, No.3, (March, 2005), pp. 325–327, ISSN 1613-6810

Daniel, M.C. & Astruc, D. (2004). Gold Nanoparticles: Assembly, Supramolecular Chemistry, Quantum-Size-Related Properties, and Applications Toward Biology, Catalysis, and Nanotechnology. *Chemical Reviews*, Vol.104, No.1, (January 2004), pp. 293–346, ISSN 0009-2665

Devaraj, N.K.; Keliher, E.J.; Thurber, G.M.; Nahrendorf, M. & Weissleder, R. (2009). ^{18}F-Labeled Nanoparticles for In Vivo PET/CT Imaging. *Bioconjugate Chemistry*, Vol.20, No.2, pp. 397-401, (February 2009), ISSN 1520-4812

Dumortier, H.; Lacotte, S.; Pastorin, G.; Marega, R.; Wu, W.; Bonifazi, D.; Briand, J.P.; Prato, M.; Muller, S. & Bianco, A. (2006). Functionalized Carbon Nanotubes are Non-Cytotoxic and Preserve the Functionality of Primary Immune Cells. *Nano Letters*, Vol.6, No.7, (July 2006), pp. 1522–1528, ISSN 1530-6984

Erathodiyil N. & Ying J.Y. (2011). Functionalization of Inorganic Nanoparticles for Bioimaging Applications. *Accounts of Chemical Research*, DOI: 10.1021/ar2000327, (June 2011), ISSN 1968-12010

Ferro-Flores, G.; Arteaga de Murphy, C.; Rodriguez-Cortes, J.; Pedraza-Lopez, M. & Ramirez-Iglesias, M.T. (2006). Preparation and Evaluation of ^{99m}Tc-EDDA/HYNIC-[Lys^{3}]-bombesin for Imaging of GRP Receptor-Positive Tumours. *Nuclear Medicine Communications*, Vol.27, No.4, (April 2006), pp. 371-376, ISSN 0143-3636

Ferro-Flores, G.; Ramirez, F. de M.; Melendez-Alafort, L. & Santos-Cuevas, C.L. (2010a). Peptides for In Vivo Target-Specific Cancer Imaging. *Mini Reviews in Medicinal Chemistry*, Vol.10, No.1, (January, 2010), pp. 87-97, ISSN 1389-5575

Ferro-Flores, G.; Ocampo-Garcia B.E.; Ramirez F. de M.; Gutierrez-Wing C.; Arteaga de Murphy C. & Santos-Cuevas C.L. (2010b). Gold Nanoparticles Conjugated to Peptides, In: *Colloids in Biothechnology*, M. Fanun, (Ed.), 231-252, CRC Press/Taylor & Francis, ISBN: 978-143-983-080-2, Boca Raton, FL, United States of America

Gao, X.H.; Cui, Y.Y.; Levenson, R.M.; Chung, L.W.K.; Nie, S.M. (2004). *In Vivo* Cancer Targeting and Imaging with Semiconductor Quantum Dots. *Nature Biotechnology*, Vol.22, No.8, (August 2004), pp.969-966, ISSN 1087-0156

Giljohann, D.A.; Seferos, D.S.; Daniel, W.L.; Massich, M.D.; Patel, P.C. & Mirkin, C. A. (2010). Gold Nanoparticles for Biology and Medicine. *Angewandte Chemie International Edition*, Vol.49, No.19, (April 2010), pp.3280-3294, ISSN 0570-0833

Glaus, C.; Rossin, R.; Welch, M.J. & Bao, G. (2010). In Vivo Evaluation of ^{64}Cu-Labeled Magnetic Nanoparticles as a Dual-Modality PET/MR Imaging Agent. *Bioconjugate Chemistry*, Vol. 21, No.4, (April 2010), pp. 715–722, ISSN 1043-1802

Guo, J.; Zhang, X.; Li, Q. & Li, W. (2007). Biodistribution of Functionalized Multiwall Carbon Nanotubes in mice. *Nuclear Medicine and Biology*, Vol.34, No.5, (May 2007), pp. 579-583, ISSN 0969-8051

Hata, K.; Futaba, D.N.; Mizuno, K.; Namai, T.; Yumura M. & Iijima S. (2004). Water-Assisted Highly Efficient Synthesis of Impurity-Free Single-Walled Carbon Nanotubes. *Science*, Vol.306, No.5700, (November 2004), pp.1362-1364, ISSN 0036-8075

Hong, H.; Zhang, Y.; Sun, J. & Cai, W. (2009a). Molecular Imaging and Therapy of Cancer with Radiolabeled Nanoparticles. *Nanotoday*, Vol.4., No.5, (October 2009), pp. 399-413, ISSN 1748-0132

Hong, H.; Gao, T. & Cai, W. (2009b). Molecular Imaging with Single-Walled Carbon Nanotubes. *Nanotoday*, Vol.4, No.3, (July 2009), pp.252-261, ISSN 1748-0132

Huang, X.; Neretina, S. & El-Sayed, M.A. (2009). Gold Nanorods: From Synthesis and Properties to Biological and Biomedical Applications. *Advanced Materials*, Vol.21, No.48, (December 2009), pp. 4880–4910, ISSN 0935-9648

Hwang, D.W.; Ko, H.Y.; Kim, S.K.; Kim, D.; Lee, D.S. & Kim, S. (2009). Development of a Quadruple Imaging Modality by Using Nanoparticles. *Chemistry- A European Journal*, Vol.15, No.37, (September 2009), pp. 9387-9393, ISSN 1521-3765

Jadzinsky, P.D.; Calero, G.; Ackerson, C.J.; Bushnell, D.A. & Komberg, R.D. (2007). Structure of a Thiol Monolayer-Protected Gold Nanoparticle at 1.1 A Resolution. *Science*, Vol.318, No.5849, (September 2007), pp. 430-433, ISSN 0036-8075

Jarrett, B.R.; Gustafsson, B.; Kukis, D.L. & Louie, A.Y. (2008). Synthesis of ^{64}Cu-Labeled Magnetic Nanoparticles for Multimodal Imaging. *Bioconjugate Chemistry*, Vol.19, No.7, (July 2008), pp.1496–1504, ISSN 1043-1802

Kam, N.W.S.; O'Connel,l M.; Wisdom, J.A. & Dai, H. (2005). Carbon Nanotubes as Multifunctional Biological Transporters and Near-infrared Agents for Selective Cancer Cell Destruction. *Proceedings of the National Academy of Sciences of the United States of America*, Vol.102, No.33, (August 2005), pp.11600–11605, ISSN 0027-8424

Kogan, M.J.; Olmedo, I.; Hosta, L.; Guerrero, A R.; Cruz L.J. & Albericio F. (2007). Peptides and Metallic Nanoparticles for Biomedical Applications. *Nanomedicine*, Vol.2, No.3, (June 2007), pp.287-306, ISSN 1743-5889

Kubas, H.; Schafer, M.; Bauder-Wust, U.; Eder, M.; Oltmanns, D.; Haberkorn, U.; Mier, W. & Eisenhut, M. (2010). Multivalent Cyclic RGD Ligands: Influence of Linker Lengths on Receptor Binding. *Nuclear Medicine and Biology*, Vol.37, No.8, (November 2010), pp. 885–891. ISSN 0969-8051

Kucka, J.; Hruby, M.; Konak, C.; Kozempel, J. & Lebeda, O. (2006). Astatination of Nanoparticles Containing Silver as Possible Carriers of ^{211}At. *Applied Radiation and Isotopes*, Vol.64, No. 2, (February 2006), pp. 201-206, ISSN 1872-9800

Lee, H.Y.; Li, Z.; Chen, K.; Hsu, A.R.; Xu, C.; Xie, J.; Sun, S. & Chen, X. (2008). PET/MRI Dual-Modality Tumor Imaging Using Arginine-Glycine-Aspartic (RGD)-Conjugated Radiolabeled Iron Oxide Nanoparticles. *Journal of Nuclear Medicine*, Vol.49, No.8, (April 2008), pp. 1371–1379, ISSN 0161-5505

Levy, R.; Thanh, N.T.K.; Doty, R.C.; Hussain, I.; Nichols, R.J.; Schiffrin, D.J.; Brust M. & Ferning, D.G., (2004). Rational and Combinatorial Design of Peptide Capping Ligands for Gold Nanoparticles. *Journal of American Chemical Society*, Vol.126, No.32, (July 2004), pp. 10076-10084, ISSN 0002-7863

Liang, S.; Wang, Y.; Yu, J.; Zhang, C.; Xia, J. & Yin, D. (2007). Surface Modified Superparamagnetic Iron Oxide Nanoparticles: As a New Carrier for Bio-Magnetically Targeted Therapy. *Journal of Materials Science: Materials in Medicine*, Vol.18, No.12, (December 2007), pp. 2297-2302, ISSN 0957-4530

Liu, S. (2008). Bifunctional Coupling Agents for Radiolabeling of Biomolecules and Target-specific Delivery of Metallic Radionuclides. *Advanced Drug Delivery Reviews*, Vol.60, No.12, (September 2008), pp. 1347-1370, ISSN 0169-409x

Liu, S. (2009).Radiolabeled cyclic RGD Peptides as Integrin $\alpha_{\upsilon}\beta_3$-Targeted Radiotracers: Maximizing Binding Affinity Via Bivalency. *Bioconjugate Chemistry*, Vol.20, No.12, (December 2009), pp.2199-2213, ISSN 1520-4812

Liu, Z.; Cai, W.; He, L.; Nakayama, N.; Chen, K.; Sun, X.; Chen, X. & Dai, H. (2007). In vivo Biodistribution and Highly Efficient Tumor Targeting of Carbon Nanotubes in Mice. *Nature Nanotechnology*, Vol.2, No.1, (January 2007), pp.47-52, ISSN 1748-3395

Madsen, M.T. (2007). Recent Advances in SPECT Imaging. *Journal of Nuclear Medicine*, Vol.48, No.4, (April 2007), pp. 661-673, ISSN 0161-5505

Maeda, H.; Wu, J.; Sawa, T.; Matsumura, Y. & Hori, K. (2000). Tumor vascular permeability and the EPR effect in macromolecular therapeutics: a review. *Journal of Controlled Release*, Vol.65, No.1-2, (March 2000), pp. 271-284, ISSN 0168-3659

Massoud, T.F. & Gamghir, S.S. (2003). Molecular Imaging in Living Subjects: Seeing Fundamental Biological Processes in a New Light. *Genes and Development*, Vol.17, No.5, (May 2003), pp. 545-580, ISSN 0890-9369

McDevitt, M.R.; Chattopadhyay, D.; Kappel, B.J.; Jaggi, J.S.; Schiffman, S.R.; Antczak, C.; Njardarson, J.T.; Brentjens, R. & Scheinberg D.A. (2007). Tumor Targeting with Antibody-Functionalized Radiolabeled Carbon Nanotubes. *Journal of Nuclear Medicine*, Vol.48, No.7, (July 2007), pp. 1180-1189, ISSN 0161-5505

Mendoza-Sanchez, A.N.; Ferro-Flores, G.; Ocampo-Garcia, B.E.; Morales-Avila, E.; Ramirez, F. de M.; De Leon-Rodriguez, L.M.; Santos-Cuevas, C.L.; Medina, L.A.; Rojas-Calderon, E.L. & Camacho-Lopez M.A. (2010). Lys^3-Bombesin Conjugated to ^{99m}Tc-Labelled Gold Nanoparticles for In Vivo Gastrin Releasing Peptide-Receptor Imaging. *Journal of Biomedical Nanotechnology*, Vol.6, No.4 (August 2010), pp. 375-384, ISSN 1550-7033

Montet, X.; Funovics, M.; Montet-Abou, K.; Weissleder, R. & Josephson, L. (2006). Multivalent Effects of RGD Peptides Obtained by Nanoparticle Display. *Journal of Medicinal Chemistry*, Vol.49, No.20, (September 2006), pp. 6087-6093, ISSN 0022-2623

Morales-Avila, E.; Ferro-Flores, G.; Ocampo-Garcia, B.E.; De Leon, L.M.; Santos-Cuevas, C.L.; Medina, L.A. & Gomez-Olivan L. (2011). Multimeric System of ^{99m}Tc-labeled Gold Nanoparticles Conjugated to c[RGDfK(C)] for Molecular Imaging of Tumour $\alpha_v\beta_3$ expression. *Bioconjugate Chemistry*, Vol.22, No.5, (May 2011), pp. 913-922, ISSN 1043-1802

Ocampo-Garcia, B.E.; Ferro-Flores, G.; Morales-Avila, E. & Ramirez, F. de M. (2011a). Kit for Preparation of Multimeric Receptor-Specific ^{99m}Tc-Radiopharmaceuticals Based on Gold Nanoparticles. *Nuclear Medicine Communications*, Vol. 32, No.11 (November 2011), pp. 1095-1104, ISSN 0143-3636

Ocampo-Garcia, B.E.; Ramirez, F. de M.; Ferro-Flores, G.; Leon-Rodriguez, L.M.; Santos-Cuevas, C.L.; Morales-Avila, E.; Arteaga de Murphy, C.; Pedraza-Lopez, M.; Medina, L.A. & Camacho-Lopez, M.A. (2011b). ^{99m}Tc-labeled Gold Nanoparticles Capped with HYNIC Peptide/Mannose for Sentinel Lymph Node Detection. *Nuclear Medicine and Biology*, Vol.38, No.1, (January 2011), pp. 1–11, ISSN 0969-8051

Pissuwan, D.; Valenzuela, S.M. & Cortie, M.B. Therapeutic possibilities of plasmonically heated gold nanoparticles. *Trends in Biotechnology*, Vol.24, No.2, (February 2006), pp. 62-67, ISSN 0167-7799

Porta, F.; Speranza, G.; Krpetic, Z.; Santo, V.D.; Francescato, P. & Scari, G. (2007). Gold Nanoparticles Capped by Peptides. *Materials Science and Engineering: B*, Vol.140, No.3 (June 2007), pp. 187-194, ISSN 0921-5107

Qingnuan, L.; Yan, X.; Xiaodong, Z.; Ruili, L.; Qieqie, D.; Xiaoguang, S.; Shaoliang, C. & Wenxin, L. (2002). Preparation of ^{99m}Tc-$C_{60}(OH)_x$ and its Biodistribution Studies. *Nuclear Medicine and Biology*, Vol.29, No.6, (June 2002), pp. 707-710, ISSN 0969-8051

Santos-Cuevas, C.L.; Ferro-Flores, G.; Arteaga de Murphy, C. & Pichardo-Romero, P. (2008) Targeted Imaging of GRP Receptors with ^{99m}Tc-EDDA/HYNIC-[Lys^3]-Bombesin: Biokinetics and Dosimetry in Women. *Nuclear Medicine Communications*, Vol.29, No.8, (August 2008), pp. 741-747, ISSN 0143-3636

Santos-Cuevas, C.L.; Ferro-Flores, G.; Rojas-Calderon, E.L.; Garcia-Becerra, R.; Ordaz-Rosado, D.; Arteaga de Murphy, C. & Pedraza-Lopez, M. (2011). ^{99m}Tc-N_2S_2-Tat(49-57)-Bombesin Internalized in Nuclei of Prostate and Breast Cancer Cells: Kinetics, Dosimetry and Effect on Cellular Proliferation. *Nuclear Medicine Communications*, Vol.32, No.4, (April 2011), pp. 303-313, ISSN 0143-3636

Singh, R.; Pantarotto, D.; Lacerda, L.; Pastorin, G.; Klumpp, C.; Prato, M.; Bianco, A.; Kostarelos, K. (2006). Tissue Biodistribution and Blood Clearance Rates of Intravenously Administered Carbon Nanotube Radiotracers. *Proceedings of the National Academy of Sciences of the United States of America*, Vol.103, No.9, (February 2006), pp. 3357–62, ISSN 0027-8424

Stelter, L.; Pinkernelle, J.G.; Michel, R.; Schwartlander, R.; Raschzok, N.; Morgul, M.H.; Koch, M.; Denecke, T.; Ruf, J. & Baumler, H. (2009). Modification of Aminosilanized Superparamagnetic Nanoparticles: Feasibility of Multimodal Detection Using 3T MRI, Small Animal PET, and Fluorescence Imaging. *Molecular Imaging and Biology*, Vol.12, No.1, (January 2009), pp. 25-34, ISSN 1536-1632

Sun, Y. & Xia, Y. (2002). Shape-Controlled Synthesis of Gold and Silver Nanoparticles. *Science*, Vol. 298, No.5601, (December, 2002), pp. 2176-2179, ISSN 0036-8075

Surujpaul, P.P.; Gutierrez-Wing, C.; Ocampo-Garcia, B.E.; Ramirez, F. de M.; Arteaga de Murphy, C.; Pedraza-Lopez, M.; Camacho-Lopez, M.A. & Ferro-Flores, G. (2008). Gold nanoparticles conjugated to [Tyr^3]octreotide peptide. *Biophysical Chemistry*, Vol.138, No.3, (December 2008), pp. 83-90, ISSN 0301-4622

Takagi, K.; Uehara, T.; Kaneko, E.; Nakayama, M.; Koizumi, M.; Endo, E. & Arano, Y. (2004). ^{99m}Tc-labeled Mannosyl-Neoglycoalbumin for Sentinel Lymph Node Identification.

Nuclear Medicine and Biology, Vol.31, No.7, (October 2003), pp. 893–900, ISSN 0969-8051

Torchilin, V.P. (2006). Multifunctional nanocarriers. *Advanced Drug Delivery Reviews*, Vol.58, No.14, (December 2006), pp. 1532-1555, ISSN 0169-409X

Torres Martin de Rosales, R.; Tavare, R.; Glaria, A.; Varma, G.; Protti, A. & Blower P.J. (2011). ^{99m}Tc-Bisphosphonate-Iron Oxide Nanoparticle Conjugates for Dual-Modality Biomedical Imaging. *Bioconjugate Chemistry*, Vol.22, No.3, (March 2010), pp. 455-465, ISSN 1043-1802

Vera, D.R.; Wallace, A.M.; Hoh, C.K. & Mattrey, R.F. (2001). A Synthetic Macromolecule for Sentinel Node Detection: ^{99m}Tc-DTPA-Mannosyldextran. *Journal of Nuclear Medicine*, Vol.42, No.6, (June 2001), pp. 951–959, ISSN 0161-5505

Wang, Z.; Levy, R.; Fernig, D.G. & Brust, M. (2005). The Peptide Route to Multifunctional Gold Nanoparticles. *Bioconjugate Chemistry*, Vol.16, No.3, (April 2005), pp. 497-500, ISSN 1043-1802

Xie, H.; Diagaradjane, P.; Deorukhkar, A.A.; Goins, B.; Bao, A.; Phillips, W.T.; Wang, Z.; Schwartz, J. & Krishnan, S. (2011). Integrin $\alpha_v\beta 3$-Targeted Gold Nanoshells Augment Tumor Vasculature-Specific Imaging and Therapy. *International Journal of Nanomedicine*, Vol. 6, (January 27), pp. 259–269, ISSN 1178-2013

Xie, J.; Chen, K.; Huang, J.; Lee, S.; Wang, J.; Gao, J. & Li, X. (2010). PET/NIRF/MRI Triple Functional Iron Oxide Nanoparticles. *Biomaterials*, Vol.31, No.11, (April 2010) pp.3016–3022, ISSN 0142-9612

Xie, R.; Chen, K.; Chen, X. & Peng, X. (2008). InAs/InP/ZnSe Core/Shell/Shell Quantum Dots as Near-Infrared Emitters: Bright, Narrow-Band, Non-Cadmium Containing, and Biocompatible. *Nano Research*, Vol.1, No 6, (October 2008), pp. 457–464, ISSN 1931-7573

Yang, X.; Hong, H.; Grailer, J.J.; Rowland, I. J.; Javadi A.; Hurley, S.A.; Xiao, Y.; Yang, Y.; Zhang, Y.; Nickles, R. J.; Cai, W. & Steeber, D.A. (2011). cRGD-Functionalized, DOX-Conjugated, and ^{64}Cu-labeled Superparamagnetic Iron Oxide Nanoparticles for Targeted Anticancer Drug Delivery and PET/MR Imaging. *Biomaterials*, Vol.32, No. 17, (June 2011), pp. 4151-4160, ISSN 0142-9612.

Yu, W.W.; Wang, Y.A. & Peng, X.G. (2003). Formation and Stability of Size-, Shape-, and Structure-Controlled CdTe Nanocrystals: Ligand Effects on Monomers and Nanocrystals. *Chemistry of Materials*, Vol.15, No.22, (October 2003), pp. 4300-4308, ISSN 1520-5002

Zhang, L.X.; Sun, X.P.; Song, Y.H.; Jiang, X.; Dong, S.J. & Wang, E.A. (2006). Didodecyldimethylammonium Bromide Lipid Bilayer-Protected Gold Nanoparticles: Synthesis, Characterization, and Self-Assembly. *Langmuir*, Vol.22, No.6, (March, 2006), pp. 2838-2843, ISSN 1520-5827

Zhang, G.; Yang, Z.; Lu, W.; Zhang, R.; Huang, Q.; Tian, M.; Li, L.; Liang, D. & Li, C. (2009). Influence of Anchoring Ligands and Particle Size on the Colloidal Stability and *in vivo* Biodistribution of Polyethylene Glycol-Coated Gold Nanoparticles in Tumor-Xenografted Mice. *Biomaterials*, Vol.30, No.10, (April 2009), pp. 1928-1936, ISSN 1878-5905.

Zhou, M.; Zhang, R.; Huang, M.; Lu, W.; Song, S.; Melancon, M.P.; Tian, M.; Liang, D. & Li, C. (2010). A Chelator-Free Multifunctional [^{64}Cu]CuS Nanoparticle Platform for Simultaneous Micro-PET/CT Imaging and Photothermal Ablation Therapy. *Journal of American Chemical Society*, Vol.132, No.43, (October 2010), pp.15351–15358, ISSN 0002-7863

3

Fluorescent X-Ray Computed Tomography Using Synchrotron Radiation Towards Molecular Imaging

Tetsuya Yuasa[1] and Tohoru Takeda[2]
[1]*Yamagata University,*
[2]*Kitasato University,*
Japan

1. Introduction

Presently, nuclear imaging techniques such as positron emission tomography (PET), and single photon emission CT (SPECT) are quite vital tools in clinical medicine as molecular imaging modalities to investigate the cause, diagnosis and therapy of diseases, e.g., Alzheimer's disease, Parkinson's disease, ischemic heart disease, cardiomyopathy and cancer, from the viewpoint of molecule. On the other hand, recent advance in genetic engineering have generated rodent models of human diseases that afford important clues to their causes, diagnoses and treatment. Studies using mouse and rat as the animal models have become important in most areas, such in molecular biology, toxicology, and drug discovery research. Hypotheses about the onset of disease and the effectiveness of treatment can be tested with the animals before terminal studies for human. Mice and rats have become key animal models for the study of development of human disease. They offer the possibility to manipulate their genome and produce accurate models of many human disorders resulting in significant progress in the understandings of human diseases. Also here, the molecular imaging techniques are quite important tools for observing the physiological and pathological status in vivo. However, they still suffer from insufficient spatial resolution. In addition, they must require radio-active imaging agency, resulting in being an intractable measurement method. So, the invention of a novel molecular imaging technique using non-radioactive imaging agencies with high-contrast and high spatial resolutions has been eagerly waited for.

X-ray fluorescence analysis (XRF) is one of the most sensitive physicochemical analysis methods to identify trace elements with high sensitivity and high quantitativeness by detecting the fluorescent x-ray emitted from them. Use of synchrotron x-ray as the light source empowers it to detect trace elements with much higher sensitivity, because synchrotron x-ray has some excellent properties for XRF. Then, fluorescent x-ray scanning tomography (FXST) has been developed based on XRF to investigate a 2-dimensional distributions of specific elements. SR-FXST at the first stage was employed in planar mode to evaluate very low contents of medium- or high-atomic-number trace elements up to the pictograms range (Iida & Gohshi, 1991; Takeda, et al., 1995). However, this method is usually limited to scanning either the surface of the object or thin slices of samples with a perpendicular x-ray beam. Fluorescent x-ray computed tomography (FXCT) method combining SR-XRF with computed tomography technique bypasses this restriction. Hogan et al. (Hogan et al., 1991) theoretically discussed this approach and we were the first to implement it by using synchrotron radiation (Takeda, et al., 1996; –, 1998).

SR-FXCT enables us to establish a low-invasive or non-destructive cross-sectional imaging method for biomedical use at high sensitivity and at high spatial resolution. The SR-FXCT is being developed to depict the distribution of specific elements inside the biomedical object (Takeda, et al., 2000; –, 2001). So far, we have successfully imaged myocardinal fatty acid metabolism of cardiomyopathic animal model ex vivo (Thet-Thet-Lwin, et al., 2007; –, 2008), and cerebral perfusion of small rodents ex vivo (Takeda et al., 2009) after injecting non-radioactive iodine labeled cerebral perfusion agent (IMP), and fatty acid metabolic agent (BMIPP), respectively.

Although SR-FXCT allows sub-millimeter resolution, this approach is hampered by the long measurement time required, as conventional FXCT is based on the first generation type of computed tomography (CT), which acquires a set of projections by translational and rotational scans using pencil-beam geometry. In order to complete the measurements during the course of anesthesia, the number of projections and the data acquisition time for each data point need to be reduced, resulting in a reduction in image quality. Thus, just a few slices can be obtained for in vivo imaging of a rat head, while under anesthesia (Takeda, et al., 2009). Therefore, conventional FXCT cannot substitute for PET or SPECT, which can obtain 3-D tomographic images. In order to overcome the difficulty, the parallel data acquisition scheme has been proposed (Huo, et al., 2008; –, 2009).

This chapter is organized as follows. In Section 2, we present some background materials on SR-FXCT. Section 3 first describes SR-FXCT of the first generation based on pencil-beam geometry in its imaging protocol, reconstruction method, and applications, then points out the difficulty to prevent the SR-FXCT from being a molecular imaging modality. A novel type of SR-FXCT based on sheet-beam geometry for overcoming the difficulty is presented in Sections 4. Section 5 discusses the imaging properties of the SR-FXCT based on experimental results. Finally, some concluding remarks are given in Section 6.

2. Backgrounds

In this section, we will introduce the fundamental items indispensable for discussion in the following sections.

2.1 Fluorescent X-ray

When materials are exposed by short-wavelength x-rays or gamma rays, photoelectric effect will take place. The photoelectric effect is a phenomenon in which electrons are emitted from matter after the absorption of energy from electromagnetic radiation. With the removal of an electron in this way, the electronic structure of the atom is unstable, and electrons in higher orbitals "fall" into the lower orbital to fill the hole left behind. In falling, energy is released in the form of a photon, the energy of which is equal to the energy difference of the two orbitals involved. Thus, the fluorescence x-rays will be emitted isotropically (Fig. 1).

There are a limited number of ways in which this can happen, L→K transition is called K_α, an M→K transition is called K_β, an M→L transition is called L_α, and so on (Fig. 2). Since each element has characteristic energy of electronic orbitals, the kind of elements can be investigated by analyzing fluorescent x-ray energy. Furthermore, the intensity of each characteristic radiation is proportional to the amount of elements, so the amount of elements can be investigated from the intensity.

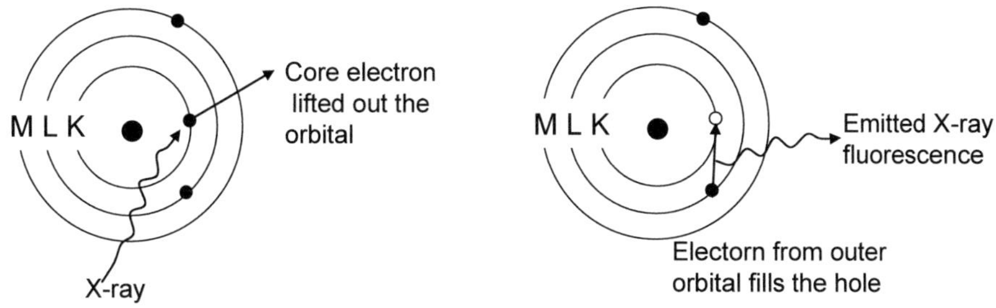

Fig. 1. Emission of fluorescent x ray

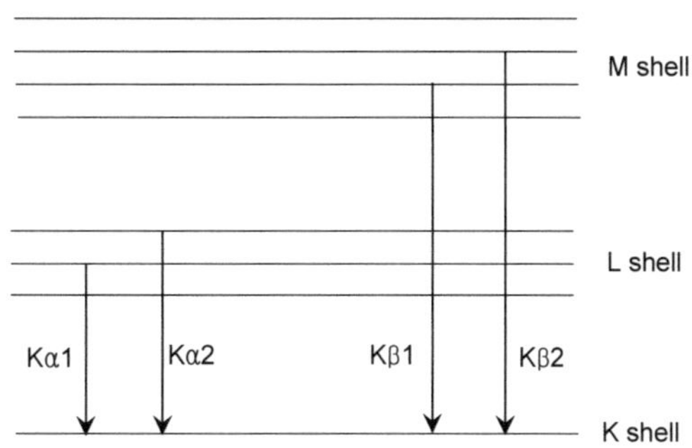

Fig. 2. Characteristics of fluorescent x rays

X-ray fluorescence analysis (XRF) is one of the most sensitive physicochemical analysis methods to identify trace elements with high sensitivity by detecting the fluorescent x ray emitted from them. Use of synchrotron x ray as the light source empowers it to detect trace elements with much higher sensitivity, because synchrotron x-ray has some excellent properties for XRF. In addition, combining XRF with computed tomography technique enable us to establish a low-invasive or non-destructive cross-sectional imaging method for biomedical use at high sensitivity and at high spatial resolution.

2.2 Synchrotron radiation

Synchrotron radiation is electromagnetic radiation from electrons accelerated to high speed in several stages to achieve a final energy that is typically in the GeV range. Then, the electrons are forced to travel in a closed path in a storage ring by strong magnetic fields of a few T. The synchrotron radiation is projected at a tangent to the electron storage ring and captured as beamlines. These beamlines may originate at bending magnets, which mark the corners of the storage ring; or insertion devices, which are located in the straight sections of the storage ring. Beamline is consisted by some optical devices which control the bandwidth, photon flux, beam dimensions, focus, and collimation of the rays.

The synchrotron radiation has some excellent properties as follows:

A. High brightness and high intensity, many orders of magnitude larger than those of x-rays produced by conventional x-ray tubes.
B. High level of polarization (linear or elliptical).
C. High collimation, i.e. small angular divergence of the beam.
D. Low emittance, i.e. the product of source cross section and solid angle of emission is small.
E. Wide tunability in energy/wavelength by monochromatization (sub eV up to the MeV range).
F. High brilliance, exceeding other natural and artificial light sources by many orders of magnitude.

The major applications of synchrotron light are in condensed matter physics, materials science, biology and medicine.

2.3 Computed tomography

In 1972, the first viable computed tomography (CT) scanner was invented by Honsfield using x rays, which can be used to investigate the structures inside bodies with various planes or even as volumetric (3D) representations. Here, we consider a 2-dimensional case using parallel incident beams. We introduce the typical coordinate systems for CT measurements. The *xy*- and *st*-coordinate systems are fixed to the object and the incident ray, as shown in Fig. 3, respectively. Here, the *st*-coordinate system is obtained by rotating the *xy*-coordinate system by θ about the origin in the counter-clockwise direction. X-ray CT is a technique for probing the attenuation coefficient of an object by use of multiple x rays. Each ray is assumed to travel through the object without changing its direction. Measured quantity at each point is described as

$$I_t(s,\theta) = I_o\, e^{\int_{R(s,\theta)} \mu(x,y)\, dl} \tag{1}$$

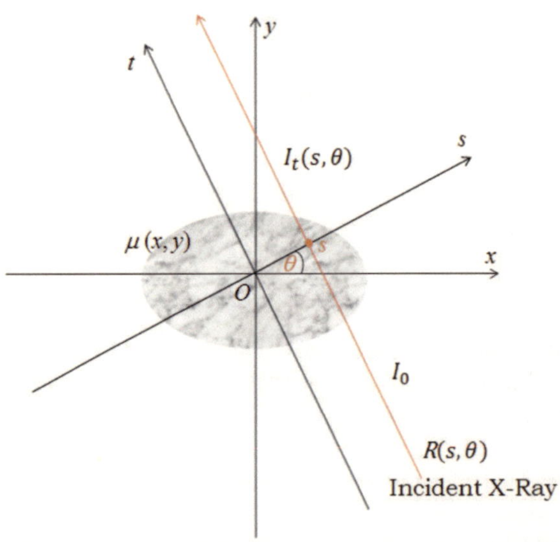

Fig. 3. CT geometry

using the Beer's law. Here, I_t and I_o are the transmitted and the incident x-ray intensities, respectively: μ is a distribution of linear attenuation coefficients, and the shoulder of exponential function means a line integral of μ along the linear trajectory of the incident x ray, $R(s,\theta)$.

In order to reconstruct 2-D function $\mu(x, y)$, we need the line integral along the x-ray path with respect to r and θ. By taking logarithm against Eq. (1), we obtain line integrals, i.e., projections. Projections along multiple x rays in multiple directions are measured. Then, applying a reconstruction algorithm to the projections, such as the filtered backprojection method, the distribution of the attenuation coefficient $\mu(x, y)$ is to be estimated. Here, we notice that the measurements required for CT reconstruction are not x-ray transmittance but the line integral. Therefore, CT measurement is a measurement protocol to systematically collect a series of line integrals of quantity of interest from multiple directions.

2.4 Fluorescent X-ray computed tomography using synchrotron radiation

Fluorescent x-ray computed tomography is a hybrid technique between XRF, which is a physicochemical analysis with high sensitivity and high quantitativeness, and CT, which obtains inside information non-destructively. We give a rough sketch of FXCT here, while the quantitative consideration is given in the next section.

Suppose that a beam of monochromatic x ray is incident on an object containing specific element such as iodine. The advantageous properties of synchrotron radiation for fluorescent x-ray analysis are its broad energy spectrum that allows beam energy tunableness, its high brightness, and its natural forwardly collimation, as described in section 2.2. Thereby, we obtain a high-quality parallel monochromatic beam as an incident beam. The atoms locating on the beam path isotropically emit fluorescent x-ray photons having energy peculiar to the element according to their concentration. Since the amount of fluorescent x-ray photons from each site on the beam path depends on the concentration of the element, we can obtain the line integral of the concentration by acquiring the fluorescent photons efficiently and precisely. For this purpose, we must consider the problem where and how the detector should be set.

We aggressively utilize a linear polarization property of SR. SR is linearly polarized in the plane of the electron storage ring. Ideally, Compton scattered radiation, which is dominant as noise source in hard x-ray regions, is not emitted in a direction at a right angle to the incident beam in the polarization plane (Yuasa et al., 1997; —, 1997). Therefore, the polarized nature of SR allows the maximal reduction of the spectral background originating from Compton scattering in the plane of the storage ring by positioning the detector at 90 degrees to the beam in the plane of the polarization. Preparing an ideal detector having a detective surface with infinitely thin height and infinitely long width, we achieve the objective.

As aforementioned, we can collect the fluorescent x-ray photons with high signal to noise ratio using SR as an incident beam. Projections are acquired at constant angular steps using a translation-rotation motion of the object over 180 degrees.

3. SR-FXCT based on pencil beam geometry

The x-ray fluorescence analysis method has been used in tracer element detection studies, with sensitivities reaching one picogram per gram of certain elements (Iida & Gohshi, 1991).

However, these measurements require a thin sample and, therefore, are limited to measurements near the surface. Then, fluorescent x-ray scanning tomography was developed in order to investigate spatial distributions of specific elements. Fluorescent x-ray scanning tomography employing an x-ray tube has been used to study iodine in samples of several millimeters in diameter (Cesareo & Mascarenhas, 1989), while x-ray fluorescence scanning microtomography employing synchrotron radiation has been used in studies of Fe and Ti in 8-mm samples and in the detection of iron in a bee head (Boisseau & Grodzins, 1987). However, 2-dimensionally scanning a sample is time-consuming. In addition, since the scanning tomography also requires a thin sample, spatial distributions of specific elements in a massive sample cannot be measured (Recently, in order to obtain 3-dimensional tomogram, scanning tomography using a confocal collimator was proposed (Chukalina, et al., 2007)). In order to overcome the problems, Hogan et al. proposed an imaging scheme based on CT concept (Hogan, et al., 1991).

3.1 SR-FXCT imaging system with pencil beam geometry

The schematic diagram of a typical SR-FXCT system of the first generation is shown in Fig. 4. A white x-ray beam from a source is monochromatized using a monochromator, which in our system is a two-crystal Bragg–Bragg device employing Si crystals. It is collimated into a thin beam using a slit before impinging on the subject. Fluorescent x ray is emitted isotropically by the de-exciting contrast atoms along the line of the incident beam, with intensity proportional to the product of the iodine concentration in the incident beam and the incident x-ray flux rate. It is detected in a solid state detector (an HPGe detector) operating in a photon-counting mode. While in this article FXCT from a single kind of imaging agent is discussed, different FXCT images from multiple kinds of imaging agents can be simultaneously obtained by setting the corresponding energy windows (Yu, et al., 2001; Golosio, et al., 2003; Deng, et al., 2007; –, 2011). The detector is collimated to reduce the amount of stray radiation being detected, and is positioned perpendicular to the incident

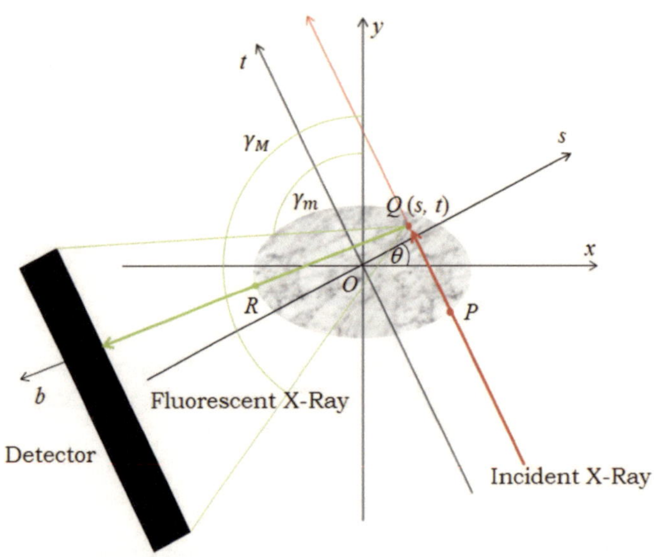

Fig. 4. CT geometry

beam for reducing the Compton scattering background in the spectrum. The energy of the incident beam is carefully tuned so that the fluorescent spectral line does not overlap with the Compton scatter peak. Despite these precautions, the detected signal contains some scattered photons.

In studies of phantom and plant (Simionovici, et al., 2000; —, 2001) and sediment particles, micro-FXCT images were obtained with a spatial resolution of less than 0.01 mm. Our FXCT system, designed for biomedical study, improved the spatial resolution from 1 mm to 0.025 mm. Compared with recent molecular imaging techniques such as micro-PET (positron emission tomography) and micro-SPECT (single photon emission computed tomography), FXCT has the advantage of not requiring the use of a radioactive agent limiting easy preparation of the object (Takeda, et al., 2001). In addition, FXCT has high quantitativeness.

3.2 Principle and formulation

The principles of the fluorescent X-ray CT is depicted in Fig. 4 (Hogan, et al., 1991; Yuasa, et al., 1997). The coordinate system (x, y) is fixed in the reference frame of the sample. The system (s, t) is represents the rotating coordinate system associated with the specimen, and they are related to system (x, y) by a rotation of an angel θ. The two coordinate systems are connected in the relationship as follows:

$$\begin{aligned} s &= x\cos\theta + y\sin\theta \\ t &= -x\sin\theta + y\cos\theta \end{aligned} \tag{2}$$

The points P, Q, and R represent the intersection of the incident x-ray beam with the object's surface, the point of interest, and an intersection of a single emitted fluorescent x-ray with the object's surface, respectively. An incident x-ray with an initial intensity I_0 travels through the point P, and arrives at the point Q, and then fluorescent emitted isotropically x ray from the iodine atoms excited at the point Q. The interaction of the beam with the object can be depicted with three steps in the following:

Step 1: Incident radiation travels from P to Q while receiving attenuation by the object. The process for a single ray at position s and projection angle θ can be given by

$$I_1(s,\theta) = I_0 \exp(-\int_{-\infty}^{t} \mu^I(s,t')dt') \tag{3}$$

where I_0 is the intensity of incident beam and $\mu^I(s,t)$ is the linear absorption coefficient for the energy of the incident x-ray. The integration proceeds along the line segment PQ.

Step 2: The fluorescent x-ray fluxes are emitted isotropically at position Q in quantity proportional to the product of the incident intensity and the concentration of imaging agents $d(s, t)$. The fluorescent x-ray emitted fluxes from the point Q, I_2 can be given by

$$I_2 = \mu_{ph} \cdot \omega \cdot \Omega(s,t) \cdot I_0 \exp(-\int_{-\infty}^{t} \mu^I(s,t')dt')d(s,t)\Delta t \tag{4}$$

where μ_{ph} is the photoelectric linear attenuation coefficient, ω is the fluorescent yield of the K_α emission, Ω is the solid angle from the source to the detector and Δt is the differential of t.

Step3: The fluorescent flux travels from Q to the detective surface while receiving attenuation by the object. It reaches the detector with a flux rate give by

$$\mu_{ph}\cdot\omega\cdot\Omega(s,t)\cdot I_0\exp(-\int_{-\infty}^{t}\mu^I(s,t')dt')d(s,t)$$
$$\cdot\exp\left(-\int_0^{\infty}\mu^F(s-b\cos\gamma,s+b\sin\gamma)db\right)\Delta t \tag{5}$$

γ ($\gamma_m\le\gamma\le\gamma_M$) denotes the angle between a single ray inside the fan-shaped emitted fluorescence photon and the *t*-axis (Fig. 4) and $\mu^F(s,t)$ is the linear attenuation coefficient of fluorescent x rays. Integration from γ_m to γ_M with respect to γ yields the flux rate of the fluorescent x ray I_3, detected by a detector is given by

$$I_3=\mu_{ph}\omega\Omega(s,t)I_0\exp(-\int_{-\infty}^{t}\mu^I(s,t')dt')d(s,t)$$
$$\cdot\int_{\gamma_m}^{\gamma_M}\exp\left(-\int_0^{\infty}\mu^F(s-b\cos\gamma,s+b\sin\gamma)db\right)d\gamma\Delta t \tag{6}$$

The total fluorescent flux to the detective surface *I*, is obtained by integrating I_3 with respect to *t* from negative infinity to positive infinity.

$$I(\theta,s)=\mu_{ph}\cdot\gamma\cdot\Omega\cdot I_0\int_{-\infty}^{+\infty}\exp(-\int_{-\infty}^{u}\mu^I(s,t')dt')\cdot d(s,t)$$
$$\cdot\int_{\gamma_m}^{\gamma_M}\exp(-\int_0^{\infty}\mu^F(s-b\cos\gamma,s+b\sin\gamma)db)d\gamma dt \tag{7}$$
$$=\int_{-\infty}^{+\infty}f(\theta,s,t)\cdot g(\theta,s,t)\cdot d(s,t)dt$$

where,

$$f(\theta,s,t)=I_0\exp(-\int_{-\infty}^{u}\mu^I(s,t')dt') \tag{8}$$

and

$$g(\theta,s,t)=\mu_{ph}\omega\int_{\gamma_m}^{\gamma_M}\exp\left[-\int_0^{\infty}\mu^F(s-b\cos\gamma,s+b\sin\gamma)db\right]d\gamma \tag{9}$$

The $f(\theta,s,u)$ represents the incident radiation intensity attenuated reaches the point Q, and $g(\theta,s,u)$ represents the fluorescent radiation intensity attenuated were detected by a detector, respectively. The goal of image reconstruction in FXCT is to solve the $d(s, u)$. We can estimate the $d(s, u)$ from eq. (7) when the distributions of the linear attenuation coefficients of the object at the energies of the incident and fluorescent x-ray, $\mu^I(s,u)$ and $\mu^F(s,u)$ are known.

3.3 Reconstruction

As seen in the previous section, the measurement process is relatively complicated. So, analytical solutions may not be available without some approximation (Hogan, et al., 1991;

Brunetti, et al., 2001; La Riviere, 2004; Miqueles, et al. 2010). To numerically solve (7), we need to discretize it. The object is assumed to be two dimensional. Here, we adopt the *xy*-coordinate system fixed to the object for discretization. Three matrices, d_j, μ^I_j and , μ^F_j (j = 1, 2, ..., N) fixed to the *xy*-coordinate system are prepared, corresponding to the functions $d(s, t)$, $\mu^I(s, t)$ and $\mu^F(s, t)$, where j (j = 1, 2, ..., N) is the index identifying the pixel. Note that μ^I_j and μ^F_j are known. Also, let us number each incident x-ray S_i with the index i that runs from 1 to M. S_i is then the set consisting of the indexes identifying pixels which are intersected by the ith ray (Fig. 5). Taking note of the jth pixel being struck by beam S_i, let us follow the process described in the previous section using Fig. 6.

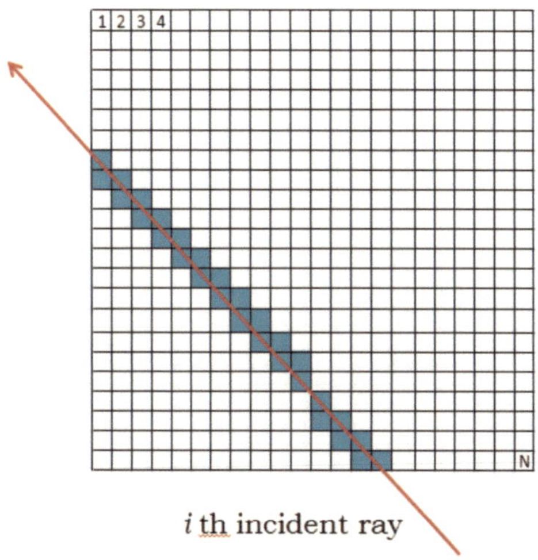

Fig. 5. Example of a set S_i defined for the ith incident X-ray.

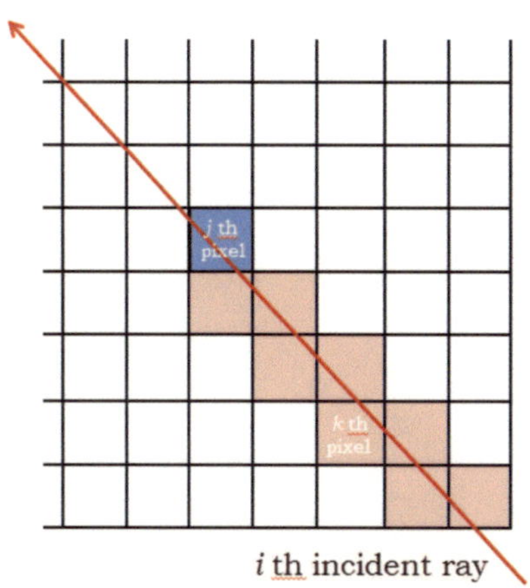

Fig. 6. Example of a set S_{ij} defined for the ith incident X-ray and the jth pixel.

Step 1: The incident x-ray is attenuated by the shaded pixels in Fig. 6. Here, S_{ij} is defined as the set of the indices denoting these pixels, which is apparently the subset of the set S_i. Defining the length of the line segment such that the ith xray is intersected with the kth pixel ($k \in S_{ij}$) as L^I_{ik}, the incident x-ray dose in front of the ith pixel is written in the form

$$f_{ij} = I_0 \exp\left(-\sum_{k \in S_{ij}} \mu_k^I L_{ik}^I \right) \tag{10}$$

which corresponds to (8).

Step 2: The fluorescent x-ray is radiated isotropically, whose absorbed flux rate is in proportion to the product of the flux rate of the x-ray entering the *j*th pixel and concerning this phenomenon, $\omega\, \mu_{ph}\, f_{ij}\, L^I_{ij}$, and the iodine concentration, d_j. Let us define the angle at which the *j*th pixel is viewed by the detector as δ (Fig. 7). The x-ray absorbed flux rate corresponding to (4) is $(\delta / 2\pi)\, \omega\, \mu_{ph} f_{ij}\, L^I_{ij}\, d_j$.

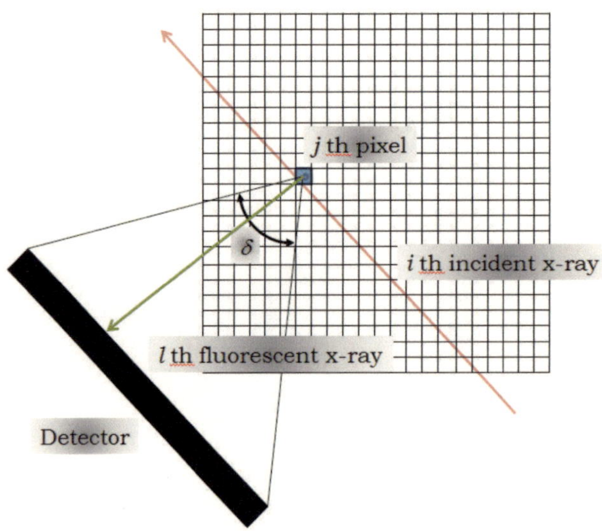

Fig. 7. Definition of angle δ.

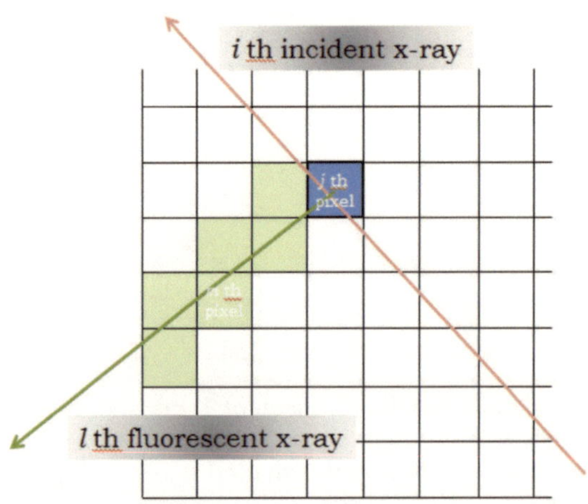

Fig. 8. Example of a set T_{ijl} defined for the *i*th incident X-ray and the *j*th pixel and the *l*th fluorescent X-ray.

Step 3: We consider the attenuation process up to the detector. For a predefined integer, K, let $\Delta\delta = \delta / K$. Here, the fan-shaped fluorescent x-ray is approximated by K individual x-rays. We define the index identifying the angle of the fluorescent x-rays as l ($1 \le l \le K$). Considering the jth pixel ($j \in S_i$) and the lth fluorescent x-ray, we consider the attenuation from the lth ray from the jth pixel to the detector (Fig. 8). Let T_{ijl} be a set of indexes consisting of the pixels which are intersected with the lth fluorescent x-ray. These pixels, denoted as the shaded pixels in Fig. 8, attenuate the lth fluorescence x-ray before they reach the detector. Let L^F_{ijm} be the length of the line segment such that the lth ray is intersected with the mth pixel ($m \in T_{ijl}$). The lth ray is subject to the attenuation by

$$\exp\left(- \sum_{m \in T_{ijl}} \mu^F_m L^F_{ijm} \right)$$

Hence, the discretized representation corresponding to (9) is

$$g_{ij} = \mu_{ph} \omega \frac{\Delta\delta}{2\pi} \sum_{l=1}^{K} \exp\left(- \sum_{m \in T_{ijl}} \mu^F_m L^F_{ijm} \right) \tag{11}$$

Accordingly, the discretization of (7) yields

$$\begin{aligned} I_i &= \sum_{j \in S_i} f_{ij} g_{ij} L^I_{ij} d_j \\ &= \sum_{j \in S_i} h_{ij} d_j \end{aligned} \tag{12}$$

where

$$h_{ij} = f_{ij} g_{ij} L^I_{ij} \tag{13}$$

The matrix representation of (12) is

$$\boldsymbol{I} = \boldsymbol{Hd} \tag{14}$$

where

$$\boldsymbol{H} = \left(h_{ij} \right) \quad \left(1 \le i \le M, 1 \le j \le N \right) \tag{15}$$

$$\boldsymbol{I} = \left(I_i \right) \quad \left(1 \le i \le M \right) \tag{16}$$

and

$$\boldsymbol{d} = \left(d_j \right) \quad \left(1 \le j \le N \right) \tag{17}$$

As a result, in order to reconstruct a cross section, you should solve the matrix equation. A variety of approaches were proposed (Chukalina, et al., 2002; Golosio, et al., 2003; Miqueles, et al., 2011; La Riviere, et al., 2010). If data amount is not so huge, you may solve it through a direct matrix calculation. If so, you should take an iterative reconstruction method. In addition, if a signal to noise ratio is not high, you should select a statistical reconstruction method such as EM algorithm (Rust, et al., 1998). On the other hand, while we discussed reconstruction when distributions of μ^I and μ^F are known, in order to obtain these distributions additional CT measurements are required. Approaches to circumvent this problem have been proposed (Schroer, et al., 2001; La Riviere, et al., 2006; —, 2006;).

3.4 Imaging experiments

Here, we introduce the actual experimental results, which show that SR-FXCT has high sensitivity and spatial resolution as well as quantitativeness, and offers useful knowledges to biomedical sciences.

3.4.1 Imaging setup

The experiment was carried out at the bending magnet beam line BLNE-5A in KEK, Japan (Fig. 9). The photon flux rate in front of the subject was approximately 10^8 photons/mm^2/sec at a beam current of 40 mA with 6.5 GeV. The FXCT system consists of a

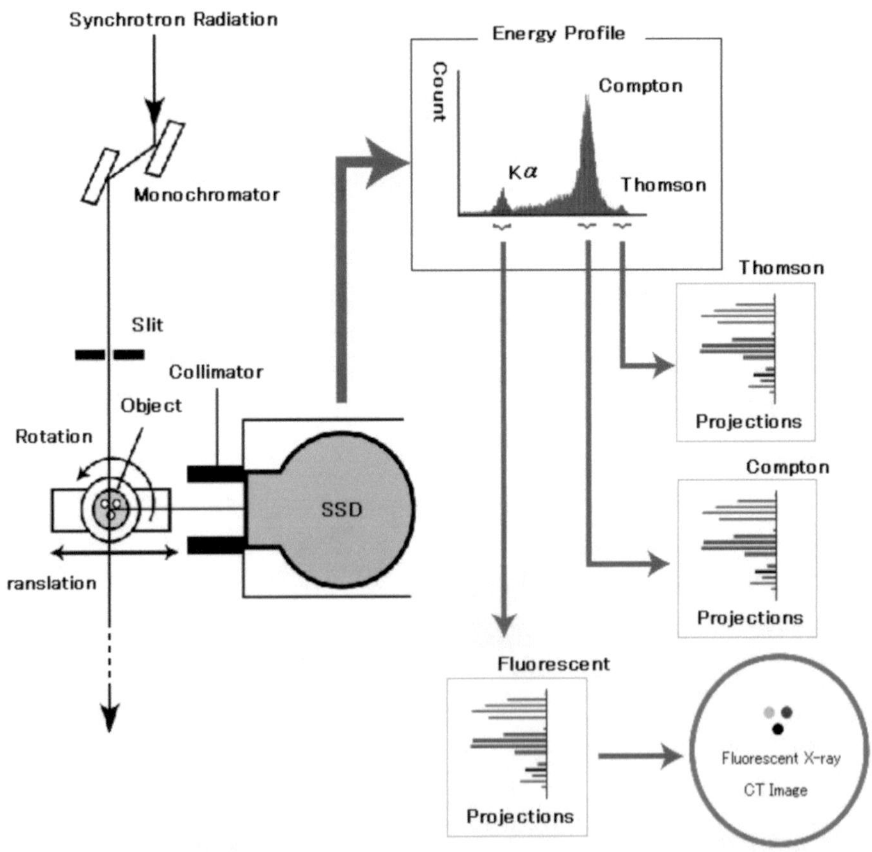

Fig. 9. Schematic of fluorescent x-ray CT system

silicon (220) double-crystal monochromator, an x-ray slit system, a scanning table for the target object, a highly purified germanium (HPGe) detector (IGRET, EG&G Ortec, USA) with a parallel collimator, two pindiode detectors and a computer system. The white x-ray beam was monochromated at 37 keV using the silicon double-crystal monochromator. The incident monochromatic x-ray beam was collimated into a pencil beam with square cross section (0.25 mm × 0.5 mm) using the x-ray slit system. Fluorescent x-rays were detected by the HPGe detector in photon-counting mode. To reduce the amount of Compton radiation captured by the detector, the HPGe detector was positioned perpendicular to the incident monochromatic x-ray beam. The data-acquisition time of the HPGe detector was set a few seconds. An example of energy profile acquired at a data point by the imaging system is shown in Fig. 10. We can observe three peaks, i.e., the iodine-fluorescence, the Compton, and the Thomson peaks. The net counts in an energy window centered at the characteristic x-ray fluorescent spectral line of 28.3 keV at each projection point constitute the CT projections. Projections are acquired at constant angular steps using a translation-rotation motion of the subject over 180 degrees in a conventional CT configuration. Also, the imaging setup can simultaneously obtain Compton scatter CT image as well as FXCT image, because the measurement process of Compton scatter is the same as that of fluorescent x-ray (Yuasa, et al., 1997; Golosio, et al., 2003). Although through this article synchrotron x ray is supposed as incident beam, currently a bench-top FXCT system using a diagnostic energy range polychromatic (i.e. 110 kVp) pencil-beam source is being developed (Cheong, et al., 2010; Jones, et al., 2011).

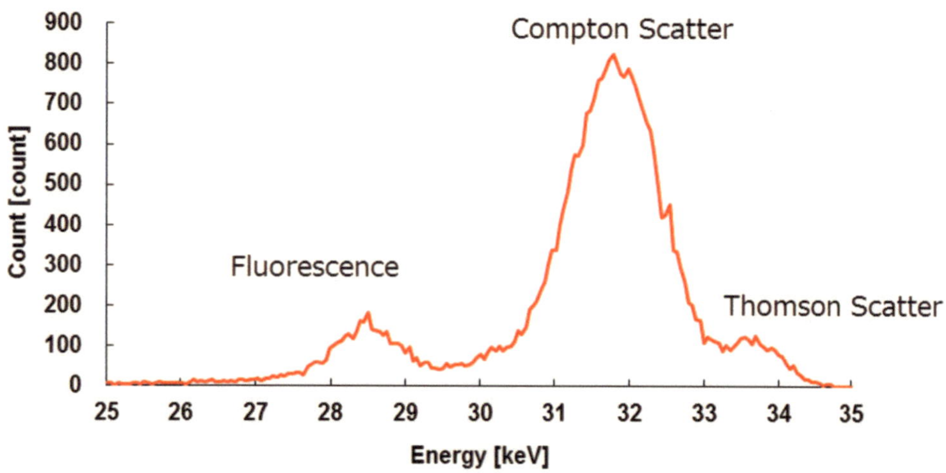

Fig. 10. Schematic of fluorescent x-ray CT system

The experiments for evaluating quantitativeness of SR-FXCT were performed using a 10 mm-diameter acrylic phantom with 3 mm holes to evaluate the contrast detectability corresponding to iodine concentrations of 200, 100, 50, 25 and 15 mg ml^{-1} (Fig. 11). Using the contrast-resolution phantom, we confirmed that the FXCT could visualize a 0.005 mg ml^{-1} iodine solution at 0.25 mm in-plane spatial resolution and 0.5 mm slice thickness. There was an excellent linear correlation between pixel value in the FXCT image and the iodine concentration (Fig. 12). From this graph we observed satisfactory quantitativeness and thus estimated the iodine concentration for a given image count.

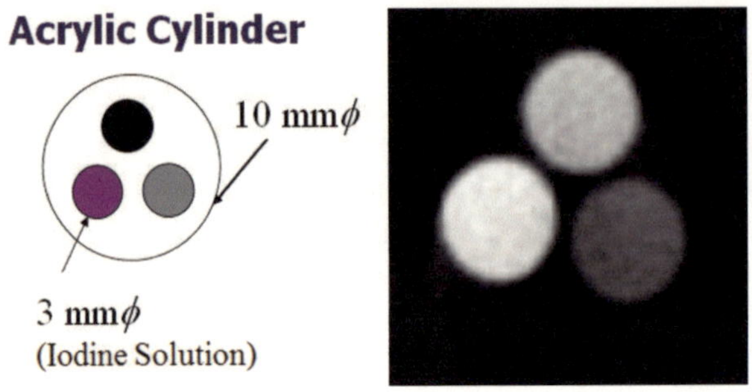

Fig. 11. Acrylic phantom and an example of FXCT image.

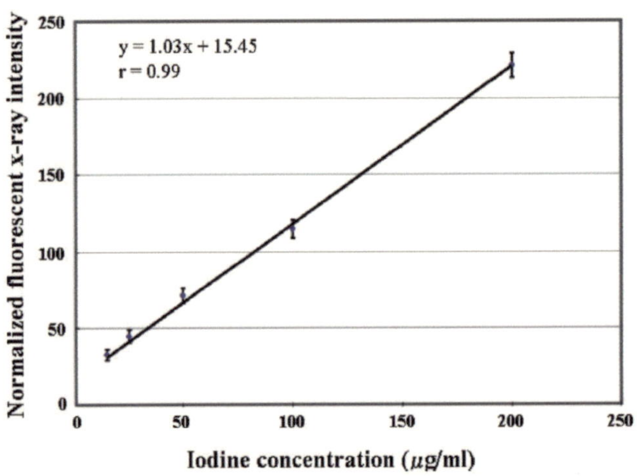

Fig. 12. Relationship between actual iodine concentration and FXCT pixel value.

3.4.2 Ex Vivo imaging of hamster's heart

With FXCT using synchrotron radiation, we successfully imaged the myocardial fatty acid metabolism in normal rat and cardiomyopathic hamster with BMIPP (^{127}I-BMIPP) labelled with non-radioactive iodine, where the BMIPP is a potential tracer for detecting the fatty acid metabolism in current clinical SPECT imaging (Thet-Thet-Lwin, et al., 2007; —, 2008). In this study the myocardial fatty acid metabolism in cardiomyopathic hamster and age-matched normal hamster were quantitatively analyzed using FXCT images, and the FXCT images were compared with optical microscope images with Masson's trichrome (MT) stain.

A 20 week J2N-k cardiomyopathic hamster and an age matched J2N-n normal hamster were imaged in this study. Under anesthesia (pentobarbital 40 mg kg^{-1} weight), hearts were extracted after 5 min intravenous injection of ^{127}I-BMIPP (0.08 mg g^{-1} weight). The hearts labeled with BMIPP were fixed by formalin and then imaged by FXCT, placing them in an acrylic cell under the same data acquisition parameters as for the phantom study. Here, five short-axis slices of heart in cardiomyopathy and three short-axis slices in normal hamster were imaged by FXCT. After FXCT imaging, specimens were cut into 0.02 mm thick slices. The degree of fibrosis and its area were evaluated by optical microscopy (Biozero, Keyence Co., Japan) with MT stain, because fibrotic tissue does not uptake BMIPP.

FXCT images revealed that BMIPP was distributed homogeneously in normal myocardium, whereas it was distributed heterogeneously in cardiomyopathic myocardium. In normal hamster, the mean BMIPP uptake value of each slice was not statistically different among the three short-axis images: 177.2 ± 18.5, 180.1 ± 17.9 and 179.1 ± 18.0. In cardiomyopathic hamster, the mean BMIPP uptake value of each slice was also not statistically significant among the five short-axis images: 151.1 ± 26.5, 164.6 ± 25.8, 157.8 ± 23.1, 150.0 ± 24.7 and 149.0 ± 25.6. The mean BMIPP uptake value of each slice in cardiomyopathic hamster heart was lower than that in normal heart and its standard deviation was larger than that of normal heart. Short-axis images of the mid-ventricular level in normal and cardiomyopathic hamsters (Figs. 13 (a) and (b)) were analyzed in detail for regions of each slice. In these images the mean BMIPP uptake in normal myocardium was 1.2 times higher than that in cardiomyopathic myocardium (177.2 ± 18.5 mg ml^{-1} versus 151.1 ± 26.5 mg ml^{-1}). In the same slices as used for the FXCT image, optical microscopy with MT stain depicted no fibrosis in normal myocardium and only a slight interstitial fibrosis in cardiomyopathic myocardium (Figs. 13 (c) and (d)). An area of 12.0% was observed as interstitial fibrosis in the whole short-axis slice of the mid-left ventricle. Areas of this interstitial fibrosis partially corresponded to that of reduced BMIPP uptake in the FXCT images (Table 1). In addition, morphological structures such as papillary muscle, wall thickness and left ventricle diameter were also approximately visualized in the FXCT images. Ventricular dilatation and mild thinning of the myocardial wall were observed in the cardiomyopathic myocardium cases.

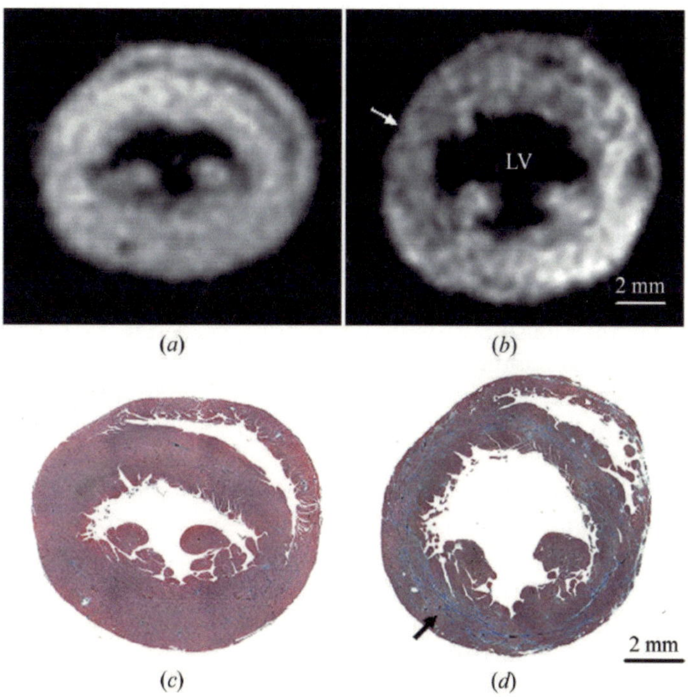

Fig. 13. FXCT images of (a) normal myocardium and (b) cardiomyphathic myocardium. Optical microscope pictures with MT stain of (c) normal and (d) cardiomyopathic myocardium (Thet-Thet-Lwin, et al., 2007; –, 2008).

State	Left-ventricle regions Anterior wall	Lateral wall	Inferior wall	Septum
Normal ($\mu g\ ml^{-1}$)	176.3 ± 13.4	174.3 ± 12.5	179.2 ± 15.2	181.1 ± 14.3
Cardiomyopathy ($\mu g\ ml^{-1}$)	167.5 ± 24.1	156.8 ± 22.7	134.5 ± 19.5	147.1 ± 28.2
Uptake − 2SD of normal myocardium (%)	18.3	20.7	75.5	41.3
Percentile fibrosis area (%)	6.9	15.3	11.5	12.3

Table 1. Mean BMIPP uptake, and percentile area of reduced BMIPP uptake and fibrosis for each myocardinal region of the mid-left ventricle (Thet-Thet-Lwin, et al., 2007; −, 2008).

3.4.3 Ex Vivo and In Vivo imaging of mouse's brain

Using x-ray fluorescent computed tomography (FXCT), the in vivo and ex vivo cerebral distribution of a stable-iodine-labeled cerebral perfusion agent, iodoamphetamine analog (^{127}I-IMP), has been recorded in the brains of mice (Takeda et al., 2009). In vivo cerebral perfusion in the cortex, hippocampus and thalamus was depicted at 0.5 mm in-plane spatial resolution. Ex vivo FXCT images at 0.25 mm in-plane spatial resolution allowed the visualization of the detailed structures of these regions. The quality of the FXCT image of the hippocampus was comparable with the ^{125}I-IMP autoradiogram. These results highlight the sensitivity of FXCT and its considerable potential to evaluate cerebral perfusion in small animals without using radioactive agents.

We obtained images from seven living mice, weighing 20–24 g with heads of diameter about 20 mm, after we employed a 10 mm-diameter contrast-resolution acrylic phantom to assess the contrast resolution in an ex vivo brain. The phantom consisted of three 5 mm-diameter axial cylindrical channels filled with three different iodine solutions, their concentrations ranging from 0.005 to 0.1 mg ml^{-1}. We used non-radioactive ^{127}I-labeled N-isopropyl-p-iodoamphetamine (^{127}I-IMP containing 0.38 mg iodine) for in vivo imaging of the brain, while radioactive ^{123}I-IMP is commonly employed to evaluate cerebral perfusion in clinical SPECT studies. Imaging started 5 min after intravenously injecting ^{127}I-IMP into a mouse anesthetized with pentobarbital; this dose is similar to that used by others in animal SPECT studies. The head of the mouse was set in the vertical direction to the pencil beam, fixed by an animal head holder to suppress any movement. Since the amount of IMP in the brain declined gradually with the approximate half-life time of 1.5 h, we surgically removed the *brain* of another mouse for the ex vivo experiments 5 min after intravenously injecting the ^{127}I-IMP and fixed it in the formalin. Then it was set within a formalin-filled acrylic cell, and imaged by FXCT at 0.5 mm and 0.25 mm in-plane spatial resolution. The FXCT image of the phantom was obtained at 0.25 mm in-plane spatial resolution. For comparison, we obtained autoradiograms with radioactive ^{125}I-IMP from two other mice. Their brains were removed surgically 5 min after injecting ^{125}I-IMP (15 kBq kg^{-1}), fixed in formalin, and cut into 0.02 mm slices. These samples were exposed on an imaging plate (IP) for 48 h, and the plate was read by a BAS 5000 (Fuji) IP reader at 0.05 mm scan steps and 16-bit depths.

The in vivo FXCT image at a 0.5 mm in-plane spatial resolution revealed the cerebral perfusion of ^{127}I-IMP throughout the brain of the mouse (Fig. 14), whereas absorption-contrast x-ray transmission CT (XTCT) discriminated only between the soft tissue and the bony structures of the skull. Cerebral perfusion in the cortex and hippocampus was more clearly visualized in the 0.5 mm in-plane spatial resolution FXCT image than in the 1 mm in-plane resolution image, while the anatomical features of the skull bone were clearly demonstrated by XTCT. Furthermore, the superimposed image (FXCT and XTCT) demonstrated the correspondence between anatomical features and cerebral perfusion (Zeniya, et al., 2001). The measured SNR of the FXCT image in cerebral cortex, hippocampus and thalamus was about 12.3, 11.7 and 21.1, respectively. We calculated that the mouse experienced a radiation-absorbed dose of about 0.36 Gy for the FXCT imaging experiment.

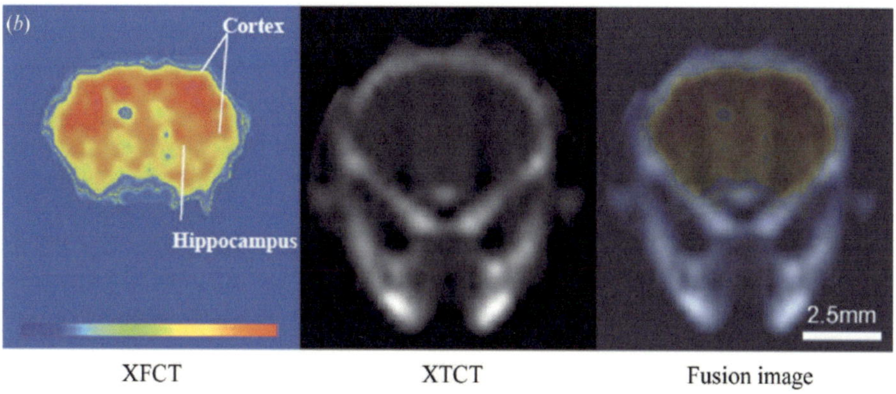

Fig. 14. In vivo FXCT, TCT and superimposed images of normal mouse brains obtained at 0.5 mm in-plane spatial resolution (Takeda et al., 2009).

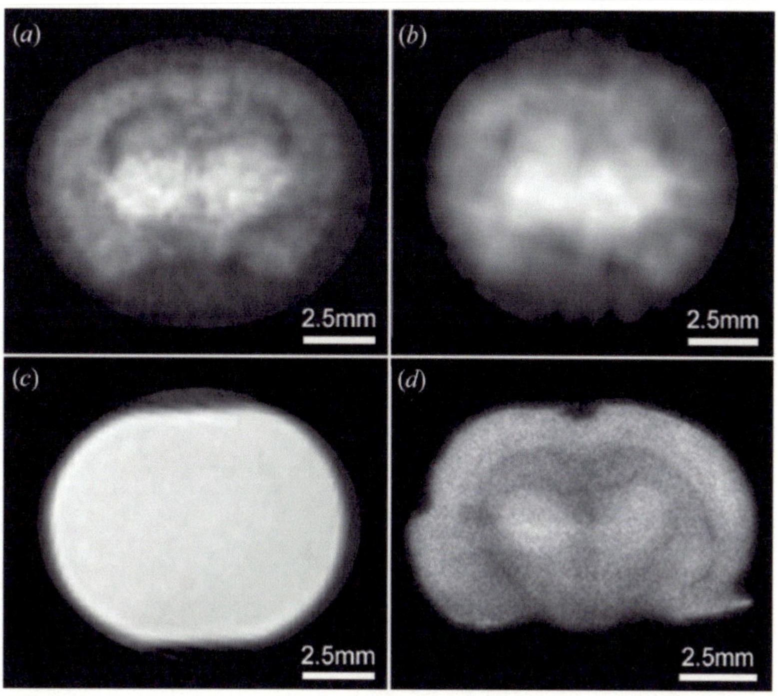

Fig. 15. FXCT image of formalin-fixed (ex vivo) mouse brain set within an acrylic cell filled with formalin (a, b, c), and autoradiogram with ^{125}I-IMP (d) (Takeda et al., 2009).

FXCT clearly imaged the formalin-fixed brain in an acrylic cell both at a 0.5 mm and a 0.25 mm in-plane spatial resolution, while, in contrast, the XTCT image discriminated only the margin of the acrylic cell, and failed to distinguish the rain from its surrounding solution (Fig. 15). An ex vivo FXCT image was obtained in the same slice level; however, the FXCT image at 0.25 mm in-plane spatial resolution clearly differentiated the detailed structures, such as the cortex, hippocampus and thalamus, with almost the same quality as an autoradiogram with radioactive ^{125}I-IMP. The IMP dose was approximately 27.3, 23.8 and 50.3 mg g^{-1} in the cortical surface, hippocampus and thalamus, respectively.

4. SR-FXCT based on sheet beam geometry

As for *in vivo* imaging, FXCT has a problem: the conventional FXCT takes a huge amount of measurement time to acquire a single tomographic image because it adopts the sequential data collection scheme with a pencil beam, which is the first generation of data acquisition scheme in CT. Although it is desirable to collect as much data as possible for a high-quality image, the whole measurement must be completed under anesthesia and then the number of data points is severely restricted. Therefore, we have not yet attained the potential spatial resolution for *in vivo* imaging.

4.1 SR-FXCT imaging system with sheet beam geometry

The long measurement time of conventional FXCT based on pencil beam geometry is due to sequential data acquisition, and for faster measurements simultaneous or parallel acquisition of a single projection is indispensable. Figure 16 shows a schematic diagram of the proposed imaging geometry (Huo, et al., 2008; –, 2009). An incident monochromatic sheet beam, where the photon fluxes are parallel to one another, impinges on the object as it covers the width of the object cross section. Contrast agents, such as iodine, are thus excited and then isotropically emit x-ray fluorescence photons on de-excitation. A linear array of detectors, where *N* solid-state detectors operating in a photon counting mode with energy resolution are equally spaced, is positioned perpendicular to the beam propagation in the plane of polarization for the lowest Compton scatter contribution in the spectrum, due to the property of linear polarization. A long slit-like collimator is installed in front of each

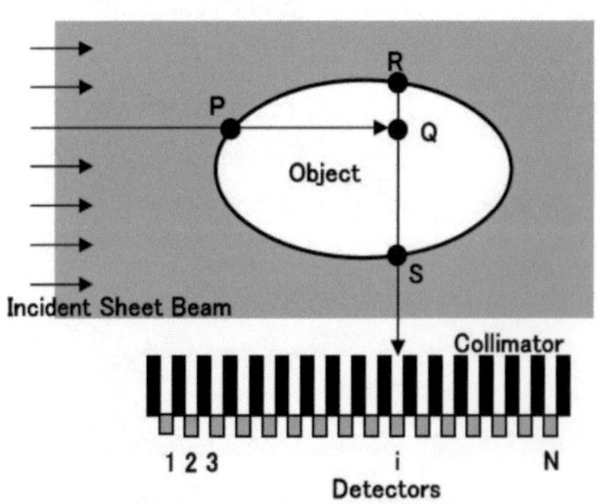

Fig. 16. FXCT based on sheet-beam geometry (Huo, et al., 2008).

detector element in order to restrict the regions emitting x-ray fluorescence incident on the detector surface and to reduce the amount of stray radiation being detected. As a result, the detector array from the 1st to the *N*th detectors simultaneously acquires projection data in a direction perpendicular to the beam propagation. Translational scans are therefore no longer required during the collection of a set of projections, though some translational scans may still be necessary to obtain a single complete projection, because each detector is partitioned by a collimator and no data are obtained at the collimator's septal walls. The overall measurement time will still be drastically reduced, as a set of projections can be collected through rotational and fewer translational scans.

4.2 Formulation and reconstruction

We set the x_1x_2-coordinate fixed to the object, and suppose that the sheet beam accompanied with the detectors array is rotated around the origin O, where the collimators in front of the array are omitted so as to see easily the diagram. The hatched region means the incident sheet-beam irradiation. We derive the formula representing fluorescent x-ray photons measured by a single detector, or the *i*th detector among *N* detectors of the array. First, we pay attention to a single incident ray among the sheet beam. The points, P, Q, S and R in Fig. 17 represent the intersection of the single incident ray with the object's surface, the point of interest, an intersection of a single emitted fluorescent x ray with the object's surface, and an intersection of line QS with the object's surface, respectively. We denote the iodine concentration distribution to be estimated, the distribution of the linear attenuation coefficient for the energy of the incident X-ray, and that of the fluorescent X-ray as $d(x)$, $a_I(x)$ and $a_F(x)$ must be known in advance by the usual x-ray CT using the CCD camera. Next, let us consider the process in which a single incident ray with an initial intensity I_0, at the point, P, arrives at the point, Q, and the fluorescent subsequently emitted x ray from the iodine atoms excited at the point, Q, reaches the *i*th detector. We partitioned the process into three steps. Here, $\theta \in S^1$ and $\theta^{\perp} \in S^1$ are unit vectors parallel and vertical to the single ray of interest.

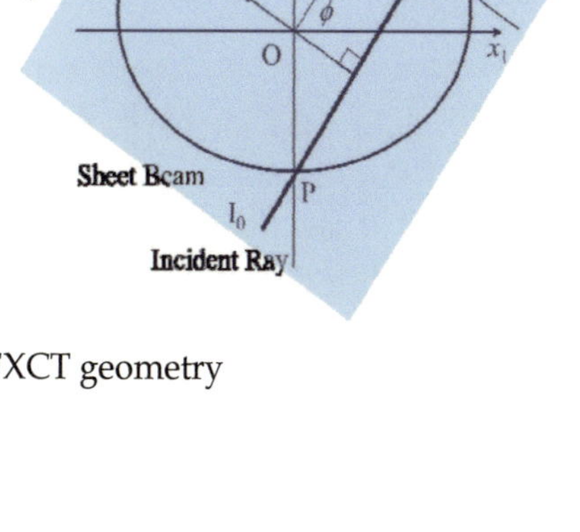

Fig. 17. Sheet-beam based FXCT geometry

Step 1: The x-ray flux rate, $I(x)$, reaching the point, Q, is given by

$$I(x) = I_0 \exp[-(Da_I)(x,\theta)] \tag{18}$$

where

$$(Da_I)(x,\theta) = \int_0^\infty a_I(x - t\theta)dt \; .$$

Step 2: The fluorescent x-ray is emitted isotropically with an intensity proportional to the product of the absorbed x-ray flux rate at the point, Q, μ_{ph} $I(x)$ Δv and the iodine concentration, $d(x)$, where μ_{ph} is the photoelectric linear attenuation coefficient of iodine, and Δv is the differential volume at Q. Accordingly, the flux rate of the fluorescent x ray emitted from the point, Q, and reaching the *i*th detector, $f(x)$, is given by

$$f(x) = I(x)d(x)\mu_{ph}\omega\Delta v \, \Omega/_{4\pi} \tag{19}$$

where ω and Ω are the yield of the fluorescent x ray and the solid angle at which the point, Q, is viewed by the ith detector, respectively.

Step 3: Following a fluorescent x-ray emitted from the point, Q, crossing the object toward the *i*th detector, it is attenuated along the line segment QS; it reaches the *i*th detector with a flux rate given by

$$I_d(x) = \exp\left[-(Da_F)(x,\theta^\perp)\right] f(x) \tag{20}$$

where

$$(Da_F)(x,\theta^\perp) = \int_0^\infty a_F(x + t\theta^\perp)dt \; .$$

Here, we obtained the contribution from the single incident ray into the *i*th detector. The formula holds for other rays among the sheet beam. The total flux rate of the fluorescent x-ray reaching the ith detector for the sheet beam x-ray is obtained by integrating with respect to x along line RS, $x \bullet \theta = s$, where s is a distance between origin O and line RS:

$$\left(R_a f\right)(\theta,s) = \int_{x\theta=s} \exp\left[-(Da_F)(x,\theta^\perp)\right] f(x)\, dx \tag{21}$$

Thus, the measurement process by the FXCT based on sheet beam geometry leads to the attenuated Radon transform. The inversion for $g = R_a f$ was given by Natterer (Natterer, 2001) as

$$f(x) = \frac{1}{4\pi} \mathrm{Re}\; div \int_{S^1} \theta \exp\left[-(Da_F)(x,\theta^\perp)\right]\left(e^{-h} H e^{h} g\right)(\theta, x\theta)\, d\theta \tag{22}$$

where $h = 1/2(I + iH)Ra_F$, and H and R are the Hilbert transform and Radon transform, respectively. We can obtain the exact iodine density $d(x)$ by first applying the exact inversion formula straightforwardly to Eq. (22), and then by applying Eq. (19) to the resulting $f(x)$. In the sheet-beam geometry, the analytical solution is exactly feasible.

4.3 Preliminary experiments

In order to prove the concept of this imaging protocol, we constructed a preliminary imaging system for simulating the proposed imaging geometry using a single HPGe SSD.

4.3.1 Imaging setup

The preliminary imaging system was constructed at the BLNE-5A bending-magnet beam line (6.5 GeV), KEK in Japan. A white x-ray beam from a source was monochromatized using a Si (220) monochromator at 37 keV. The photon flux rate in front of the object was approximately 9.3 $\times 10^7$ photons/mm^2/s for a beam current of 40 mA. The monochromatized beam was shaped to a sheet beam of 2.0 cm wide × 1.0 mm thick using an x-ray slit. Figure 18 shows the schematic of the preliminary detection system for simulating a sheet-beam geometry, consisting of an HPGe detector operating in photon counting mode to detect emitted fluorescent photons and a long Pb slit collimator installed in front of the detector surface. We prepared two types of collimators: one coarse (1.0 mm height × 0.5 mm width × 100 mm long) and the other fine (1.0 mm height × 0.25 mm width × 100 mm long). The distance between the sample surface and the collimator tip was set at 12 mm. First the sample was scanned translationally along the beam direction and, after the translational scan, the sample was rotated. Although the data collection scheme is sequential, the dataset finally obtained corresponds to that acquired using a linear array of detectors. Projection data at the data point was generated from the K_α peak by summing the fluorescent-photon counts in the energy window with the center at 28.3 keV and width of 2 keV.

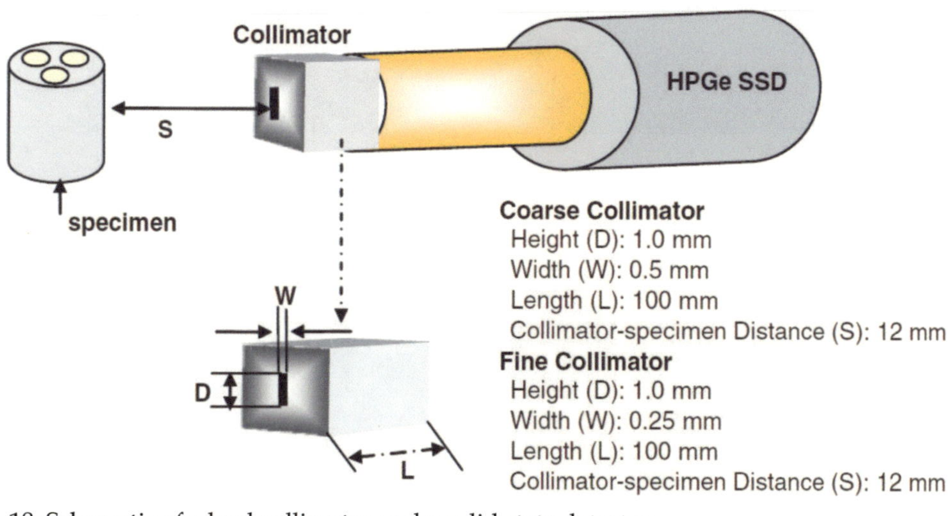

Fig. 18. Schematic of a lead collimator and a solid state detector.

4.3.2 Phantom imaging

To confirm the efficacy, we performed an imaging experiment using a physical phantom, which is a 10-mm-diameter acrylic cylinder with three 3-mm-diameter holes filled with iodine solutions at different concentrations (200, 100, and 50 µg/ml). The sample was imaged twice. First, it was scanned using the coarse collimator translationally and rotationally at 0.5-mm steps and 2° steps over 180°, respectively. The measurement time for a data point was 5 s, and dead-time rate was less than 10%. Second, it was done using the fine collimator translationally and rotationally at 0.25-mm steps and 2° step over 180°, respectively. The measurement time for a data point was 5 s and dead-time rate was less than 5%. The reconstructed images for the coarse and fine collimators are shown in Figs. 19 (a) and (b), respectively. In both the images, the three circles corresponding to the regions including the iodine solution are successfully delineated, but the image for the coarse collimator is more blurred than that for the fine collimator. Figure 19 suggests that pixel values in the iodine regions depend on the actual iodine concentration. So, we investigated the imaging scheme quantitatively using the physical phantom. For this, we imaged the phantom while changing the iodine concentrations, and then compared the actual iodine concentrations with the average pixel values in the iodine regions set in the reconstructed images. Figure 20 shows the relationship. A good correlation was observed between the pixel value in the reconstructed image and the iodine concentration (R = 0.99). We can use the result as the calibration line for quantitative measurement.

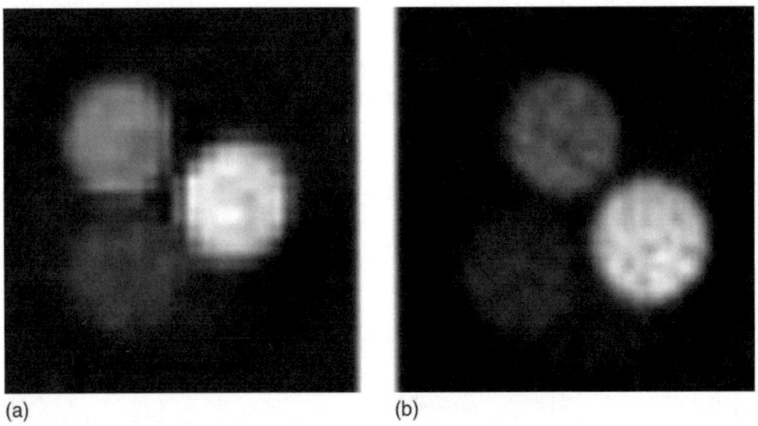

Fig. 19. FXCT image of a 10-mm-diameter acrylic cylindrical phantom which has three channels (3 mmϕ) filled with three different concentrations of iodine solution: (a) coarse collimator, (b) fine collimator (Huo, et al., 2009).

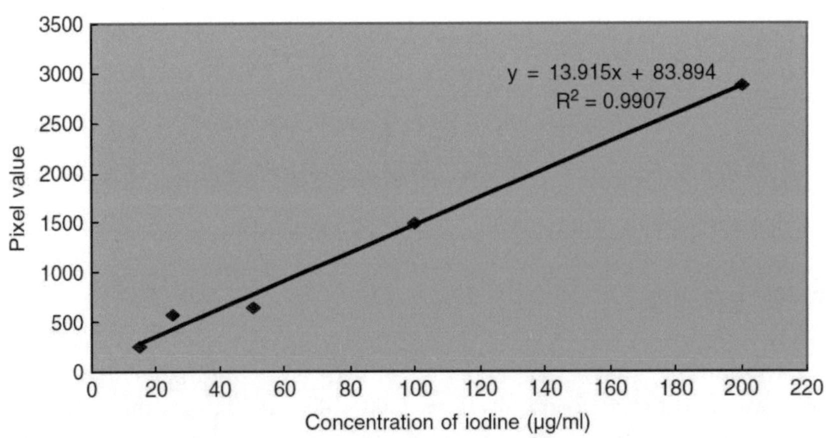

Fig. 20. Relationship between actual iodine concentration and FXCT pixel value.

4.3.3 Ex Vivo imaging of mouse's brain

We imaged a normal mouse brain *ex vivo* in order to confirm the suitability of the technique for biomedical imaging. Under anesthesia, the brain of a mouse was extracted after 5 min intravenous injection of non-radioactive iodine labeled ^{127}I-IMP (about 0.05 mg/ml) and fixed by formalin. This experiment was approved by the Medical Committee for the Use of Animals in Research of the University of Tsukuba, Japan. The brain was fixed in an acrylic cylinder filled with formalin and was put on the stage (Fig. 21). The sample was imaged twice. First, it was scanned using the coarse collimator translationally and rotationally at 0.5-mm steps and 2° step over 180°, respectively. The measurement time for a data point was 20 s and dead-time rate was less than 10%. Second, it was done using the fine collimator translationally and rotationally at 0.25-mm steps and 2° step over 180°, respectively. The measurement time for a data point was 20 s and dead-time rate was less than 5%. The reconstructed images for the coarse and fine collimators are shown in Figs. 22 (a) and (b), respectively. The reconstructed image for the coarse collimator is more blurred than that for the fine collimator. However, in the both images, the cortex and thalamus can be identified anatomically, and the iodine content of the brain is estimated to be about 20.0 μg/ml on average using the calibration line in Fig. 20. The iodine content approximately coincides with that obtained using the system based on a pencil-beam geometry. From these results we can conclude that the proposed scheme can also offer quantitative biomedical information related to cerebral perfusion at a high spatial resolution.

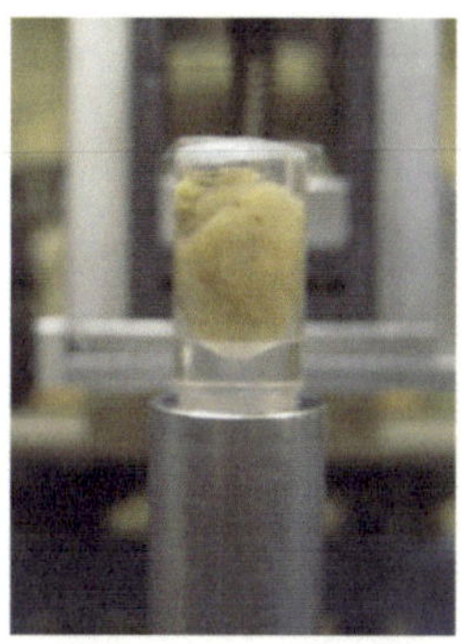

Fig. 21. Extracted mouse brain put in an acrylic cylinder filled with formalin.

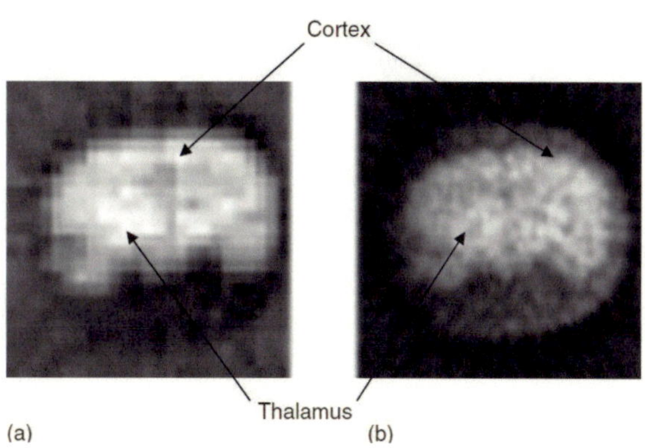

Fig. 22. Ex vivo FXCT images of normal mouse brain: (a) coarse collimator, and (b) fine collimator (Huo, et al., 2009).

5. Considerations

Here, we investigate the differences between FXCTs based on pencil-beam and sheet-beam geometries in their imaging properties by considering each measurement process in detail. As shown in Fig. 23 (a), in the pencil-beam geometry a thin incident beam impinges on an object and excites imaging agents on the incident beam line, and then fluorescent x-ray photons are isotropically emitted from the imaging agents. Pay attention to the point Q inside the object in order to consider the measurement process in a more detail. The measurement process is broadly divided into three steps in the following:

A. The incident flux travels from P to Q while being attenuated by the object.
B. The fluorescent flux of X-ray photons is isotropically emitted at Q in proportion to the product of the incident intensity and the concentration of imaging agents at Q. Of the photons, only those that propagate toward the detective surface ST are detected.
C. The fluorescent flux travels from Q to the detector surface ST while being attenuated by the object. Here, the amount of attenuation depends on the propagation direction. For example, while the fluorescent flux reaching points W and X on the detector surface ST is attenuated by segments QU and QV, respectively, the amount of attenuation is different.

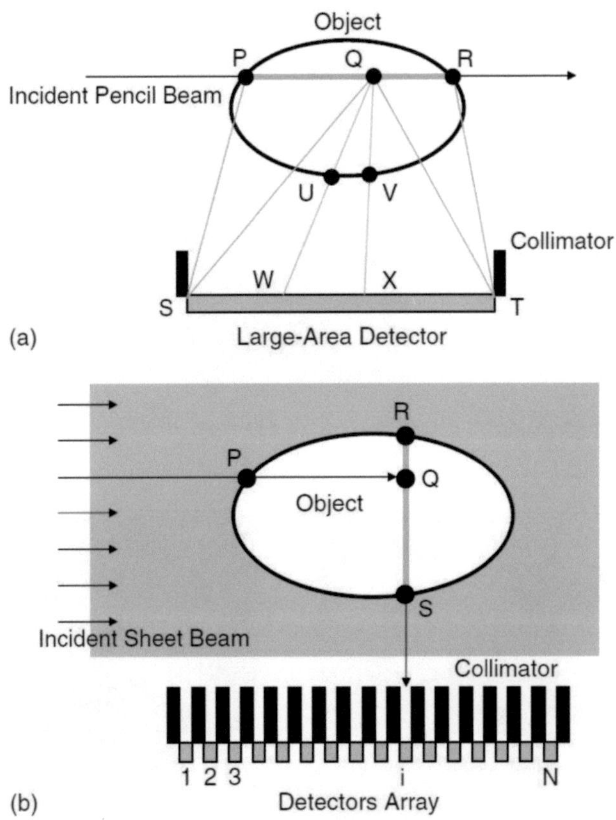

Fig. 23. Schematics of measurement process: (a) pencil-beam geometry, and (b) sheet-beam geometry.

Since the fluorescent flux obtained above is a contribution from the point Q, the total detected photons can be obtained by integration through PR. The measurement process of the pencil beam geometry is very complex, and hence the attenuation correction also is very complex. In sheet-beam geometry, concerning the measurement by the *i*th detector along path P→Q→S in Fig. 23 (b), the measurement process is divided into three steps:

A. The incident flux is attenuated by an object during the propagation from points P to Q.
B. The x-ray fluorescence photons are isotropically emitted at point Q, whose number is proportional to both the incident flux rate and the iodine quantity at point Q.
C. The fluorescent flux travels toward the detector while being attenuated by the object during the propagation from point Q to S.

As each point on line RS is similarly subjected to the above process, the number of fluorescent photons detected by the *i*th detector is obtained by integrating the contributions from all the points on RS. The measurement process of the sheet-beam geometry is very simple, and therefore the attenuation correction is relatively simple.

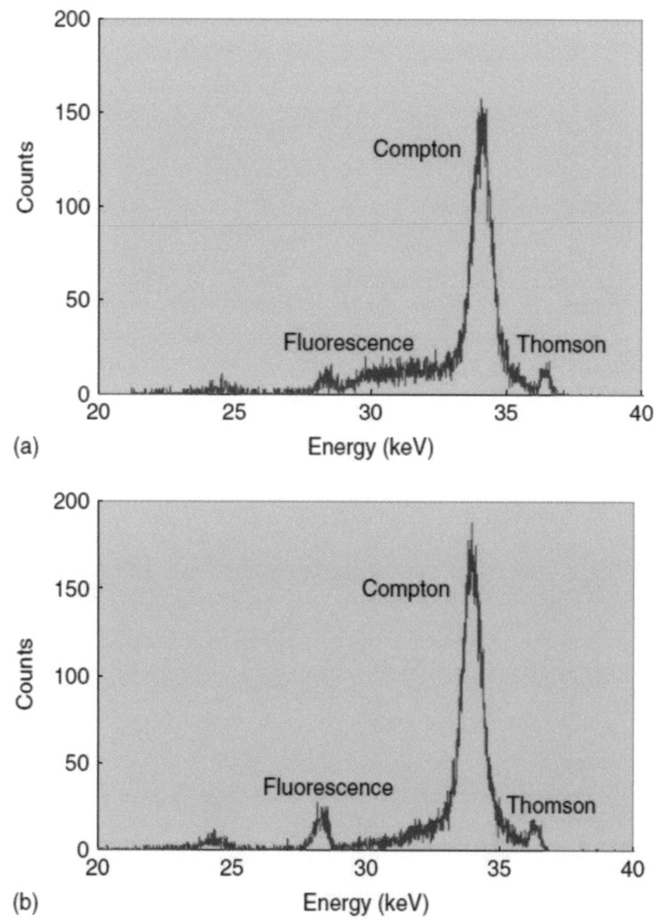

Fig. 24. Example of energy profile: (a) pencil-beam geometry, and (b) sheet-beam geometry (Huo, et al., 2009).

First, we consider signal quality based on the above specification on the measurement process. Figures 24 (a) and (b) show the energy profile obtained from the identical physical phantom using the systems based on pencil- and sheet-beam geometry, respectively. In both the figures, fluorescence, Compton scatter, and Thomson scatter peaks are observed from the left to the right. The first point to notice is that the counts in a region between the fluorescent and the Compton peaks, which correspond to multiple scatter components, in the pencil-beam geometry is more than those in the sheet-beam geometry, although the energy profiles are very similar in appearance. In the pencil-beam geometry, the detector collects a great deal of multiply scattered components from various directions because of the use of a large area of the detector surface. On the other hand, in the sheet-beam geometry, the detection efficiency of fluorescence is remarkably low because of the use of the slit-like collimator. However, the collimator in turn suppresses the scattered components maximally. Therefore, the system based on sheet-beam geometry can measure fluorescence under less dead-time ratio of the detector, and thus it can collect data more reliably than the system based on pencil-beam geometry.

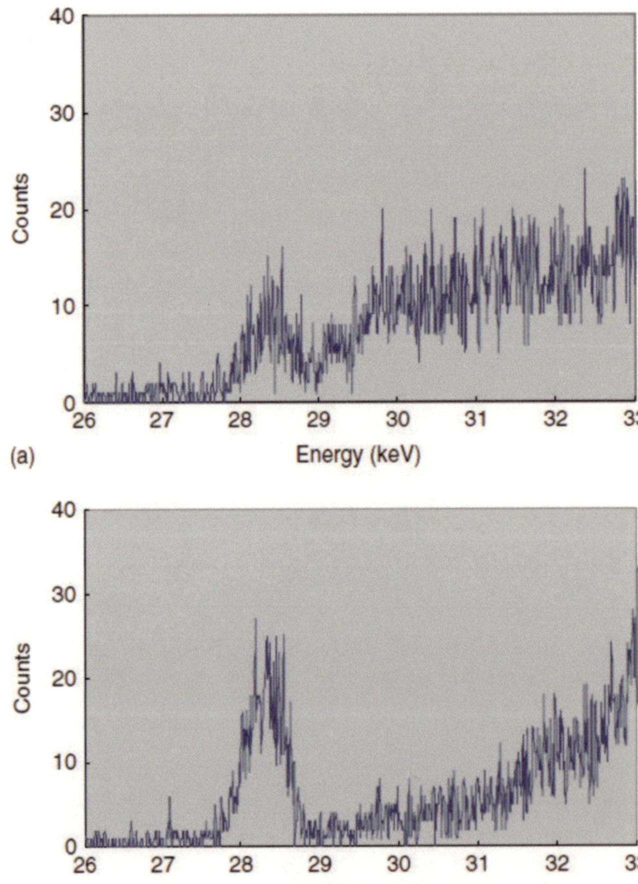

Fig. 25. Example of energy profile around the fluorescent peak: (a) pencil-beam geometry, and (b) sheet-beam geometry (Huo, et al., 2009).

Figures 25 (a) and (b) show the enlarged energy profiles around the fluorescent peaks for the pencil- and sheet-beam geometry, respectively, where Figs. 25 (a) and (b) are respectively generated from Figs 24 (a) and (b). From Fig. 25 (a), in the pencil-beam geometry, we can see that the multiply scattered components overlap with the fluorescent peak. In contrast, the background noise in the fluorescence region is not observed in Fig. 25 (b). Therefore, we can conclude that the system based on the sheet beam geometry can detect data at a higher signal-to-noise ratio than that on the pencil-beam geometry. The higher quantitative results described earlier can be attributed to the above factors.

Next, we consider a relationship between the spatial resolution and the measurement time. In the sheet-beam geometry, the spatial resolution of the reconstructed image mainly depends on the slit width of the collimator installed in front of the detector, as discussed earlier. In principle, the measurement time depends less on the resolution, because a single projection is obtained simultaneously or in parallel. On the other hand, in the pencil beam geometry, the resolution depends on the cross section of the thin incident beam. Reduction of the beam cross section for higher resolution leads to reduction of the translational step, and therefore the measurement time to acquire a single projection increases. Therefore, the sheet-beam geometry is indispensable for compatibility of the measurement time with the resolution.

Finally, we estimate the measurement time. Using an array of 100 energy-resolved detectors, each with a detector surface 0.25 mm in width and arrayed equally 0.25 mm apart, three translations at steps of 0.25 mm can produce a single complete projection of 25 mm in width. On the assumption that the time for a single measurement is 5 s and the rotational step is 2° over 180°, the total time is 900 (= 5 × 2 × 90) s, plus the time required for the mechanical scans. Thus, we can image a single object in about 15 min. If the detector elements are two-dimensionally arrayed, we can obtain a 3-D CT image by piling up the 2-D tomographic images.

6. Conclusion

In this chapter, we first introduced FXCT of the first generation based on pencil-beam, which offers excellent imaging properties, such as high spatial resolution, high sensitivity, and high quantitativeness. Especially, spatial resolution can be improved up to the microns range by decreasing cross-section of incident-beam. However, the measurement time increases because a decrease in beam cross-section causes a reduction of step size in translationally scanning incident beam, leading to an increase in the number of data, and further an increase in the measurement time. Therefore, in FXCT based on pencil-beam the measurement time and the spatial resolution have a trade-off relationship, since it collects data sequentially. Long measurement time is fatal to in vivo imaging, i.e., molecular imaging.

Then, in order to circumvent the above problem, we proposed the parallel data-acquisition scheme based on sheet-beam geometry. This method collects a set of data in a single projection at once, and thus drastically reduces the total measurement time. We experimentally proved the feasibility by demonstrating reconstructed images of a physical phantom and a biomedical sample using a preliminary system constructed at KEK, Japan.

The proposed method based on sheet-beam geometry also preserves the excellent imaging properties. Also, we take notice of the fact that the sheet-beam geometry offers the exact analytical solution. In addition, the FXCT system can acquire not only functional information but also morphological one. If the CCD camera is placed downstream of the object, we can simultaneously obtain a transmission image which can provide auxiliary data for attenuation correction and morphological information. The proposed FXCT can, therefore, simultaneously obtain both morphological and functional information, while PET/CT requires separate measurements to obtain the two kinds of images.

7. A view to the future

The problem left is how to reconstruct 3-D image. PET and SPECT produce 3-D images. If FXCT gives only 2-D images in spite of a good spatial resolution, FXCT ranks with PET and SPECT. However, the problem can be solved using 2-D detectors array and a volumetric parallel incident beam. If we treat the volumetric beam as an accumulation of sheet beams in a vertical direction, we can apply the proposed data-acquisition scheme and the reconstruction algorithm to each supposed sheet-beam straightforwardly. Finally, we construct a 3-D image by accumulating the reconstructed 2-D images in a vertical direction. The measurement time in 3-D case is the same as that in 2-D case. For this purpose, we need a 2-D detectors array with energy resolution. However, presently it is still too expensive, and has an insufficient size of each detector element. Advent of 2-D detectors array with energy resolution and with each detective surface area sufficiently fine will accelerate development of the FXCT system for molecular imaging.

8. Take-home-message

FXCT is a hybrid from x-ray fluorescent analysis and computed tomography. FXCT imaging system has excellent properties as follows:

1. use of non-radioactive imaging agent, i.e., non-inner exposure inspection,
2. non-destructive measurement,
3. high sensitivity,
4. high spatial resolution,
5. high quanatitativeness, and
6. simultaneous acquisition of functional and morphological information.

9. Acknowledgment

We would like to thank Professor Emeritus Takao Akatsuka (Yamagata University) for adequate advice through the research for long years. Also, we thank Kazuyuki Hyodo PhD, Thet-Thet-Lwin MD, Jin Wu MD, Qingkai Huo PhD, Naoki Sunaguchi PhD, Quanwen Yu PhD, Masahiro Akiba PhD, and Tsutomu Zeniya PhD for their scientific and technical supports. This research was partially supported by a Grant-In-Aid for Scientific Research (No. 21390339 & 23602002) from the Japanese Ministry of Education, Science and Culture, and performed under the auspices of the National Laboratory for High Energy Physics (2010G055).

10. References

Boisseau, P. & Grodzins, L. (1987), Fluorescence tomography using synchrotron radiation. Hyperfine Interactions, Vol. 33, pp. 283–292

Brunetti, A. & Golosio, B. (2001). Software for X-ray fluorescence and scattering tomographic reconstruction. *Computer Physics Communications*. Vol. 141, No. 3, pp. 412-425

Cesareo, R. & Mascarenhas, S. (1989). A new tomographic device based on the detection of fluorescent X-rays. Nucl. Instrum. Mech., Vol. A277, pp. 669–672

Cheong, S. K.; Jones, B. L.; Siddiqi, A. K.; Liu, F; Manohar, N & Cho, S. H. (2010). X-ray fluorescence computed tomography (XFCT) imaging of gold nanoparticle-loaded objects using 110 kVp x-rays. *Physics in Medicine and Biology*, Vol. 55, Iss. 3, pp. 647-662

Chukalina, M.; Simionovici, A; Snigirev, A. & Jeffries, T (2002). Quantitative characterization of microsamples by x-ray fluorescence tomography. *X-Ray Spectrometry*, Vol. 31, Iss. 6, pp. 448-450

Chukalina, M.; Simionovici, A.; Zaitsev, S. & Vanegas, C. J. (2007). Quantitative comparison of X-ray fluorescence microtomography setups: Standard and confocal collimator apparatus. *Spectrochimica ACTA Part B - Atomic Spectroscopy*, Vol. 62, Iss. 6-7, pp. 544-548

Deng, B. A.; Yang, Q.; Xie, H. L. .; Du, G. H. & Xiao, T. Q. (2011). First X-ray fluorescence CT experimental results at the SSRF X-ray imaging beamline. *Chinese Physics C*, Vol. 35, Iss. 4, pp. 402-404

Deng, B; Yu, X. H.; Li, A. G.& Xu, H. J (2007). Nondestructive analysis by combined X-ray tomography on a synchrotron radiation facility. *Nuclear Science and Techniques*, Vol. 18, Iss. 5, pp. 257-260

Golosio, B.; Simionovici, A.; Somogyi, A.; Lemelle, L.; Chukalina, L. M. & Brunetti, A. (2003). Internal elemental microanalysis combining x-ray fluorescence, Compton and transmission tomography. *J. Appl. Phys.*, Vol. 94, No. 1, pp. 145-156

Golosio, B.; Simionovici, A.; Somogyi. A; Camerani, C. & Steenari, B. M. (2003). X-ray fluorescence tomography of individual waste fly ash particles. *Journal de Physique IV*, Vol. 104, pp. 647-650

Hogan, J. P.; Gonsalves, R. A. & Krieger, A. S. (1991). Fluorescent computer tomography: A model for correction of X-ray absorption. *IEEE Trans. Nuc. Sci.*, Vol. 38, pp. 1721–1727

Huo, Q.; Yuasa, T.; Akatsuka, T.; Takeda, T.; . Wu, J.; Thet-Thet-Lwin; Hyodo, K. & Dilmanian, F. A. (2008). Sheet beam geometry for in vivo fluorescent x-ray computed tomography : Proof-of-concept experiment in molecular imaging. *Opt. Lett.*, Vol. 33, Iss. 21, pp. 2494-2649

Huo, Q.; Sato, H.; Yuasa, T.; Akatsuka, T.; Wu, J.; Thet-Thet-Lwin; Takeda, T. & Hyodo, K. (2009). First experimental result with fluorescent X-ray CT based on sheet-beam geometry. *X-Ray Spectrometry*, Vol. 38, pp. 429-445

Iida, A & Gohshi, Y. (1991). Tracer element analysis by X-ray fluorescent, In: *Handbook on Synchrotron Radiation*, vol. 4, S. Ebashi, M. Koch, and E. Rubensein, (Eds.), 307–348, , North-Holland: Elsevier, Amsterdam, Netherlands

Jones, B. L. & Cho, S. H. (2011). The feasibility of polychromatic cone-beam x-ray fluorescence computed tomography (XFCT) imaging of gold nanoparticle-loaded objects: a Monte Carlo study. *Physics in Medicine and Biology*, Vol. 56, pp. 3719-3730

La Riviere, P. J. (2004). Approximate analytic reconstruction in x-ray fluorescence computed tomography. *Physics in Medicine and Biology*, Vol. 49, pp. 2391-2405

La Riviere, P. J. & Vargas, P. A. (2006). Monotonic penalized-likelihood image reconstruction for X-ray fluorescence computed tomography. *IEEE Trans. Med. Imaging*, Vol. 25, Iss. 9, pp. 1117-1129

La Riviere, P. J.; Billmire, D; Vargas, P; Ri ers, M & Sutton, S. R. (2006). Penalized-likelihood image reconstruction for x-ray fluorescence computed tomography. *Optical Engineering*, Vo. 45, Iss. 7, 077005

La Riviere, P.; Vargas, P.; Xia, D. & Pan, X. C (2010). Region of Interest Reconstruction in X-Ray Fluorescence Computed Tomography for Negligible Attenuation. *IEEE Trans. Nuclear Science*, Vol. 57, Iss. 1, pp. 234-241

Miqueles, E. X. & De Pierro, A. R. (2010). Exact analytic reconstruction in x-ray fluorescence CT and approximated versions. *Physics in Medicine and Biology*, Vol. 55, No. 4, pp. 1007-1024

Miqueles, E. X. & De Pierro, A. R. (2011). Iterative Reconstruction in X-ray Fluorescence Tomography Based on Radon Inversion. *IEEE Trans. Medical Imaging*, Vol. 30, Iss. 2, pp. 438-450

Natterer, F. (2001). Inversion of attenuated Radon transform. *Inverse Problem*, Vol. 17, pp. 113-119

Rust, G. F. & Weigelt, J. (1998). X-ray fluorescent computer tomography with synchrotron radiation. *IEEE Trans. Nucl. Sci.*, Vol. 45, Iss. 1, pp. 75-88

Schroer, C. G. (2001). Reconstructing x-ray fluorescence microtomograms. *Appl. Phys. Lett.*, Vol. 79, No. 12, pp. 1912-1914

Simionovici, A.; Chukalina, M.; Schroer, C.; Drakopoulos, M.; Snigirev, A.; Snigireva, I.; Lengeler, B.; Janssens, K. & Adams, F. (2000). High-resolution X-ray fluorescence microtomography of homogeneous samples. *IEEE Trans. Nucl. Sci.*, Vol. 47, Iss. 6, pp. 2736-2740

Simionovici, A.; Chukaline, M.; Gunzler, F.; Schroer, C.; Snigirev, A.; Snigireva, I.; Tummler, J. & Weitkamp, T. (2001). *Nucl. Instr. Meth. A*, 467–468, pp. 889-893

Takeda, T.; Maeda, T.; Yuasa, T.; Akatsuka, T.; , Ito, K.; Kishi, K.; Kazama, M.; Hyodo, K. & Itai, Y. (1995). Fluorescent scanning X-ray tomography with synchrotron radiation. *Rev. Sci. Instrum.*, Vol. 66, no. 2, pp.1471–1473

Takeda, T.; Akiba, M.; Yuasa, T.; Kazama, M.; Hoshino, A.; Watanabe, Y.; Hyodo, K.; Dilmanian, F. A.; Akatsuka, T. & Itai, Y. (1996). Fluorescent x-ray computed tomography with synchrotron radiation using fan collimator. *Proc. SPIE*, Vol. 2708, pp. 685–695

Takeda, T.; Kazama, M.; Zeniya, T.; Yuasa, T.; Akiba, M.; Uchida, A.; Hyodo, K.; Akatsuka, T.; Ando, M. & Itai, Y. (1998). Development of a monochromatic X-ray computed tomography with synchrotron radiation for functional imaging, In: *Medical Applications of Synchrotron Radiation*, M. Ando, C. Uyama, (Eds.), pp. 103-107, Springer-Verlag, Tokyo, Japan

Takeda, T.; Momose, A.; Yu, Q.; Yuasa, T.; Dilmanian, F. A.; Akatsuka, T. & Itai, Y. (2000). *Cell. Mol. Biol.*, Vol. 46, No. 6, pp. 1077-1088

Takeda, T.; Yu, Q.; Yashiro, T.; Zeniya, T.; Wu, J.; T.; Hasegawa, Y.Thet-Thet-Lwin; Hyodo, K.; Yuasa, T.; Dilmanian, F. A.; Itai, Y. & Akatsuka, T. (2001). Iodine imaging in thyroid by fluorescent X-ray CT with 0.05 mm spatial resolution. *Nucl. Instrum. Methods A*, Vol. 467–468, pp. 1318-1321

Takeda, T.; Yu, Q.; Yashiro, T.; Zeniya, T.; Wu, J.; Hasegawa, Y.; Thet- Thet-Lwin; Hyodo, K.; Yuasa, T.; Dilmanian, F. A.; Akatsuka, T. & Itai, Y. (2001). Iodine imaging in thyroid by fluorescent X-ray CT with 0.05 mm spatial resolution. *Nucl. Instrum. Methods A*, Vol. 467–468, pp. 1318-1321

Thet-Thet-Lwin; Takeda, T.; Wu, J.; Sunaguchi, N.; Murakami, T.; Mouri, S.; Nasukawa, S.; Huo, Q.; Yuasa, T.; Hyodo, K. & T. Akatsuka. (2007). Preliminary quantitative analysis of myocardial fatty acid metabolism from fluorescent X-ray computed tomography imaging. *J. Synchrotron Radiat.*, Vol. 14, No. 1, pp. 158-162

Thet-Thet-Lwin; Takeda, T.; Wu, J.; Huo, Q.; Yuasa, T.; Hyodo, K. & Akatsuka, T. (2008). Visualization of age-dependent myocardial metabolic impairment in cardiomyopathic model hamster obtained by fluorescent X-ray computed tomography using I-127 BMIPP. *J. Synchrotron Radiat.*, Vol. 15, No. 5, pp. 528-531

Takeda, T.; Wu, J.; Thet-Thet-Lwin; Huo, Q.; Yuasa, T.; Hyodo, K.; Dilmanian, F. A. & Akatsuka, T. (2009). X-ray fluorescent CT imaging of cerebral uptake of stable-iodine perfusion agent iodoamphetamine analog IMP in mice. *J. Synchrotron Radiat.*, Vol. 16, No. 1, pp. 57-62

Yu, Q.; Takeda, T.; Yuasa, T.; Hasegawa, Y.; Wu, J.; Thet-Thet Lwin; Hyodo, K.; Dilmanian, F. A.; Itai, Y. & Akatsuka, T. (2001). Preliminary experiment of fluorescent X-ray computed tomography to detect dual agents for biological study. *J. Synchrotron Radiat.*, Vol. 8, pp. 1030-1034

Yuasa, T.; Akiba, M.; Takeda, T.; Kazama, M.; Hoshino, A.; Watanabe, Y.; Hyodo, K.; Dilmanian, F. A.; Akatsuka, T. & Itai, Y. (1997). Reconstruction method for fluorescent x-ray computed tomography by least squares method using singular value decomposition. *IEEE Trans. Nucl. Sci.*, Vol. 44, pp. 54–62

Yuasa, T.; Akiba, M.; Takeda, T.; Kazama, M.; Hoshino, A.; Watanabe, Y.; Hyodo, K.; Dilmanian, F. A.; Akatsuka, T. & Itai, Y. (1997). Incoherent-scatter computed tomography with monochromatic synchrotron x ray: feasibility of multi-CT imaging system for simultaneous measurement-of fluorescent and incoherent scatter x rays. *IEEE Trans. Nucl. Sci.*, Vol. 44, pp. 1760-1769

Zeniya, T.; Takeda, T.; Yu, Q.; Hasegawa, Y.; Hyodo, K.; Yuasa, T.; Hiranaka, Y.; Itai, Y. Akatsuka, T. (2001). Integrated image presentation of transmission and fluorescent X-ray CT using synchrotron radiation, *Nucl. Instrum. Methods A*, Vol. 467–468, pp. 1326-1328

4

Investigating the Conformation of HER Membrane Proteins in Cells via Single Molecule and FLIM Microscopy

Marisa L. Martin-Fernandez et al.*
Central Laser Facility, Research Complex at Harwell, Rutherford Appleton Laboratory, Didcot, Oxford, UK

1. Introduction

Understanding how signal inputs and outputs are organised in membrane protein signalling networks is an important question in biology. The current goal is to derive methods that would allow the 'watching' of these network proteins in action and at atomic resolution to see details of their structure. This requires the addition of a 'time' dimension to structural biology so that the spatio-temporal parameters of all atoms in each protein can be described in detail. This is a huge challenge that in cell-free systems has begun to be partially addressed through dynamic experiments combined with molecular simulations. However, in cells, the functions of particular structural motifs are not just constrained by Brownian motions, energy landscapes and thermodynamics, but also by the local availability of partners in subcellular compartments and the boundary constraints imposed by cell environments, for example in the plasma membrane, with its 2D dimensionality, local curvature and electric fields. To understand protein function in cells, observations have to be made in the only physiologically-relevant 'laboratory', the cell. This adds levels of complexity to an already vast challenge.

Using molecular biology techniques in combination with optical methods, we can now annotate individual genes and gene products, screen for protein-protein, protein-DNA and small molecule interactions, and quantify dynamic changes. However, only the combination of fluorescence imaging, fluorescence resonance energy transfer (FRET) and single molecule detection currently offers sensitive spatio-temporal detection in cells for low abundance protein interactions. This is beginning to bridge the gap between protein structure and function by allowing real-time quantitative observations of structural details,

---

*David T. Clarke[1], , Michael Hirsch[1], Sarah R. Needham[1], Selene K. Roberts[1], Daniel J. Rolfe[1], Chris J. Tynan[1], Stephen E.D. Webb[1], Martyn Winn[2], and Laura Zanetti Domingues[1]
[1]*Central Laser Facility, Research Complex at Harwell, Rutherford Appleton Laboratory, Didcot, Oxford, UK,*
[2]*Computational Science and Engineering Department, Science and Technology Facilities Council, Daresbury Laboratory, Warrington, UK*

conformational intermediates, association and dissociation constants, diffusion rates, and rare events. Previous information on complex protein networks, such as the human epithelial growth factor receptor (HER) bio-system, has been derived generally from high-throughput screens and/or single cell models using ensemble (averaged) technologies such as biochemical extraction followed by mass spectrometric analysis. Here we describe examples of how single molecule and ensemble fluorescence microscopy methods can offer the means to understand and predict in cells the structure-function relationships of proteins in the input layer of the HER signalling network, from the changes in complex interactions between their microscopic molecular components to their response to perturbations.

2. The human epidermal growth factor receptor (HER) family

HER molecules are prototypical examples of the growth factor receptor tyrosine kinase (RTK) super-family, which also comprises 18 sub-groups of cell surface receptors for many growth factors, cytokines and hormones (Schlessinger 2000). The HER family consists of four homologous receptors, known in cells of human origin as HER1, HER2, HER3 and HER4 (Citri & Yarden 2006). The HER1 molecule (also known as Epidermal Growth Factor Receptor (EGFR)) is the founding member of the RTK family (Fig. 1). In other mammals HER molecules are known as ErbB receptors (ErbB1-4). This name originates from an oncogenic erythroblastosis retrovirus (v-erbB) which encodes a mutated homologue of HER1 (Downward et al. 1984).

HER molecules are encoded as single pass trans-membrane proteins (Fig. 1). The primary structure of HER1, which is shared with all receptor tyrosine kinases, consists of a single polypeptide chain (1,186 amino acids) of 170 kD, containing a heavily glycosylated 622-amino acid residue amino-terminal extracellular ligand binding domain that is connected to the cytoplasmic domain by a single transmembrane (TM) helix of 23 residues. The 542-residue cytoplasmic domain contains a conserved 250-amino acid tyrosine kinase core (Ullrich et al. 1984). The kinase domain is the locus of the enzymatic activity of the receptor and at the core of its signalling function in the cell.

Mature HER molecules are translocated to the plasma membrane lipid bilayer, which is the outer boundary of the cell separating the extracellular and intracellular environments (Hillier & Hoffman 1953), were they are able to accept signalling cues from their environment (Fig. 1). In the HER family signalling cues are provided by 13 potential ligands (reviewed in Yarden & Sliwkowski 2001; Citri et al. 2003; Citri & Yarden 2006). These ligands, known as epidermal growth factor (EGF)-related peptides, can be classified in three functional groups according to their specific binding targets (Olayioye et al. 2000): EGF, transforming growth factor alpha (TGFα), amphiregulin and epigen bind HER1; betacellulin, epiregulin and heparin binding EGF-like growth factor bind HER1 and HER4; neuregulins 1 to 4 (NRG, also known as heregulins), bind either both HER3 and HER4 (NRG-1 and NRG-2) or HER4 alone (NRG-3 and NRG-4). HER2 is thought to be an orphan receptor, with none of the EGF family of ligands discovered so far being able to bind and activate it (Baselga & Swain 2009; Olayioye et al. 2000).

EGF-related peptide growth factors are synthesised as cell membrane associated precursors in the plasma membrane. The extracellular domains of membrane-bound growth factors are subsequently shed via the action of members of a family of proteases known as a disintegrin

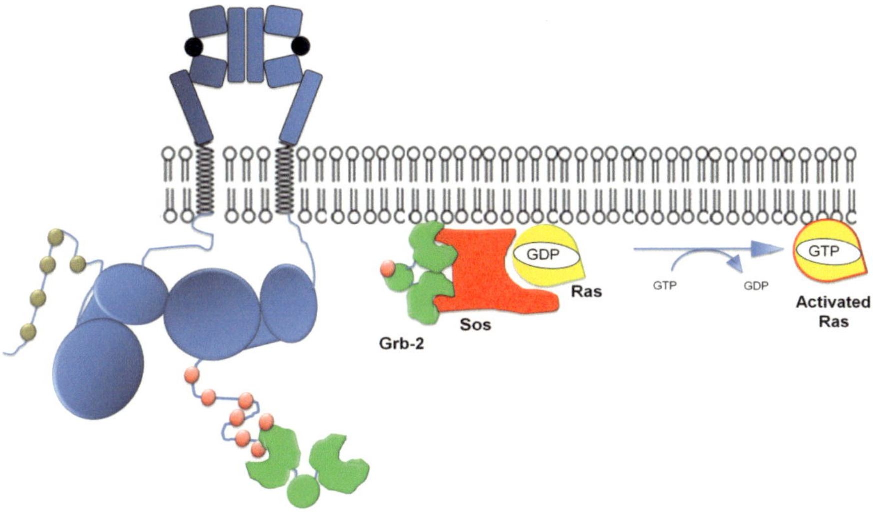

Fig. 1. A cartoon of a 2:2 EGF/HER1 dimer complex showing the initial stages of effector recruitment and signalling. Shown are the external domains of HER1 bound to EGF (black spheres) derived from crystallographic data (Garret et al. 2002; Ogiso et al. 2002; Ferguson et al. 2003). In the cytoplasm the two tyrosine kinase domains of the HER1 dimer form an asymmetric dimer (Zhang et al. 2006). Following recruitment and phosphorylation of effectors like Grb2, recruitment of Sos leads to the activation of Ras via exchange of GTP for GDP to activate the Ras mediated signalling pathway (Zhang & Liu 2002).

and metalloproteases (ADAMs) family. As indicated by their name, these proteolytic enzymes are zinc-dependent trans-membrane metalloproteases (Zhou et al. 2005). Other members of the ADAMs family also shed extracellular domains of other cytokines and receptors (Edwards et al. 2008). Growth factor shedding is critical for the production of soluble functional HER ligands that can activate cell signalling via paracrine and autocrine mechanisms. Growth factors that remain membrane-bound can bind HER molecules on adjacent cells leading to juxtacrine signalling (Riese & Stern 1998).

3. Ligand-induced receptor dimerisation

An essential step in HER activation and signalling is achieved via ligand-induced receptor dimerisation (Schlessinger 2000). Ligand molecules bind the extracellular region of their cognate receptor in specific sites promoting dimerisation and interactions between two receptor monomers (Fig. 1). If two receptors are of the same type (e.g. HER1-HER1 dimer) the process is known as homo-dimerisation. For receptors of two different types (e.g. HER1-HER3) the process is known as hetero-dimerisation. Inactive receptors are believed to exist mainly as monomers, although unliganded (inactive) HER dimers have also been detected in cells (Martin-Fernandez et al. 2002; Clayton et al. 2005).

A defining characteristic of the HER family is that only HER1 and HER4 can bind ligands and also signal autonomously via homo-dimerisation and trans-activation of their tyrosine kinases (Yarden & Sliwkowski, 2001). In contrast, HER2 and HER3 are not autonomous. As discussed above, HER2 lacks the intrinsic ability to interact with known ligands, whereas the kinase of HER3 is defective (reviewed in Citri et al. 2003). HER2 and HER3 can therefore only initiate signals through hetero-dimer formation. The following interacting pairs have been reported in the literature: HER1-HER1, HER4-HER4, HER1-HER2, HER1-HER3, HER1-HER4, HER2-HER3, HER2-HER4 and HER3-HER4 (reviewed in (Bublil & Yarden 2007)). HER2-HER2 and HER3-HER3 homo-dimers may also exist, but this is less certain. Despite having no soluble ligand, HER2 is important because it is the preferred hetero-dimerisation partner of the other ligand-bound family members (GrausPorta et al. 1997). In addition, there are also reports of higher order homo-oligomers of HER1 (such as tetramers) (Clayton, et al. 2005; Clayton et al. 2008).

4. HER signalling in cancer

Aberrant behaviour of HER family members has been implicated in many cancers (Sharma et al. 2007). Research has shown that in adulthood, excessive HER signalling upsets the balance between cell growth and apoptosis resulting in the development of a wide variety of solid tumours (reviewed in Bublil & Yarden 2007). In particular, the level of expression and/or activation of HER1 and HER2 are altered in many tumours of epithelial origin, and clinical studies indicate that HER1 and HER2 have important roles in tumour aetiology and progression (Hynes & Lane 2005). For example, deregulated signalling by cell surface HER1 receptors (e.g. via activating mutations in the *HER1* gene) is implicated in a substantial percentage of lung cancers (Paez et al. 2004). Gene amplification leading to HER1 overexpression is also often found in other human cancers like glioblastoma and esophageal squamous cell carcinoma (Ohgaki et al. 2004; Sunpaweravong et al. 2005). As activation of HER molecules has been shown to result in the growth and progression of the malignancy, the HER family is an important target of the pharmaceutical industry and there have been considerable research efforts directed toward the development of effective inhibitors of HER signalling. Two important types of HER inhibitor are in clinical use: Humanized antibodies directed against the extracellular domain of HER1 or HER2, which elicit an immune response and/or block ligand-binding and dimerisation, and small-molecule tyrosine-kinase inhibitors (TKIs) that compete with ATP in the tyrosine-kinase domain of the receptor inhibiting its intrinsic tyrosine kinase activity (Hynes & Lane 2005). Some of these TKIs have already demonstrated substantial clinical activity against several cancers (e.g. targeting of HER1 and HER2 are in different stages of pre-clinical and clinical trials) (Bublil & Yarden 2007; Citri & Yarden 2006; Hynes & Lane 2005).

5. Structural insights on the HER family: The extracellular domain

The original paradigm proposed for the activation of HER molecules was that the binding of ligand induced the dimerisation of monomeric unliganded receptors via ligand-crosslinking of two receptor moieties (Schlessinger 2000). Contrary to these expectations, crystallographic studies of HER1 ectodomain fragments bound to two types of ligands, EGF and TGFα, have shown quasi-symmetric 2:2 ligand-receptor dimers where each ligand binds simultaneously to subdomains I and III of one of the monomers (Fig. 2). These HER1 dimer structures therefore clearly showed that the dimerisation of this receptor was not directly mediated by the binding of ligand but achieved exclusively via receptor-receptor contacts via subdomain II (Garrett et al. 2002; Ogiso et al. 2002) (Fig. 2).

Crystal structures of unliganded HER1, HER3 and HER4 monomers show that these are held in a closed conformation by an intramolecular tether formed by loops in subdomains II and IV (Bouyain et al. 2005; Ferguson et al. 2003; Hyun-Soo & Leahy 2002). These data suggest that ligand binding and dimerisation involves major extracellular structural rearrangements in HER1, HER3 and HER4 molecules because in ligand-occupied receptor dimers the intramolecular tether is broken and the receptor is opened into an extended conformation which interacts with another monomer to form a back-to-back dimer (Burgess et al. 2003; Ferguson, et al. 2003). Interestingly, unliganded HER2 has an extended configuration that resembles the structure of ligand-bound 'activated' HER1 (Cho et al. 2003). This may explain the unique properties of HER2, which has no known ligand and can cause cell transformation (and tumorigenesis) by simple overexpression (Yu & Hung 2000). The latter appears to force the equilibrium towards spontaneous HER2 homodimer formation, which leads to receptor activation in the absence of ligands. This is the situation observed in a variety of human cancers.

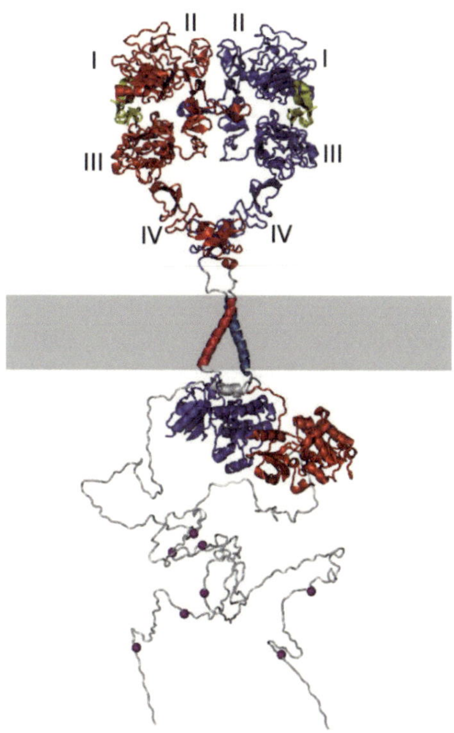

Fig. 2. A structural model of the 2:2 EGF/HER1 complex. Shown are the four subdomains (I–IV) of the HER1 ectodomain (Garret et al. 2002; Ogiso et al. 2002; Ferguson et al. 2003) and the TM helices. In the cytoplasm, the two tyrosine kinase domains form an asymmetric dimer (Zhang et al. 2006). The EGF ligands are shown in yellow. Fragments known from crystallography or NMR are coloured, while the pale grey sections denote regions of uncertain structure, including the extracellular JM linker, the intracellular JM domain (Jura et al. 2009a; Brewer et al. 2009), and the C-terminal tails. On the latter, purple spheres indicate known auto-phosphorylation sites. Figures have been prepared using visual molecular dynamics (Humphrey el al. 1996).

The typical high-resolution representation of ligand-bound HER1 dimeric holoreceptors is depicted in Fig. 2. This generally accepted model has been derived by putting together the available structural information on extracellular and intracellular fragments (Garrett et al. 2002; Ogiso et al. 2002; Ferguson et al. 2003; Brewer et al. 2009; Jura et al. 2009a; Jura et al. 2009b; Zhang et al. 2006). In this model, the extracellular domains are oriented with respect to the membrane based on the historical view that receptors are protruding from the plasma membrane as antennae.

6. Structural insights into the HER family: The intracellular domain

Ligand binding and the dimerisation of HER1 extracellular domain leads across the plasma membrane to the formation of an asymmetric dimer by the two associated intracellular kinases (Zhang et al. 2006) that is stabilised by the inner juxtamembrane (JM) region (Brewer et al. 2009; Jura et al. 2009a) (Fig. 2). Kinase activation follows through an allosteric mechanism in which the C-lobe of one kinase (activator) "pushes" the N-lobe of the other kinase (receiver) in an interaction that is highly reminiscent of the activation of CDK2 by binding of cyclin A (Jeffrey et al. 1995). Active kinases in the homodimer (and possibly heterodimer) then proceed to phosphorylate *in trans* tyrosine residues in the C-terminal tail of the partner receptor (Zhang et al. 2006). Fig. 2 depicts the C-termini of a HER1-HER1 dimer (for which there is no structural data), showing the location of tyrosine amino acid residues. These tyrosine residues are phosphorylated by the addition of a phosphate group (PO_4^{3-}). When phosphorylated these sites act as docking sites for a large repertoire of intracellular adaptors and enzymes containing Src homology 2 (SH2) domains (Pawson 2004). These include Grb2 (Fig. 1), GAP, Shc (Pai & Tarnawski 1998), phospholipase Cγ (PLCγ) (Katan 1998), and phosphatidylinositol 3′-kinase (PI3K) (Vanhaesebroeck et al. 2001), which regulate Ras/Rho-like GTPases (Ridley 2001), Ca^{2+} second messenger production (Defize et al. 1989), and the Ras-activated MAP/SAP kinase pathways (Zhang & Liu 2002). In this way, HER molecules start the intracellular signalling cascades that lead to cell proliferation, changes in cell morphology, trafficking, and the termination of signals via endocytosis of the receptor-ligand complexes (Carpenter 2000; Sorkin 2001).

The pattern of phosphorylated tyrosine motifs is specific to each HER homo and hetero pair (Schulze, Deng, & Mann 2005a). This is the way by which intracellular effector proteins can selectively be recruited by different HER pairs at the plasma membrane to initiate different signalling events and cascades in the cell (reviewed in (Citri & Yarden 2006)). The combinatorial variety of homo/hetero HER1-4 complexes therefore provides a mechanism by which different cell responses can be induced via recruitment of different combinations of signalling effectors to phosphorylated homo and hetero HER complexes, activating intracellular pathways for signal attenuation (receptor desensitisation, down-regulation, endocytosis and trafficking), signal amplification and cell growth, death signals (apoptosis) and other signal processing pathways (Yarden & Sliwkowski 2001). This may explain how subtle differences in the expression pattern of HER1-4 and their ligands may ultimately regulate development and homeostasis in many tissue types.

7. Towards a systems biology perspective

A glimpse of the true complexity in the HER network has only been obtained recently in the light of high-throughput screens and proteomic assays. These have added hundreds of putatively assigned new interactions and several new signal regulators in different cellular compartments to an already complicated picture, making the network increasingly difficult to describe. The burgeoning of data is facilitating the emergence of a cellular systems level perspective (Jones et al. 2006; Schulze, Deng, & Mann 2005b) which is beginning to uncover non-intuitive features of HER signalling, such as the high biological potency of a low-affinity mutant of EGF (Schoeberl et al. 2002). The emerging view is that of a complex 'fail-safe' robust network system (Citri & Yarden 2006), which is able to maintain some degree of function through embedded layers of functional degeneracy, modularity, redundancy, buffering and signalling controls, even if some components are damaged. The robustness of the HER signalling network is underlined by its bi-stability (ligand-regulated ON/OFF states) and its 'bow-tie' configuration, in which multiple positive cues (ligand binding) and negative cues (receptor trafficking) are fanned out through an intermediate core processing unit. The core consists of multiple isoforms of interconnected effector units and signalling cascades, intertwined with densely coupled subnetworks (e.g. the phosphoinositide and Ca^{2+} networks and the endocytic machinery; see (Sorkin 2001)). The number of intracellular proteins that form part of this core is vast, including not only the HER1 effectors outlined above, but also entire families of adaptors and enzymes of (e.g. Grb2 and Shc) (Pai & Tarnawski 1998), ubiquitin ligases (e.g. the E3 ubiquitin ligase c-Cb) (reviewed (Thien & Langdon 2005)), lipid and protein kinases (e.g. PI3K, Akt; reviewed (Vanhaesebroeck, et al. 2001)), GTPases (Ridley 2001) (e.g. Ras, Rho) and phospholipases (e.g. PLC-γ (Katan 1998)). More recently, the activation of the small RhoGTPase Cdc42 by HER1 signalling has also been established (El-Sibai et al. 2007; Feng et al. 2006; Kurokawa et al. 2004). HER signalling also results in the specific induction of outputs through transcription factors (Grandis et al. 1998) (e.g. STAT3) which, depending on the exact combination recruited through the core and the cellular context, ultimately lead to different cell fates, including proliferation, survival, adhesion, migration and differentiation (Oda et al. 2005).

8. Multi-colour labelling of signalling proteins in the HER network

Because of the complexity of the HER signalling network (Oda, et al. 2005), the systems-level perspective provides a useful framework to describe network behaviour and to expose and predict the fragility of network activity centres. However, the bottleneck in mathematical 'Systems' modelling is incomplete biological understanding. This is mainly due to the difficulties of obtaining quantitative kinetic/dynamic data and structure-function relationships in the cellular environment. To gain a better understanding of HER signalling that can facilitate a systems perspective it is necessary, for example, to devise better means of obtaining structural data on the input layer of the HER signalling network. It is also necessary to obtain much more information on the dynamic rules of engagement between HER network proteins in vivo and to understand the positive and negative feedback-loops regulating the HER network that allow functioning under perturbation.

Fluorescence microscopy methods provide a convenient approach to study protein conformation and dynamic interactions between HER network members at the plasma membrane of living cells. This method is non-invasive and allows several types of proteins to be specifically tagged and observed simultaneously. For example, heteromeric pan-HER interactions can in principle be measured in living cells by using a combination of fluorophores to label each of the four members of the HER family with a different colour tag

(Fig. 3) and then employing FRET and/or multicolour single molecule tracking to follow their interactions in real-time (see below). These methods can in principle be extended in cells bio-engineered to express specific combinations of interacting fluorescent ligand/HER1-4/adaptor/inhibitor variants.

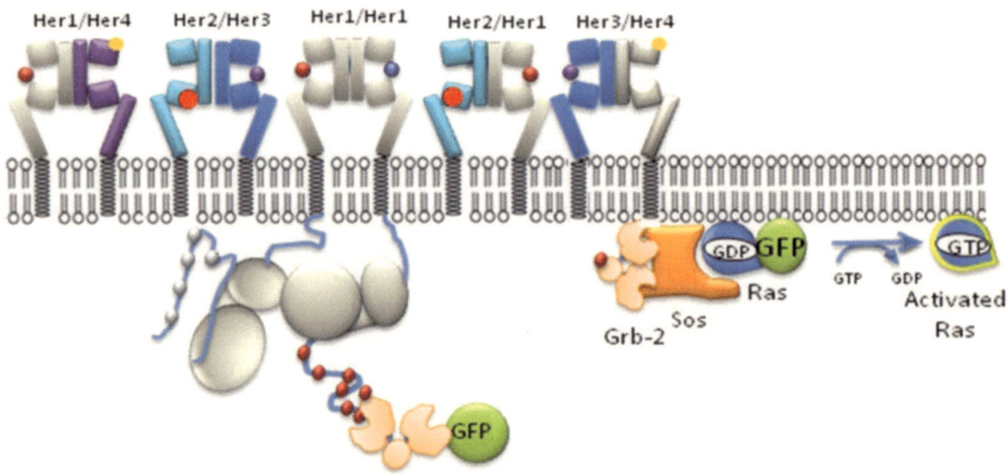

Fig. 3. A cartoon showing the HER1 homo-dimer and hetero-dimers at the plasma membrane. (The intracellular domains of hetero-dimers are not shown for simplicity). Different colour labels are targeted to the extracellular domains (small colour spheres). Intracellular proteins can be labelled using fluorescence proteins such as GFP.

One strategy to label HER molecules is to use their cognate ligands (e.g. EGF or small affibodies) as delivery vehicles for the fluorophores (Fig. 3). For this, fluorophores of different colours can be bound in a 1:1 ratio to different activating and non-activating ligands, each specific for one of the receptor types. Once these ligands bind their cognate receptors, each receptor type will be tagged with a different colour molecule. This means that each receptor type is colour-coded and will appear in a different colour channel. Other strategies include chemical synthesis of fluorescent ACP- (a 6 kDa, acyl carrier protein), MCP- (a mutant version of ACP), SNAP- and CLIP-tag substrates, fluorescence protein fusions to HER C-termini, N/C-termini of scaffolds and effectors (Fig. 2) and cell permeant benzylguanine (BG) or benzylcytosine (BC) dye derivatives (Banala, Arnold, & Johnsson 2008), including BG and BC conjugated to TMRstar (which can fluorescently label any O6-alkylguanine-DNA alkyltransferase (AGT)-tagged, i.e. SNAP or CLIP tagged, intracellular proteins in live cells).

The remainder of this chapter shows steps taken in our laboratory towards the development of an integrated experimental approach that can provide data on multi-molecular interactions towards a system-focused approach. These steps have so far consisted of developing the tools to extract structural and dynamic information on the HER bio-system in the cellular context by gathering information on conformational changes, receptor interactions and the dynamic rules of engagement in HER signalling.

9. Investigating HER protein-protein interactions by FRET

FRET is a phenomenon by which the excited-state energy of an optically excited fluorescent molecule (donor) is transferred to a neighbouring fluorescent molecule (acceptor) non-radiatively via intermolecular Van der Waals (dipole-dipole) interactions (Stryer & Haugland 1967). For FRET to occur the electronic levels of donors and acceptors must overlap. FRET depends on the distance between donors and acceptors as the inverse of the sixth power and is therefore very sensitive to short inter-molecular distances in the range ~2-8 nm. It can therefore be a useful tool to investigate molecular interactions.

FRET observations can be made either in the steady-state, by detecting the quenching of the fluorescence emitted by the donor as energy is transferred to the acceptor, or time-resolved, by measuring the shortening of the fluorescence lifetime of the donor. FRET imaging between fluorescent EGF derivatives bound to HER1 molecules in cells has been widely employed to investigate HER1 homo-dimerisation (Gadella & Jovin 1995; Sako et al. 2000; Martin-Fernandez et al. 2002; Clayton et al. 2005; Clayton et al. 2008). A popular strategy for this was to measure the efficiency of FRET between donor and acceptor fluorophores bound to the N-termini of receptor-bound EGF ligands. Although distances shorter than ~8 nm (averaged over the receptor population) were ubiquitously reported by FRET in these conditions in cells, it should be noted that the preferred (back-to-back) crystallographic dimer shows N-terminal inter-ligand distances of >11 nm (Fig. 3). This distance is too large to be detected by FRET and will remain so even when extreme deformations are applied to this crystal structure; for example, by changing the angle between domains I and III and domain II and/or applying extreme perturbations along low frequency normal modes. The FRET results therefore suggest that other interfaces between receptor monomers not yet found by crystallographic methods must also occur at the plasma membrane of cells.

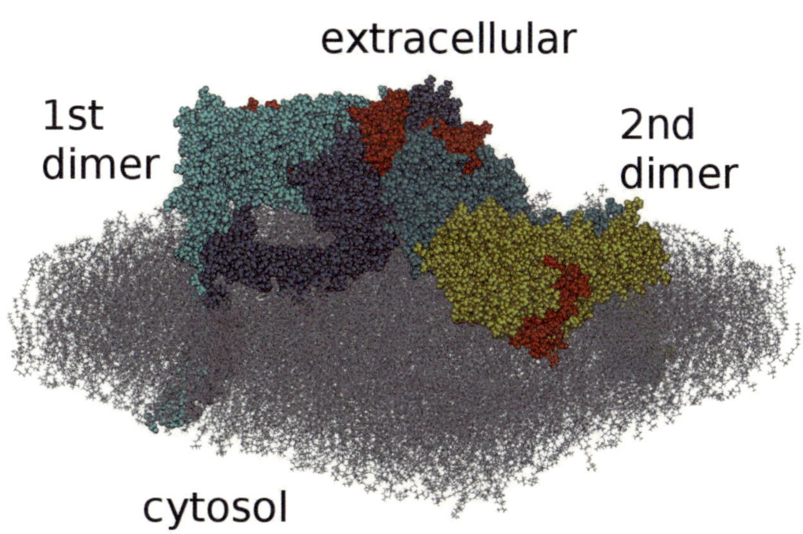

Fig. 4. The back-to-back / head-to-head / back-to-back tetramer on the plasma membrane (Kästner et al. 2009). The grey- stick models are the atomistically modelled lipid molecules of the membrane. EGF ligands are shown in red.

Attempts to understand the origin of FRET between donor/acceptor EGF ligands bound to HER1 include the pioneering work by Clayton et al. in intact BaF/3 cells, a murine interleukin-3 dependent pro-B cell line which do not overexpress ErbB1 (the mammal HER1 equivalent). Using fluorescence correlation microscopy, this work showed the presence in cells of tetramers of activated cell surface EGF/ErbB1 complexes. FRET in turn showed the presence of very short distances (< 4 nm) between ErbB1-bound EGF ligands (Clayton, et al. 2005). It was postulated that these short distances could explain the presence of FRET in the context of a tetramer formed by two back-to-back crystallographic dimers. These short distances between EGF ligands bound to HER1 were subsequently found in human A431 epithelial cells by single pair FRET imaging (Webb et al. 2008). This work provided additional evidence for HER1-HER1 interfaces in cells other than that described in the back-to-back crystallographic structure.

The work of Clayton et al. 2005 and Webb et al. 2008 set the basis for two new models of HER1 activation: In one model tetramers were generated through side-by-side contacts between two adjacent back-to-back dimers; however, there is no crystallographic evidence yet for this arrangement. In the second model (Fig. 4) tetramers were made of two back-to-back dimers joined by a weak, asymmetric "head-to-head" interface seen in crystal structures (Garret et al. 2002). This interface also results in short distances between the N-termini of the two bound EGF molecules of < 4 nm. Molecular dynamics (MD) simulations showed that the head-to-head interaction stabilises appreciably when the tetramer is relaxed on the membrane (its interface area increased from 443 Å^2 seen in the crystal structure to 604 Å^2) (Kastner, et al. 2009). In this tetramer the two dimers remained stable but lost the approximate 2-fold symmetry of the crystal structure. The average dimerisation interface area rose from 1,197 Å^2 to 1,483 Å^2, largely as a result of additional interactions between the N-terminus and the dimerisation arm, while the two ligands buried 1,166 Å^2 and 1,211 Å^2 at distinct binding sites.

Interestingly, the ligand-membrane distances predicted by the tetramer in Fig. 4 are significantly shorter than those predicted by the crystallographic back-to-back dimers standing upright from the membrane (Fig. 3), a hypothesis that can be tested using FRET (see section 11). Initial measurements by Webb et al. (2008) were consistent with the short ligand-membrane distances proposed by the model in Fig. 4 (see section 11).

10. Investigating the origin of ligand - Binding heterogeneity to HER1

Possibly the main disappointment of the HER crystal structures is that they did not explain a 30-year old puzzle in the HER signalling field, namely the origin of the characteristic heterogeneity in EGF-binding affinity to cell-surface HER1 molecules. This heterogeneity was first detected in EGF binding kinetic experiments in cells, as these display characteristic concave-up Scatchard plots (Magun et al. 1980; Shoyab et al. 1979). As HER1 is expressed as a single translation product (Ullrich & Schlessinger 1990), the concave-up EGF-binding Scatchard plots were interpreted as indicating the presence of two receptor populations: a small minority of high-affinity receptors with dissociation constants (K_D) of <1 nM that mediate most signalling events, and a majority of low affinity receptors with K_D of >1 nM (Defize et al. 1989; Friedman et al. 1984). When crystallographic structural data became available ~ 10 years ago, the high- and low-affinity populations were initially expected to be extended HER1 dimers and tethered HER1 monomers, respectively; however, in this model stabilization of the extended dimer configuration by one ligand molecule would facilitate the binding of a second ligand to the remaining unliganded receptor in the dimer, resulting in positive cooperativity and therefore concave-down Scatchard plots (Mattoon et al. 2004).

Using global modelling of ligand-binding data as a function of receptor number, Macdonald and Pike subsequently showed that EGF-binding heterogeneity could be accounted for by negative cooperativity in HER1 dimers (Macdonald & Pike 2008). However, negative cooperativity requires that ligand binding to one subunit of the HER1 dimer decreases the ligand affinity of the other subunit. This would, in turn, require the interactions between ligand and the two subunits of the receptor dimer to be asymmetric, inconsistent with the symmetry observed in the back-to-back structure of HER1. A series of recent crystallographic structures recently showed that in the drosophila counterpart of HER1 (known as drosophila EGFR or dEGFR) the extracellular domain asymmetry is induced by the binding of the first ligand growth factor to the dEGFR dimer, which structurally restrains the unoccupied binding site, reducing the affinity for binding of the second ligand (Alvarado et al. 2010). Interestingly, concave-up Scatchard plots were observed in preparations of the isolated extracellular region of the dEGFR, in direct contrast with its human counterpart, in which concave-up plots are observed only when ligands bind to full-length receptors in cells. These differences suggest that other receptor regions, conformations, and/or other unknown cellular components must be involved in the regulation of ligand affinity in HER1 in the cellular environment. A better understanding of the conformation of HER1 in the plasma membrane environment is therefore required to understand the origin of the heterogeneity of EGF-binding.

11. Using FRET microscopy to report *in situ* protein conformation

Besides ligand-ligand interactions, FRET can also be employed to investigate the conformation of proteins at the plasma membrane, for example by measuring the distance from a specific site in the protein of interest (e.g. the binding site of a growth factor ligand) to the cell surface (Fig. 5). Protein-membrane distances can be determined from the variation of the efficiency of FRET between fluorescent donors attached to the protein of interest and acceptors labelling the cell surface, measured as a function of acceptor surface density (Fig. 5). When crystal structures of the protein and/or protein fragments are available, protein-membrane distances derived from FRET can be used to constrain the disposition of protein structures with respect to the plasma membrane to inform on protein conformation *in situ*.

Analytical expressions describing the energy transfer process between random distributions of donors (e.g. in specific sites in proteins) and acceptors on lipid membrane surfaces have been derived for a number of geometries (see for example Wolber & Hudson 1979). The solutions to these equations are the distance of closest approach between the protein-bound fluorescent donor probe and a lipid acceptor chromophore at the plasma membrane. Examples using this FRET method include an investigation to derive the mean distance between the EGF binding site of HER1 and the plasma membrane of cells in suspension (Carraway et al. 1990), changes in conformation of α4-Integrin during activation (Chigaev et al. 2003), and the minimum separation between the protein portion of GPI-anchored proteins to the bilayer surface (Lehto & Sharom 2002).

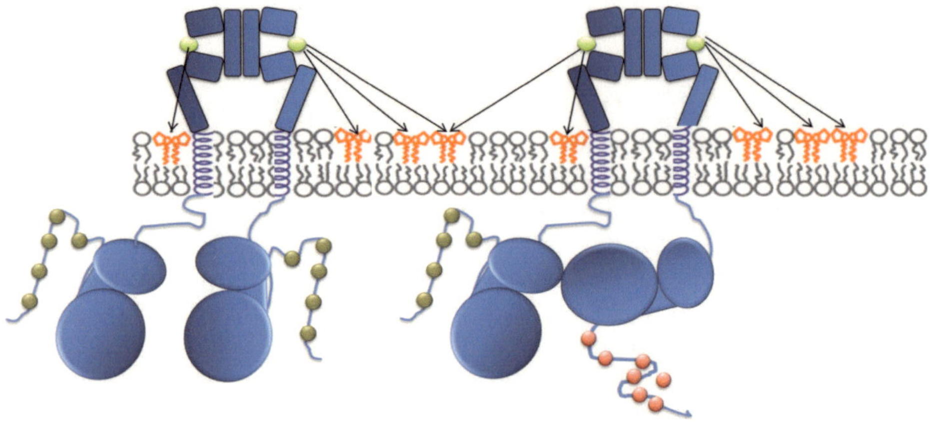

Fig. 5. A cartoon illustrating the FRET problem in two dimensions. Two receptor dimers are depicted bound to donor-labelled EGF (green spheres). The plasma membrane is labelled with lipid acceptors (red). Many distances are possible between each donor and the acceptors in the membrane. By varying the concentration of acceptors at the plasma membrane the vertical distance from donors to the cell surface can be calculated (Tynan et al. 2011).

The three examples cited were derived from cell-averaged steady-state intensity measurements (e.g., flow cytometry). The efficiency of FRET between a random distribution of donors and acceptors can also be determined using fluorescence lifetime imaging microscopy (FLIM). This method images with optical resolution the shortening of the fluorescence decay time of donor-labelled EGF induced by the lipid acceptors. Being a time-resolved assay, FLIM has the advantage of being able to directly measure the time between the absorption and emission of individual photons in the FRET donor fluorophores, providing results largely free from artefacts such as photobleaching and radiative transfer which can increase the errors in the measurement (Martin-Fernandez et al. 2002).

Using the combination of FLIM and FRET to measure protein-membrane distances, Webb et al obtained initial evidence for two types of EGF/HER1 complexes, tilted and upright with respect to the cell surface, that are associated to high-affinity and low-affinity EGF binding, respectively (Webb, et al. 2008). Subsequently, using MD simulations Kästner et al. showed that, with minor rearrangements, the HER1 back-to-back dimer can be aligned almost flat on the cell membrane, leading to conformational changes which further stabilize the extracellular dimer (Kästner et al. 2009). This work also showed that alignment on the cell surface and the interactions between the HER1 dimer and the upper leaflet of the membrane that follow break the pseudo-2-fold symmetry of the HER1 extracellular region, resulting in a highly asymmetric HER1 dimer structure.

12. HER1 can adopt key features of dEGFR asymmetry

To investigate the relevance of the MD-derived asymmetric model of the HER1 dimer relaxed on the membrane (Kastner et al. 2009) to EGF-binding heterogeneity and negative cooperativity (Macdonald & Pike 2008)), Tynan et al extended the FLIM-FRET assay previously reported (Webb et al. 2008) to include FRET titrations as a function of acceptor concentration together with a data analysis method based on Monte-Carlo simulations (Tynan et al. 2011). This method allowed full quantification of the distance of closest approach between HER1-bound ligands and the surface of adherent epithelial cells, the assessment of the variation associated to the distance measurement, and also the rejection of potential sources of artifacts resulting from non-uniform distributions of FRET donors and acceptors.

Given the known flexibility regions in the accepted crystallographic HER1 ectodomain dimer structure, the FRET-derived distance data obtained from HER1 that display high-affinity for EGF (< 4 nm) could only be reconciled with HER1 structural data if receptors are aligned flat on the membrane (Fig. 6). MD simulations of doubly-liganded, singly-liganded and unliganded HER1 dimers aligned on a model membrane under the same conditions revealed that the asymmetry resulting from alignment on the membrane shares a number of key features with the equivalent doubly-liganded and singly-liganded structures observed recently in soluble dEGFR (Alvarado et al. 2010). These results suggest that the structural basis for negative cooperativity is conserved from invertebrates to humans but that in HER1 the extracellular region asymmetry requires interactions with the plasma membrane.

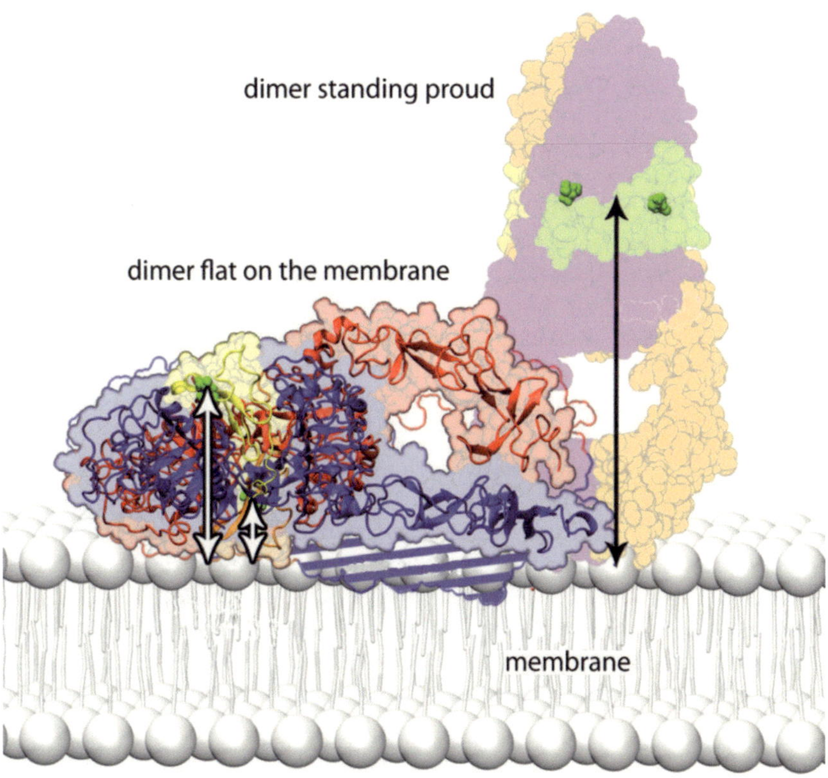

Fig. 6. The EGFR ectodomain dimer with two bound ligands, modelled on crystallographic structures (Garret et al. 2002; Ogiso et al. 2002; Ferguson et al. 2003) and placed in the membrane. Darker green spheres indicate the N termini of the ligands to which donor dyes are attached. Configurations standing upright and lying down are compared.

13. Imaging membrane protein interactions at the nanoscale

Understanding the structure-function relationships of biological macromolecules ultimately requires us to determine molecular structure at a range of resolutions. These include: Atomic resolutions (~1 Å) for detailed protein structure, derived from x-ray crystallography (Vrielink & Sampson 2003); 1-10 nm for measurement of conformations and inter-molecular distances, a range covered by electron microscopy (Agronskaia et al. 2008) and FRET (Stryer & Haugland 1967); and 10-20 nm for measurement of inter-unit separation and therefore the oligomerisation states of protein complexes. Given the importance of HER homo and hetero-oligomerisation in signalling, access to distances in the 10-20 nm range is crucial in investigation of HER interactions because, as discussed above, structural studies indicate that the inter-unit separation in the preferred receptor dimer should be in the region of 10-15 nm (Fig. 3) (Garrett et al. 2002; Ogiso et al. 2002). However, measurements in this range are challenging because these distances fall in a "resolution gap" between FRET and optical microscopy, which is diffraction-limited around 200 nm at best.

In recent years, a number of so-called "super-resolution" optical methods have been developed, that break the diffraction limit for light microscopy. These include stimulated emission depletion (STED) microscopy (Hell 2003) near-field scanning optical microscopy (NSOM) (Dunn 1999), photo-activated localization microscopy (PALM) (Betzig et al. 2006), fluorescence imaging with one-nanometre accuracy (FIONA) (Yildiz & Selvin 2005), single-molecule high resolution imaging with photobleaching (SHRImP) (Balci et al. 2005), nanometre-localized multiple single-molecule (NALMS) microscopy (Qu et al. 2004) and single-molecule high resolution co-location (SHREC) (Churchman et al. 2005). Theoretically, many of these techniques have the potential to measure distances in the required range. However, there are challenges in applying them to the cellular environment. NSOM is not well-suited to the wet conditions required for living or lightly fixed cells. STED and PALM are essentially ensemble imaging techniques that are not easily applied to the measurement of the distance between two or more specific molecules in the crowded cell environment. SHRImP, SHREC, and NALMS can measure distances between molecules with better than 10 nm resolution. Like PALM, all these methods "beat" the diffraction limit by imaging single molecules, fitting the point spread function (PSF) of the microscope, and locating its centre with nanometre accuracy. NALMS uses single molecule detection to count discrete steps in traces of fluorescence intensity vs time from diffraction limited spots, each step corresponding to the activation or bleaching of a single fluorophore, and measuring the change in the PSF of the spot before and after a step. In SHRImP, global fitting is carried out on spots before and after bleaching, producing nearly identical results to the sequential NALMS method. SHREC again uses PSF fitting, but two different fluorophores with different spectral characteristics are used, imaged in distinct channels which must be very accurately registered to determine intra-molecular distance. In all these techniques, spatial resolution is ultimately limited by the signal-to-noise ratio of the data, which determines the precision with which the centre of the PSF can be determined. For this reason, SHRImP, SHREC, and NALMS have so far been demonstrated only in "clean" samples such as purified, immobilised molecules on glass, and in the presence of antifade reagents.

The environment of mammalian cells is not conducive to the collection of high signal-to-noise data. The main source of background noise is intracellular autofluorescence, arising from molecules such as NADPH and flavins (Monici 2005). A common approach to reduce background when looking at membrane proteins is to use total internal reflection (TIRF) excitation (Fig. 1) (Axelrod 1989). TIRF creates an evanescent field on the coverslip on which the cells are cultured. The field reduces exponentially with depth, and only penetrates approximately 300 nm into the sample. Thus, fluorescence is not excited in the bulk of the cell, reducing autofluorescence. This enables single molecule detection, as shown in Fig. 7 (left panel). Single molecules are clearly visible, but there is also a contribution from background noise. This results from residual autofluorescence, scattered light, and fluorescence from out-of-focus fluorophores.

In our laboratory we are developing new methods to improve the accuracy of intra-molecular distance measurement in cells and tissues. We currently achieve sub-10 nm positioning resolution in cells by using new data fitting algorithms that perform well in the noisy environment of cells (manuscript in preparation). Crucially, our techniques give robust estimates of errors, allowing the significance of distance measurements to be properly determined. Fig. 7 (right panel) shows typical single molecule traces and accompanying position measurement from labelled HER1 complexes in fixed epithelial cervical carcinoma HeLa cells.

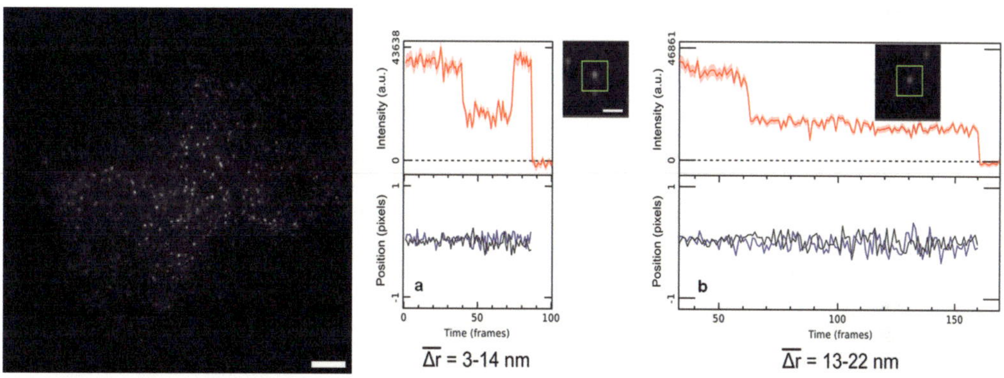

Fig. 7. ***Left:*** Single molecule TIRF image of EGFR in the plasma membrane of HeLa cells. EGFR are labelled with their ligand EGF, conjugated with the fluorophore Atto 647N (bar 8 μm). ***Right:*** Traces of single molecule fluorescence intensity (red) vs time for two example spots in fixed HeLa cells labelled with EGF-Atto 647N. a) shows a relatively short intra-molecular distance, b) a longer distance. Fluorophore x and y positions are plotted in black and blue, respectively.

14. Determining dynamic interactions from diffusion at the membrane

HER molecules interact with each other and with other network proteins while being embedded in the lipid bilayer of the plasma membrane, which is composed of neutral, charged, saturated and unsaturated lipids (Fig. 1). The lipids in the membrane consist of a hydrophilic charged region, the phospholipids heads, which form the extreme outer and inner leaflets of the membrane, and hydrophobic C-H chains of different lengths (typically from C_{12} to C_{20}) that forms the core of the bilayer (van Meer 2005). Water molecules concentrate on the inner and outer surfaces of the plasma membrane at the boundaries with the extracellular and intracellular regions and can occasionally enter the bilayer through surface defects created by lipid mismatch. Hydrophilic protein regions are excluded from the hydrophobic inner part of the lipid bilayer and stick out from the plasma membrane.

The simplest membrane model consists of a 2-D liquid model surrounded by a 3-D solvent (Singer & Nicolson 1972). In this simple model, membrane proteins diffuse freely in the lipid bilayer which is modelled as a viscous liquid. Proteins interact with the surrounding lipid 2-D 'liquid' and diffuse with a speed that depends on lipid viscosity. However, it is observed experimentally that the lateral mobility of proteins in biological membranes can be orders of magnitude slower than in synthetic membranes. Reasons for this include:

i. The presence of lipid rafts: The plasma membrane is composed of different lipids (e.g. phospholipids, sphingolipids and cholesterol) that can form microdomains of different viscosity. These rafts microdomains concentrate certain proteins (including HER molecules) and exclude others (see for example (Kusumi et al. 2005; Nagy et al. 2002).
ii. Intra-membrane barriers: Biological membranes are quite crowded with 15-35% of surface area occupied by many different types of proteins which can interact with each other affecting diffusion mobility (Scheuring & Sturgis 2005).
iii. Skeletal interactions: Proteins are able to interact with protein scaffolds and the cytoskeletal network beneath the plasma membrane in the intracellular side, which have the effect of corralling the membrane proteins in some regions and not others (reviewed in Costa et al. 2011).

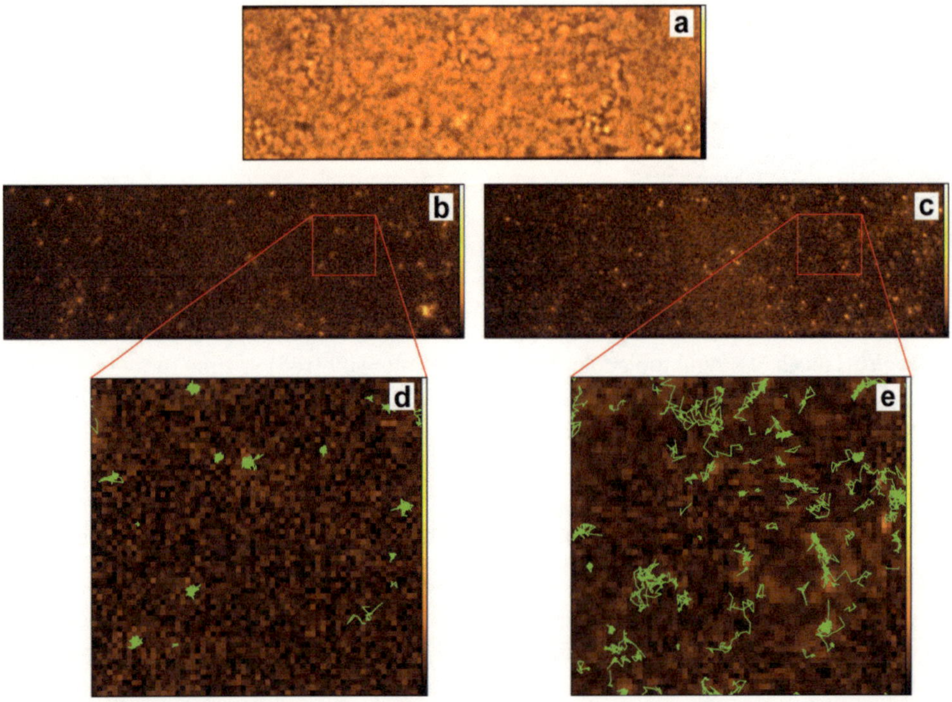

Fig. 8. Two-colour single molecule tracking of T47D cells. a) White light transmission image; b) cells labelled with 0.1 nM anti-ErbB2 affibody-Atto 647N; c) cells labelled with 2 nM anti-EGFR affibody-Alexa 488; d and e) single molecule tracks (green) from the spots located within the boxes marked in b and c.

The role of membrane microdomains, intra-membrane barriers and skeletal interactions in HER signalling is not yet understood. This role can be investigated using single molecule tracking. Advantages of a single molecule approach include the ability to observe dynamic, stochastic behaviour, such as compartmentalized diffusion (Andrews et al. 2008; Dahan et al. 2003; Fujiwara et al. 2002) that would be masked in ensemble measurements, and the ability for localisation of molecules with a precision well below the diffraction limit of light (see section 11).

To investigate protein diffusion and protein-membrane interaction in the HER bio-system we have used, for example, a two colour tracking system (Clarke et al. 2011) to follow the movements of HER1 and HER2 at the plasma membrane of live T47D cells, a human ductal breast epithelial tumour cell line cell model that expresses the four HER receptor types at a level between 10,000-30,000 receptors per cell. Fig. 8 shows single molecule images of HER1, and HER2 in living cells in their basal state. The receptors are labelled with an anti-HER1 affibody (Nordberg et al. 2010) conjugated with Alexa 488 an anti-HER2 affibody (Tran et al. 2007) conjugated with Atto 647N. The data were analysed using Bayesian segmentation algorithms and other data analysis methods described in (Rolfe et al. 2011). The resulting tracks indicate that HER1 displays in these cells higher mobility at the plasma membrane than HER2. We are now developing the methods to extract from these data the different mean displacements of each receptor in the plasma membrane from which their co-localisation kinetics can be derived.

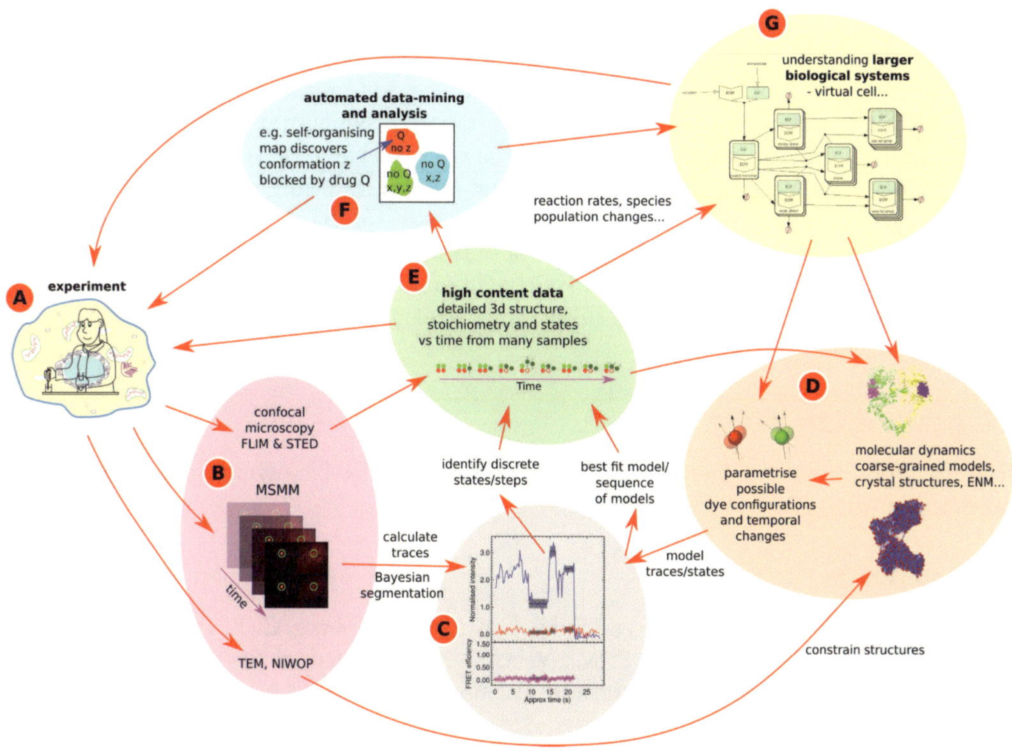

Fig. 9. Experimental and computational methods to investigate the HER signalling network

15. Towards an integrated approach

Ultimately, our goal is to use a cross-disciplinary portfolio of experimental and data analysis techniques to describe the HER signalling network not just in cell models but also in the real world setting. To achieve this we aim at deriving models of ligand-induced behaviour exploiting combined single molecule imaging, ensemble FLIM analysis and systems predictions. We also aim at establishing how HER signalling is influenced by feed-back loops and internal and external perturbations, e.g. HER mutations (seen in human subjects), RTK inhibitors and function-blocking antibodies. We also plan to combine experimental approaches with molecular dynamics and coarse-grained simulations and to explore data mining techniques for exploiting this rich data (Fig. 9).

16. View to the future: Potential clinical applications and take home message

We ultimately aim to refine single molecule fluorescence detection to be applicable to human tissues. We have already demonstrated single-molecule fluorescence imaging of HER receptors in fixed and frozen tissue sections from mouse tumour xenografts and human tissue biopsies (manuscript in preparation). This work is being done in collaboration with Prof. Peter Parker and colleagues at King's College London/Guy's & St Thomas' NHS Foundation Trust. Our aim is to extend the use of fluorescently labelled ligands, affibodies, anti-HER monoclonal antibodies (mAbs) and function blocking antibodies from cultured cell models to investigations of HER signalling on normal primary cells and tissue sections. We also plan to study naturally occurring somatic mutations (e.g. in human lung adenocarcinoma, see review on HER1 mutations in: Lynch et al. 2004) and also study cross-talk interactions with other non-HER receptors in lung and breast cancer tissue. It is hoped that these experiments will allow us to obtain further insights into the HER network and assess predictions made by our models. Once the methods have been optimised, studies will be extended to include other carcinoma cells and tissues, including matched normal tissue. Downstream targets of receptor activation will be assessed by western blotting to set the baseline population behaviour and ensure specificity of reagents. It is hoped that results from these experiments will provide novel insight on how the HER network operates at the tissue level and the supra-molecular rules and controls that are necessary to ensure normal network function.

17. Acknowledgements

The authors gratefully acknowledge funding from the UK Biotechnology and Biological Sciences Research Council (BB/G006911/1).

18. References

Agronskaia, A. V., Valentijn, J. A., van Driel, L. F., Schneijdenberg, C. T., Humbel, B. M., van Bergen en Henegouwen, P. M., Verkleij, A. J., Koster, A. J., and Gerritsen, H. C. (2008). Integrated fluorescence and transmission electron microscopy. *Journal of structural biology* 164, 183-9.

Alvarado, D., Klein, D. E., and Lemmon, M. A. (2010). Structural Basis for Negative Cooperativity in Growth Factor Binding to an EGF Receptor. *Cell* 142, 568-579.

Andrews, N. L., Lidke, K. A., Pfeiffer, J. R., Burns, A. R., Wilson, B. S., Oliver, J. M., and Lidke, D. S. (2008). Actin restricts Fc epsilon RI diffusion and facilitates antigen-induced receptor immobilization. *Nature cell biology* 10, 955-963.

Axelrod, D. (1989). Total internal reflection fluorescence microscopy. *Methods Cell. Biol.* 30, 245-70.

Balci, H., Ha, T., Sweeney, H. L., and Selvin, P. R. (2005). Interhead distance measurements in myosin VI via SHRImP support a simplified hand-over-hand model. *Biophys J* 89, 413-7.

Banala, S., Arnold, A., and Johnsson, K. (2008). Caged substrates for protein labeling and immobilization. *Chembiochem* 9, 38-41.

Baselga, J., and Swain, S. M. (2009). Novel anticancer targets: revisiting ERBB2 and discovering ERBB3. *Nature Reviews Cancer* 9, 463-475.

Betzig, E., Patterson, G. H., Sougrat, R., Lindwasser, O. W., Olenych, S., Bonifacino, J. S., Davidson, M. W., Lippincott-Schwartz, J., and Hess, H. F. (2006). Imaging intracellular fluorescent proteins at nanometer resolution. *Science* 313, 1642-5.

Bouyain, S., Longo, P. A., Li, S., Ferguson, K. M., and Leahy, D. J. (2005). The extracellular region of ErbB4 adopts a tethered conformation in the absence of ligand. *Proceedings of the National Academy of Sciences of the United States of America* 102, 15024-9.

Brewer, M. R., Choi, S. H., Alvarado, D., Moravcevic, K., Pozzi, A., Lemmon, M. A., and Carpenter, G. (2009). The Juxtamembrane Region of the EGF Receptor Functions as an Activation Domain. *Molecular cell* 34, 641-651.

Bublil, E. M., and Yarden, Y. (2007). The EGF receptor family: spearheading a merger of signaling and therapeutics. *Curr Opin Cell Biol* 19, 124-34.

Burgess, A. W., Cho, H. S., Eigenbrot, C., Ferguson, K. M., Garrett, T. P., Leahy, D. J., Lemmon, M. A., Sliwkowski, M. X., Ward, C. W., and Yokoyama, S. (2003). An open-and-shut case? Recent insights into the activation of EGF/ErbB receptors. *Mol Cell* 12, 541-52.

Carpenter, G. (2000). The EGF receptor: a nexus for trafficking and signaling. *Bioessays* 22, 697-707.

Carraway, K. L., Koland, J. G., and Cerione, R. A. (1990). Location Of The Epidermal Growth-Factor Binding-Site On The EGF Receptor - A Resonance Energy-Transfer Study. *Biochemistry* 29, 8741-8747.

Chigaev, A., Buranda, T., Dwyer, D. C., Prossnitz, E. R., and Sklar, L. A. (2003). FRET detection of cellular alpha 4-integrin conformational activation. *Biophysical journal* 85, 3951-3962.

Cho, H. S., Mason, K., Ramyar, K. X., Stanley, A. M., Gabelli, S. B., Denney, D. W., and Leahy, D. J. (2003). Structure of the extracellular region of HER2 alone and in complex with the Herceptin Fab. *Nature* 421, 756-760.

Churchman, L. S., Okten, Z., Rock, R. S., Dawson, J. F., and Spudich, J. A. (2005). Single molecule high-resolution colocalization of Cy3 and Cy5 attached to macromolecules measures intramolecular distances through time. *Proceedings of the National Academy of Sciences of the United States of America* 102, 1419-1423.

Citri, A., Skaria, K. B., and Yarden, Y. (2003). The deaf and the dumb: the biology of ErbB-2 and ErbB-3. *Exp Cell Res* 284, 54-65.

Citri, A., and Yarden, Y. (2006). EGF-ERBB signalling: towards the systems level. *Nature Reviews Molecular Cell Biology* 7, 505-516.

Clarke, D.T., Botchway, S. W., Needham S. R., Roberts, S. K., Rolfe, D. J., Tynan, C. J., Ward, A. D., Webb, S.E.W., Yadav, R., Zanetti-Domingues, L. and Martin-Fernandez, M.L. (2011). Octopus: A multi-laser facility for combined single molecule and ensemble microscopy. *Rev. Sci. Ins.* (In press).

Clayton, A. H., Walker, F., Orchard, S. G., Henderson, C., Fuchs, D., Rothacker, J., Nice, E. C., and Burgess, A. W. (2005). Ligand-induced dimer-tetramer transition during the activation of the cell surface epidermal growth factor receptor-A multidimensional microscopy analysis. *J Biol Chem* 280, 30392-9.

Clayton, A. H. A., Orchard, S. G., Nice, E. C., Posner, R. G., and Burgess, A. W. (2008). Predominance of activated EGFR higher-order oligomers on the cell surface. *Growth Factors* 26, 316-324.

Costa, M. N., Radhakrishnan, K., and Edwards, J. S. (2011). Monte Carlo simulations of plasma membrane corral-induced EGFR clustering. *Journal of biotechnology* 151, 261-70.

Dahan, M., Levi, S., Luccardini, C., Rostaing, P., Riveau, B., and Triller, A. (2003). Diffusion dynamics of glycine receptors revealed by single-quantum dot tracking. *Science* 302, 442-445.

Defize, L. H. K., Boonstra, J., Meisenhelder, J., Kruijer, W., Tertoolen, L. G. J., Tilly, B. C., Hunter, T., Henegouwen, P., Moolenaar, W. H., and Delaat, S. W. (1989). Signal Transduction By Epidermal Growth-Factor Occurs Through The Subclass Of High-Affinity Receptors. *Journal of Cell Biology* 109, 2495-2507.

Downward, J., Parker, P., and Waterfield, M. D. (1984). Autophosphorylation Sites On The Epidermal Growth-Factor Receptor. *Nature* 311, 483-485.

Dunn, R. C. (1999). Near-field scanning optical microscopy. *Chemical Reviews* 99, 2891-2927.

Edwards, D. R., Handsley, M. M., and Pennington, C. J. (2008). The ADAM metalloproteinases. *Molecular Aspects of Medicine* 29, 258-289.

El-Sibai, M., Nalbant, P., Pang, H., Flinn, R. J., Sarmiento, C., Macaluso, F., Cammer, M., Condeelis, J. S., Hahn, K. M., and Backer, J. M. (2007). Cdc42 is required for EGF-stimulated protrusion and motility in MTLn3 carcinoma cells. *Journal of cell science* 120, 3465-3474.

Feng, Q. Y., Baird, D., Peng, X., Wang, J. B., Ly, T., Guan, J. L., and Cerione, R. A. (2006). Cool-1 functions as an essential regulatory node for EGF receptor-and Src-mediated cell growth. *Nature cell biology* 8, 945-956.

Ferguson, K. M., Berger, M. B., Mendrola, J. M., Cho, H. S., Leahy, D. J., and Lemmon, M. A. (2003). EGF activates its receptor by removing interactions that autoinhibit ectodomain dimerization. *Molecular cell* 11, 507-17.

Friedman, B. A., Frackelton, A. R., Ross, A. H., Connors, J. M., Fujiki, H., Sugimura, T., and Rosner, M. R. (1984). Tumor Promoters Block Tyrosine-Specific Phosphorylation Of The Epidermal Growth-Factor Receptor. *Proceedings of the National Academy of Sciences of the United States of America-Biological Sciences* 81, 3034-3038.

Fujiwara, T., Ritchie, K., Murakoshi, H., Jacobson, K., and Kusumi, A. (2002). Phospholipids undergo hop diffusion in compartmentalized cell membrane. *Journal of Cell Biology* 157, 1071-1081.

Gadella, T. W., Jr., and Jovin, T. M. (1995). Oligomerization of epidermal growth factor receptors on A431 cells studied by time-resolved fluorescence imaging microscopy. A stereochemical model for tyrosine kinase receptor activation. *The Journal of cell biology* 129, 1543-58.

Garrett, T. P., McKern, N. M., Lou, M., Elleman, T. C., Adams, T. E., Lovrecz, G. O., Zhu, H. J., Walker, F., Frenkel, M. J., Hoyne, P. A., Jorissen, R. N., Nice, E. C., Burgess, A. W., and Ward, C. W. (2002). Crystal structure of a truncated epidermal growth factor receptor extracellular domain bound to transforming growth factor alpha. *Cell* 110, 763-73.

Grandis, J. R., Drenning, S. D., Chakraborty, A., Zhou, M. Y., Zeng, Q., and Tweardy, D. J. (1998). Requirement of Stat3 but not Stat1 activation for epidermal growth factor receptor-mediated cell growth in vitro. *Journal of Clinical Investigation* 102, 1385-1392.

GrausPorta, D., Beerli, R. R., Daly, J. M., and Hynes, N. E. (1997). ErbB-2, the preferred heterodimerization partner of all ErbB receptors, is a mediator of lateral signaling. *Embo Journal* 16, 1647-1655.

Hell, S. W. (2003). Toward fluorescence nanoscopy. *Nat. Biotechnol.* 21, 1347-55.

Hillier, J., and Hoffman, J. F. (1953). On The Ultrastructure Of The Plasma Membrane As Determined By The Electron Microscope. *Journal of Cellular and Comparative Physiology* 42, 203-247.

Humphrey, W., Dalke, A. and Schulten, K. (1996). VMD: Visual molecular dynamics. *J. Mol. Graphics.* 14, 33-38.

Hynes, N. E., and Lane, H. A. (2005). ERBB receptors and cancer: the complexity of targeted inhibitors. *Nature reviews. Cancer* 5, 341-54.

Hyun-Soo, C., and Leahy, D. J. (2002). Structure of the extracellular region of HER3 reveals an interdomain tether. *Science* 297, 1330-1333.

Jeffrey, P. D., Ruso, A. A., Polyak, K., Gibbs, E., Hurwitz, J., Massague, J., and Pavletich, N. P. (1995). Mechanism Of CDK Activation Revealed By The Structure Of A Cyclina-CDK2 Complex. *Nature* 376, 313-320.

Jones, R. B., Gordus, A., Krall, J. A., and MacBeath, G. (2006). A quantitative protein interaction network for the ErbB receptors using protein microarrays. *Nature* 439, 168-174.

Jura, N., Endres, N. F., Engel, K., Deindl, S., Das, R., Lamers, M. H., Wemmer, D. E., Zhang, X. W., and Kuriyan, J. (2009a). Mechanism for Activation of the EGF Receptor Catalytic Domain by the Juxtamembrane Segment. *Cell* 137, 1293-1307.

Jura, N., Shan, Y., Cao, X., Shaw, D. E., and Kuriyan, J. (2009b). Structural analysis of the catalytically inactive kinase domain of the human EGF receptor 3. *Proceedings of the National Academy of Sciences of the United States of America* 106, 21608-13.

Kastner, J., Loeffler, H. H., Roberts, S. K., Martin-Fernandez, M. L., and Winn, M. D. (2009). Ectodomain orientation, conformational plasticity and oligomerization of ErbB1 receptors investigated by molecular dynamics. *Journal of structural biology* 167, 117-28.

Katan, M. (1998). Families of phosphoinositide-specific phospholipase C: structure and function. *Biochimica Et Biophysica Acta-Molecular and Cell Biology of Lipids* 1436, 5-17.

Kurokawa, K., Itoh, R. E., Yoshizaki, H., Ohba, Y., Nakamura, T., and Matsuda, M. (2004). Coactivation of Rad1 and Cdc42 at lamellipodia and membrane ruffles induced by epidermal growth factor. *Molecular Biology of the Cell* 15, 1003-1010.

Kusumi, A., Ike, H., Nakada, C., Murase, K., and Fujiwara, T. (2005). Single-molecule tracking of membrane molecules: plasma membrane compartmentalization and dynamic assembly of raft-philic signaling molecules. *Semin Immunol* 17, 3-21.

Lehto, M. T., and Sharom, F. J. (2002). Proximity of the protein moiety of a GPI-anchored protein to the membrane surface: A FRET study. *Biochemistry* 41, 8368-8376.

Lynch TJ, Bell DW, Sordella R, Gurubhagavatula S, Okimoto RA, Brannigan BW, Harris PL, Haserlat SM, Supko JG, Haluska FG, Louis DN, Christiani DC, Settleman J, Haber DA. (2004). Activating mutations in the epidermal growth factor receptor underlying responsiveness of non-small-cell lung cancer to Gefitinib. *N. Eng. J. Med.* 350:2129-39.

Macdonald, J. L., and Pike, L. J. (2008). Heterogeneity in EGF-binding affinities arises from negative cooperativity in an aggregating system. *Proceedings of the National Academy of Sciences of the United States of America* 105, 112-117.

Magun, B. E., Matrisian, L. M., and Bowden, G. T. (1980). Epidermal Growth-Factor - Ability Of Tumor Promoter To Alter Its Degradation, Receptor Affinity And Receptor Number. *Journal of Biological Chemistry* 255, 6373-6381.

Martin-Fernandez, M., Clarke, D. T., Tobin, M. J., Jones, S. V., and Jones, G. R. (2002). Preformed oligomeric epidermal growth factor receptors undergo an ectodomain structure change during signaling. *Biophysical journal* 82, 2415-27.

Mattoon, D., Klein, P., Lemmon, M. A., Lax, I., and Schlessinger, J. (2004). The tethered configuration of the EGF receptor extracellular domain exerts only a limited control of receptor function. *Proceedings of the National Academy of Sciences of the United States of America* 101, 923-928.

Monici, M. (2005). *Cell and tissue autofluorescence research and diagnostic applications*.

Nagy, P., Vereb, G., Sebestyen, Z., Horvath, G., Lockett, S. J., Damjanovich, S., Park, J. W., Jovin, T. M., and Szollosi, J. (2002). Lipid rafts and the local density of ErbB proteins influence the biological role of homo- and heteroassociations of ErbB2. *Journal of cell science* 115, 4251-4262.

Nordberg, E., Ekerljung, L., Sahlberg, S. H., Carlsson, J., Lennartsson, J., and Glimelius, B. (2010). Effects of an EGFR-binding affibody molecule on intracellular signaling pathways. *International Journal of Oncology* 36, 967-972.

Oda, K., Matsuoka, Y., Funahashi, A., and Kitano, H. (2005). A comprehensive pathway map of epidermal growth factor receptor signaling. *Molecular systems biology* 1,

Ogiso, H., Ishitani, R., Nureki, O., Fukai, S., Yamanaka, M., Kim, J. H., Saito, K., Sakamoto, A., Inoue, M., Shirouzu, M., and Yokoyama, S. (2002). Crystal structure of the complex of human epidermal growth factor and receptor extracellular domains. *Cell* 110, 775-87.

Ohgaki, H., Dessen, P., Jourde, B., Horstmann, S., Nishikawa, T., Di Patre, P. L., Burkhard, C., Schuler, D., Probst-Hensch, N. M., Maiorka, P. C., Baeza, N., Pisani, P., Yonekawa, Y., Yasargil, M. G., Lutolf, U. M., and Kleihues, P. (2004). Genetic pathways to glioblastoma: A population-based study. *Cancer research* 64, 6892-6899.

Olayioye, M. A., Neve, R. M., Lane, H. A., and Hynes, N. E. (2000). The ErbB signaling network: receptor heterodimerization in development and cancer. *Embo Journal* 19, 3159-3167.

Paez, J. G., Janne, P. A., Lee, J. C., Tracy, S., Greulich, H., Gabriel, S., Herman, P., Kaye, F. J., Lindeman, N., Boggon, T. J., Naoki, K., Sasaki, H., Fujii, Y., Eck, M. J., Sellers, W. R.,

Johnson, B. E., and Meyerson, M. (2004). EGFR mutations in lung cancer: Correlation with clinical response to gefitinib therapy. *Science* 304, 1497-1500.

Pai, R., and Tarnawski, A. (1998). Signal transduction cascades triggered by EGF receptor activation - Relevance to gastric injury repair and ulcer healing. *Digestive Diseases and Sciences* 43, 14S-22S.

Pawson, T. (2004). Specificity in signal transduction: from phosphotyrosine-SH2 domain interactions to complex cellular systems. *Cell* 116, 191-203.

Qu, X. H., Wu, D., Mets, L., and Scherer, N. F. (2004). Nanometer-localized multiple single-molecule fluorescence microscopy. *Proceedings of the National Academy of Sciences of the United States of America* 101, 11298-11303.

Ridley, A. J. (2001). Rho family proteins: coordinating cell responses. *Trends in cell biology* 11, 471-477.

Riese, D. J., and Stern, D. F. (1998). Specificity within the EGF family ErbB receptor family signaling network. *Bioessays* 20, 41-48.

Rolfe. D. J., McLachlan, C. I., Hirsch, M., Needham, S. R., Tynan C. J., Webb, S. E. D., Martin-Fernandez, M. L., and Hobson M. P. (2011). *Eur. Biophys. J.* (In press)

Sako, Y., Minoghchi, S., and Yanagida, T. (2000). Single-molecule imaging of EGFR signalling on the surface of living cells. *Nature cell biology* 2, 168-72.

Scheuring, S., and Sturgis, J. N. (2005). Chromatic adaptation of photosynthetic membranes. *Science* 309, 484-487.

Schlessinger, J. (2000). Cell signaling by receptor tyrosine kinases. *Cell* 103, 211-25.

Schoeberl, B., Eichler-Jonsson, C., Gilles, E. D., and Muller, G. (2002). Computational modeling of the dynamics of the MAP kinase cascade activated by surface and internalized EGF receptors. *Nature biotechnology* 20, 370-375.

Schulze, W. X., Deng, L., and Mann, M. (2005a). Phosphotyrosine interactome of the ErbB-receptor kinase family. *Molecular systems biology* 1, 2005 0008.

Schulze, W. X., Deng, L., and Mann, M. (2005b). Phosphotyrosine interactome of the ErbB-receptor kinase family. *Molecular systems biology* 1,

Sharma, S. V., Bell, D. W., Settleman, J., and Haber, D. A. (2007). Epidermal growth factor receptor mutations in lung cancer. *Nature reviews. Cancer* 7, 169-81.

Shoyab, M., Delarco, J. E., and Todaro, G. J. (1979). Biologically-Active Phorbol Esters Specifically Alter Affinity Of Epidermal Growth-Factor Membrane-Receptors. *Nature* 279, 387-391.

Singer, S. J., and Nicolson, G. L. (1972). Fluid Mosaic Model Of Structure Of Cell-Membranes. *Science* 175, 720-&.

Sorkin, A. (2001). Internalization of the epidermal growth factor receptor: role in signalling. *Biochemical Society transactions* 29, 480-484.

Stryer, L., and Haugland, R. P. (1967). Energy transfer: a spectroscopic ruler. *Proceedings of the National Academy of Sciences of the United States of America* 58, 719-26.

Sunpaweravong, P., Sunpaweravong, S., Puttawibul, P., Mitarnun, W., Zeng, C., Baron, A. E., Franklin, W., Said, S., and Varella-Garcia, M. (2005). Epidermal growth factor receptor and cyclin D1 are independently amplified and overexpressed in esophageal squamous cell carcinoma. *Journal of Cancer Research and Clinical Oncology* 131, 111-119.

Thien, C. B. F., and Langdon, W. Y. (2005). c-Cbl and Cbl-b ubiquitin ligases: substrate diversity and the negative regulation of signalling responses. *Biochemical Journal* 391, 153-166.

Tran, T., Engfeldt, T., Orlova, A., Sandstrom, M., Feldwisch, J., Abrahmsen, L., Wennborg, A., Tolmachev, V., and Karlstrom, A. E. (2007). Tc-99m-maEEE-Z(HER2 : 342), an affibody molecule-based tracer for the detection of HER2 expression in malignant tumors. *Bioconjugate Chemistry* 18, 1956-1964.

Tynan, C. J., Roberts, S. K., Rolfe, D. J., Clarke, D. T., Loeffler, H. H., Kastner, J., Winn, M. D., Parker, P. J., and Martin-Fernandez, M. L. (2011). Human-EGFR aligned on the plasma membrane adopts key features of Drosophila-EGFR asymmetry. *Molecular and cellular biology* 31, 2241-2252.

Ullrich, A., Coussens, L., Hayflick, J. S., Dull, T. J., Gray, A., Tam, A. W., Lee, J., Yarden, Y., Libermann, T. A., Schlessinger, J., and et al. (1984). Human epidermal growth factor receptor cDNA sequence and aberrant expression of the amplified gene in A431 epidermoid carcinoma cells. *Nature* 309, 418-25.

Ullrich, A., and Schlessinger, J. (1990). Signal transduction by receptors with tyrosine kinase activity. *Cell* 61, 203-12.

van Meer, G. (2005). Cellular lipidomics. *Embo Journal* 24, 3159-3165.

Vanhaesebroeck, B., Leevers, S. J., Ahmadi, K., Timms, J., Katso, R., Driscoll, P. C., Woscholski, R., Parker, P. J., and Waterfield, M. D. (2001). Synthesis and function of 3-phosphorylated inositol lipids. *Annual review of biochemistry* 70, 535-602.

Vrielink, A., and Sampson, N. (2003). Sub-Angstrom resolution enzyme X-ray structures: is seeing believing? *Current Opinion in Structural Biology* 13, 709-715.

Webb, S. E., Roberts, S. K., Needham, S. R., Tynan, C. J., Rolfe, D. J., Winn, M. D., Clarke, D. T., Barraclough, R., and Martin-Fernandez, M. L. (2008). Single-molecule imaging and fluorescence lifetime imaging microscopy show different structures for high- and low-affinity epidermal growth factor receptors in A431 cells. *Biophysical journal* 94, 803-19.

Wolber, P. K., and Hudson, B. S. (1979). Analytic Solution To The Forster Energy-Transfer Problem In 2 Dimensions. *Biophysical journal* 28, 197-210.

Yarden, Y., and Sliwkowski, M. X. (2001). Untangling the ErbB signalling network. *Nature reviews. Molecular cell biology* 2, 127-37.

Yildiz, A., and Selvin, P. R. (2005). Fluorescence imaging with one nanometer accuracy: application to molecular motors. *Accounts of chemical research* 38, 574-82.

Yu, D., and Hung, M. C. (2000). Overexpression of ErbB2 in cancer and ErbB2-targeting strategies. *Oncogene* 19, 6115-21.

Zhang, W., and Liu, H. T. (2002). MAPK signal pathways in the regulation of cell proliferation in mammalian cells. *Cell Research* 12, 9-18.

Zhang, X., Gureasko, J., Shen, K., Cole, P. A., and Kuriyan, J. (2006). An allosteric mechanism for activation of the kinase domain of epidermal growth factor receptor. *Cell* 125, 1137-49.

Zhou, B. B. S., Fridman, J. S., Liu, X. D., Friedman, S. M., Newton, R. C., and Scherle, P. A. (2005). ADAM proteases, ErbB pathways and cancer. *Expert Opinion on Investigational Drugs* 14, 591-606.

5

Nucleic Acid Aptamers for *In Vivo* Molecular Imaging

Vittorio de Franciscis[1], Anna Rienzo[2] and Laura Cerchia[1]
[1]*Istituto per l'Endocrinologia e l'Oncologia Sperimentale del CNR "G. Salvatore", Naples,*
[2]*School of Physics and Astronomy, University of Nottingham,*
[1]*Italy*
[2]*UK*

1. Introduction

New drug compounds discovery has moved at an accelerated pace in recent years, with a considerable focus on the transition from *in vitro* to *in vivo* models. As a result, there has been a significant increase in the need to adapt and develop novel non-invasive, high resolution *in vivo* imaging approaches for studying disease development and quantitatively determining molecular and cellular events in vivo. Non-invasive imaging methods allow continuous monitoring of disease development *in vivo*. For example, real time spatial-temporal analysis of tumour growth can reveal the dynamics of cancer progression. Furthermore, the effects of therapy can be evaluated non-invasively *in vivo*. These approaches offer the ability to perform repetitive observations and interventions of the biological processes underlying disease development and progression.

Thus, the development of imaging agents with high sensitivity, high specificity, and low toxicity is necessary to obtain biochemical functional information for the early characterization of the molecular alterations and, in turn, to improve diagnosis and therapy for clinical applications.

Despite significant progress in developing rapid and accurate *ex-vivo* medical diagnostic tests, it is still essential to investigate approaches for *in vivo* non-invasive imaging because many human diseases and the outcomes of therapy not always and not easily can be determined by the analysis of blood samples or biopsies. For instance, whether a tumor shrinks during cancer therapy has to be determined by bioimaging modalities. In addition, non-invasive imaging techniques enable the examination of cellular and biomolecular events in locations that are difficult to access by any other means.

Thus, the development of imaging agents with high sensitivity, high specificity, and low toxicity is necessary to improve diagnosis and therapy for clinical applications.

In this perspective an emerging attractive class of targeting molecules is represented by short single-stranded oligonucleotides ligands, named aptamers, being able to bind with high affinity to specific protein or non-protein targets by folding into complex tertiary structures. They discriminate between closely related targets and are characterised by high specificity and low toxicity thus representing a valid alternative to antibodies for *in vivo* cell recognition. Owing to their relatively small size in comparison to antibodies, aptamers should be better-suited for rapid target tissue penetration and blood clearance. In addition, different from antibodies, aptamers are chemically synthesized at low cost with high batch fidelity, are sufficiently stable and can be readily chemically modified to further enhance their stability, bioavailability and pharmacokinetics. Moreover, aptamer immunogenicity has never been reported. These properties indicate a great potential of aptamers as imaging agents, especially when compared to antibodies.

The present chapter will be dedicated to aptamer-based molecular imaging modalities by reviewing the recent application of aptamers as ligands for inflammation imaging, thrombus imaging and tumour imaging.

2. *In vivo* non-invasive imaging

The functional imaging techniques developed in the past decades have given raised to powerful biomedical imaging tools that permit repeated non-invasive assessment and quantification of specific biological and pharmacological processes at the molecular level in human and animal (Lyons, 2005).

By employing medical image modalities one can assess the physiological activities within a certain tissue or organ choosing among the imaging platforms available: positron-emission tomography (PET), single photon emission computed tomography (SPECT), nuclear magnetic resonance imaging (NMRI), optical imaging (OI) and computed tomography (CT).

2.1 The emission tomography

The emission tomography is based on the decay process of a specific radioactive element to detect the isotope distribution within the body as function of the time. The radionuclide concentration changes with time as consequence of the decay events as well as for the biochemical processes kinetics. Moreover the concentrations of tracer imaged the given tissue metabolic activity, in terms of the specific molecules of interest uptake (Massoud et al. 2003). Differently from radio-diagnostics methods, more directed towards a morphologic analysis, emission tomography hold an essential rule in field of diagnostic and functional analysis (heart attack, epilepsy, cardiopathy, Parkinson disease).

The compound tracer-ligand, which is of interest for its chemical binding properties to certain types of tissues, is injected into the body and depending on the nature of the radionuclide the decay product can be a photon (SPECT) or a positron (PET).

The radioactivity profiles obtained are processed by an electronic calculator by means of appropriate reconstruction algorithms for the reconstruction of the tomographic image of the studied section.

SPECT imaging is a quite new survey technique by which it is possible to reconstruct scintigraphic images related to the spatial and temporal distribution of a radioactive substance. SPECT equipment consists of one or more rotational gamma chambers which detect gamma rays, in the energy range between 80 KeV and 300 KeV, emitted from gamma-emitting radioisotopes (^{99m}Tc, ^{111}I, ^{123}I, ^{131}I, ^{125}I), previously injected into the patient. The use of targeted radiolabeled ligands to determine the tissue distributions of receptors allows the detection of disease upon imaging with a gamma-camera. Multiple 2D image projection can be acquired at different angles resulting in the visualization of the 3D biodistribution of the radionuclides. The spatial resolution of the reconstructed image depends on the number of angular and linear samples selected besides on the collimator and the tomographic reconstruction parameters.

PET is the most extensively used technique in the field of clinical oncology, neurology and cardiology (Cantore et al., 2011). In the same way of SPECT, this technique is based on the use of radio labelled compounds which are injected into the living subject (usually into blood circulation). Especially useful to assess the degree of changes in the cellular metabolism as well as in their anatomic structure and in the dimension of the tumor mass, it plays a fundamental role in the screening, early detection, diagnosis and treatment of neoplasms (Langen et al., 2011). This powerful technique supplies the most advanced and outstanding tools on monitoring the early results of a tumor treatment plan giving the evidence on the success of the treatment itself and so avoiding useless chemotherapy cycles.

Radionuclides used in PET scanning, typically isotopes with short half-lives (^{11}C, ^{13}N, ^{15}O , ^{18}F) which undergo positron emission decay, are incorporated either into compounds normally used by the body such as, glucose, water, ammonia, or into molecules that bind to receptors. PET apparatus is made up of a detector block (scintillator crystal and photomultiplier) and a detectors ring which detects the two 511 keV gamma photons emitted in coincidence at 180 degrees to each other further to positron-electron annihilation events. By this means it is possible to localize their source along a straight line of coincidence. Following the radiotracers journey inside the body or the organs it is possible to trace its biological pathway and collect data for analysis. During the scan a record of tissue concentration is made as the tracer decays. The radiological image obtained is a fingerprint of the functionality of the examined organs. Even though PET and SPECT are similar there are remarkable differences in terms of efficiency and resolution. Due to the detection methodology, since emissions are detected "coincident" in time, PET scanner provides more radiation events and localization information, thus giving higher resolution images than SPECT, about 4-5mm against 7-8mm. In terms of efficiency only 1 to 10 photons upon 10.000 emitted can be detected with SPECT while PET efficiency is about 100 times higher (pmoles vs nanomoles).

Small animals SPECT can provide resolutions up to 200 micrometer (Acton & Kung, 2003). Sensitivity, resolution, and field of view are dependent upon the pinhole collimator of the instrument. On the other end small animals PET scanner can provide lower spatial resolution (0.6 mm). PET is best suited for small molecules and molecules with fast kinetics. Moreover PET tracers have lower specific activity, shorter half-lives and are more difficult to synthesize. Finally PET radiation dose is 10 fold higher than SPECT (Larobina et al., 2006).

2.2 Nuclear magnetic resonance imaging

NMRI is a medical imaging technique based on nuclear magnetic resonance to image nuclei of atoms inside the body and is able to distinguish pathologic tissue from normal tissue (Schellenberger, 2004). This technique is widely used in radiology as it provides good contrast between the different soft tissues of the body in addition to a high images quality. Based on the use of strong magnetic fields and non-ionizing radiation, radio frequency range, NMRI is completely harmless to the patient.

Differences of nuclei behavior subject to a strong magnetic field gradient can be recorded to construct an image of the scanned area of the body resulting in the visualization of detailed internal structures. In the classical representation of an atom nucleus is depicted as a rotational sphere along an axis. This rotational motion is associated with a physical quantity called: angular momentum (spin). Because of the nuclear composition the so called rotational sphere is positively charged resulting in the generation of a magnetic field as a consequence of charge motion. By this means nuclei possess an intrinsic angular momentum (spin) associated to a magnetic momentum. The spin of a charged particle is associated with a magnetic dipole momentum by a proportional factor called gyromagnetic factor. The g-factor is a characteristic of each nucleus. Allowed values of spin are 0, 1/2, 1, 3/2, 2, etc., which corresponds to certain magnetic momentum values according to a specific proportional relationship. The sensitivity by which a nucleus can be detected with NMR depends on the g-factor. Nuclei with a high gyromagnetic ratio will be easily examined. Nuclei with spin value equal to zero, null magnetic momentum, are "transparent" to external magnetic field so they can not be analyzed with NMR. Therefore only atoms with an odd number of nucleons (protons and/or neutrons) resulting in a nonzero nuclear spin can be chosen for this methodic. In the presence of a magnetic field sample nuclear spins, randomly arranged, will align along the external field lines (polarization), absorbing and re-emitting electromagnetic radiation at a specific resonance frequency which depends on the strength of the magnetic field and on the magnetic properties of the sample atoms. For a set value of magnetic field applied, different nuclei give rise to distinct resonant frequencies depending on the strength of applied field. If a sample is placed in a non-uniform magnetic field then the resonance frequencies of the sample's nuclei depend on where in the field they are located. In the NMRI techniques the polarization of the magnetic nuclear spins is achieved by exposing the sample to a constant static magnetic field. The following step is the perturbation of this alignment by employing an electro-magnetic, usually radio frequency (RF), pulse. The required perturbing frequency is dependent upon the static magnetic field and the nuclei of observation. When the RF pulse is turned off nuclear spins at different locations relaxes to the equilibrium state with consequent emission of characteristic frequencies detectable by the scanner. The electromagnetic signals shifts induced by strong field gradients are recorded to construct tridimensional images of studied area. To maximize the NMR signal strength the two fields are usually chosen to be perpendicular to each other.

NMRI uses intense applied magnetic fields in order to achieve dispersion and very high stability to deliver spectral resolution. The spatial resolution of the imaging technique depends on the magnitude of magnetic field gradient. Very high resolution images, on the order of one tenth of millimeter, can be achieved with a 3 Tesla scanners.

For mouse MRI imaging can achieve 10-100 micrometer spatial resolution, with preferably at least 7.0 Tesla. To enhance the appearance of blood vessels, tumors or inflammation, contrast agents, properly modified, may be injected intravenously acting as specific molecular probe. This opens the possibility to monitor *in vivo* cellular functions as well as get information on the spatial distribution of a specific molecular target (Percy et al., 2011).

The employment of stable isotopes as contrast agents, diversely from PET methodology, gives to this technique the great advantage of supervising metabolic pathways or receptors dynamic for infinite time.

2.3 Optical Imaging

This non-ionizing imaging technique is based on the use of electromagnetic radiation in the near-infrared and visible field to observe single-molecule in living cells. Cost-effective, rapid, easy to use, optical imaging can be readily applied to studying disease processes and biology *in vivo* (Luker & Luker, 2008). A charge-coupled device camera (CCD camera) detects light emitted allowing for real time 2D imaging and 3D reconstruction. The key feature is the different behavior of light interaction with tissues such as adsorption, emission, excitation, scattering, fluorescence and luminescence.

Molecular targets labeled with nanodiamonds, fluorescent dyes, quantum dots, as well as bioluminescent, chemiluminescent and fluorescent reporters, would enable biomolecule tracking inside cells (Rong Tong et al., 2010). Fluorescently labeled antibodies or biomarkers can target and identify tumors or other diseases in *in vivo* modalities (van der Meel et al., 2010). Molecular and biochemical events such as transgene expression, transforming phenotype and enzyme activity can be detected by means of fluorescent probes. Tumor cells, stem cells, immunological cells can be transfected to overexpress luminescent or fluorescent proteins (Pomper, 2005). Widely used in animal models trial for low costs and good sensitivity (pmol concentrations, few cells), optical labeling technology scanner has an anatomical resolution relatively poor (1mm) due to scattering of light in tissue (Hickson, 2009). OI has a minimal use in clinic owing to limited depth profiling (couple of centimeters in tissue depth) (Leblond et al., 2010).

2.4 Computed tomography

X-ray computed tomography (CT) is a radiological technique which provides high spatial resolution (less than 1 mm) of morphological imaging; three-dimensional anatomical images. Axial sections of well-defined depth are imaged upon differential x-ray absorption by different tissues. CT is based on detection of an X-ray beam by means of detectors system which converts the attenuated beam intensity into electric pulse of equivalent value.

By interaction with electrons of the material probed, photons are removed from the incident beam. The total energy of the resulting beam is then attenuated. The higher the electron density, the more interaction of X-ray with the sample material occurs and the more attenuated is the final energy. Because of the inherent high-contrast resolution of CT, differences between tissues that differ in physical density by less than 1% can be distinguished. The CT methodology is widely use in medicine as a diagnostic tool: detailed studies of bone and joint structure, bone metastasis scans, measurement of tumor size and location, and visualization of airway structure in the lungs, can be assess with high resolution. The major drawback of the technology is the high radiation dose which can be lethal or mutagenic. For imaging systems dedicated to *in vivo* studies in animal models, the optimal resolution is 50–100 micrometer. Specimen instruments have resolutions down to less than 10 micrometer and can visualize e.g. trabecular bone structure.

3. Aptamers as excellent targeting molecules for *in vivo* imaging

Aptamers are single-stranded oligonucleotides (DNA or RNA) that like peptides or monoclonal antibodies, bind to their targets by complementary shape interactions. Indeed, aptamers function by folding into unique globular three-dimensional conformation that dictates high-affinity and specificity binding to a variety of targets, each structure being unique and determined by the sequence of the nucleic acid (Figure 1 A). As discussed in this chapter, the advantages of using nucleic acid aptamers for imaging/therapy are their favourable pharmacokinetic properties (rapid renal clearance) and their excellent affinity and specificity for their targets. These properties render aptamers useful targeting molecules for *in vivo* imaging allow obtaining high-resolution images with high signal-to-noise ratios and decreasing non-specific targeting thus reducing toxicity to non-target tissues (Tavitian et al., 1998, 2009; Perkins & Missailidis, 2007).

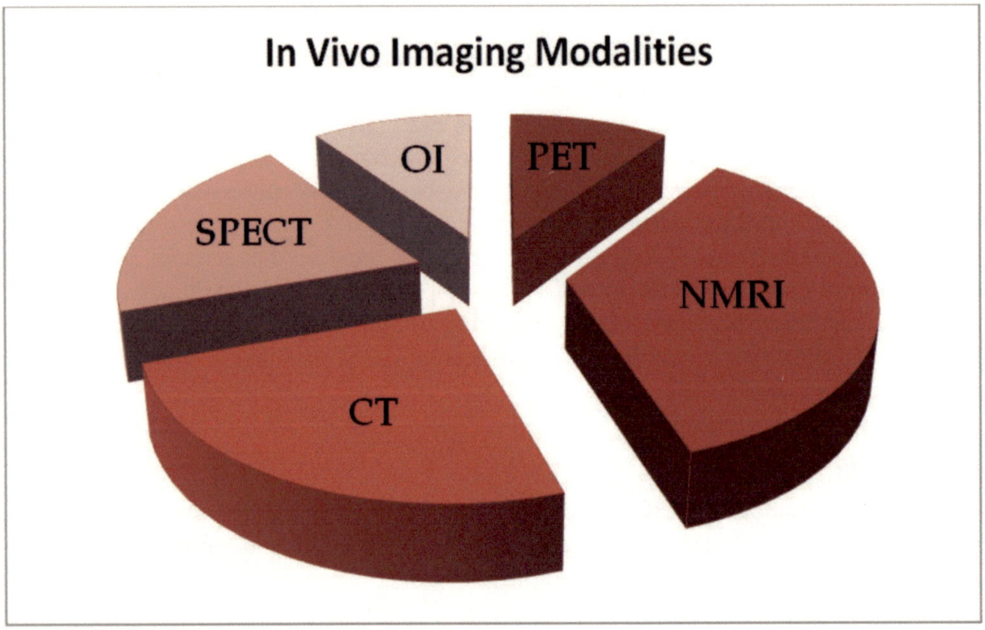

Fig. 1. The size of each slice is related to the resolution of the indicated technique; the colour scale is proportional to the cost (clockwise).

3.1 Aptamers production

Aptamers are generated by an *in vitro* evolutionary selection-amplification scheme, named SELEX (Systematic Evolution of Ligands by EXponential enrichment) from libraries of random sequence oligonucleotides of large sequence complexity (generally between 10^{13} and 10^{15} members) (Ellington & Szostak, 1990; Tuerk & Gold, 1990). As schematized in Figure 1 B, a typical SELEX experiment includes reiterated rounds of: (1) incubating the library with the target molecule; (2) partitioning nucleic acids bound specifically to the target molecule from unbound sequences; (3) dissociating the nucleic acid-protein complexes; and (4) amplifying of the nucleic acids pool enriched for specific ligands. After the final round, the PCR products are cloned and sequenced to subsequently identify the best binding sequences. Due to the fact that the specific, three-dimensional arrangements of a small number of contact points of the aptamer mediates the target-aptamer interaction, rather than a general affinity for the sugar-phosphate backbone of the nucleic acid, aptamers can achieve high target selectivity. In addition, the binding characteristics of aptamers can be influenced by the type of the experimental system used for the selection and counter-selection (depletion of aptamers that bind to non-target molecules). As a result, aptamers bind their own target with sub-nanomolar affinity thus revealing useful for many of the applications for which antibodies are already employed because of their own definite characteristics: (i) capacity to discriminate among closely related targets (e.g., will typically not bind other proteins from the same gene family); (ii) capacity to quantify the level of expression of the protein target; (iii) through binding, may act as inhibitors to block the activity of the target product. More important, they are usable not only for *in vitro* but also for *in vivo* purposes since they are sufficiently stable and can be readily chemically modified to further enhance their stability, bioavailability and pharmacokinetics (Esposito et al., 2011; Keefe et al., 2008, 2010).

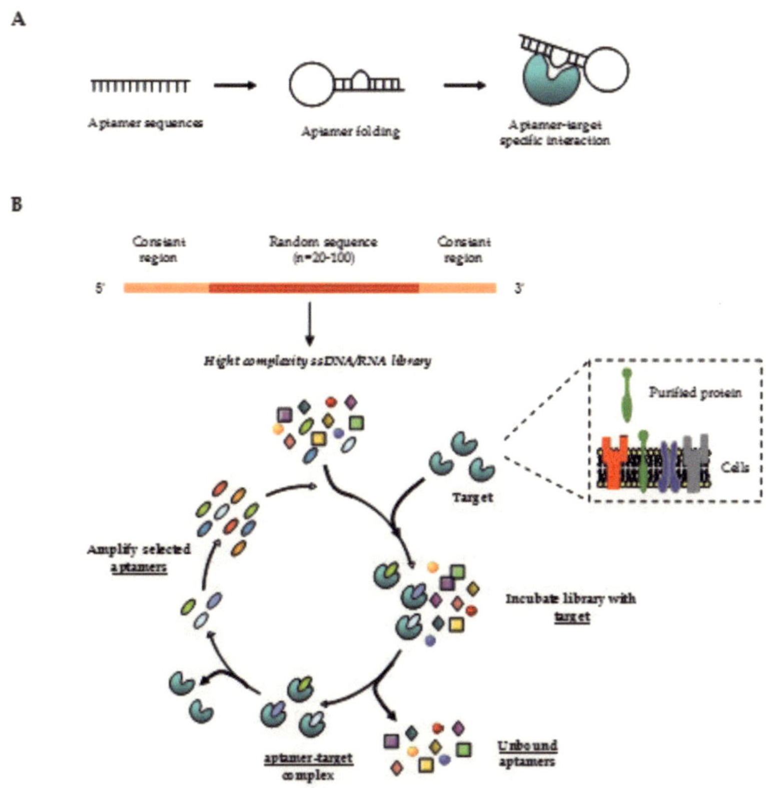

Fig. 2. Schematic representation of SELEX technology. The RNA/DNA aptamer library contains a variable region flanked by two constant regions. These constant regions include primer sites for PCR amplification and a consensus promoter for the T7-RNA polymerase (in the case of an RNA library). The library is used for the selection process. The target can be a purified recombinant protein (Protein-SELEX) or a complex target as entire living cells (cell-SELEX)

3.2 Systemic clearance of the aptamers

Furthermore, due to their relatively small size (8-15 kDa) in comparison to antibodies (150 kDa), aptamers should be better suited for rapid tissue penetration and blood clearance, two excellent characteristics for contrast agents in imaging. Indeed, when antibodies bind their target, their slow clearance may necessitate waiting for days before a significant signal emerges from the background of excess unbound ligand. This of course often results in organ toxicity and, in addition, limits the usefulness of imaging technology in diagnosing acute conditions, and precludes the use of short-lived radionuclides.

On the contrary, aptamers not conjugated to polyethylene glycol (PEG) are cleared very quickly from blood circulation because of renal excretion and hepatobiliary clearance. A typical short, nuclease-resistant oligonucleotide administered intravenously exhibits an *in vivo* half-life of <10 min, unless filtration can be blocked by either facilitating rapid distribution out of the blood stream into tissues or by increasing the apparent molecular weight of the oligonucleotide above the effective size cut-off for the glomerulus. In addition, immunogenicity has been found to be either absent or limited when 1000-fold higher doses of an aptamer (than would be required clinically) were administered to monkeys (Foy et al., 2007).

This property depends on the fact that antibodies to synthetic oligonucleotides are not generally produced and, in addition, the innate immunity response against non-self RNAs does not hinder aptamer therapy because 2′-modified nucleotides abrogate Toll-like receptors responses (Yu et al., 2009).

3.3 Stability of the aptamers

Prerequisites for a successful *in vivo* application of aptamers as molecular target imaging agents are represented by high affinity and selectivity to their target as well by adequate stability against *in vivo* degradation. Since oligonucleotides, especially RNAs, are rapidly degraded by nucleases in whole organisms, resulting in a very short half-life in the blood, a variety of approaches have been addressed to increase the stability of natural nucleic acids in biological media (Keefe & Cload, 2008).

The most effective modifications to circumvent this limitation are the substitutions at the 2′-ribose of the pyrimidines that are mainly affected by serum nuclease degradation. Initially, attention is focused on 'post-SELEX modifications', however, due to the fact that folding rules for single-stranded oligonucleotide regions change when these modifications are introduced, the binding properties of an aptamer selected in the presence of standard nucleotides might be completely different when the same sequence is synthesized with nucleotides containing a different 2′-substituent (Blank et al., 2001; Usman & Blatt, 2000; Aurup et al., 1992). To circumvent this limitation selections can be performed directly in the presence of 2′-modified nucleotides, as long as the modified nucleotides are accepted by T7 RNA polymerase for the *in vitro* reaction steps of the selection (Aurup et al., 1992; Ruckman et al., 1998). RNA-aptamers containing 2′-fluoro and 2′-amino pyrimidine (2′-F-Py, 2′-NH2-Py, respectively) can be generated performing the selection in the presence of 2′-modified nucleotides (Chelliserrykattil et al., 2004).Analogously, aptamers containing 2′-O-Metyl purines (2′-O-Me) have also been developed through post-SELEX modification steps or by starting from 2′-O-Me-containing random sequence libraries during the SELEX process itself (Burmeister et al., 2004; Chelliserrykattil & Ellington, 2004).

Even if 2′-modified nucleotides-containing aptamers show considerable increase in serum stability also in the absence of other modifications, changes in the internucleotide linkages (such as the use of phosphorothioate) and in the nucleobases (for example, the substitution of 5-position of uridine) as well the capping at the oligonucleotide 3′-terminus, have been reported (Keefe & Cload, 2008).

Conformation flexibility is hypothesized to be a major factor limiting the affinity and specificity of interactions due to the entropic penalty upon binding. Furthermore, since single-stranded regions are the primary site of nuclease attack, the conformational flexibility would render the aptamer more accessible to nucleolytic degradation and thus, reduction of flexibility would be a key prerequisite for successful *in vivo* application. One way to stabilize aptamers is to increase thermal stability of double-stranded areas located within non-binding regions. In this respect, the use of locked nucleic acids (LNA), containing a methylene bridge to connect the 2′-O to the 4′-C, increases the stability of base pairing stabilizing the duplex and enhancing the resistance to nuclease. For example the introduction of LNA-modifications in the anti-tenascin C (TN-C) aptamer significantly improves its plasma stability of approximately 25% and enhances the tumor uptake (Schmidt et al., 2004).

An interesting application of the SELEX process is based on the selection of RNA aptamers binding to the mirror-image of an intended target molecule (e.g. an unnatural D-amino acid peptide), followed by the chemical synthesis of the mirror-image of the selected sequence (Eulberg & Klussmann, 2003). As a consequence of molecular symmetry, the mirror-image aptamer (made from L-ribose) binds to the natural target molecule. Because of the substitution of the natural D-ribose with L-ribose, the mirror-image aptamer (named Spiegelmer) is totally stable. NOX-A12 and NOX-E36 are two spiegelmers actually in clinical trials for the treatment of hematologic tumors and complications of type 2 diabetes, respectively (Esposito et al., 2011; Ellington, 2010).

4. Inflammation imaging with aptamers

The assessment of precise and reliable methods for the diagnosis of inflammatory processes is an important goal in medicine for the effective management of inflammation-related diseases. Acute inflammatory diseases are characterized by a significant increase in the lymphocytes and neutrophils count in the peripheral blood while chronic inflammatory diseases are characterized by infiltration of the target organ by mononuclear cells, such as lymphocytes, plasma cells, and macrophages (Weiss, 1989).

Some inflammatory processes, such as organ-specific autoimmune disorders, are difficult to diagnose because they either are asymptomatic or have non-specific symptoms. The possibility of diagnosing inflammatory processes during the early stage may allow for early therapeutic intervention and possible prevention of the disease.

During inflammation, levels of several proteolytic enzymes are significantly increased including neutrophil elastase that is released by neutrophils accumulated at the site of inflammation (Doring, 1994). Aptamers as specific irreversible inhibitors of neutrophil elastase have been isolated by 'blended SELEX', a modification of the basic SELEX technology that allows to confer high-affinity binding to a weak, covalent inhibitor of an enzyme (Smith et al., 1995; Charlton et al., 1997).

In this process, a randomized nucleic acid library attached covalently to an inhibitory compound of elastase (a valyl diphenyl ester phosphonate) was used to select for a secondary, stabilizing contact for the target molecule. By iterative selection and amplification steps, the nucleic acid sequences that best promote the covalent reaction of the valyl phosphonate moiety with the active-site serine of elastase were identified. In addition to inhibiting elastase free in solution, these aptamers were highly effective at blocking degradation of elastin particles by activated neutrophils. Further, a truncated DNA aptamer version, named NX21909, was tested in a rat model of lung inflammation and was found to inhibit neutrophil infiltration by 53% at a dose of 40 nmol (Bless et al., 1997). Using fluorescent flow cytometry, the aptamer revealed able to bind preferentially to activated neutrophils (Charlton et al., 1997).

The first example of the use of aptamers as *in vivo* imaging probes is represented by the use of NX21909 for diagnostic imaging of inflammation in a rat model of the reverse passive Arthus reaction induced by immune complex deposition (Charlton et al., 1997). The aptamer was labelled with ^{99m}Tc and given by intravenous injection 3.5-4 h after induction of inflammation. Rats were imaged on a gamma camera in 10 min frames continuously for 40 min and additional 10 min frames were taken every hour up to 4 h after administration of imaging agent.

Remarkably, a better signal-to-noise ratio was achieved by the aptamer compared to a clinically used IgG-based inflammation imaging agent used as a positive control (for the aptamer, a ratio of 4.3 ± 0.6 was achieved at 2 h; for IgG, a ratio of 3.1 ± 0.1 was achieved at 3 h). This ratio was achieved primarily by the rapid clearance of the aptamer from the peripheral circulation. thus indicating that the aptamer technology may be successfully applied to diagnostic imaging.

5. Thrombus imaging with aptamers

Thrombin is the last enzyme in the clotting cascade functioning to cleave fibrinogen to fibrin which forms the fibrin gel of a hemostatic plug or a pathologic thrombus. In addition to its role in blood coagulation, it also triggers important anticoagulant and antifibrinolytic pathways (Petäjä, 2011). The crystal structure of thrombin has been determined (Bode et al., 1992; Stubbs & Bode, 1993) thus giving important insight into its structure-function relationship. DNA aptamers have been generated that bind to different domains of the protein. ODN1 binds to exosite 1, the thrombin substrate binding site, thus competing with fibrin for binding to the same site on thrombin (Bock et al., 1992; Wu et al., 1992). Conversely, ODN2 reacts with exosite 2, the heparin binding site on thrombin (Tasset et al., 1997). These aptamers have been extensively characterised for their binding to thrombin and ODN1, is currently being evaluated in phase II clinical trials by ARCA Biopharma/Archemix Corp. as an anticoagulant for use during acute coronary artery bypass surgery. Being unmodified and unstable *in vivo* the aptamer, designated as Nu172, has to be administered by continuous intravenous infusion (Esposito et al., 2011).

To generate thrombin-dependent images in aptamer-mediated thrombus imaging approaches, the radiolabeled aptamer must form a ternary complex with thrombin bound to the fibrin matrix. For this reason ODN 2, but not ODN 1, has been used for thrombus imaging (Dougan et al., 2003).

In vitro experiments showed that ODN2 can form a ternary complex (with thrombin and fibrin) in clots, a necessity for thrombus imaging, thus indicating that allosteric interference from the fibrin binding site (exosite 1) did not impede ODN 2 binding at exosite 2. Thrombin-dependent uptake of ODN 2 was observed with *in situ* labeling of clots and by labeling of preformed clots. Further, the retention of [^{125}I]ODN 2 increased as the thrombin content of thrombi was increased whereas the rate of release of ODN 2 out of preformed thrombi decreased. Then, the aptamer was tested *in vivo*, in a rabbit jugular vein model using thrombus supplemented with human thrombin,. The labeled aptamer was introduced internally with the portion of rabbit blood, or else externally to a preformed unlabeled clot via the truncated facial vein and the thrombus area was imaged with a 2D scintigraphic camera, or excised for counting. Despite the clearly promising effect *in vitro* when ODN 2 was tested *in vivo*, the uptake was equal to the ovalbumin control and did not reflect thrombin content. A possible explanation of the failure of the *in vivo* thrombin-dependent imaging was attributed to the rapid clearance of ODN 2 from blood, combined with slow mass transfer in the thrombus. It is conceivable that nucleic acid analogs with extended lifetimes in circulation might help overcome this problem. For instance, the clearance rates of aptamers can be altered to keep them in circulation by anchoring them to liposome bilayers, by coupling them to inert large molecules such as PEG or to other hydrophobic groups (Willis et al., 1998; Healy et al., 2004).

It is noteworthy that the Food and Drug Administration (FDA)-approved aptamer, Macugen, as well as all the aptamers in clinical trials, except for Nu172, have been conjugated with PEG to enhance their half-life *in vivo* (Esposito et al., 2011).

6. Aptamers as *in vivo* imaging reagents in cancer

The aim of this section is to give a detailed overview on the aptamers developed for tumour imaging. Pointing out the attention on the structural modification as well as the bioconjugation with specific tags, we will focus on the experimental results emphasizing the essential requirements for potential application of aptamers as imaging probes for *in vivo* studies: high target specificity and affinity, rapid pharmacokinetics, exclusion of toxic side effects, tumour penetration, chemical stability, and high signal-to-noise ratio.

Five modalities (PET, SPECT, NMRI, CT and OI) are available to the scientist for oncological investigations in animals (Lewis et al., 2002; Tavitian, 2003). PET and NMRI technologies offer deep tissue penetration and high spatial resolution, but compared with non-invasive small animal optical imaging, these techniques are very costly and time consuming to implement. Aptamers have been successfully coupled to different targeted radiolabeled ligands and contrast agents to generate probes for *in vivo* medical imaging by using the five modalities previously described.

6.1 Aptamers conjugated with ^{99m}Tc for SPECT

The TTA1 aptamer against TN-C has been generated by a crossover SELEX experiment that involves crossing from cell-SELEX on TN-C-positive U251 glioblastoma cells to protein-SELEX against purified recombinant TN-C (Hicke et al., 2001).

To improve stability against plasma nucleases, therefore guarantee a good blood persistence leading to sufficient signal-to-noise ratios for imaging, aptamer backbone (2′-F-Py containing RNA, 39mer) has been modified with the addition of maximal 2′-OMe purine substitutions, a thymidine cap at the 3′ end and LNA in not binding critical stem (Shimdt et al., 2004). This TTA1 derivative has been further conjugated with mercapto-acetyl diglycine (MAG2) chelate via an hexyl-aminolinker at the 5′ end and labelled with ^{99m}Tc for performing single photon emission computed tomography (Hicke et al., 2006) .

To assess the degree of stability, an essential feature to achieve a sufficient targeting and blood clearance, combined to low background activity in non-target organs, tumour to blood and tissue distribution of ^{99m}Tc-labeled aptamer have been examined in murine xenograft models of glioblastoma and breast cancer (Hicke et al., 2006). Images of glioblastoma and breast tumors were taken at various times after intravenous injection in mice using a γ-camera. After 3 h post injection the tumor mass was visible as well as liver and bladder. At 18h post injection the two major clearance pathways were entirely clean from any radioactivity, as predicted by biodistribution analysis (Table1), and the tumor was clearly visualized as blazing structure (Hicke et al., 2006). Data show a rapid renal and hepatobiliary clearance, 0.2 %ID/g and 1.5 %ID/g at 3h, respectively and a rapid tumor penetration (6% injected dose at 60 min). Tumor retention is durable (2.7% injected dose at 60 min) and the tumor-to-blood signal is significantly high (Hicke et al., 2006).

Substitution of DTPA-^{111}In or insertion of a $PEG_{3,400}$ linker have also been tested for biodistribution analysis showing a dramatic alteration of tissue uptake and clearance patterns, indicating that simple changes to chelator can have significant effects on tissue uptake and clearance patterns.

DNA-aptamers that target cell-surface mucin 1 glycoprotein (MUC1), generated by Protein-SELEX against purified MUC1 peptides (Ferreira et al., 2006), have also been labeled with ^{99m}Tc (Ferreira et al., 2006). The aptamers, named AptA and AptB, have been selected against the protein core or the glycosylated protein, respectively. Various chelating agents have been conjugated to the aptamers and multi aptamer complexes have shown increased retention of the complex in circulation without increasing the immunogenicity of the complex or adversely altering its tumor penetration properties. The biodistribution data of the labeled products have shown differences that depend on the size of the conjugate and the type of ligand (Borbas et al., 2007). Four types of chelators have been coupled to anti-MUC1 aptamers to generate a novel complex for diagnostic imaging with improved properties: MetCyc, MAG_3, DOTA and 4 (Figure 3).

Differently from the monomeric Tc-MetCyc-Apt and Tc-MAG3-Apt, the tetrameric compounds, DOTA and 4, conjugate with ^{99m}Tc are able to grab four aptamer molecules modified at 5′ by insertion of amine groups to facilitate coupling with the ligands carboxylic terminations and 3′ ends to protect against nuclease degradation. Both tetrameric and monomeric aptamers were tested in nude mice bearing xenografted MCF7 breast cancer tumor. Compared to the monomeric biomarker composites, DOTA and 4 showed an increased retention in the circulation by means of their largest molecular weight. Despite the tetrameric complexes showed improved tumor retention and pharmacokinetic properties compared to the monomeric compounds, biodistribution studies have exhibited presence of free technetium in the stomach and large intestine highlighting some kind of lack in the Tc-aptamer binding (Borbas et al., 2007).

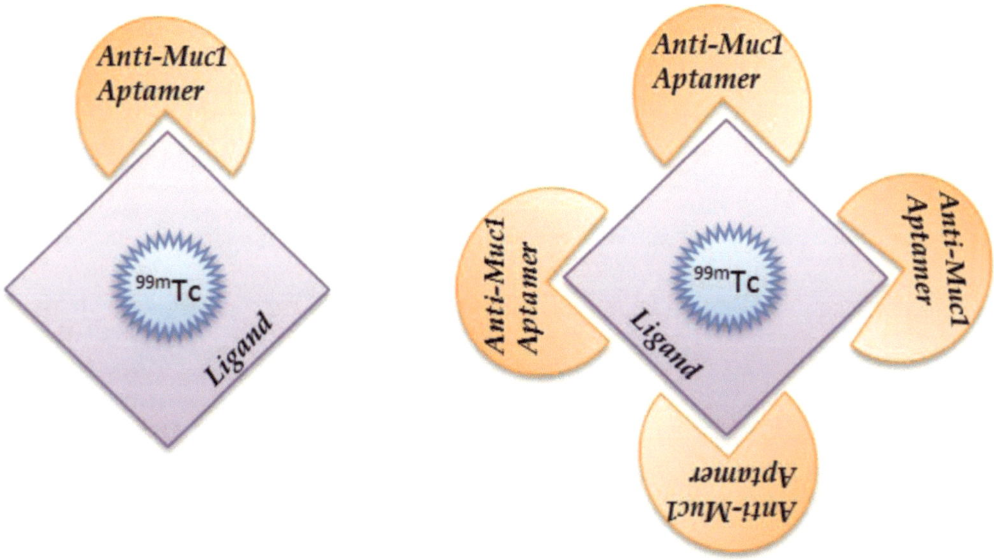

Fig. 3. Schematic representation of monomeric and tetrameric aptamer bioconjugates (see text for details).

Anti-MUC1 aptamers have also been successfully conjugated to MAG2chelator and the complexes have been labeled with ^{99m}Tc (Pieve et al., 2009). Analysis of two aptamer-radionuclide conjugates, AptA and AptB, biodistribution properties in MCF7 xenograft-bearing nude mice shows strong ^{99m}Tc binding properties (70-80% for AptA and ≥80% for AptB) and high stability *in vivo*, in terms of nuclease degradation and leaking of the metal (Table 1). Both aptamers show a maximum tumor uptake after 5h post injection, even though Apt B has higher accumulation rate, 0.12 %ID/g (for AptA) and 0.14 %ID/g (for AptB), followed by a decrease at 16h, 0.033 %ID/g (for AptA) and 0.016 %ID/g (for AptB) and 22h, 0.008 %ID/g (for AptA) and 0.013 %ID/g (for AptB). As pointed out by these data AptB releases quicker from the target keeping his activity constant between 16h and 22h, whilst AptA activity decreases constantly in time. The activity discrepancy is consequence of a different kinetic behaviour upon binding with the molecular target. AptB, in fact, internalized in the cancer cell quicker than AptA. Table 1 shows tumour-to-blood ratios values, taken at different times post injection, of both oligonucleotide carriers, confirming the assumption of Missailidis's group. The maximum levels of tumour uptake and clearance has reached at 5h post injection for AptA and AptB (table 1) but whiles the tumour-to-blood ratio trend of AptB, after 5h, is constant in time, AptA decreases drastically at 16 h, reaching his minimum value, and increases again at 22h, suggesting that the bound aptamer was not internalized.

Even if the radiolabeled aptamers demonstrate good tumor uptake and clearance, they require further optimization before diagnostic use.

Target	TNC	MUC1	
Aptamer	TTA1/2'Fy-RNA	AptA/DNA	AptB/DNA
Length(nt)	39	25	25
K_d *(nM)*	5	5	5
Tag	^{99m}Tc	^{99m}Tc	^{99m}Tc
Tumour (%ID/g)			
10 min	5.9±0.6		
1h	2.69±0.30		
3h	1.88±0.10	0.051±0.022	0.044±0.008
5h		0.12±0.046	0.14±0.040
16h		0.033±0.034	0.016±0.005
22h		0.008±0.001	0.013±0.005
Blood (%ID/g)			
10 min	2.27±0.25		
1h	0.11±0.00		
3h	0.03±0.00	0.027±0.002	0.024±0.001
5h		0.14±0.04	0.19±0.04
16h		0.005±0.001	0.009±0.001
22h		0.004±0.001	0.007±0.004
T/Blood			
10 min	2.6		
1h	24.0		
3h	62.6	1.8	1.8
5h		0.8	0.7
16h		6.6	1.8
22h		2	1.8

Table 1. *In vitro* characteristics and pharmacokinetics in mice for anti-TNC and anti- MUC1 aptamers.

6.2 Nanoparticle-aptamer conjugates for OI and NMRI

Aptamers were also used to functionalize nanoparticles surface for a potential *in vivo* cell imaging applications (Farokhzad et al., 2004; Javier et al., 2008; Chu et al., 2006; Rong et al., 2010; Savla et al., 2011).

Much work has been made by using the two 2'fluoro-pyrimidine (2'Fy)-RNA aptamers (A9 and A10) that have been generated against the extracellular domain of PSMA (prostate-specific membrane antigen), (Lupold et al., 2002). These aptamers bind with high affinity to the acinar epithelial cells of prostate cancer tissue. They have been used to deliver nanoparticles, quantum dots (QDs), toxin, or siRNA to prostate cancer cells (Cerchia & de Franciscis, 2010).

Poly(D,L-lactic acid) (PLA)-PEG-COOH nanoparticles and microparticles, conjugated with the A10 RNA aptamer have been developed to target the (PSMA) cells *in vivo* (Farokhzad et al., 2004).

PLA derivatives exhibit a desirable characteristic by means of their neutral to slightly negative surface charge, preserving the aptamers binding characteristic by specific interaction with them. On the opposite, particles with a positive surface charge may interact non specifically with the negatively charged aptamers affecting their binding properties.

Moreover the incorporation of PEG containing a terminal hydroxyl and carboxylic acid functional groups results essential to maximize nanoparticle circulating half-life and to allow the covalent coupling with 3'-NH2–modified aptamer.

To examine the presence of the aptamer-nanoparticle conjugates on the surface of PSMA-positive cells, the A10 aptamer has been labeled at 5'end with FITC and uptake by LNCaP cells has been evaluated by fluorescent microscopy. Images taken after 2 h and 16 h of incubation, showed a massive internalization just after 2h of nanoparticle-aptamer compound versus control group (aptamer-treatment of PSMA-negative PC3 cells).

These aptamer-nanoparticles conjugates have been loaded with docetaxel, anti-cancer therapeutic and successfully used for targeted delivery to PSMA-positive cells (Farokhzad et al., 2006).

PSMA has been also labelled using aptamer-quantum dots conjugates (Chu et al., 2006). A different anti-PSMA aptamer, A9, has been selected and conjugated to luminescent CdSe and CdTe nanocrystals for cell labelling.

Quantum dots (QD) represent the most promising fluorescent markers and delivery vehicles. These semiconductor particles have nanometre size and offer revolutionary fluorescence performance over traditional fluorescence dyes such as long-term photostability for live-cell imaging and dynamics studies, brilliant colors for simple, single-excitation multicolor analysis, fixability for follow-up immunofluorescence after in vivo studies, narrow and symmetrical emission spectra for low interchannel crosstalk.

Before conjugation the synthesized aptamer was biotinylated at its 3'-end by periodate oxidation and conjugation to biotin hydrazide (Qin & Pyle, 1999).

Labeling experiments were carried out for fixed and live cells and live cells embedded in a collagen matrix. The A9 aptamer-QD conjugates showed specific in vitro labeling for the selected target exhibited a good capacity to penetrate keep into tissues.

QD has also been conjugated with MUC1 aptamer and doxorubicin (QD-MUC1-DOX), via acid labile hydrazine bond, for in vivo imaging and drug delivery (Salva et al., 2011). In vitro and in vivo studies confirmed that the complex QD-MUC1-DOX accumulate predominately in the tumor and effectively release inside cancer cells (Salva et al., 2011).

A novel, multifunctional, thermally cross-linked superparamagnetic iron oxide nanoparticle (TCL-SPION) which can detect prostate cancer (PCa) cells and deliver targeted chemotherapeutic drugs has been developed (Wang et al., 2008). TCL-SPION nanoparticle has been conjugated with A10 aptamer and the complex so obtained has been tested for PCa imaging, using a single-sided NMR probe, and therapy, loading the bioconjugate with DOX.

NMR studies confirm the potential of the TCL-SPION-Apt complex as a targeted MR contrast showing that the bioconjugate can detect PSMA-expressing PCa cells with high sensitivity. The Dox-loaded TLC-SPION-Apt compound has been tested for antiproliferative activity against both the LNCaP and PC3 cell lines. Results showed selective delivery to PSMA-expressing cells without loss in cytotoxicity (Wang et al., 2008).

Further, PLA nanoparticles containing stably incorporated cyanine dyes have been tested for *in vitro* and *in vivo* imaging applications (Tong et al., 2010). Cy5-PLA/A10 aptamer nanoparticles have been found to only bind to and get internalized by LNCaP and canine prostate adenocarcinoma cells (PSMA-positive), but not to PC3 cells (PSMA-negative). Then, conjugates have been intravenously administered to balb/c mice and *in vivo* biodistribution evaluated by using the LI-COR Odyssey scanner. Accumulation of Cy5-PLA NP within visceral organs allows for greater than >10-fold increase in fluorescent intensity in comparison with background autofluorescence. Splenic accumulation of Cy5-PLA NP is the greatest for all visceral organs examined (spleen, liver, kidney, lung, and heart).

Another application of the anti-PSMA A9 aptamer as molecular-specific contrast agents for prostate cancer imaging has been developed by Javier et al (Javier et al., 2008). The aptamer has been conjugated by using an extended aptamer design where the extension is complementary to an oligonucleotide sequence attached to the surface of gold nanoparticles. Binding of nanoparticle-aptamer bioconjugates to prostate LNCaP cells has been valuated by reflectance imaging of the labeled cells with confocal microscopy in reflectance mode.

More recently, *in vivo* imaging of tumor has been performed by using the DNA aptamer sgc8, generated by cell-SELEX on human acute lymphoblastic leukaemia cells and identified to interact with protein tyrosine kinase-7 (PTK7) (Shi et al., 2011). The aptamer has been modified in order to generate an activatable probe consisting of the binding site of the aptamer (A-strand), a poly-T linker and a short DNA sequence complementary to a part of the A-strand, with a fluorophore and a quencher attached at either terminus. In the absence of binding, the aptamer is in a hairpin structure resulting in a quenched fluorescence. When the probe binds to cell-surface receptors, it changes conformation resulting in an activated fluorescence signal. This molecule was intravenously injected into tumor-bearing mice and fluorescence images were collected. Compared to always-on aptamer probes, the activatable aptamer showed significantly enhanced image contrast and shortened diagnosis time to 15 min.

6.3 Nanoparticle-aptamer conjugates for *in vivo* multimodal imaging

Recently, a multimodal cancer-targeted imaging system capable of simultaneous *in vivo* fluorescence imaging, radionuclide imaging and magnetic resonance imaging in mice, has been reported by using the AS1411 aptamer as targeting molecule (Hwang et al., 2010). AS1411 aptamer is a 26-mer guanine-rich oligonucleotide (GRO), which in solution folds into quadruplex structures, that make it very stable and resistant to degradation by serum enzymes. This aptamer that binds to nucleolin, a protein that is often over-expressed on the surface of cancer cells, is currently in Phase II of clinical development (Bates et al., 1999, 2009; Mongelard & Bouvet, 2010). In this study, the aptamer was conjugated with a cobalt-ferrite nanoparticle surrounded by fluorescent rhodamine, and the resulting particle was bound with 2-(p-isothio-cyanatobenzyl)-1,4,7-triazacyclonane-1,4,7-triacetic acid (p-SCN-bn-NOTA) chelating agent and further labeled with radionuclide gallium citrate Ga-67.

The purified nanoparticles, designated MFR-AS1411, were intravenously injected into a mice xenografted with nucleolin-expressing C6 rat glioma cells and radionuclide images were acquired at 1, 6, and 24 h after injection. Scintigraphic images of C6 tumors in mice that received MFRAS1411 showed that tumors had accumulated MFR-AS1411 at 24 h after injection whereas the mutant, not functional, MFR-AS1411 administration revealed rapid clearance via the bloodstream.

Further, bioluminescence images analysed using IVIS200 system in the C6 cells, stably expressing the luciferase gene, illustrated the *in vivo* distribution. MR images of the same mice injected with MFR-AS1411 showed dark T2 signals inside the tumor region, compared with the MRI signal of the tumor region injected with mutant MFR-AS1411 particles.

Taken together, the above results by means of multifunctional imaging modality platforms demonstrate that MFR-AS1411 specifically targeted cancer cells.

7. Future perspectives

To date only few aptamers have been developed as targeting agents in imaging modalities, as discussed in the present chapter and schematized in figure 4, nevertheless, their low immunogenicity, good tumor penetration, rapid uptake and fast systemic clearance, indicate a great potential of these molecules as imaging agents especially when compared to antibodies. Given the nature of the aptamers and their discrimination and targeting capacities, the majority of the aptamers not bound to the target tissues is cleared rapidly from the system. In comparison, intact radiolabelled antibodies remain in circulation for a very long time, often resulting in organ toxicity.

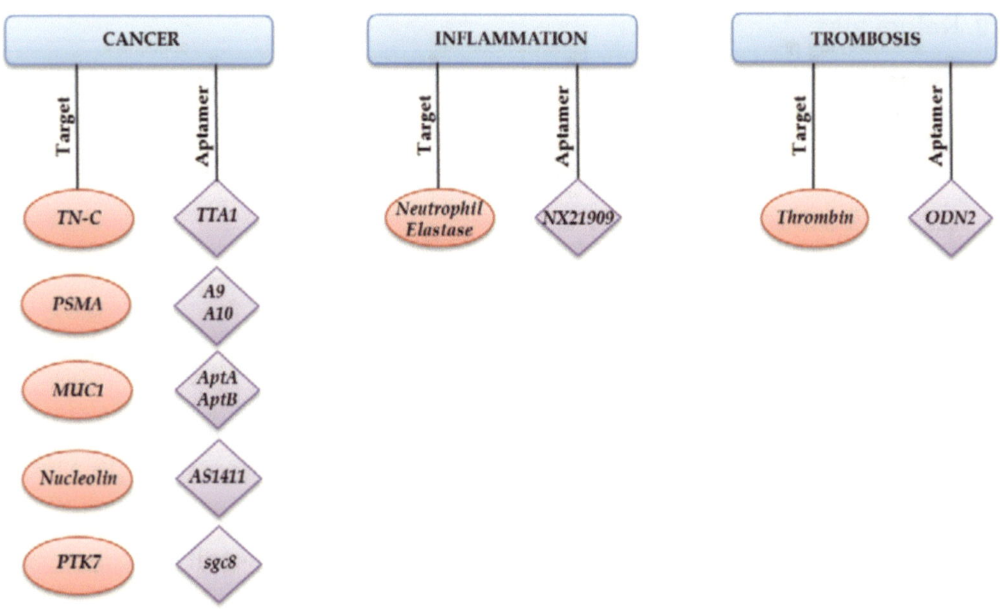

Fig. 4. Aptamers to date developed as ligands for tumour imaging, inflammation imaging and thrombus imaging

Further, the continuous advances in SELEX technology allow now to easily generate aptamers against virtually any protein and it is plausible speculate that the global market demand for nucleic acid aptamers will increase in the next few years opening the aptamer field for development for therapy, diagnosis and drug development imaging.

8. Take-home-message

Some molecule, most notably those found in nature, have the ability to reach out and grab other molecules and bound to them. Aptamers appear to fulfill this criterion and have been identified as excellent candidates for targeting specific epitopes in clinical diagnosis and therapy of different diseases. Further, because of their high specificity and low toxicity aptamers may reveal as the compound of choice for *in vivo* cell recognition as delivery agents for nanoparticles, small interfering RNAs bioconjugates, chemotherapeutic cargos and molecular imaging probes (Cerchia & de Franciscis, 2010).

There have been significant technological advances in cell-SELEX and *in vivo*-SELEX strategies. Although aptamers are relatively new to the clinic, the fact that they can act as specific recognition ligands to target cells *in vivo* suggests that these molecules will have a considerable impact in patient care in the near future.

9. Acknowledgments

This work was supported by funds from C.N.R., the Italian Ministry of Economy and Finance to the CNR for the Project FaReBio di Qualita', AICR No 11-0075 (L.C.), MIUR grant, MERIT RBNE08YFN3_001 (VdF), AIRC No 4971 (L.C.) and EU grant EMIL No 503569.

10. References

Acton, P.D. & Kung, H.F. (2003). Small animal imaging with high resolution SPECT. *Nuclear Medicine and Biolog*, Vol.30, pp. 889-895

Aurup, H.; Williams, D.M. & Eckstein, F. (1992). 2'-Fluoro- and 2'-amino-2'-deoxynucleoside 5'-triphosphates as substrates for T7 RNA polymerase. *Biochemistry*, Vol.31, No.40, pp. 9636-9641

Bates, P.J.; Kahlon, J.B.; Thomas, S.D.; Trent, J.O. & Miller, D.M. (1999). Antiproliferative activity of G-rich oligonucleotides correlates with protein binding. *Journa of Biological Chemistry*, Vol.274, No.3, pp. 26369-26377

Bates, P.J., Laber, D.A.; Miller, D.M.; Thomas, S.D. & Trent, J.O. (2009). Discovery and development of the G-rich oligonucleotide AS1411 as a novel treatment for cancer. *Experimental and Molecular Pathology*, Vol.86, No.3, pp. 151-164

Blank, M.; Weinschenk, T.; Priemer, M. & Schluesener, H. (2001). Systematic Evolution of a DNA Aptamer Binding to Rat Brain Tumor Microvessels. Journal of Biology Chemistery, Vol.276, pp. 16464-16468

Bless, N.M.; Smith, D.; Charlton, J.; Czermak, B.J.; Schmal, H.; Friedl, H.P. & Ward, P.A. (1997). Protective effects of an aptamer inhibitor of neutrophil elastase in lung inflammatory injury. *Current Biology*, Vol.7, No.11, pp. 877-880

Bode, W.; Turk, D. & Karshikov, A. (1992). The refined 1.9-Angstrom X-ray crystal-structure of D-Phe-Pro-Arg chloromethylketone-inhibited human alpha-thrombin-structure-analysis: Overall structure, electrostatic properties, detailed active site geometry, and structure-function relationships. *Protein Science,* Vol.1, No.4, pp. 426–471

Bock, L.C.; Griffin, L.C.; Latham, J.A.; Vermaas, E.H. & Toole, J.J. (1992). Selection of single-stranded DNA molecules that bind and inhibit human thrombin. *Nature,* Vol.355, No.6360, pp. 564–566

Borbas, K.E.; Ferreira, C.S.; Perkins, A.; Bruce, J.I. & Missailidis, S. (2007). Design and synthesis of mono- and multimeric targeted radiopharmaceuticals based on novel cyclen ligands coupled to anti-MUC1 aptamers for the diagnostic imaging and targeted radiotherapy of cancer. *Bioconjugate Chemistry,* Vol.18, No.4, pp. 1205-1212

Burmeister, P.E.; Lewis, S.D.; Silva, R.F; Preiss, J.R.; Horwitz, L.R.; Pendergrast, P.S.; McCauley, T.G.; Kurz, J.C.; Epstein, D.M.; Wilson, C. & Keefe, A.D. (2004). Direct *In Vitro* Selection of a 2′-*O*-Methyl-Stabilized Aptamer Against VEGF. *Chemistry& Biology,* Vol.12, No.1, pp. 25-33

Cantore, M.; Capparelli, E.; Berardi, F.; Perrone, R. & Colabufo, N.A. (2011). Clinical Pharmacokinetic and Metabolism of PET Radiotracers for Imaging P-glycoprotein in Chemoresistant Tumor of Colorectal Cancer. *Current Drug Metabolism.* Epub ahead of print.

Cerchia, L. & de Franciscis, V. (2010). Targeting cancer cells with nucleic acid aptamers. *Trends Biotechnol,*Vol.28, No10, pp.517-525.

Charlton, J.; Sennello, J. & Smith, D. (1997). In vivo imaging of inflammation using an aptamer inhibitor of human neutrophil elastase. *Chemistry* & *Biology,* Vol.4, No.11, pp. 809-816

Charlton, J.; Kirschenheuter, G.P. & Smith, D. (1997). Highly potent irreversible inhibitors of neutrophil elastase generated by selection from a randomized DNA-valine phosphonate library. *Biochemistry,* Vol.36, No.10, pp. 3018-3026

Chelliserrykattil, J. & Ellington, AD. (2004). Evolution of a T7 RNA polymerase variant that transcribes 2'-O-methyl RNA. *Nature Biotechnol*ogy, Vol.22, No.9, pp. 1155-1160

Chu, T.C.; Shieh, F.; Lavery, L.A.; Levy, M.; Richards-Kortum, R.; Korgel, B.A. & Ellington, A.D. (2006). Labeling tumor cells with fluorescent nanocrystal-aptamer bioconjugates. *Biosensors and Bioelectronics,* Vol.21, No.10, pp. 1859-1866

Doring, G. (1994). The role of neutrophil elastase in chronic inflammation. *American Journalof Respiratory and Critical Care Medicine,* Vol.150, No.6 Pt 2, pp. S114-11

Dougan, H.; Weitz, J.I.; Stafford, A.R.; Gillespie, K.D.; Klement, P.; Hobbs, J.B. & Lyster, D.M. (2003). Evaluation of DNA aptamers directed to thrombin as potential thrombus imaging agents. *Nuclear Medicine and Biology,* Vol.30, No.1, pp. 61-72

Ellington, A.D. & Szostak, J.W. (1990). In vitro selection of RNA molecules that bind specific ligands. *Nature,* Vol.346, No.6287, pp. 818-822

Esposito, C.L.; Catuogno, S.; de Franciscis, V. & Cerchia, L. (2011). New insight into clinical development of nucleic acid aptamers. *Discov. Med.,* Vol. 11, No.61, pp.487-496

Eulberg, D. & Klussmann, S. (2003). Spiegelmers: biostable aptamers. *ChemBioChem,* Vol.4, No.10, pp. 979-983

Farokhzad, O.C.; Jon, S.; Khademhosseini, A.; Tran, T.N.; Lavan, D.A. & Langer, R. (2004). Nanoparticle-aptamer bioconjugates: a new approach for targeting prostate cancer cells. *Cancer Research,* Vol.64, No.21, pp. 7668-7672

Farokhzad, O.C.; Cheng, J.; Teply, B.A.; Sherifi, I.; Jon, S.; Kantoff, P.W.; Richie, J.P. & Langer, R. (2006). Targeted nanoparticle-aptamer bioconjugates for cancer chemotherapy in vivo. *Proceeding of the National Academy of Sciences of the United State of American,* Vol.103, No.16, pp. 6315-6320

Ferreira, C.S.; Matthews, C.S. & Missailidis, S. (2006). DNA aptamers that bind to MUC1 tumour marker: design and characterization of MUC1-binding single-stranded DNA aptamers. *Tumour Biology,* Vol.27, No.6, pp. 289-301

Foy, J.W.; Rittenhouse, K.; Modi, M. & Patel, M. (2007). Local tolerance and systemic safety of pegaptanib sodium in the dog and rabbit. *Journal Ocular Pharmacology and Therapeutics,* Vol.23, No.5, pp. 452-466

Healy, J.M.; Lewis, S.D.; Kurz, M.; Boomer, R.M.; Thompson, K.M.; Wilson, C. & McCauley, T.G. (2004). Pharmacokinetics and biodistribution of novel aptamer compositions. Pharmaceutical Research, Vol.21, No.12, pp. 2234-2246

Hicke, B.J.; Marion, C.; Chang, Y.F.; Gould, T.; Lynott, C.K.; Parma, D.; Schmidt, P.G. & Warren, S. (2001). Tenascin-C aptamers are generated using tumor cells and purified protein. *Journal of Biological Chemistry,* Vol. 276, No.52, pp. 48644-48654

Hicke, B.J.; Stephens, A.W.; Gould, T.; Chang, Y.F.; Lynott, C.K.; Heil, J.; Borkowski, S.; Hilger, C.S.; Cook, G.; Warren, S. & Schmidt, P.G. (2006). Tumor targeting by an aptamer. *Journal of Nuclear Medicine,* Vol.47, No.4, pp. 668-678

Hickson, J. (2009). In vivo optical imaging: preclinical applications and considerations. *Urologic Oncolgy,* Vol.27, No.3, pp. 295-297

Hwang, do W.; Ko, H.Y.; Lee, J.H.; Kang, H.; Ryu, S.H.; Song, I.C.; Lee, D.S. & Kim, S. (2010). A nucleolin-targeted multimodal nanoparticle imaging probe for tracking cancer cells using an aptamer. *Journal of Nuclear Medicine,* Vol.51, No.1, pp. 98-105

Hui Shi, Xiaoxiao He, Kemin Wang1, Xu Wu, Xiaosheng Ye, Qiuping Guo, Weihong Tan, Zhihe Qing, Xiaohai Yang, and Bing Zhou. (2011). Activatable aptamer probe for contrast-enhanced in vivo cancer imaging based on cell membrane protein-triggered conformation alteration *PNAS,* Vol.108, No.10, pp. 3900-3905

Javier, D.J.; Nitin, N.; Levy, M.; Ellington, A. & Richards-Kortum, R. (2008). Aptamer-targeted gold nanoparticles as molecular-specific contrast agents for reflectance imaging. *Bioconjugate Chemistry,* Vol.19, No.6, pp. 1309-1312

Keefe, A.D. & Cload, S.T. (2008). SELEX with modified nucleotides. *Current Opinion in Chemical Biology,* Vol.12, No.4, pp. 448-456

Keefe, A.D.; Pai, S. & Ellington, A. (2010). Aptamers as therapeutics. *Nature Reviews Drug Discovery,*Vol.9, No.7, pp. 537-550

Langen, K.J.; Bartenstein, P.; Boecker, H.; Brust, P.; Coenen, H.H.; Drzezga, A.; Grünwald, F.; Krause, B.J.; Kuwert, T.; Sabri, O.; Tatsch, K.; Weber, W.A. & Schreckenberger, M. (2011). German guidelines for brain tumour imaging by PET and SPECT using labelled amino acids. *Nuklearmedizin,* Vol.50, No.4. Epub ahead of print.

Larobina, M.; Brunetti, A. & Salvatore, M (2006). Small animal PET: a review of commercially available imaging systems. *Current Medical Imaging Reviews;* Vol.2, No.2, pp. 187-192

Leblond, F.; Davis, S.C.; Valdés, P.A. & Pogue, B.W. (2010). Pre-clinical whole-body fluorescence imaging: Review of instruments, methods and applications. *Journal of Photochemistry and Photobiology B: Biology,* Vol.98, No.1, pp. 77-94

Lewis, J.S.; Achilefu, S.; Garbow, J.R.; Laforest, R. & Welch, M.J. (2002). Small animal imaging. current technology and perspectives for oncological imaging. *European Journal of Cancer,* Vol.38, No.16, pp. 2173-88

Luker, G.D. & Luker, K.E. (2008). Optical imaging: current applications and future directions. *The Journal of Nuclear Medicine*, Vol.49, No.1, pp. 1-7

Lupold, S.E; Hicke, B.J.; Lin, Y. & Coffey, D.S. (2002). Identification and characterization of nuclease-stabilized RNA molecules that bind human prostate cancer cells via the prostate-specific membrane antigen. *Cancer Research*, Vol.62, No.14, pp. 4029-4033

Lyons, S.K. (2005). Advances in imaging mouse tumour models in vivo. *Journal of Pathology*, Vol. 205, No. 2, pp. 194-205

Massoud, T.F. & Gambhir, S.S. (2003). Molecular imaging in living subjects: seeing fundamental biological processes in a new light. *Gene & Development*, Vol. 17, No. 5, pp. 545-580, ISSN 0890-9369

Mongelard, F. & Bouvet, P. (2010). AS-1411, a guanosine-rich oligonucleotide aptamer targeting nucleolin for the potential treatment of cancer, including acute myeloid leukemia. *Current Opinion in Molecular Therapeutics*, Vol.12, No.1, pp.107-114

Percy, D.B.; Ribot, E.J.; Chen, Y.; McFadden, C.; Simedrea, C; Steeg, P.S.; Chambers, A.F. & Foster, P.J. (2011). In Vivo Characterization of Changing Blood-Tumor Barrier Permeability in a Mouse Model of Breast Cancer Metastasis: A Complementary Magnetic Resonance Imaging Approach. *Investigative Radiology*. Epub ahead of print.

Perkins, A.C. & Missailidis, S. (2007). Radiolabelled aptamers for tumour imaging and therapy. *Quarterly Journal of Nuclear Medicine and Molecular Imaging*, Vol.51, No.4, pp. 292-296

Petäjä, J. (2011). Inflammation and coagulation. An overview. *Thrombosis Research*, Vol.127 Suppl 2, pp. S34-37

Pieve, C.D.; Perkins, A.C. & Missailidis, S. (2009). Anti-MUC1 aptamers: radiolabelling with (99m)Tc and biodistribution in MCF-7 tumour-bearing mice. *Nuclear Medicine and Biology*, Vol.36, No.6, pp. 703-710

Pomper, M.G. (2005). Translational molecular imaging for cancer. *Cancer Imaging*, Vol.5, No.A, pp. S16-26

Qin, P.Z. & Pyle, A.M. (1999). Site-specific labeling of RNA with fluorophores and other structural probes. Methods, Vol.18, No.1, pp. 60-70

Ruckman, J.; Green, L.S.; Beeson, J.; Waugh, S.; Gillette, W.L.; Henninger, D.D.; Claesson-Welsh, L. & Janjic, N. (1998). 2'-Fluoropyrimidine RNA-based aptamers to the 165-amino acid form of vascular endothelial growth factor (VEGF165). Inhibition of receptor binding and VEGF-induced vascular permeability through interactions requiring the exon 7-encoded domain. *Journal Biology Chemistry*,Vol.273, No.32, pp. 20556-20567

Savla, R.; Taratula, O.; Garbuzenko, O. & Minko, T. (2011). Tumor targeted quantum dot-mucin 1 aptamer-doxorubicin conjugate for imaging and treatment of cancer. *Journal of Controlled Released*, Vol.153, No.1, pp. 16-22

Schellenberger, E.A.; Sosnovik, D., Weissleder, R. & Josephson, L. (2004). Magneto/optical annexin V, a multimodal protein. *Bioconjugate Chemistry*, Vol.15, No.5, pp. 1062-1067

Schmidt, K.S.; Borkowski, S.; Kurreck, J.; Stephens, A.W.; Bald, R.; Hecht, M.; Friebe, M.; Dinkelborg, L. & Erdmann, V.A. (2004). Application of locked nucleic acids to improve aptamer in vivo stability and targeting function. *Nucleic Acids Research*, Vol.32, No.19, pp. 5757-5765

Schmidt, K.S.; Borkowski, S.; Kurreck, J.; Stephens, A.W.; Bald, R.; Hecht, M.; Friebe, M.; Dinkelborg, L. & Erdmann, V.A. (2004) Application of locked nucleic acids to improve aptamer in vivo stability and targeting function. *Nucleic Acid Research*, Vol.32, No.19, pp. 5757-5765

Smith, D.; Kirschenheuter, G.P.; Charlton, J.; Guidot, D.M. & Repine, J.E. (1995). *In vitro* selection of RNA-based irreversible inhibitors of human neutrophil elastase. *Chemistry & Biology*, Vol.2, No.11, pp. 741-750

Stubbs, M.T. & Bode, W. (1993). A player of many parts: the spotlight falls on thrombin's structure. *Thrombosis Research*, Vol.69, No.1, pp. 1–58

Tasset, D.M.; Kubik, M.F. & Steiner, W. (1997). Oligonucleotide inhibitors of human thrombin that bind distinct epitopes. *Journal of Molecular Biology*, Vol.272, No.5, pp. 688–698

Tavitian, B.; Terrazzino, S.; Kühnast, B.; Marzabal, S.; Stettler, O.; Dollé, F.; Deverre, J.R.; Jobert, A.; Hinnen, F.; Bendriem, B.; Crouzel, C. & Di Giamberardino, L. (1998). In vivo imaging of oligonucleotides with positron emission tomography. *Nature Medicine*, Vol.4, No.4, pp. 467-471

Tavitian, B. (2003). In vivo imaging with oligonucleotides for diagnosis and drug development. *Gut*, Vol.52 Suppl 4, pp. iv40-7

Tavitian, B.; Ducongé, F. ; Boisgard, R. & Dollé, F. (2009). In vivo imaging of oligonucleotidic aptamers. *Methods in Molecular Biology*, Vol.535, pp. 241-259

Tong, R.; Coyle, V.J.; Tang, L.; Barger, A.M.; Fan, T.M. & Cheng, J. (2010). Polylactide nanoparticles containing stably incorporated cyanine dyes for in vitro and in vivo imaging applications. *Microscopy Research Techinique*, Vol.73, No.9, pp. 901-909

Tuerk, C. & Gold, L. (1990). Systematic evolution of ligands by exponential enrichment: RNA ligands to bacteriophage T4 DNA polymerase. *Science*, Vol.249, pp. 505-510

Usman, N. & Blatt, LM. (2000). Nuclease-resistant synthetic ribozymes: developing a new class of therapeutics. *Journal of Clinical Investigation*, Vol.106, No.10, pp. 1197-1202

van der Meel, R.; Gallagher, W.M.; Oliveira, S.; O'Connor, A.E.; Schiffelers, R.M. & Byrne, A.T. (2010). *Drug Discovery Today*, Vol.15, No.3-4, pp. 102-114

Wang, A.Z.; Bagalkot, V.; Vasilliou, C.C.; Gu, F.; Alexis, F.; Zhang, L.; Shaikh, M.; Yuet, K.; Cima, M.J.; Langer, R.; Kantoff, P.W.; Bander, N.H.; Jon, S.; & Farokhzad, O.C. (2008). Superparamagnetic Iron Oxide Nanoparticle–Aptamer Bioconjugates for Combined Prostate Cancer Imaging and Therapy. *Chem. Med. Chem.* Vol.3, pp.1311-1315

Weiss, S.J. (1989). Tissue destruction by neutrophils. *N. Engl. 1. Med.* Vol.320, pp.365-376

Willis, M.C.; Collins, B.D.; Zhang, T.; Green, L.S.; Sebesta, D.P.; Bell, C.; Kellogg, E.; Gill, S.C.; Magallanez, A.; Knauer, S.; Bendele, R.A.; Gill, P.S.; Janjic, N. & Collins, B. (1998). Liposome-anchored vascular endothelial growth factor aptamers. *Bioconjugate Chemistry*, Vol.9, No.5, pp. 573-582

Wu, Q.; Tsiang, M. & Sadler, J.E. (1992). Localization of the single-stranded DNA binding site in the thrombin anion-binding exosite. *Journal of Biological Chemistry*, Vol.267, No.34, pp. 24408–24412

Yu, D.; Wang, D.; Zhu, F.G.; Bhagat, L.;Dai, M.; Kandimalla, E.R. & Agrawal, S. (2009). Modifications incorporated in CpG motifs of oligodeoxynucleotides lead to antagonist activity of toll-like receptors 7 and 9. *Journal of Medicinal Chemistry*, Vol.52, No.16, pp. 5108-5114

6

3D Optical Imaging of Fluorescent Agents in Biological Tissues

Manuel Freiberger and Hermann Scharfetter
Graz University of Technology
Austria

1. Introduction

Fluorescence diffuse optical tomography (fDOT) is an imaging modality which goes beyond well-established techniques such as 2D fluorescence imaging and fluorescence microscopy. Being a 3D tomographic modality, it seeks to overcome limitations of 2D systems as are: (i) the determination of the depth of fluorescent objects and (ii) a correction of the broadening of the fluorescence signal due to the massive scattering of photons.

Compared to high-resolution tomography systems such as CT and MRI, fDOT has the particular advantage that the optical activity of many fluorophores is influenced by the chemical milieu in which they are located and, thus, by the biological surrounding. Researchers have already shown the dependency on the oxygenation of the tissue (Longmuir & Knopp (1976); Shives et al. (2002)), the pH value (Gannot et al. (2004); Mordon et al. (1992)), or the temperature (Chen & Wood (2009)), for example. This influence on metabolic processes and states offers information beyond the visualization of anatomical structures and, therefore, is termed *functional imaging*.

In comparison to 2D in-vivo imaging, 3D sensing of fluorescent particles in biological specimen imposes additional problems:

- Light of lower wavelength (blue and green) is absorbed by many biologically relevant materials such as hemoglobin. In order to excite deep fluorophore-structures, excitation light in the far red and near infrared (NIR) range has to be used, which requires suitable (i.e. NIR-excitable) fluorescent targets.
- Visible and NIR-light is heavily scattered in biological tissue. This compromises the achievable resolution especially in comparison to CT and MR and requires special treatment during image reconstruction.
- The light intensity decays exponentially with the probing depth, which infers a depth-dependent maximum resolution.

The outline of this chapter is as follows: In section 2 the optical properties of tissue will be introduced. Section 3 deals with possible hardware setups for 3D sensing. Mathematical models for light propagation are described in section 4. In section 5 nonlinear image reconstruction methods are compared. An overview about clinical and pre-clinical applications is given in section 6 and section 7 concludes with an outlook.

2. Optical properties of tissue

For the determination of the 3D distribution of fluorescent particles inside biological samples, it is necessary to describe light propagation in tissue with mathematical models. This in turn requires to quantify typical light-tissue interaction processes in terms of measurable quantities. The most common processes are certainly absorption and scattering of photons as well as fluorescence and phosphorescence phenomena.

2.1 Absorption

Absorption is the extinction of a photon, whose energy is stored by the absorbing medium via excitation of an electron or in rotational or vibrational states of atoms. This physical processes are stochastic in their nature and therefore should be described by a probability density measure. However, for most models it is sufficient to give the average occurrence rate of an absorption event per photon path length. This leads to the definition of the absorption coefficient μ_a given in units of inverse length; frequently in cm^{-1} or mm^{-1}. It specifies the average number of photons being absorbed when traveling a given distance inside an absorbing medium. An absorption coefficient of $0.2\,\mathrm{cm}^{-1}$ would mean an average of two absorption events per 10 cm which the photon travels inside the object. In other words, a photon can on average travel μ_a^{-1} ($= 5\,\mathrm{cm}$ for the former example) without being absorbed. The latter quantity is called the *mean absorption-free path length*.

2.2 Scattering

Scattering is the deflection of a photon out of its original trajectory into a new direction. In analogy to absorption, the scattering coefficient μ_s gives the average number of scattering events per length of travel. The inverse μ_s^{-1} is the average length a photon can propagate in tissue without being scattered and is thus known as *mean scattering-free path length*. To fully quantify the scattering behavior of some medium, it is not sufficient to know only how often scattering happens but also the direction into which the photon will be deflected is of importance. The latter is given by the scattering phase function $\Theta(\hat{s}, \hat{s}')$, which is the probability for a photon arriving from direction $\hat{s}$ to be scattered into a new direction $\hat{s}'$. Two possible scattering phase functions are depicted in Figure 1. If every scattered direction $\hat{s}'$ has the same probability, the scattering is said to be *isotropic*. This ideal case is not valid in biological media, where scattering is usually strongly forward biased as displayed on the right in Figure 1. At this point, it is also worth noticing that most tissue types are much more scattering than absorbing. Exceptions to this rule are well perfused tissues such as liver and highly transparent liquids as liquor, for example.

2.3 Scattering anisotropy factor

For many real-world applications the description of the scattering distribution by the scattering phase function is much too complicated to be useful. Instead, one seeks to approximate the anisotropic scattering with a scattering coefficient μ_s through an isotropic model with another scattering coefficient μ_s'. To this end, the scattering anisotropy factor g is introduced which is the mean value of the cosine of the scattering angle. This factor is in the range from -1 to 1. Positive values indicate a preference for forward-scattering while negative values indicate an imbalance towards photons which are back-scattered. In the isotropic case g is equal to 0.

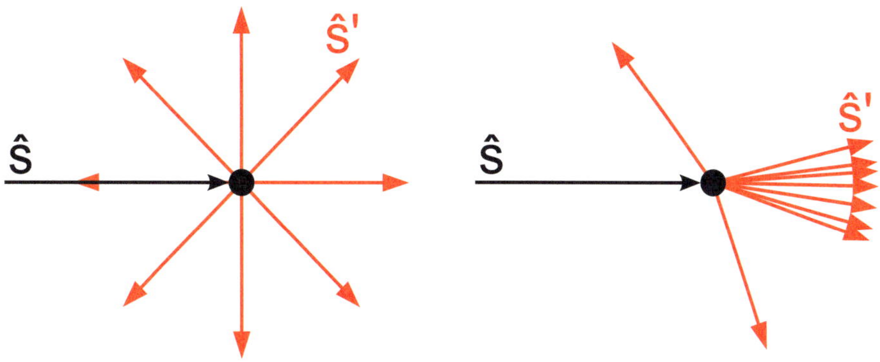

Fig. 1. Visualization of two scattering phase functions. The incoming photons with direction $\hat{s}$ are drawn in black, the scattered ones having a direction $\hat{s}'$ in red. Left: The scattering angles are equally distributed; the scattering is isotropic. Right: Nearly all photons are scattered in a forward direction which is true for most biological tissues.

With the definition of the anisotropy coefficient, one can define the reduced scattering coefficient μ_s' as $\mu_s' := (1-g)\mu_s$. The idea is to approximate anisotropic (forward-directed) scattering with probability μ_s and anisotropy g by isotropic scattering with a smaller scattering coefficient μ_s'. This working principle is illustrated in Figure 2. The true path of a scattered photon is sketched with small arrows. If the anisotropy coefficient of the tissue was $g = 0.875$, every $(1-0.875)^{-1} = 8$ anisotropic steps would be combined into one isotropic step. Thus, the number of scattering events per length of travel decreases and the mean scattering-free path length increases. The approximated scattering can be assumed to be isotropic.

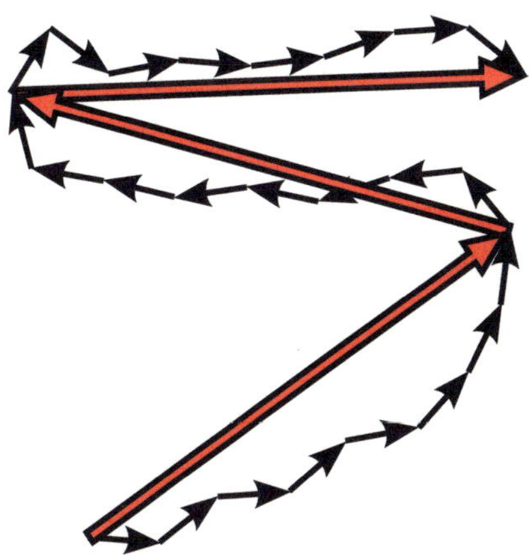

Fig. 2. Principle of the anisotropy coefficient: The short arrows represent the path of a scattered photon in tissue. Each arrow is of length μ_s^{-1}, which is the mean scattering-free path length. Assuming $g = 0.875$, every eight anisotropic scattering events are approximated by one isotropic scattering event which is drawn with red arrows. The isotropic scattering has a reduced scattering coefficient $\mu_s' = (1-g)\mu_s$, i.e. the isotropic mean scattering-free path length is larger than the anisotropic one.

2.4 Diagnostic window

The tissue's ability to absorb photons is a highly wavelength-dependent property. In the so called *diagnostic window* around 650–1300 nm, most tissues are sufficiently weak absorbers and light can penetrate deepest. The lower wavelength boundary of this wavelength range is made up by oxygenated and de-oxygenated hemoglobin; the upper boundary is due to the absorption of water.

3. Hardware

Since the early days of fDOT a number of different systems has been built, most of them for research purposes, but meanwhile also commercial systems are available. Regarding the details of implementation the systems differ considerably, for a good review see e.g. Leblond et al. (2010). A basic distinction can be made concerning the operation mode in terms of its temporal behavior. For some applications the reconstruction of intensity images is sufficient and then the system can operate in continuous-wave (CW) mode, thus leading to CW fluorescence tomography (CWFT). If, however, also the fluorescence lifetime ought to be imaged, the response of the sample to either very short light pulses (usually shorter than 100 ps) or harmonically modulated light with modulation frequencies between several tens of MHz up to several GHz must be acquired. The respective technologies are termed *time domain fluorescence tomography* (TDFT) or *frequency domain fluorescence tomography* (FDFT). All three modes can also be used spectroscopically, which requires in addition a dispersive element or a tunable filter at the detector side.

While the idea of TDFT is intuitively clear (direct measurement of the decay of the light signal), FDFT is more indirect. It relies on the fact that the complete time domain information can be recovered from quasi-stationary measurements with sinusoidally modulated light at many modulation frequencies—thus sampling in Fourier space—and transforming back to time domain by an inverse Fourier transform. However, the relevant bandwidth of the time domain signals is up to several GHz (Gibson et al. (2005)) and frequency domain systems allow sufficiently accurate operation only up to approximately 1 GHz (Chance et al. (1998)). Thus, currently the equivalence cannot be exploited from the instrumentation point of view. Typical modulation frequencies range from less than 100 MHz up to little more than 1 GHz (Durduran et al. (2010); Masciotti et al. (2009); Reynolds et al. (1997)). Assuming a mono-exponential fluorescence decay the lifetime can be recovered from measurements at a single frequency because a single exponential is Fourier transformed to a low pass of first order and thus the knowledge of modulus and phase of the light signal is sufficient.

All systems realized so far share three main components: A light source, a sample holder and a light detection system.

3.1 Light sources

The light source can have a wide spectral range (e.g. xenon arc lamps) in combination with filters but narrowband sources like lasers and LEDs are increasingly popular due to their versatility and the relative ease of producing either short pulses or properly modulated light. As for standard tomography the light should be concentrated to different locations on the sample surface, collimated beams are required, which favors the use of lasers. In any case the spectrum of the light source should be matched to the absorption spectrum of the fluorophore, but in the case of e.g. small Stokes shifts the excitation wavelength may be chosen somewhat below the absorption maximum in order to account for the limited steepness of excitation and emission filters. In order to keep the hardware flexible, usually filter wheels with selectable cutoff wavelengths are provided in case of wideband sources so as to adapt the system to different fluorophores.

For CWFT practically any light source with appropriate power and spectral content can be used. As FDFT typically requires modulation up to several 100 MHz, classical wideband sources require a fast optical shutter (electro-optic or acousto-optic, see e.g. Lakowicz (2006)) but such technologies are increasingly replaced by laser diodes which can be easily modulated up to 1 GHz in a useful power range (typically several tens of mW for in vivo applications). Even wideband sources based on lasers (supercontinuum lasers) and tunable diode lasers with external cavity are now available. The highest demands on the source are posed by TDFT. Currently the short light pulses are typically generated by Ti:sapphire lasers but also diode lasers are available which can deliver sufficiently short pulses (Lakowicz (2006)). Ti:sapphire lasers provide the unique feature of being tunable, see e.g. Kumar et al. (2008), where 150 fs-pulses are generated with a repetition rate of 80 MHz in a tuning range between 750 nm and 850 nm. In the same publication the spectral range could still be extended to 500 nm by the use of a super-continuum source based on a poly-crystalline fiber. The 80 MHz repetition rate is widely used and has also been adopted for pulsed laser diodes, e.g. in Soloviev et al. (2009).

3.2 Detectors

On the detector side also a large variety of different realizations can be found. Again a major difference exists between CWFT, TDFT and FDFT. While there is no special restriction in CW operation, TDFT requires very fast and precise time-gating of the detector or single photon counting and precise time correlation between excitation and detection (so called time correlated single photon counting, TCSPC).

The most sensitive and versatile devices are certainly photomultiplier tubes (PMTs), photomultipliers with microchannel plates (MCP-PMTs) and image intensifiers based on MCPs with either optical readout on a phosphor screen or electrical readout on a multi-anode grid. Though comparatively expensive, all these variants of photomultiplier devices offer wide dynamic range and frequently also single photon counting capabilities thus enabling TDFT with TCSPC. The possible photon counting rate is primarily limited by the recovery time after arrival of one pulse which may last several ns.

Avalanche photodiodes (APDs) are also useful detectors but have some limitations: The aperture is small compared to that of PMTs, therefore yielding poorer light collection properties. As APDs exhibit a long tail in their pulse response special active quenching of the avalanche process is necessary in order to arrive at high counting rates. So called single photon avalanche photodiodes (SPADs) are able to detect single photons and most recently imaging arrays have been developed for time-resolved optical imaging with a time resolution of about 100 ps (Li et al. (2010); Niclass et al. (2004); Pavia et al. (2011)).

A very appealing but somewhat exotic detector is the streak camera which, in principle, is a PMT with an electron deflection stage and a phosphor screen. This allows to distribute narrowly spaced subsequent pulses on the screen and thus provides an unrivaled high effective counting rate. Such devices have been used in some instances for spectrally resolved

TCSPC in phase fluorometers but also to generate tomographic slice images in diffuse optical tomography (Hebden et al. (1997)).

Several research groups (e.g. Nothdurft et al. (2009); Patwardhan & Culver (2008); Soloviev et al. (2009); Zhang & Badea (2009)) are using ultrafast time-gated image intensified CCD cameras (ICCD) which allow to sample photons within 300 ps at repetition rates up to 110 MHz. Such cameras can acquire a sequence of time-delayed frames from which the time spread function can be approximately reconstructed. The time resolution is not as good as with TCSPC but the data quality is sufficient for many applications. As reported by Patwardhan & Culver (2008), the Fourier transform can then provide the equivalent frequency domain data up to modulation frequencies of more than 1 GHz.

The detectors also differ in their spectral sensitivity. While most PMTs have a high quantum efficiency at the shorter wavelengths of the visible spectrum (VIS) and even at UV they perform comparatively poorly in the NIR range, especially above 850 nm. APDs based on silicon technology are typically more sensitive in the NIR range and can be used up to 1100 nm.

Both TDFT and FDFT require special electronics after the detectors. FDFT is less demanding and uses either heterodyne or homodyne demodulation of the radio-frequency (RF) signal which can be achieved with a fast detector (e.g. PMT) and subsequent downmixing in an RF stage (for basic concepts see Chance et al. (1998)). Alternatively, the downmixing can also be accomplished directly in the detector by modulating its gain with the local oscillator frequency. This approach is the method of choice when using image intensifiers with phosphor screen because due to the afterglow they are too slow for transmitting the high frequencies. Gain modulation, however, is easily possible at the photocathode, though precautions have to be made with respect to modulation depth because many photocathodes exhibit significant heating at high frequencies due to ohmic losses. Systems operating with this concept usually apply homodyne demodulation (see e.g. Godavarty et al. (2003); Reynolds et al. (1997); Sevick-Muraca & Rasmussen (2008)). Also slow detectors in combination with an electro-optic or acousto-optic shutter can be thought of, but their poorer modulation characteristics usually precludes the use of this technique.

The design of a TSCPC circuitry is non-trivial and comprises two input stages for the reference light pulse and the sample pulse. The arrival times of the pulses are determined by a so-called constant fraction discriminators (CFD) and then passed to a time to voltage converter which is read out by a subsequent analog/digital converter. Only pulses within a certain peak height window are counted, thus excluding pulses arising from thermal emission and cosmic rays. TSCPC boards are commercially available and nowadays fairly compact, even for multidimensional TSCPC with up to 16 channels at prices in the range of several tens of k$, depending on the specification. The currently fastest commercial boards are specified with useful count rates up to 20 MHz. As in single photon counting the excitation light levels are chosen in a way that no more than 1 % of the excitation pulses lead to a detected photon, the limit is currently posed by the laser pulse repetition rate which is typically 80 MHz. The required count rate is then at least 800 000 per second, thus current TSCPC speed is more than sufficient.

Especially older tomographic systems employ PMTs or PMTs with multiple anodes, (e.g. Schmidt et al. (2000)) and fiber-optic coupling to the specimen. Also fiber-coupling and cameras as detectors was reported (Godavarty et al. (2003)). However, the coupling is a significant source of systematic errors and thus the trend goes towards so-called free-space systems without any physical contact to the sample (Schulz et al. (2004)). An early hybrid solution was reported by Graves et al. (2003) where only the excitation side was fiber-coupled. Free-space systems can still be based on single PMTs, but the light is then collected via collimators or focusing lenses at a distance of several cm from the object surface (Kepshire et al. (2009)). Most instruments, however, employ cameras together with an external or built-in image intensifier. Due to the large number of pixels available on the camera chip, the number of possible detectors is much higher than in PMT-based systems and hence the information content in the data is enhanced.

3.3 Sample holder/manipulation stages

Steering of the light beam can be achieved in different ways. The most common ones are galvanometer-controlled mirrors (galvo scanners, see e.g. Zhang et al. (2009)), movable laser diode assemblies or bundles of optically multiplexed fibers (Davis et al. (2008)). While fibers require a more or less direct coupling with the surface of the object/animal, galvo scanners and movable laser diodes provide free-space scanning. Fiber-based systems usually do not move the animal but many free-space systems employ rotational and/or linear stages to move the animal so as to image it from different sides. A recently developed free-space system (Li et al. (2009)) includes a conical mirror which partially encloses the sample and thus collects significantly more light than a camera alone or systems with flat mirrors (see e.g. Chaudhari et al. (2005) in a non-fluorescent application). The conical mirror makes a rotational stage unnecessary because light can be collected from nearly all sides of the sample at once. The excitation beam is coupled to the sample via a galvo scanner and auxiliary optics. In addition, some systems include a laser-based surface scanner in order to provide the outer boundary shape of the animal under investigation (e.g. Li et al. (2009); Zavattini et al. (2006)).

3.4 Multispectral imaging

Multi- and hyperspectral imaging can improve the depth resolution of fDOT systems due to the strong wavelength dependence of absorption and scattering properties of tissue (Zavattini et al. (2006)). *Multispectral* means the collection of several (e.g. up to 10) different wavelengths while *hyperspectral* means the acquisition at many (e.g. 100) different wavelengths (Chaudhari et al. (2005)). Also excitation spectroscopy, i.e. the use of many excitation wavelengths, has been proposed and is even considered as preferable because the dependence of the absorption coefficient on the wavelength is stronger at shorter wavelengths, i.e. on the excitation side (Chaudhari et al. (2009)). While many fDOT systems developed so far operate at more than one excitation wavelength, spectroscopic detection is still not very widespread in tomographic systems. Recent examples were published by Zavattini et al. (2006), Li et al. (2009) and Zacharakis et al. (2011). Culver et al. (2003) developed a hybrid CW/frequency domain fDOT system for breast cancer imaging. This system needs a matching fluid and coupling of 45 detector fibers to the volume under investigation. Excitation is achieved with four selectable laser diodes with the wavelengths 650, 690, 786 and 830 nm, each of which can be modulated sinusoidally at 70 MHz. Nine fibers carry light to a PMT based demodulation stage while simultaneously a transmission image is captured with a CCD camera in CW mode. Li et al. (2009) published a CW system with two excitation lasers at 650 and 785 nm. Detection is possible at 9 spectral bands, which are spaced between 680 nm to 840 nm and have a width of 20 nm, thus allowing for excitation spectroscopy. Zavattini et al. (2006)

described a CW system with one moving excitation laser at 640 nm and a CCD camera based spectrograph. The spectrograph consists of a grating and an entrance slit which allows for a spectral resolution of 3 nm. The camera provides x-λ images, i.e. spatial information along one dimension (x) and spectral information between 400 nm to 1000 nm. A translational stage allows scanning along the second spatial dimension (y). Another recently published CW system comprises a CCD camera and a Czerny-Turner spectrograph as detection unit while exciting the animal at relatively short wavelengths, i.e. the 488 and 514 nm lines of an Argon laser (Zacharakis et al. (2011)). Zhang & Badea (2011) presented an improvement of the system developed by Zhang et al. (2009), thus not only allowing for time-gated time domain acquisition but also for multi-wavelength-excitation by the introduction of a tunable Ti:sapphire laser. The tuning range from 690 to 1040 nm provides the unique possibility of time resolved excitation spectroscopy, though in Zhang & Badea (2011) still no use was made of the tuning option.

3.5 Hybrid systems: Combining high resolution modalities with fDOT

fDOT images exhibit low resolution due to the massive scattering of photons in most biological tissues. The integration of good regularizing priors based on anatomical data, provided by e.g. CT or MRI, can lead to significant improvement of the image quality (Panagiotou et al. (2009); Zhang et al. (2009)) and is mandatory when following recent trends. This motivates the development of bimodal imaging systems which combine fDOT with high-resolution methods.

A laboratory system was described in da Silva et al. (2007); Silva et al. (2009), comprising an X-ray generator and a flat panel detector as well as a krypton laser (752 nm) and a CCD camera. The sample is rotated and translated in order to form the projections. In addition, the laser beam is steered via a movable mirror. A similar concept was used by Aguirre et al. (2008), i.e. a single laser diode with 675 nm a CCD camera, an X-ray source and flat panel detector as well as a galvo scanner. In contrast to (da Silva et al. (2007)) all components were mounted on a rotating gantry with 360° angular steering range.

More recently the optical units were integrated into commercial micro-CT devices: Schulz et al. (2010) reported a hybrid fDOT-CT system, which employs a free-space CW-fDOT equipment on the rotating gantry of a micro-CT device. Two fiber-coupled laser diodes (670 and 750 nm) are used as sources, the animal is scanned with an x-y-stage. The detector is a cooled CCD camera with a 50 mm macro-lens.

Yang et al. (2010) developed an fDOT-CT dual-modality system with a flat panel detector-based micro-CT for small animals. The CW-fDOT part relies on a 748 nm diode laser and a cooled CCD camera mounted orthogonally to the micro-CT and the projection images were acquired without rotation of the sample. Similarly, Lin et al. (2010) employed an X-ray CT system with 2 lasers at 785 and 803 nm as well as a cooled CCD camera on a rotating gantry.

All these XCT-fDOT systems operate only in CW-mode.

Only a few attempts have been made so far to build hybrid devices employing MRI as the high-resolution modality. Some pioneering work was already done in the field of DOT, e.g. by Ntziachristos et al. (2000) involving a fiber-optic interface for the investigation of the human breast inside of an MRI scanner. The optical instrumentation comprised a PMT-based single-photon counting system. Masciotti et al. (2009) published an 9.4 T MRI small animal scanner with an animal coil (38 mm diameter) and a fiber-optic interface with 13 source fibers and 27 detection fibers. The system comprises two lasers at 757 and 828 nm, which can be modulated up to about 1 GHz. Homodyne demodulation is performed with a modulated ICCD. Davis et al. (2008) designed a spectroscopic CW fDOT unit, which is coupled to the animal bed inside a 3 T-MRI body scanner via fibers (8 detectors, 16 sources). The excitation laser operates at 690 nm. The animal bed is placed inside a specially designed rodent coil for MR-acquisition.

3.6 Advanced hardware concepts

As scanning time is an important issue in fDOT, reducing the required time for data acquisition is a challenging task. Wang et al. (2010) applied spatial encoding of the excitation light in order to reduce the time needed to create different excitation patterns. Several laser diodes are switched on in a particular pattern and moved in axial direction during the scanning process.

A completely different approach avoids source multiplexing completely, thus reducing hardware complexity significantly. In contrast to usual spatial encoding by various combinations of source/detector locations, only a single macro-illumination light source with a broad spectrum and a tunable excitation filter is used. The required spatial encoding is achieved by varying the excitation wavelength and exploiting the frequency-dependent sensitivity distribution inside of the target for the image reconstruction. A prototype (Klose & Pöschinger (2011)) consists of a commercial 2D-small animal imager with a white light source, a tunable filter and a cooled CCD camera. The excitation wavelength was varied in nine steps from 590 to 660 nm with a bandwidth of 10 nm per step. Fluorescence light was collected at 700 nm. The price paid for the simpler hardware setup is a more complex reconstruction algorithm which must contain a valid model of frequency-dependent light propagation in moderately absorbing tissues, which requires extensions of the popular diffusion approximation of the radiative transfer equation.

3.7 Comparison of technologies

It is intuitively clear that CW systems do not allow fluorescence lifetime imaging (FLIM) but besides it is also not possible to separately identify the absorption and scattering coefficients of the medium under investigation (Arridge & Lionheart (1998)). More sophisticated investigations thus require either the use of FDFT or TDFT. As the instrumentation is significantly less expensive and demanding for FDFT it would be desirable to contrast the two approaches in the context of information content and data quality. As mentioned, the information content is theoretically equal for both modalities when the same sources and detectors are applied and when the number of frequencies in FD corresponds to the number of time steps in TD. However, in time domain spectroscopy there are two apparent advantages from the instrumentation point of view. These are in particular: (i) Dark noise and PMT gain noise can be eliminated very effectively which is not the case for FDFT. (ii) Artifacts arising from e.g. reflections can be frequently sorted out prior to any subsequent data processing just by time-gating.

A rigorous comparison of the methods is difficult because it should include adequate noise models and cutting-edge reconstruction techniques, which exploit all the information available in the data for both modalities. Moreover, parameters like the effective aperture of the detectors, power of the light sources and effective measurement time must be taken into account for a fair comparison. One attempt was made for diffuse optical tomography (DOT) by Nissilä et al. (2006) where the authors compared the time domain system of the University College London (UCL) (Schmidt et al. (2000)) and a frequency domain system developed at Helsinki University of Technology (HUT) (Nissilä et al. (2005)). Both systems are fiber-coupled but differ in the number of source and detector positions. Both systems operate in the NIR range at very similar wavelengths, i.e. 780 and 815 nm (UCL) and 760 and 830 nm (HUT), respectively. As the HUT system operates only at one single modulation frequency of 100 MHz a comparison can only be made in the context of time harmonic image reconstruction, i.e. in terms of magnitude and phase. Considering this limitation the noise data of both systems are similar, yielding an amplitude noise of 1.7 % and 0.5 % and a phase noise of 0.2 and 0.5°, respectively at a detected light power of 1 pW. However, the laser power was different (8 mW for HUT and 40 mW for UCL) and the acquisition speed was somewhat shorter in the HUT system. The authors of the article also list some data of other frequency domain systems and show that the HUT and UCL systems, at that time, had comparatively good noise performance and could thus serve as reference systems. The analysis also comprises image reconstruction results from data generated with both systems, but only based on a frequency domain approach. Therefore, this comparison cannot be generalized because it neither takes into account the full information content of time domain data nor the specific advantages of optimized time domain reconstruction algorithms. A more rigorous and comprehensive comparison including realistic noise models and adequate solvers for all modalities is still lacking.

4. Mathematical description of light transport

Before we can discuss reconstruction methods to find the fluorophore distribution inside an object, it is necessary to describe mathematical methods to model how light spreads inside an object. Nowadays, three models are commonly used which are—with decreasing accuracy—the Monte Carlo method, the radiative transport equation and its diffusion approximation.

4.1 Random-walk Monte Carlo method

Random-walk Monte Carlo (MC) methods for solving the forward model have a rather long tradition in optics and have been implemented in different flavors. In the most simple form, the path of a single photon throughout the tissue is simulated in every run. As most of the physical processes like the change of the polarization state or the absorption of photons by electron excitation are stochastic in their nature, MC methods are well suited to model these effects. Furthermore, it is comparatively easy to incorporate tissue inhomogeneities, reflection and refraction at internal boundaries due to variations in the index of refraction, anisotropic scattering phase functions and so on.

The drawback of MC methods is their slow convergence which is proportional to the square root of the number of runs. In order to achieve reliable results for three dimensional objects, it is often necessary to simulate the propagation of millions of photons. The convergence is also poor when a certain physical process has a very low probability, say it occurs only once in one thousand trials.

A series of strategies for speeding up the simulations has been developed, for example, simulating photon packets rather than individual particles (Wang et al. (1995)) and running photons in parallel using modern graphics hardware (Fang & Boas (2009)). Still, the comparatively high computational effort limits the applicability of Monte Carlo methods for reconstructing fluorophore properties.

4.2 Transport equation

A deterministic solution for light propagation can be found in Boltzmann's transport equation which is also frequently called the *radiative transport equation* (RTE). Rather than modeling each particle independently, which can be done with Monte Carlo methods, the RTE deals with an ensemble of photons in an infinitesimal volume. To be more precise, the RTE is a balance equation for the number of photons per unit volume (i.e. the photon density) $\Phi(\vec{x}, \hat{s}, t)$ at a spatial location $\vec{x}$ traveling into an infinitesimal solid angle around a direction $\hat{s}$ at a time instance t. The transport equation reads

$$\frac{1}{v}\frac{\partial \Phi(\vec{x}, \hat{s}, t)}{\partial t} + \hat{s} \cdot \nabla \Phi(\vec{x}, \hat{s}, t) + (\mu_a(\vec{x}) + \mu_s(\vec{x}))\, \Phi(\vec{x}, \hat{s}, t) = q_{int}(\vec{x}, \hat{s}, t) + \mu_s(\vec{x}) \int_{S^2} \Theta(\hat{s}', \hat{s}) \Phi(\vec{x}, \hat{s}', t)\, d\hat{s}' \qquad \text{in } \Omega, \qquad (1)$$

together with the boundary condition

$$\Phi(\vec{x}, \hat{s}, t) = q_{bc}(\vec{x}, \hat{s}, t) \qquad \forall \hat{s} : \hat{s} \cdot \hat{n} < 0 \qquad \text{on } \Gamma, \qquad (2)$$

where v is the speed of light in the tissue, μ_a and μ_s are the absorption and scattering coefficients, respectively, and $\Theta(\hat{s}', \hat{s})$ is the scattering phase function which states the probability that a photon traveling in direction $\hat{s}'$ will be deflected into direction $\hat{s}$. In this equation, S^2 is the surface of the unit sphere and thus the integral is taken over all possible directions. The term q_{int} models sources inside the domain.

The left-hand side of equation (1) models the decrease in photon density due to movement and absorption, while the right-hand side incorporates the photon gain caused by scattering and an internal source.

The boundary condition imposes restrictions on the solution only for inward-pointing directions, i.e. for all $\hat{s}$ with $\hat{s} \cdot \hat{n} < 0$ where $\hat{n}$ is the outward-pointing unit normal of the domain. It states that no light can enter the domain from the outside except at locations where a boundary source is present, i.e. where $q_{bc}(\vec{x}, \hat{s}, t) \neq 0$.

A limitation of the transport equation is that it cannot handle wave effects. As a consequence, the wavelength of the light must be much smaller than the dimensions of the structures in the domain (Gibson et al. (2005)). Furthermore, varying indices of refraction are not included in equation (1) but can be incorporated.

Despite these insufficiencies, the transport equation would be well suited for biomedical optics. It is able to handle many different types of tissue whether they are highly scattering like muscle, as absorbing as the liver or as transparent as liquor, for example. Furthermore, the boundary equation is physically meaningful.

The reason why the RTE is frequently avoided is the high computational effort required for calculating an accurate solution. The photon density $\Phi(\vec{x}, \hat{s}, t)$ has to be discretised in the spatial and angular domain which requires five variables for a 3D problem (three coordinates and two angles). If too little angular directions are chosen for the discretisation, the resultant photon field favors propagation along these directions resulting in star-like patterns, where one would expect a radial symmetric distribution instead. To illustrate the influence of the angular discretisation on the computational effort, imagine a rather coarse discretisation of only 32 divisions for both the azimuth and the inclination. This results in 1024 angular directions, which have to be multiplied by the number of mesh points used for the spatial discretisation.

4.3 Diffusion approximation

Due to the shortcomings of the previously mentioned models, the most common description for photon migration is the diffusion approximation. This is a reduced form of the RTE which first expands the direction-dependent quantities Φ, Θ, q_{int} and q_{bc} into spherical harmonics. Then, all spherical harmonics except the first one are neglected, i.e. only the isotropic propagation of photons is considered. Some additional constraints are imposed on the photon flux and the scattering phase function Θ. A thorough derivation is found in the review article by Arridge (1999). The model is valid in the regime where photon propagation is diffuse, which is the case in tissues which are much more scattering than absorbing, at a sufficient distance from the source. Problems arise if the tissue is either strongly absorbing such as in the liver or nearly transparent as in liquor. Furthermore, the model is inaccurate near the light source, where the photon propagation is not yet diffuse due to the small number of scattering events, and at places where the optical properties jump which might be the case at the boundary of organs, for example (Gibson et al. (2005)).

In its frequency domain form, the diffusion approximation is a partial differential equation (PDE) which reads

$$-\nabla \cdot (\kappa(\vec{x})\nabla\varphi(\vec{x})) + \left(\mu_a(\vec{x}) + \frac{i\omega}{\nu}\right)\varphi(\vec{x}) = q_{int}(\vec{x}), \qquad \text{in } \Omega, \tag{3}$$

$$\varrho\varphi(\vec{x}) + \kappa(\vec{x})\hat{n}\cdot\nabla\varphi(\vec{x}) = \begin{cases} \varrho\, q_{bc}(\vec{x}), & \text{on } \Gamma_{bc}, \\ 0, & \text{on } \Gamma \setminus \Gamma_{bc}, \end{cases} \tag{4}$$

where φ is the fluence, $\kappa = \left(3\left(\mu_s' + \mu_a\right)\right)^{-1}$ the diffusion coefficient of the tissue, μ_s' the reduced scattering coefficient and μ_a the absorption coefficient. ω is the modulation frequency of the excitation light source with the special case of $\omega = 0\,\text{s}^{-1}$ for CW excitation with a constant intensity. The injected light can be modeled by an internal source q_{int} ,which is frequently used for collimated beams, or a boundary source q_{bc}, which is suitable for spatially extended sources on a part Γ_{bc} of the boundary Γ. ϱ is a reflection coefficient to incorporate the reflections at the boundary Γ of the domain Ω due to the differences in the indices of reflection.

4.4 Diffusion approximation for fDOT

For fDOT, the diffusion approximation has to be extended as now two different photon distributions with different wavelengths have to be simulated: (i) excitation light due to the illumination of the sample and (ii) emission light which has been generated by a fluorophore inside the sample by conversion from the excitation wavelength. As the optical parameters of tissue vary with the chosen wavelength, we distinguish them by sub-scripts x and m for excitation and emission, respectively. Furthermore, these coefficients have to depend on the

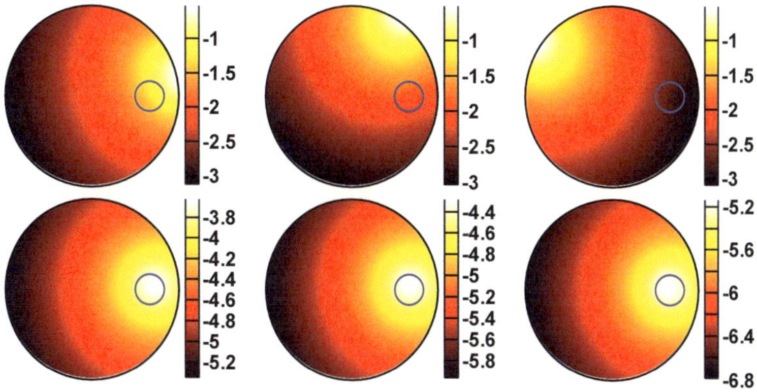

Fig. 3. Simulation of the fluences $\varphi_x(\vec{x})$ (top row) and $\varphi_m(\vec{x})$ (bottom row) due to three different boundary sources positioned at angles of 11.25° (left), 56.25° (middle) and 146.25° (right). The color encodes the logarithm of the amplitude of the photon densities.

fluorophore concentration $c(\vec{x})$ which one seeks to reconstruct from measurements in a known manner. If the concentration is fairly small, it can be seen as an additional absorber and the effective absorption coefficients can be written in the form

$$\mu_x(\vec{x}) := \mu_{a,0,x}(\vec{x}) + \epsilon_x\, c(\vec{x}) + \frac{i\omega}{\nu} \quad \text{and} \tag{5}$$

$$\mu_m(\vec{x}) := \mu_{a,0,m}(\vec{x}) + \epsilon_m\, c(\vec{x}) + \frac{i\omega}{\nu}, \tag{6}$$

where $\mu_{a,0,i}$, $i \in \{x, m\}$, is the background absorption of the tissue in the absence of fluorescent agent and ϵ_x, ϵ_m are the molar extinction coefficients which relate the fluorophore's concentration to its absorption coefficients. With these definitions the diffusion approximation for fDOT can be written as a two-state model (Sevick-Muraca et al. (2003)):

$$-\nabla \cdot (\kappa_x(\vec{x})\nabla\varphi_x(\vec{x})) + \mu_x(\vec{x})\varphi_x(\vec{x}) = q_{int}(\vec{x}), \qquad \text{in } \Omega, \tag{7}$$

$$-\nabla \cdot (\kappa_m(\vec{x})\nabla\varphi_m(\vec{x})) + \mu_m(\vec{x})\varphi_m(\vec{x}) = \frac{\eta}{1+i\omega\tau}\epsilon_x\, c(\vec{x})\varphi_x(\vec{x}), \qquad \text{in } \Omega, \tag{8}$$

with the boundary conditions

$$\varrho_x\varphi_x(\vec{x}) + \kappa_x(\vec{x})\hat{n}\cdot\nabla\varphi_x(\vec{x}) = \begin{cases} \varrho_x q_{bc}(\vec{x}), & \text{on } \Gamma_{bc}, \\ 0, & \text{on } \Gamma \setminus \Gamma_{bc}, \end{cases} \tag{9}$$

$$\varrho_m\varphi_m(\vec{x}) + \kappa_m(\vec{x})\hat{n}\cdot\nabla\varphi_m(\vec{x}) = 0, \qquad \text{on } \Gamma. \tag{10}$$

The conversion efficiency of the fluorophore is denoted by the constant η and its fluorescent lifetime by τ. A typical simulation result is depicted in Figure 3.

The measurement data is gathered by illuminating the sample with differently positioned light sources and recording the photons leaving the boundary. The simplest type of measurement is to record the photons leaving the boundary at a certain location, i.e. to integrate the photon flux over a detector area χ:

$$-\int_\Gamma \kappa_m(\vec{x})\hat{n}\cdot\nabla\varphi_m(\vec{x})\chi(\vec{x})\,d\vec{x} \stackrel{(10)}{=} \varrho_m \int_\Gamma \varphi_m(\vec{x})\chi(\vec{x})\,d\vec{x}. \tag{11}$$

The detector function χ can also incorporate linear transfer characteristics of the system such as a weighting due to an oblique viewing angle when using a camera. Other types of measurements based on the logarithm of the intensity, for example, have been reported in e.g. Arridge (1995); Arridge & Schweiger (1993); Sevick & Chance (1991).

As for a tomographic measurement N_s light sources and N_d detectors are used, the data can be written in a matrix $\mathcal{M}$ of size $N_d \times N_s$. The emission field φ_m depends on the fluorophore concentration c, which makes the measurement matrix dependent on c and we write $\mathcal{M}(c)$ to emphasize this fact.

5. Image reconstruction

The aim of fluorescence tomography is to reconstruct the fluorophore concentration and/or the fluorophore's lifetime inside a 3D object from intensity measurements performed on the object's boundary. In the previous section, methods have been described to simulate the photon propagation inside an object, where the tissue and fluorophore properties are known exactly. This is called the *direct* or *forward problem*. The estimation of the fluorophore distribution from measurement data is known as the *inverse problem* of fluorescence tomography. An overview about the whole reconstruction process is displayed in Figure 4. In the following, more details will be provided for solving this problem. For the sake of simplicity, the focus is put on FDFT-systems, whose mathematics is easier to grasp. Furthermore, one can Fourier-transform time domain data and apply FDFT-algorithms. Last but not least, CW-reconstructions are a special case of FDFT-reconstructions with a modulation frequency of $\omega = 0\,\mathrm{s}^{-1}$.

Mathematically the problem can be formulated as follows: Let $\mathcal{M}^\delta$ denote a light measurement taken at the object's surface, which is usually perturbed by noise bounded by δ coming from different origins, e.g. detector noise, discretisation errors and modeling errors. Then, one seeks to find a fluorophore concentration c such that the data mismatch $\left\|\mathcal{M}(c) - \mathcal{M}^\delta\right\|^2$ is minimized.

5.1 Ill-posedness of the inverse problem

Fiber-coupled fDOT systems usually result in a limited amount of data. Configurations with approximately 16 sources and 16 detectors are common which gives a set of 256 measurements. The inverse problem is under-determined in this case: there is much less measurement data than the number of voxels (typically in the order of ten-thousands) in which we would like to compute the fluorophore concentration.

The situation is different for the free-space arrangement. The camera can take images of the whole surface (which depends quadratically on the object's dimension d). If also the excitation beam can be positioned everywhere at the surface, one would get measurement combinations in the order of $d^2 \times d^2 = d^4$ but needs to reconstruct only d^3 voxels. In this case more measurement data is available than there are unknown parameters and the problem is said to be over-determined.

However, we cannot expect to reconstruct high-resolution images similar to CT from fluorescence tomography data. In CT the X-ray beams pass the object under investigation in nearly straight lines as illustrated in Figure 5(a). If the X-ray hits an absorbing object (the small

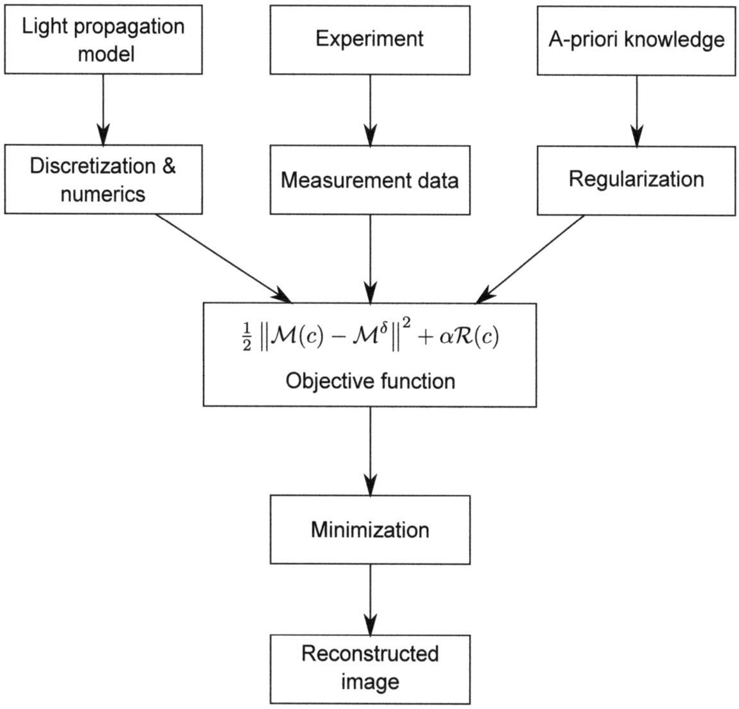

Fig. 4. Typical image reconstruction process: With the help of appropriately discretized mathematical models the simulated measurement data $\mathcal{M}(c)$ is computed. The simulated measurements have to be close to the true data $\mathcal{M}^{\delta}$ gathered from experiments. A regularization term $\mathcal{R}(c)$ has to be created from a-priori knowledge, which is needed to stabilize the algorithm. Finally, the image is reconstructed by minimizing the sum of the data mismatch and the penalty term.

ball), it is partly absorbed which casts a "shadow" in the recorded intensity projection I. In fDOT the photons are massively scattered and spread throughout the whole object. Figure 5(b) shows the distribution of the light emitted by a fluorescent ball when a small part of the surface at the top is illuminated with light. A camera looking at the object's bottom records a much more diffuse light intensity pattern compared to the CT detector. The interface between the fluorescent object and the background cannot be determined from these measurements directly.

An important quantity for the solution of the inverse problem is the so-called *sensitivity*. It measures the influence of a change in an image voxel onto a detector datum. This concept is illustrated for CT and fDOT in Figure 6: The sensitive area of an X-ray beam which is generated by a source S and detected by D consists of all voxels along the line which the X-ray passes. Analogously, an fDOT measurement is sensitive in that region which photons generated by the source S and recorded by the detector D traverse. Due to the massive scattering, the resulting fDOT sensitivity profile is much broader than the one from CT. In other words, a single fDOT measurement incorporates information from nearly the whole sample volume, while a CT datum only measures along a line.

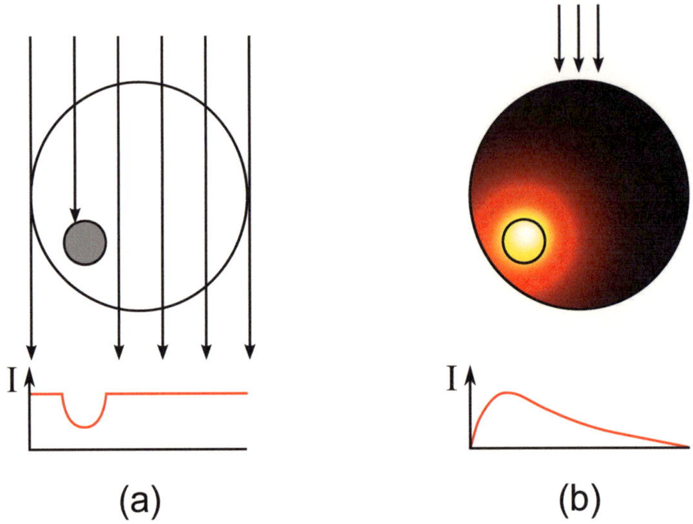

Fig. 5. Comparison between CT (a) and fDOT (b). In a CT system the X-ray beams pass the sample in nearly straight lines. The intensity *I* decreases if an absorbing object is encountered resulting in a "shadow" projection. In fDOT the emission light (shown in color) spreads throughout the sample although the surface is excited at a very small patch only. The intensity profile which a camera would record from the bottom is much more diffuse than the CT projection.

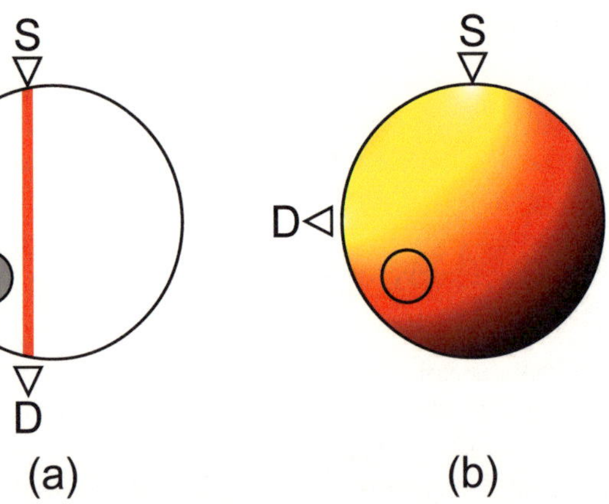

Fig. 6. Sensitivity profile for a single CT- and fDOT-measurement. (a) The voxels to which a CT measurement is sensitive lie along the line which the X-ray beam passes. (b) The photons in fDOT have a much larger coverage than an X-ray beam which leads to a broadening of the sensitivity profile.

An elegant way to compute the sensitivity mathematically is through the use of *adjoint* fields. These fields are generated by formally treating the detectors as sources which generate an adjoint photon distribution. The adjoint field is a spatially resolved measure for the detection efficiency of a sensor. The sensitivity at a certain position in the sample is then the product of the forward field (the photon distribution due to the light source) times the adjoint field (the distribution of the photon collection efficiency). It is highest at locations which are reached by many photons from the source and from which many photons are collected by the detector *at the same time.*

The adjoint system to the forward system (7)–(10) is another system of PDEs which reads

$$-\nabla \cdot (\kappa_m(\vec{x})\nabla\psi_m(\vec{x})) + \overline{\mu}_m(\vec{x})\psi_m(\vec{x}) = 0 \qquad \text{in } \Omega \tag{12}$$

$$-\nabla \cdot (\kappa_x(\vec{x})\nabla\psi_x(\vec{x})) + \overline{\mu}_x(\vec{x})\psi_x = \frac{\eta}{1-i\omega\tau}\epsilon_x\, c(\vec{x})\psi_m(\vec{x}) \qquad \text{in } \Omega \tag{13}$$

$$\varrho_m\psi_m(\vec{x}) + \kappa_m(\vec{x})\hat{n}\cdot\nabla\psi_m(\vec{x}) = \varrho_m\chi(\vec{x}) \qquad \text{on } \Gamma \tag{14}$$

$$\varrho_x\psi_x(\vec{x}) + \kappa_x(\vec{x})\hat{n}\cdot\nabla\psi_x(\vec{x}) = 0 \qquad \text{on } \Gamma. \tag{15}$$

The sensitivity of the ij-th measurement around c into direction h is given by

$$\begin{aligned}\mathcal{M}'_{ij}(c)h &:= \lim_{h\to 0}\frac{\mathcal{M}_{ij}(c+h)-\mathcal{M}_{ij}(c)}{\|h\|}\\ &= -\int_\Omega \kappa'_x h\,\nabla\varphi_x(q_j)\cdot\nabla\overline{\psi}_x(\chi_i)\,d\vec{x} - \int_\Omega \mu'_x h\,\varphi_x(q_j)\overline{\psi}_x(\chi_i)\,d\vec{x}\\ &\quad -\int_\Omega \kappa'_m h\,\nabla\varphi_m(q_j)\cdot\nabla\overline{\psi}_m(\chi_i)\,d\vec{x} - \int_\Omega \mu'_m h\,\varphi_m(q_j)\overline{\psi}_m(\chi_i)\,d\vec{x}\\ &\quad + \frac{\eta}{1+i\omega\tau}\epsilon_x\int_\Omega h\,\varphi_x(q_j)\overline{\psi}_m(\chi_i)\,d\vec{x}.\end{aligned} \tag{16}$$

In this equation, we used the notation $\varphi(q_j)$ and $\varphi(\chi_i)$ to emphasize the dependencies of the forward field on the excitation source q_j and the adjoint field on the detector χ_i, respectively.

When solving the inverse problem, one seeks to reconstruct the parameters in the sensitive area from the measurement data. Looking at Figure 6, it is intuitively clear that this task is much easier for CT, where one can simply distribute a measurement datum back along the line which the X-ray beam passed, than for fDOT, where every recording has to be distributed in the whole sample. This lack of information is valid for both fiber-based and free-space arrangements. The reconstruction problem is said to be *ill-posed*.

5.2 The role of prior information

To deal with the ill-posedness of the inverse problem, additional knowledge has to be incorporated into the reconstruction algorithm which is known as *regularization*. This means that unphysical or undesired images are penalized while images featuring certain characteristics are favored. Using regularization terms of Tikhonov-type, one can state the image reconstruction as an optimization problem, where one seeks to minimize the functional

$$\mathcal{L}_\alpha(c) := \tfrac{1}{2}\left\|\mathcal{M}(c)-\mathcal{M}^\delta\right\|^2 + \alpha\mathcal{R}(c). \tag{17}$$

In this equation, $\mathcal{R}(c)$ is a penalty for unwanted fluorophore distributions. With the parameter α it is possible to adjust between sticking to the data ($\alpha = 0$, which means no regularization at all) and reconstructing a concentration according to the prior information ($\alpha \to \infty$, which means that the simulated and the measured data can diverge arbitrarily). As the problem (17) is non-linear, one can choose e.g. Newton methods to solve it. If the Hessian (i.e. the second derivatives of the forward operator $\mathcal{M}(c)$) is neglected, one can write the iterations in the form

$$\mathrm{Re}\left\{\mathcal{M}'^{*}(c_k)\mathcal{M}'(c_k) + \alpha_k \widetilde{\mathcal{R}}''(c_k)\right\}\Delta c_k = \mathrm{Re}\left\{\mathcal{M}'^{*}(c_k)\left(\mathcal{M}^{\delta} - \mathcal{M}(c_k)\right) - \alpha_k \mathcal{R}'(c_k)\right\}, \quad (18)$$

where the parameter α can vary in every iteration. This is known as the iteratively regularized Gauß-Newton algorithm and is treated in detail elsewhere (Bakushinskiĭ (1992); Blaschke et al. (1997); Engl et al. (1996)). In this context, $\mathcal{M}'^{*}$ means the adjoint of the sensitivity operator $\mathcal{M}'$ and its exact meaning depends on the chosen discretisation. $\mathcal{R}'(c_k)$ and $\widetilde{\mathcal{R}}''(c_k)$ are the first and approximated second derivatives of the regularization term evaluated for the current concentration c_k. Besides the Gauß-Newton method, other algorithms are available such as the Levenberg-Marquardt method (Marquardt (1963)), the Newton-Landweber method (Kaltenbacher (1997)) and the truncated Newton-CG method (Hanke (1997)). Applications to the field of optical tomography are e.g. Egger & Schlottbom (2011); Jiang (1998); Joshi et al. (2004); Roy & Sevick-Muraca (1999); Schweiger et al. (2005). A good overview of reconstruction methods applied to fluorescence tomography is given by Sevick-Muraca et al. (2003).

Unfortunately, there is no one-size-fits-all-type regularization method. Instead, $\mathcal{R}(c)$ has to be chosen with respect to the application and the expected outcome. In the following, typical regularization methods are discussed.

5.2.1 Quadratic regularization terms

The probably most often used regularization term is the L^2-norm of the concentration, which is a penalty for large concentrations such as outliers. Thus, smaller values for the concentration in the whole domain are preferred. The dominance of this particular regularization term in many engineering applications is most likely not not due to its physical meaning but rather due to its simplicity and speed, both in implementation and evaluation. If we denote the identity operator with I, the regularization term and its derivatives can be written as

$$\mathcal{R}(c) = \tfrac{1}{2}\|c\|^2, \qquad \mathcal{R}'(c) = c, \qquad \mathcal{R}''(c) = I. \quad (19)$$

If one can provide an a-priori guess c_0 for the fluorophore distribution, it is advantageous to penalize the difference between the prior guess and the current concentration, i.e. to use a regularization term of the form

$$\mathcal{R}(c) = \tfrac{1}{2}\|c - c_0\|^2. \quad (20)$$

Another quadratic regularization term is based on the H^1-semi-norm instead of the L^2-norm. This semi-norm does not penalize higher concentration values but it penalizes variations in the reconstructed fluorophore distribution and thus enforces the resultant images to be smooth. From a physical point of view, this is most often more meaningful than to suppress outliers. The regularization functional is defined as

$$\mathcal{R}(c) = \tfrac{1}{2}\|\nabla c\|^2, \qquad \mathcal{R}'(c)h = \langle \nabla c, \nabla h \rangle, \qquad \langle \mathcal{R}''(c)h_1, h_2 \rangle = \langle \nabla h_1, \nabla h_2 \rangle . \tag{21}$$

5.2.2 Total-variation regularization

Although the H^1-semi-norm is physically meaningful, it faces the problem that large gradients of the fluorophore concentration are still penalized which prevents steep transitions (jumps) from an object to the background. However, if one knows a-priori that the fluorophore is well localized (e.g. inside a localized tumor) and piecewise constant, the total-variation (TV) regularization might be an option. Although this method also measures the gradient of the reconstructed image, it uses an L^1-norm rather than the L^2-norm for penalization:

$$\mathrm{TV}(c) := \int_\Omega |\nabla c(\vec{x})| \, d\vec{x}. \tag{22}$$

Using the L^1-norm, the penalty grows linearly with the gradient (instead of quadratically), i.e. larger gradients are allowed to some extent.

Unfortunately, the TV functional is not differentiable at points where $\nabla c(\vec{x}) = 0$. A possible mitigation is to use a relaxation as suggested by Acar & Vogel (1994) which reads

$$\mathcal{R}(c) = \int_\Omega \sqrt{\beta + |\nabla c(\vec{x})|^2} d\vec{x}, \qquad \mathcal{R}'(c)h = \int_\Omega \frac{\nabla c(\vec{x}) \cdot \nabla h(\vec{x})}{\sqrt{\beta + |\nabla c(\vec{x})|^2}} \, d\vec{x},$$

$$\left\langle \widetilde{\mathcal{R}}''(c)h_1, h_2 \right\rangle = \int_\Omega \frac{\nabla h_1(\vec{x}) \cdot \nabla h_2(\vec{x})}{\sqrt{\beta + |\nabla c(\vec{x})|^2}} \, d\vec{x} \tag{23}$$

where a scalar $\beta > 0$ has been introduced to smooth the square-root around the origin. Note also that $\widetilde{\mathcal{R}}''$ is just an approximation of the true Hessian, because the derivative of the denominator has been neglected.

5.2.3 Level-set method

Another possibility of regularization is through the use of level-set methods, which have been used for diffuse optical tomography (Alvarez et al. (2009); Schweiger et al. (2008)). The principle is that if the background fluorescence and the fluorescence inside and object are constant, the reconstruction problem reduces to finding the interface which separates the inclusions from the background. This interface can be described using level-set methods: The level-set function $\phi(\vec{x}), \vec{x} \in \Omega$ is negative inside the inclusion and positive outside. Thus, the separating interface consists of all points where the level-set function is zero, i.e. it is the zero-level set $\{\vec{x} : \phi(\vec{x}) = 0\}$. Applying the Heaviside function

$$H(z) := \begin{cases} 1, & z \geq 0, \\ 0, & \text{else}, \end{cases} \tag{24}$$

one can express the concentration distribution as the sum

$$c(\vec{x}) = c_{in} + H(\phi(\vec{x}))(c_{out} - c_{in}), \tag{25}$$

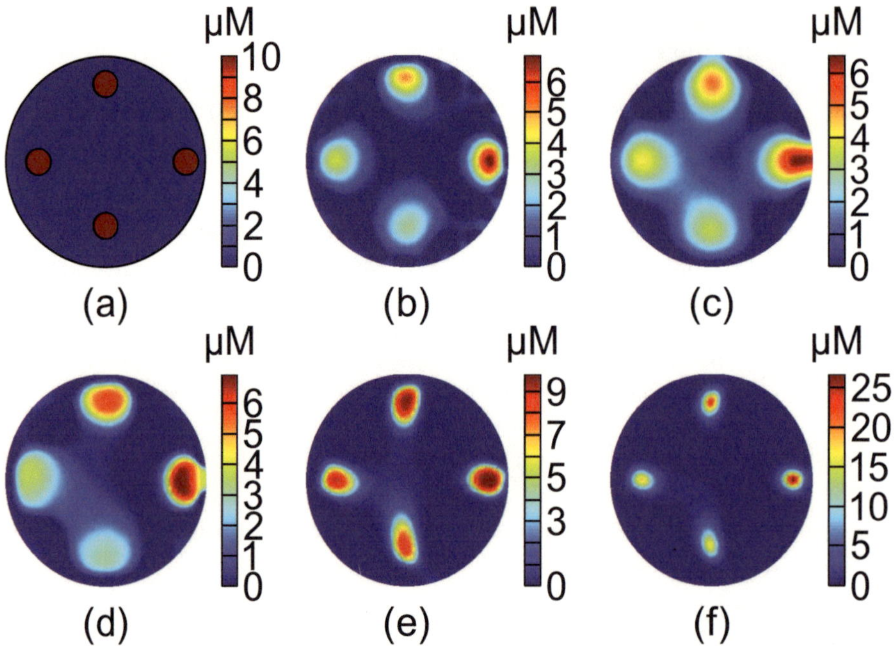

Fig. 7. Comparison of reconstructions of (a) four fluorescent objects with a concentration of 10 μM each. The reconstructions are based on (b) the L^2-norm, (c) the H^1-norm (d) the total-variation. Also the results from a method of level-set type with $c_{out} = 10\,\mu\text{M}$ are presented with two different levels for the concentration inside the object: (e) $c_{in} = 10\,\mu\text{M}$ and (f) $c_{in} = 50\,\mu\text{M}$.

where c_{out} and c_{in} are the two scalar fluorophore concentrations in the background and inside the inclusion.

Unfortunately, the numerical effort for the computation of the evolution of the level-set function is comparatively high. The reason is again the non-differentiability of the Heaviside function. A mitigation has been studied as a *method of level-set type* in Frühauf et al. (2005) and Egger & Leittão (2009). The idea is to parametrize the concentration c by a nonlinear, smooth, monotonically increasing function $H_\beta(\phi)$ and to reconstruct the level-set function ϕ which is done by minimizing the objective function

$$\mathcal{L}_\alpha^\phi = \tfrac{1}{2}\|F(H_\beta(\phi))\|^2 + \alpha\mathcal{R}(\phi). \tag{26}$$

One possible parametrization is by using the error function such that the approximated Heaviside reads

$$H_\beta(z) := \frac{c_{in} + c_{out}}{2} + \frac{c_{in} - c_{out}}{2}\,\mathrm{erf}\left(\frac{z}{\beta}\right). \tag{27}$$

This parametrization restricts the concentration by the lower and upper bounds c_{out} and c_{in}, respectively, but still allows values in between. Furthermore, it has a smooth derivative which is useful for the Gauß-Newton algorithm.

Example reconstructions using the different kinds of regularization methods, which have been presented in this chapter, are shown in Figure 7.

5.2.4 Multi-modality regularization

When combining fDOT with a high-resolution modality such as CT or MRI, it is advantageous to use information from the highly resolved anatomical images to improve the quality of fDOT-reconstructions. In the following, some attempts for incorporating this information are listed.

In the work by Davis et al. (2007), the anatomical images were segmented and the regularization term $\mathcal{R}(c)$ was constructed such that it allows larger variations between voxels from different segments but keeps variations between voxels from the same segment small.

Although only applied to DOT, Douiri et al. (2007) used a-priori edge information (which could be obtained from CT, for example) together with an anisotropic diffusion model which preserves sharp edges in the reconstructed optical properties. This method could also be extended to fDOT to constrain the leakage of fluorescent agent in the reconstruction across anatomical boundaries.

Another approach, which uses segmented images from a high-resolution modality like MRI or CT, was presented by Hyde et al. (2010). Their algorithm first uses only one fluorescence concentration for each segment (thus reducing the dimension of the reconstruction problem) and creates a spatially-varying regularization matrix from the low-dimensional reconstruction in a second step.

5.3 Regularisation parameter and stopping criterion

The choice of the regularization parameter α in equation (17) has attracted quite some interest. The basic problem is that this parameter balances the *goodness of fit*, i.e. how well the mathematical model approximates the measured data, and the stability of the inversion. For the iteratively regularized Gauß-Newton algorithm, typically exponentially decaying sequences are suggested (Blaschke et al. (1997); Engl et al. (1996)).

Another problem is the stopping criterion for the iterative reconstruction. Most often these criteria are implemented using heuristics. For example, one can set a lower limit for the regularization parameter or stop if stagnation occurs and the residual no longer changes as done by Dehghani et al. (2008). Note that for the latter approach a good choice for the step length is mandatory. Otherwise, the residual will decrease very slowly which triggers the stopping criterion even when no (local) minimum of the objective functional has been reached.

An objective stopping criterion is given by Morozov's discrepancy principle (Morozov (1966)). It states that the residual shall not be smaller than the error in the measurement. Thus, if the true measurement without any noise is denoted as $\mathcal{M}$, α should be chosen such that

$$\|\mathcal{M}(c_\alpha) - \mathcal{M}^\delta\| \approx \|\mathcal{M} - \mathcal{M}^\delta\|, \tag{28}$$

where c_α denotes the reconstructed fluorophore distribution with regularization parameter α. In other words, the difference between the simulated measurement and the noisy data should be approximately the same as the difference between the (inaccessible) measurement values and the noisy data. Unfortunately, the expression on the right-hand side cannot be evaluated in practice as the true measurements $\mathcal{M}$ are not known. Thus, one has to deduce this quantity by other means based on the distribution of the noise, for example.

6. Recent developments for pre-clinical and clinical applications

2D fluorescence imaging in pre-clinical sciences is a well-established technology. In this section, we would like to give an overview about applications of truly three-dimensional fluorescence imaging. There are many publications showing the potential of fDOT in phantoms or ex-vivo while the number of in-vivo studies is still very limited. However, as in-vivo molecular imaging is probably the most attractive future field of application, this subchapter summarizes some important in-vivo results.

From the technological point of view, we can observe two major groups of applications, the first of which serves for the non-quantitative visualization of molecular or cellular processes, mostly evaluating quantum yield data. The second group tackles the more challenging field of quantitative imaging, frequently exploiting both quantum yield and fluorescence lifetime imaging (FLIM). The reconstruction of the fluorescence lifetime is of particular interest because it yields more reliable information about the chemical interaction of the probe with its environment than the fluorophore's quantum efficiency (Lakowicz (2006)).

In the first group we find e.g. the use of a cathepsin-activatable fluorescence probe by Niedre et al. (2008) to monitor a mouse lung tumor and by Haller et al. (2008) for the visualization of pulmonary inflammation. Another example is the visualization of macrophage infiltration of infarcted mycardium in a mouse model by Sosnovik et al. (2007), who compared MRI, planar fluorescence imaging and fluorescence tomography. Kozloff et al. (2007) investigated the feasibility of localizing bone mineralization/demineralization processes with a specific fluorescent probe in mice. So-called far-red fluorescent pamidronate (FRFP) was proven to specifically bind to bone mineral sites and fDOT images made with a commercial system enabled the visualization of deep mineralizing structures including the growth plates in the femoral heads. Biswal et al. (2011) developed a 2-nitroimidazole-ICG probe for monitoring tumor hypoxia and present images of tumors of sizes of a few millimeter, however, without assessing the accuracy of the tumor location and size in the reconstructions. Tan et al. (n.d.) used fluorescence tomography to monitor stem cells in Drosophila Pupae by the expression of a DsRed reporter.

In the second group (FLIM) we find a paper by Nothdurft et al. (2009) who were the first to show in-vivo life-time tomography on mice, where they imaged agarose gel implants as well as a cypate-labeled tumor. Gaind et al. (2010) showed the feasibility of reconstructing fluorescence resonance energy transfer (FRET) parameters, including the nanometer donor-acceptor distance, also from deep tissue regions in a mouse. 3D-studies of inter- and intra-molecular FRET could be of high importance for the investigation of diseases like Alzheimer's and some cancers related to protein misfolding. McGinty et al. (2011) presented FLIM in combination with Förster resonance energy transfer (FRET). In their experiment, a mouse genetically expressed a eGFP-mCherry-FRET probe.

So far there are only very few attempts to apply fluorescence tomography in human applications. The main reasons are certainly (i) the limited penetration depth of light in tissue which precludes the application of fDOT in extended parts of the body and (ii) the lack of approval for human use of most fluorescent labels known in molecular imaging. Corlu et al. (2007) presented a proof-of-concept study utilizing fluorescence tomography for detecting breast cancer in women using ICG as fluorescent agent. An interesting recent application for breast cancer imaging was reported by Mastanduno et al. (2011). The authors combined breast DCE-MRI, diffuse optical tomography and fDOT for imaging nine healthy volunteers and one patient with breast cancer. fDOT was used for the reconstruction of autofluorescence from protoporphyrine IX, thus no extrinsic labeling agents were applied. The results, though lacking statistical power, suggest that combined application of all three modalities may provide improved information on malignancy when compared with DCE-MRI alone.

7. Trends and outlook

In this chapter, we addressed hardware-issues and reconstruction principles for fluorescence tomography and presented promising applications especially for pre-clinical sciences.

In the near future, we expect that more compact fluorescence tomography hardware will be developed e.g. through the replacement of photomultiplier tubes by silicon APDs. Another development will focus on hybrid devices such as fDOT/CT and fDOT/MRI combinations to use all the information from different modalities.

The reconstruction algorithms will on the one hand follow the hardware development, i.e. reliable strategies for the incorporation of a-priori information from CT and MRI into fDOT-images will be needed. On the other hand, the recent developments in commodity parallel computing architectures, such as modern graphics hardware with NVIDIA's CUDA toolkit or the OpenCL framework, will certainly aid the implementation of advanced algorithms including e.g. non-linear image regularization.

fDOT so far appears difficult to be used for human imaging. However, if autofluorescence could be used for producing diagnostically relevant contrasts, some niche-applications may arise. A recent example is the work by Mastanduno et al. (2011) which may open a new application window in breast imaging. Another important decisive issue is whether new fluorescent contrast agents will be approved for the use in humans.

In the field of pre-clinical imaging fDOT has been demonstrated to be feasible and the availability of commercial devices will certainly increase its use and importance. Current challenges are quantification and 3D lifetime imaging. As FLIM paves the way for 3D sensing of chemical analytes, this could be a new attractive field of research. Some pioneering work was already done by Shives et al. (2002) who showed the feasibility of FLIM-based oxygen sensing in-vitro and there is certainly potential for future developments towards in-vivo applications.

8. References

Acar, R. & Vogel, C. R. (1994). Analysis of bounded variation penalty methods for ill-posed problems, *Inv. Probl.* 10: 1217–1229.

Aguirre, J., Sisniega, A., Ripoll, J., Desco, M. & Vaquero, J. J. (2008). Design and development of a co-planar fluorescence and x–ray tomograph, *IEEE Nuclear Science Symposium Conference Record*, IEEE, pp. 5412–5413.

Alvarez, D., Medina, P. & Moscoso, M. (2009). Fluorescence lifetime imaging from time resolved measurements using a shape-based approach, *Opt. Express* 17: 8843–8855.

Arridge, S. R. (1995). Photon-measurement density functions. part I: Analytical forms, *Appl. Opt.* 34(31): 7395–7409.

Arridge, S. R. (1999). Optical tomography in medical imaging, *Inv. Probl.* 15: R41–R93.

Arridge, S. R. & Lionheart, W. R. B. (1998). Non–uniqueness in diffusion–based optical tomography, *Opt. Lett.* 23: 882–884.

Arridge, S. R. & Schweiger, M. (1993). The use of multiple data types in time-resolved optical absorption and scattering tomography (TOAST), *in* D. C. Wilson & J. N. Wilson (eds), *Mathematical Methods in Medical Imaging II*, Proc. Soc. Photo-Opt. Instrum. Eng. 2035, pp. 218–229.

Bakushinskiĭ, A. B. (1992). On a convergence problem of the iterative-regularized Gauss-Newton method, *Zh. Vychisl. Mat. i Mat. Fiz.* 32(9): 1503–1509.

Biswal, N. C., Pavlik, C., Smith, M. B., Aguirre, A., Xu, Y., Zanganeh, S., Kuhn, L. T., Claffey, K. P. & Zhu, Q. (2011). Imaging tumor hypoxia by near-infrared fluorescence tomography, *J. Biomed. Opt.* 16(6): 066009.

Blaschke, B., Neubauer, A. & Scherzer, O. (1997). On convergence rates for the iteratively regularized Gauss-Newton method, *IMA J. Numer. Anal.* 17(3): 421–436.

Chance, B., Cope, M., Gratton, E., Ramirez, N. & Tromberg, B. J. (1998). Phase measurement of light absorption and scatter in human tissue, *Rev. Sci. Instr.* 69: 3457 – 3481.

Chaudhari, A. J., Ahn, S., Levenson, R., Badawi, R. D., Cherry, S. R. & Leahy, R. M. (2009). Excitation spectroscopy in multispectral optical fluorescence tomography: methodology, feasibility and computer simulation studies, *Phys. Med. Biol.* 54(15): 4687–4704.

Chaudhari, A. J., Darvas, F., Bading, J. R., Moats, R. A., Conti, P. S., Smith, D. J., Cherry, S. R. & Leahy, R. M. (2005). Hyperspectral and multispectral bioluminescence optical tomography for small animal imaging, *Phys. Med. Biol.* 50(23): 5421–5441.

Chen, Y. Y. & Wood, A. W. (2009). Application of a temperature-dependent fluorescent dye (rhodamine b) to the measurement of radiofrequency radiation-induced temperature changes in biological samples, *Bioelectromagnetics* 30: 583–590.

Corlu, A., Choe, R., Durduran, T., Rosen, M. A., Schweiger, M., Arridge, S. R., Schnall, M. D. & Yodh, A. G. (2007). Three-dimensional in vivo fluorescence diffuse optical tomography of breast cancer in humans, *Opt. Express* 15(11): 6696–6716.

Culver, J. P., Choe, R., Holboke, M. J., Zubkov, L., Durduran, T., Slemp, A., Ntziachristos, V., Chance, B. & Yodh, A. G. (2003). Three-dimensional diffuse optical tomography in the parallel plane transmission geometry: evaluation of a hybrid frequency domain/continuous wave clinical system for breast imaging, *Med. Phys.* 30(2): 235–247.

da Silva, A., Bordy, T., Debourdeau, M., Dinten, J.-M., Peltié, P. & Rizo, P. (2007). Coupling x-ray and optical tomography systems for in vivo examination of small animals, *Conf Proc IEEE Eng Med Biol Soc* 2007: 3335–3338.

Davis, S. C., Dehghani, H., Wang, J., Jiang, S., Pogue, B. W. & Paulsen, K. D. (2007). Image-guided diffuse optical fluorescence tomography implemented with Laplacian-type regularization, *Opt. Express* 15(7): 4066–4082.

Davis, S. C., Pogue, B. W., Springett, R., Leussler, C., Mazurkewitz, P., Tuttle, S. B., Gibbs-Strauss, S. L., Jiang, S. S., Dehghani, H. & Paulsen, K. D. (2008). Magnetic resonance-coupled fluorescence tomography scanner for molecular imaging of tissue, *Rev. Sci. Instrum.* 79(6): 064302.

Dehghani, H., Eames, M. E., Yalavarthy, P. K., Davis, S. C., Srinivasan, S., Carpenter, C. M., Pogue, B. W. & Paulsen, K. D. (2008). Near infrared optical tomography using NIRFAST: Algorithms for numerical model and image reconstruction algorithms, *Commun. Numer. Methods Eng.* 25(6): 711–732.

Douiri, A., Schweiger, M., Riley, J. & Arridge, S. R. (2007). Anisotropic diffusion regularization methods for diffuse optical tomography using edge prior information, *Meas. Sci. Technol.* 18(1): 87–95.

Durduran, T., Choe, R., Baker, W. B. & Yodh, A. G. (2010). Diffuse optics for tissue monitoring and tomography, *Rep. Prog. Phys.* 73: 1 – 43.

Egger, H. & Leittão, A. (2009). Nonlinear regularization methods for ill-posed problems with piecewise constant or strongly varying solutions, *Inv. Probl.* 25: 115014.

Egger, H. & Schlottbom, M. (2011). Efficient reliable image reconstruction schemes for diffuse optical tomography, *Inv. Probl. Sci. Engrg.* 19(2): 155–180.

Engl, H. W., Hanke, M. & Neubauer, A. (1996). *Regularization of Inverse Problems*, Kluwer, Dordrecht.

Fang, Q. & Boas, D. A. (2009). Monte carlo simulation of photon migration in 3d turbid media accelerated by graphics processing units, *Opt. Express* 17(22): 20178–20190.

Frühauf, F., Scherzer, O. & Leitão, A. (2005). Analysis of regularization methods for the solution of ill-posed problems involving discontinuous operators, *SIAM J. Numer. Anal.* 43: 767–786.

Gaind, V., Kularatne, S., Low, P. S. & Webb, K. J. (2010). Deep–tissue imaging of intramolecular fluorescence resonance energy-transfer parameters., *Opt Lett* 35(9): 1314–1316.

Gannot, I., Ron, I., Hekmat, F., Chernomordik, V. & Gandjbakhche, A. (2004). Functional optical detection based on ph dependent fluorescence lifetime, *Lasers Surg. Med.* 35(5): 342–348.

Gibson, A. P., Hebden, J. C. & Arridge, S. R. (2005). Recent advances in diffuse optical imaging, *Phys. Med. Biol.* 50: R1–R43.

Godavarty, A., Eppstein, M. J., Zhang, C., Theru, S., Thompson, A. B., Gurfinkel, M. & Sevick-Muraca, E. M. (2003). Fluorescence-enhanced optical imaging in large tissue volumes using a gain-modulated ICCD camera, *Phys. Med. Biol.* 48: 1701–1720.

Graves, E. E., Ripoll, J., Weissleder, R. & Ntziachristos, V. (2003). A submillimeter resolution fluorescence molecular imaging system for small animal imaging, *Med. Phys.* 30(5): 901–911.

Haller, J., Hyde, D., Deliolanis, N., de Kleine, R., Niedre, M. & Ntziachristos, V. (2008). Visualization of pulmonary inflammation using noninvasive fluorescence molecular imaging, *J. Appl. Physiol.* 104(3): 795–802.

Hanke, M. (1997). Regularizing properties of a truncated Newton-CG algorithm for nonlinear inverse problems, *Numer. Func. Anal. Optim.* 18: 971–993.

Hebden, J. C., Arridge, S. R. & Delpy, D. T. (1997). Optical imaging in medicine: I. experimental techniques, *Phys. Med. Biol.* 42: 825–840.

Hyde, D., Miller, E., Brooks, D. & Ntziachristos, V. (2010). Data specific spatially varying regularization for multimodal fluorescence molecular tomography, *IEEE Trans. Med. Imag.* 29(2): 365–374.

Jiang, H. (1998). Frequency-domain fluorescent diffusion tomography: A finite-element-based algorithm and simulations, *Appl. Opt.* 37: 5337–5343.

Joshi, A., Bangerth, W. & Sevick-Muraca, W. M. (2004). Adaptive finite element based tomography for fluorescence optical imaging in tissue, *Opt. Express* 12: 5402–5417.

Kaltenbacher, B. (1997). Some newton-type methods for the regularization of nonlinear ill-posed problems, *Inv. Probl.* 13: 729–753.

Kepshire, D., Mincu, N., Hutchins, M., Gruber, J., Dehghani, H., Hypnarowski, J., Leblond, F., Khayat, M. & Pogue, B. W. (2009). A microcomputed tomography guided fluorescence tomography system for small animal molecular imaging, *Rev. Sci. Instrum.* 80(4): 043701.

Klose, A. D. & Pöschinger, T. (2011). Excitation-resolved fluorescence tomography with simplified spherical harmonics equations, *Phys. Med. Biol.* 56(5): 1443–1469.

Kozloff, K. M., Weissleder, R. & Mahmood, U. (2007). Noninvasive optical detection of bone mineral, *J. Bone Miner. Res.* 22(8): 1208–1216.

Kumar, A. T. N., Raymond, S. B., Dunn, A. K., Bacskai, B. J. & Boas, D. A. (2008). A time domain fluorescence tomography system for small animal imaging, *IEEE Trans. Med. Imag.* 27: 1152–1163.

Lakowicz, J. R. (2006). *Priciples of Fluorescence Spectroscopy*, Springer.

Leblond, F., Davis, S. C., Valdés, P. A. & Pogue, B. W. (2010). Pre-clinical whole-body fluorescence imaging: Review of instruments, methods and applications, *J. Photochem. Photobiol. B* 98(1): 77–94.

Li, C., Mitchell, G. S., Dutta, J., Ahn, S., Leahy, R. M. & Cherry, S. R. (2009). A three-dimensional multispectral fluorescence optical tomography imaging system for small animals based on a conical mirror design, *Opt. Express* 17(9): 7571–7585.

Li, D. U., Arlt, J., Richardson, J., Walker, R., Buts, A., Stoppa, D., Charbon, E. & Henderson, R. (2010). Real–time fluorescence lifetime imaging system with a 32x32 0.13um cmos low dark–count single-photon avalanche diode array, *Opt. Express* 18: 10257?–10269.

Lin, Y., Barber, W. C., Iwanczyk, J. S., Roeck, W., Nalcioglu, O. & Gulsen, G. (2010). Quantitative fluorescence tomography using a combined tri-modality ft/dot/xct system, *Opt. Express* 18(8): 7835–7850.

Longmuir, I. S. & Knopp, J. A. (1976). Measurement of tissue oxygen with a fluorescent probe, *J. Appl. Physiol.* 41(4): 598–602.

Marquardt, D. (1963). An algorithm for least-squares estimation of nonlinear parameters, *SIAM J. Appl. Math.* 11: 431–441.

Masciotti, J. M., Lee, J., Hielscher, A. H. & Stewart, M. (2009). Instrumentation for simultaneous magnetic resonance and optical tomographic imaging of the rodent brain, *Proc. SPIE 7171*.

Mastanduno, M. A., Davis, S. C., Jiang, S., diFlorio Alexander, R., Pogue, B. W. & Paulsen, K. D. (2011). Combined three–dimensional magnetic resonance guided optical spectroscopy for functional and molecular imaging of human breast cancer, *Proc. of SPIE-OSA Biomedical Optics, SPIE Vol. 8089*.

McGinty, J., Stuckey, D. W., Soloviev, V. Y., Laine, R., Wylezinska-Arridge, M., Wells, D. J., Arridge, S. R., French, P. M. W., Hajnal, J. V. & Sardini, A. (2011). In vivo fluorescence lifetime tomography of a FRET probe expressed in mouse, *Biomed. Opt. Express* 2(7): 1907–1917.

Mordon, S., Maunoury, V., Devoisselle, J. M., Abbas, Y. & Coustaud, D. (1992). Characterization of tumorous and normal tissue using a ph-sensitive fluorescence indicator (5,6-carboxyfluorescein) in vivo, *J. Photochem. Photobiol. B* 13(3-4): 307–314.

Morozov, V. A. (1966). On the solution of functional equations by the method of regularization, *Soviet Math. Dokl.* 7: 414–417.

Niclass, C., Rochas, A., Besse, P.-A. & Charbon, E. (2004). Toward a 3-D camera based on single photon avalanche diodes, *IEEE J. Sel. Topics Quant. Electr.* 10: 796 – 802.

Niedre, M. J., de Kleine, R. H., Aikawa, E., Kirsch, D. G., Weissleder, R. & Ntziachristos, V. (2008). Early photon tomography allows fluorescence detection of lung carcinomas and disease progression in mice in vivo, *Proc Natl Acad Sci U S A* 105(49): 19126–19131.

Nissilä, I., Hebden, J. C., Jennions, D., Heino, J., Schweiger, M., Kotilahti, K., Noponen, T., Gibson, A., Järvenpää, S., Lipiäinen, L. & Katila, T. (2006). Comparison between a time-domain and a frequency-domain system for optical tomography, *J. Biomed. Opt.* 11(6): 064015.

Nissilä, I., Noponen, T., Kotilahti, K., Katila, T., Lipiäinen, L., Tarvainen, T., Schweiger, M. & Arridge, S. (2005). Instrumentation and calibration methods for the multichannel measurement of phase and amplitude in optical tomography, *Rev. Sci. Instrum.* 76: 04432–1–04432–10.

Nothdurft, R. E., Patwardhan, S. V., Akers, W., Ye, Y., Achilefu, S. & Culver, J. P. (2009). In vivo fluorescence lifetime tomography, *J. Biomed. Opt.* 14(2): 024004–1–7.

Ntziachristos, V., Yodh, A., Schnall, M. & Chance, B. (2000). Concurrent MRI and diffuse optical tomography of breast after indocyanine green enhancement, *Proc. Natl. Acad. Sci.* 97: 2767–2772.

Panagiotou, C., Somayajula, S., Gibson, A. P., Schweiger, M., Leahy, R. M. & Arridge, S. R. (2009). Information theoretic regularization in diffuse optical tomography, *JOSA A* 26: 1277–1290.

Patwardhan, S. V. & Culver, J. P. (2008). Quantitative diffuse optical tomography for small animals using an ultrafast gated image intensifier, *J. Biomed. Opt.* 13(1): 011009.

Pavia, J. M., Charbon, E. & Wolf, M. (2011). 3d near-infrared imaging based on a singlephoton avalanche diode array sensor, *Proc. SPIE 8088, 808811.*

Reynolds, J. S., Troy, T. L. & Sevick-Muraca, E. M. (1997). Multipixel techniques for frequency-domain photon migration imaging, *Biotechnol. Prog.* 13: 669–690.

Roy, R. & Sevick-Muraca, E. M. (1999). Truncated Newton's optimization scheme for absorption and fluorescence optical tomography: Part I theory and formulation, *Opt. Express* 4: 353–371.

Schmidt, F., Fry, M., E.M.C.Hillman, Hebden, J. & Delpy, D. (2000). A 32 channel time-resolved instrument for medical optical tomography, *Rev. Sci. Instrum.* 71: 256–265.

Schulz, R. B., Ale, A., Sarantopoulos, A., Freyer, M., Soehngen, E., Zientkowska, M. & Ntziachristos, V. (2010). Hybrid system for simultaneous fluorescence and x-ray computed tomography, *IEEE Trans. Med. Imag.* 29(2): 465–473.

Schulz, R. B., Ripoll, J. & Ntziachristos, V. (2004). Experimental fluorescence tomography of tissues with noncontact measurements, *IEEE Trans. Med. Imag.* 23(4): 492–500.

Schweiger, M., Arridge, S. R. & Nissilä, I. (2005). Gauss–Newton method of image reconstruction in diffuse optical tomography, *Phys. Med. Biol.* 50: 2365–2386.

Schweiger, M., Dorn, O. & Arridge, S. R. (2008). 3-D shape and contrast reconstruction in optical tomography with level sets, *Journal of Physics: Conference Series* 124(1): 012043.

Sevick, E. M. & Chance, B. (1991). Photon migration in a model of the head measured using time and frequency domain techniques: potentials of spectroscopy and imaging, *in* B. Chance & A. Katzir (eds), *Time-Resolved Spectroscopy and Imaging of Tissues*, Proc. Soc. Photo-Opt. Instrum. Eng. 1431, pp. 84–96.

Sevick-Muraca, E. M., Kuwana, E., Godavarty, A., Houston, J. P., Thompson, A. B. & Roy, R. (2003). Near-infrared fluorescence imaging and spectroscopy in random media and tissue, *in* T. Vo-Dinh (ed.), *Biomedical Photonics Handbook*, CRC Press, Boca Raton, chapter 33.

Sevick-Muraca, E. M. & Rasmussen, J. C. (2008). Molecular imaging with optics: primer and case for near-infrared fluorescence techniques in personalized medicine, *J. Biomed. Opt.* 13(4): 041303.

Shives, E., Xu, Y. & Jiang, H. (2002). Fluorescence lifetime tomography of turbid media based on an oxygen-sensitive dye, *Opt. Express* 10: 1557–1562.

Silva, A. D., Leabad, M., Driol, C., Bordy, T., Debourdeau, M., Dinten, J.-M., Peltié, P. & Rizo, P. (2009). Optical calibration protocol for an x-ray and optical multimodality tomography system dedicated to small-animal examination, *Appl. Opt.* 48(10): D151–D162.

Soloviev, V. Y., D'Andrea, C., Valentini, G., Cubeddu, R. & Arridge, S. R. (2009). Combined reconstruction of fluorescent and optical parameters using time-resolved data, *Appl. Opt.* 48(1): 28–36.

Sosnovik, D. E., Nahrendorf, M., Deliolanis, N., Novikov, M., Aikawa, E., Josephson, L., Rosenzweig, A., Weissleder, R. & Ntziachristos, V. (2007). Fluorescence tomography and magnetic resonance imaging of myocardial macrophage infiltration in infarcted myocardium in vivo, *Circulation* 115(11): 1384–1391.

Tan, Y., Novo, M., Yao, L., Zhou, L. & Jiang, H. (n.d.). In vivo monitoring of stem cells in drosophila pupae using the radiative transfer equation-based fluorescence molecular tomography, *Mol. Imag. Biol.* pp. 1–6. 10.1007/s11307-010-0434-6.

Wang, D., Liu, X., Liu, F. & Bai, J. (2010). Full-angle fluorescence diffuse optical tomography with spatially coded parallel excitation, *IEEE Trans Inf Technol Biomed* 14(6): 1346–1354.

Wang, L.-H., Jacques, S. L. & Zheng, L.-Q. (1995). MCML - monte carlo modeling of photon transport in multi-layered tissues, *Computer Methods and Programs in Biomedicine* 47: 131–146.

Yang, X., Gong, H., Quan, G., Deng, Y. & Luo, Q. (2010). Combined system of fluorescence diffuse optical tomography and microcomputed tomography for small animal imaging, *Rev. Sci. Instrum.* 81(5): 054304.

Zacharakis, G., Favicchio, R., Simantiraki, M. & Ripoll, J. (2011). Spectroscopic detection improves multi-color quantification in fluorescence tomography, *Biomed. Opt. Express* 2(3): 431–439.

Zavattini, G., Vecchi, S., Mitchell, G., Weisser, U., Leahy, R. M., Pichler, B. J., Smith, D. J. & Cherry, S. R. (2006). A hyperspectral fluorescence system for 3d in vivo optical imaging, *Phys. Med. Biol.* 51(8): 2029–2043.

Zhang, X. & Badea, C. (2009). Effects of sampling strategy on image quality in noncontact panoramic fluorescence diffuse optical tomography for small animal imaging, *Opt. Express* 17(7): 5125–5138.

Zhang, X. & Badea, C. T. (2011). Highly efficient detection in fluorescence tomography of quantum dots using time-gated acquisition and ultrafast pulsed laser, *Proc Soc Photo Opt Instrum Eng* p. 7896.

Zhang, X., Badea, C. T. & Johnson, G. A. (2009). Three-dimensional reconstruction in free-space whole-body fluorescence tomography of mice using optically reconstructed surface and atlas anatomy, *J. Biomed. Opt.* 14(6): 064010.

7

Focal Modulation Microscopy: Principle and Techniques

Nanguang Chen, Guangjun Gao and Shau Poh Chong
National University of Singapore, Singapore

1. Introduction

Focal modulation microscopy (FMM) is an emerging single-photon fluorescence microscopy technique that can provide superior image contrast with sub-micron spatial resolutions at large penetration depths in highly scattering media such as biological tissues, mainly by preserving the signal-to-background ratio (SBR). To achieve this, FMM utilizes the coherence property of the light source, through a spatio-temporal modulation scheme to differentially phase modulate segments of the excitation beam. These segments of the beam, when being focused by the objective lens, generate an intensity modulation exclusively at the focal region. Demodulation of the collected fluorescence signal at the designated modulation frequency could allow us to discriminate the in-focus fluorescence from the multiple-scattered background, hence greatly enhance the SBR compared to confocal microscopy. More importantly, the penetration depth of FMM can be significantly improved as the degradation of the image contrast is considerably much slower, and thus could potentially revolutionize the clinical and biomedical applications of FMM for *in vivo* high-resolution visualization of biological specimens. Up to date, a penetration depth up to 600 μm has been demonstrated with biological specimens.

In this book chapter, we first highlight the major challenges of optical imaging in achieving large penetration depths when visualizing biological tissues, with further descriptions on the fundamental issues that determine the penetration depths achievable. Then, current optical techniques that are progressively important for deep imaging are briefly reviewed, in which confocal microscopy and two-photon microscopy will be emphasised, mainly due to their superior spatial resolution as well as optical sectioning capability. Distinctive technical differences between these microscopy techniques and advantages of FMM as compared to aforementioned techniques are also being outlined as guidance for readers to adopt the appropriate techniques for their applications.

Subsequently, the core principle of the FMM will be introduced through the concept of point-spread-function (PSF) based on scalar diffraction theory. The performance of FMM imaging in turbid media is also being assessed and validated through our theoretical study that includes scalar diffraction theory and Monte Carlo simulation methods. In particular, the SBR improvement as compared to confocal microscopy is presented. We then discuss the effect of aperture configurations on the modulation depths of FMM, that is crucial in optimizing FMM.

The next section of this book chapter will cover some of the implementations of FMM since it was invented in year 2008. Notably, two phase modulation schemes - double reflecting mirrors, and FMM based on acousto-optical modulators that are significantly progressive in term of stability and image performance will be described in details. Some of the images acquired using our FMM systems will also be compared side-by-side with confocal images to demonstrate the improvement in image qualities. We have tested on a wide collection of biological specimens, including but not limited to chicken chondrocytes, mouse brain vasculatures, *Drosophila* fruitfly as well as tissue phantom. Various fluorescence probes are also being utilized with FMM, proving its compatibility for the study of most fluorescence-related biological parameters.

For a concluding remark, we give a glimpse of future development of FMM, with emphasis on its applications in addressing basic problems in biomedical researches and understanding the pathophysiology of human diseases.

2. Challenges and potential impacts of deep tissue imaging

The desire to probe even deeper into biological specimens while resolving microstructural details and observing specific molecular events has grown over the last decade. This is largely because the knowledge obtained by looking at the biological system continuously over the entire entity coupled with functional information, as compared to individual snapshots via tiny-sectioned specimens, could greatly empower the understanding of cellular biology as well as diagnosis and prognosis of many diseases. However, the penetration depth that can be achieved in visualizing biological specimens is usually quite shallow compared to the total tissue volume, and is not absolutely defined mainly because image degradation by background and noise is a gradual process. Here, we briefly overview the current state of deep tissue imaging.

First and foremost, the achievable penetration depth depends largely on the optical properties of the specimen - how transparent, scattering, or opaque it is (Oheim, Beaurepaire et al. 2001). For instance in the case of zebrafish *Danio rerio*, one can see entirely through an embryo or larva with basic light and fluorescence microscopy and hence zebrafish has become a model organism in developmental genetics and neuroscience (Detrich, Westerfield et al. 2010). Similarly, other organisms that are virtually transparent, such as early-stage roundworm *Caenorhabditis elegans* and fruit fly *Drosophila melanogaster* are also popular for the *in vivo* study of many biological processes. In particular, fruit fly *Drosophila melanogaster* has been valuable in identifying genes that control embryonic development, as well as the formation of the nervous system. Nevertheless, many other organisms and their body parts are so opaque that it is impossible for the current state-of-arts microscopy techniques to achieve more than $1\,mm$ penetration depth with uncompromised image quality. As an example, one can resolve little or no cellular details within the cerebral cortex without first drilling holes on the skull of mammals. Very often, this is done with an invasive biocompatible window opened on the skull of a mouse brain to allow an imaging depth up to 600 μm (Kleinfeld, Mitra et al. 1998; Svoboda, Helmchen et al. 1999), which corresponds to the cortical layers 1-3 (Theer, Hasan et al. 2003), yet is still very shallow.

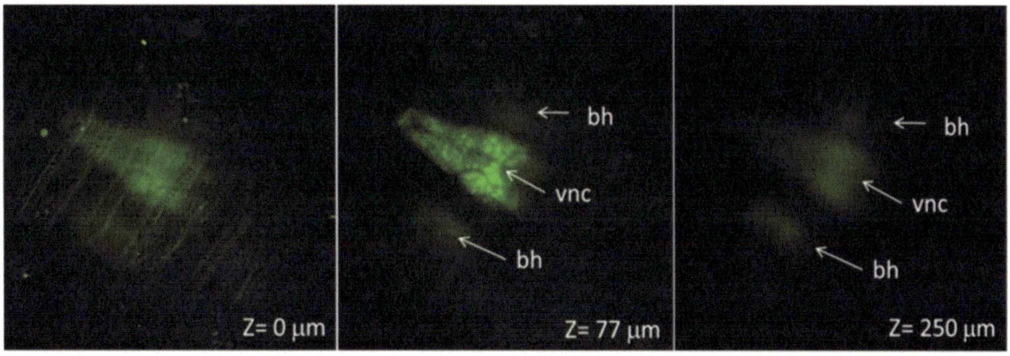

Fig. 1. Image stack of Drosophila pupa expressing elav-GFP to label CNS (brain and ventral nerve cord). The images were acquired with a confocal microscope Zeiss 5 live (10x objective).

Secondly, the imaging depth is also fundamentally limited by the onset of out-of-focus fluorescence generation due to light scattering near the top of the sample (Ying, Liu et al. 1999). At large imaging depths, this out-of-focus background fluorescence would gradually overwhelm the in-focus signal. As a consequence, a loss of image contrast will be observed (Theer, Hasan et al. 2003). Thus, it is generally difficult to preserve the quality of image when imaging at depth more than a few scattering mean free path[1](MFP). One specific example on how scattering has hindered the study of developmental biology in *Drosophila* fruitfly model is illustrated in the Fig. 1. It is clearly seen that the blurriness of brain hemispheres (bh) and ventral nerve cord (vnc) in deeper tissue sections (250 μm) in contrast to better resolving capability of the confocal microscope at shallower region (i.e. 77 μm). The poor contrast at large penetration depth is due to the attenuation of the fluorescence emission as well as multiple scattering.

This severe limitation of penetration depth of high-resolution optical imaging techniques that can only applied to physically sectioned biological samples through laborious sectioning procedures, or to natural transparent live specimens, such as organisms at very early stages of development, outlined the urgent need to improve *in vivo* visualization capability in thick biological tissues. For instance, current high-resolution intravital imaging techniques could permit visualization of tumor microstructure and vascular morphology superficially ($300 - 400\mu m$ depth), which is over volumetric regions that are a small fraction of the total tumor volume in small animal models (Vakoc, Lanning et al. 2009), thus very much limited our understanding on the tumor microenvironment over multistate and multiscale level.

High-resolution optical techniques with large penetration depth can be proved vital in biomedical applications as they allow observation of enormous biological processes within large tissue volumes especially for *in vivo* visualization of dynamic phenomenons in developing organism to address some of the basic problems in development biology, such as understanding the development phase of central nervous system in *Drosophila* fruitfly

[1] The average distance between each scattering event.

over the whole body volume, as depicted by Fig. 1. Visualization beyond penetration limit of modern microscopy techniques will not only open new pathways in understanding the signaling and interactions of tissues with drugs and environmental factors in adult model organisms but also could potentially useful for noninvasive imaging and spectroscopy of intact biological tissues of human subjects, including but not limited to nondestructive diagnosis of major human diseases such as early cancer detection (Zeng, Vangveravong et al. 2007; Pavlova, Williams et al. 2008). Specifically, the capability to visualize tissue microstructures at penetration depth up to 1 *mm* in biological tissues will be clinically important in *in vivo* diagnosis of skin melanomas in dermatology. We further highlight that deep imaging could also assist in dissecting tumor pathophysiology of intact tumor microenvironment (Jain, Munn et al. 2002; Vakoc, Lanning et al. 2009), as well as understanding how the single cells respond to the damage of the nervous system in neuropathology (Misgeld and Kerschensteiner 2006) of living animal models, just to list a few.

In summary, the development of optical techniques with large penetration depth will have great impacts in revolutionizing the usages of optical techniques in biomedical and clinical applications.

3. Current optical techniques for deep tissue imaging

This section gives a brief review of some optical microscopy techniques that are being important for observation of thick biological specimens. The principles of each technique are being described along with their advantages and disadvantages, in an attempt to give a snapshot of current capabilities in deep tissue imaging.

3.1 Confocal microscopy

The invention of confocal microscopy (CM) (Minsky 1961; Minsky 1988; Pawley 2006) has radically transformed optical imaging in biology research as it provides diffraction-limited spatial resolution with unprecedented optical sectioning capability to eliminate from images the background caused by out-of-focus light and scatter (Conchello and Lichtman 2005). This is achieved through a small pinhole (point) aperture or single-mode fiber being used in the detection/image plane which acts as a spatial filter/angular gate to block highly scattered out-of-focus light (see Fig. 2). This removal of undesired out-of-focus light not only enhanced the image contrast but more importantly also allowed three-dimensional imaging as images of thin slices can be acquired over thick specimens. The pinhole also rejects the scattered halo of light around the illumination spot if the pinhole size is small enough (i.e. about the size of Airy disk) (Conchello and Lichtman 2005), optimizing the point spread function for good resolution. In other words, the pinhole with appropriate size can effectively ensure that most of the ballistic photons contribute mostly of the signals being collected.

Nonetheless, this selective detection mechanism becomes less effective when the focal points moves deeper into the specimens or thick samples are being used, as multiple scattered stray photons will eventually leak through the pinhole (Kempe, Thon et al. 1994; Schmitt, Knuttel et al. 1994; Kempe, Rudolph et al. 1996), eroding the image contrast and signal-to-noise ratio (Dunn, Smithpeter et al. 1996). Furthermore, in most cases for deep tissue imaging, larger pinhole aperture radius are preferred to allow more photons to be collected

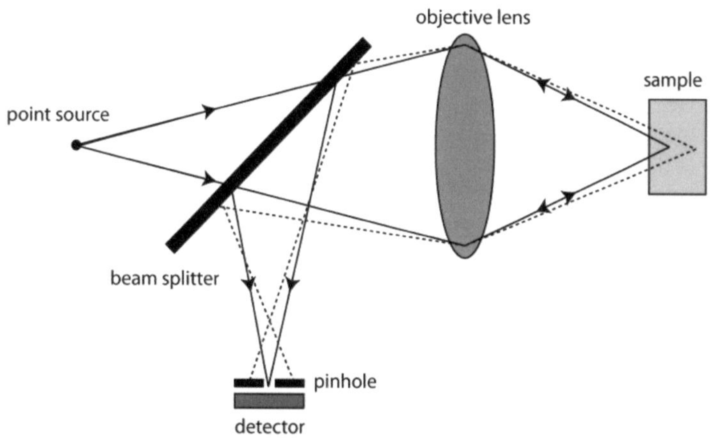

Fig. 2. Schematic diagram for a confocal reflection microscope. Dotted line represents the path for the light coming from out-of-focus areas in the sample; which will be blocked by the pinhole with appropriate size.

to compensate for the signal lost by attenuation, which could further deteriorate the imaging performance. This is because increasing the pinhole aperture size though will marginally improve the signal-to-noise ratio but will also drastically reduce the depth discrimination power (i.e. optical sectioning capability) of the microscope, leading to diminishing image contrast. Hence, very often, it is the trade-off between the signal level and background scattered-light rejection that places a fundamental limit on the sectioning capability of the microscope (Schmitt, Knuttel et al. 1994) as well as the imaging depth (Smithpeter, Dunn et al. 1998; Theer and Denk 2006). As the scattering effects gradually dominate at larger depth, image contrast of CM will eventually lost and thus limit its usefulness at near the tissue surface (less than 100 μm) (Conchello and Lichtman 2005). In fact, imaging of CM in turbid media such as living tissue is usually performed at imaging depth up to few tens of microns only due to limited contrast at higher depth aforementioned.

By combining with other mechanism to reject the multiple-scattered photons (Gan, Schilders et al. 1997), it is possible to improve the penetration depths of CM. Notably, optical coherence microscopy (OCM) combines the coherence gating mechanism of optical coherence tomography (OCT) and the pinhole effect of the CM to enhance the selection of ballistic photons for image reconstruction. Significant improvement in optical sectioning capability and penetration depths has been demonstrated (Izatt, Hee et al. 1994). Nevertheless, OCM is only sensitive to back-scattered light and not applicable for visualization of fluorescence, thus severely limited its biological applications.

In term of spatial resolution, CM could provide superior lateral ($\approx 1.4 \times$ improvement) and axial ($\approx 1.05 \times$ improvement) resolution compared to conventional widefield microscopy (Sheppard and Wilson 1980; Gu 1996). However, this improvement in spatial resolutions is only appreciable when infinitesimal pinhole is being used which preclude any signal collections. Therefore, optimal pinhole size between 60% and 80% of the diameter of the diffraction-limited spot (Sandison, Piston et al. 1995) are generally used, with further adjustment on the pinhole size to accommodate for desired optical sectioning capability and signal level.

3.2 Two-photon microscopy

Another promising optical techniques for subcellular spatial resolution *in vivo* deep tissue imaging is nonlinear two-photon fluorescence microscopy (Denk, Strickler et al. 1990; Helmchen and Denk 2005; Svoboda and Yasuda 2006). Two-photon fluorescence microscopy is very similar to CM in term of the system design except that it uses 'higher-order' light-matter interactions to generate fluorescence excitation in which two low-energy photons arrive 'simultaneously' (within ~0.5 femtoseconds, see Fig. 3A) at a fluorescence molecule combine their energies to promote the molecule to an excited state, which then proceeds along the normal fluorescence-emission pathway.

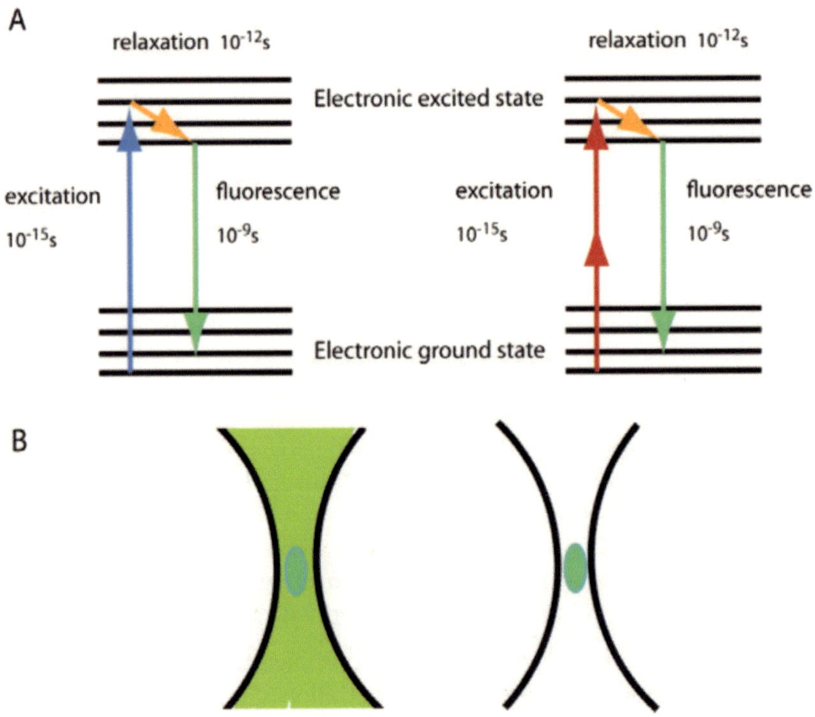

Fig. 3. Single-photon and two-photon process. A. Jablonski diagrams for one-photon excitation and two-photon excitation. B. Schematics of one-photon versus two-photon fluorescence emission.

The process of two-photon absorption requires extremely high concentration of excitation in spatial and temporal domain. Hence, very expensive pulse lasers that emit 'ultrashort' pulses in the range of hundreds femtoseconds with correspondingly high peak intensities have to be used with a high NA objective to focus the light beam into a diffraction-limited volume. A highly enhanced two-photon fluorescence system in focused laser enable vast majority of the fluorescence excitation occurs in a focal volume that can be as small as ~0.1 μm^3. This localization of excitation will limit the out-out-focus fluorescence excitation because even the excitation beam illuminated the sample like the case of CM (i.e. over the illumination cone as illustrated in Fig. 3B), the out-of-focus excitation light are too weak to generate appreciable two-photon fluorescence. Thus, intrinsic optical sectioning and high-contrast imaging can be achieved. As all the fluorescence photons are assumed generated from the focal region and can be collected as useful signals for imaging, spatial filters in the detection path (i.e. the detector pinhole in the CM) is not necessary, allowing higher collection efficiency (i.e. for greater signal level) and unprecedented imaging depths (Deng and Gu 2003). In particular, imaging up to a depth of 600 μm for vasculature and 700 μm for neuron of mouse brain has been achieved with femtosecond mode-locked Titanium: Sapphire (Ti: S) oscillators (Helmchen and Denk 2005).

It is worth to mention that these penetration depths are achieved partly due to the use of near-infrared excitation light that reduces light scattering, however, the achievable lateral and axial resolution are both slightly worse due to longer wavelength light sources are being used. Furthermore, two-photon fluorescence microscope uses very expensive pulse laser that may not be easily affordable for most research groups. Another concern for application of two-photon microscopy is the photo-damage/photobleaching at the focal volume, mainly due to the high intensity pulse laser to elicit fluorescence at the focus point. It is further claimed that the photobleaching that occurs at the focus is higher for two-photon absorptions than it is for single photon absorptions for comparable emission yields (Patterson and Piston 2000; Dittrich and Schwille 2001). This is undesirable for functional imaging as photobleaching at the focus is likely to be more detrimental than bleaching at plane above and below the focus. On top of that, the optical indicators that can be used with two-photon microscopy are only a small subset of the indicators that can be used with single-photon excitation microscopy, mainly due to the limited availability of fluorescence probes with large "two-photon absorption cross-section". This limitation could severely constrain the types of biological parameters and processes that can be studied using two-photon fluorescence microscopy.

Regardless of the superiority of nonlinear mechanism to inhibit the generation of out-of-focus fluorescence, the performance of two-photon microscopy could still be affected by multiple scattering. At extended depths, the ability of excitation light to reach the focus unscattered (ballistic excitation photons) and of emitted fluorescence to arrive at the detector, with generation of out-of-focus fluorescence near the surface, are placing a fundamental limit on how deep two-photon microscopy can probe (Theer and Denk 2006; Kobat, Durst et al. 2009). Recent efforts on improving the penetration depths of two-photon microscopy by using longer wavelength excitation (Kobat, Durst et al. 2009) or by reducing the pulse width of excitation laser (Theer, Hasan et al. 2003) (to increase two-photon fluorescence excitation yield) has been very successful with imaging depths over 1000 μm being reported (Theer, Hasan et al. 2003; Kobat, Durst et al. 2009). Still, those techniques are very selective on the availability of fluorescence probes that can be excited using near-infrared light and are still very technically demanding (Kobat, Durst et al. 2009) to be adopted by most biological research groups.

3.3 Optical coherence tomography

Coherence optical tomography (OCT) (Huang, Swanson et al. 1991; Fujimoto 2003) is an emerging biomedical optical imaging technique that is capable of considerable high resolution and cross-sectional tomographic imaging of microstructures in biological systems. Typically, OCT can provide micron-range axial resolution for an imaging depth up to $2-3\ mm$ in tissue depending on the optical scattering (Fujimoto, Brezinski et al. 1995).

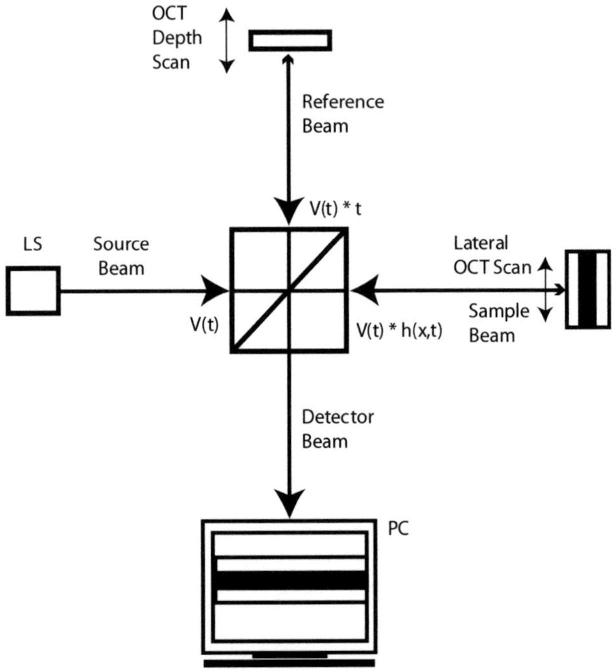

Fig. 4. Standard OCT scheme based on a low time-coherence Michelson interferometer. The intensity I_E of the interferometer exit depends on the sample response $h(x,z)$ convolved with the source coherence function $\Gamma_{source}(z)$. LS = low time-coherence light source; PC = personal computer. Adapted from (Fercher, Drexler et al. 2003).

OCT uses coherence gating (i.e. interference between the back-scattered light and a reference beam) to improve the detection of backscattered light for image reconstruction. OCT can generate good contrasts as only the backscattered light that has a well-defined optical path length and polarization state will interfere constructively with the reference beam to generate strong fringe signals for image reconstruction (see Fig. 4) (Fercher, Drexler et al. 2003). The intensity of the interferometer exit I_E can be represented by:

$$I_E(x,z) = I_s + I_R + 2Re[\Gamma_{source}(z) \times h(x,z)] \quad (1)$$

where I_s and I_R are the intensity at the sample and reference arms respectively, Γ_{source} being the source coherence function and $h(x,z)$ is the sample response function (i.e. determined by the sample geometry and reflectivity due to refractive index mismatches).

Due to its relatively larger penetration depths, OCT has found applications in ophthalmology and dermatology (Prati, Regar et al. 2010). Specifically, OCT has been heavily applied for diagnosis of various eye diseases such as age-related macular degeneration and glaucoma (Fercher 2010; Prati, Regar et al. 2010) On top of that, OCT has also been applied in functional imaging such as spectroscopic imaging of tissue properties, Doppler blood flow measurement and quantification of blood oxygenation or tissue birefringence (Fujimoto 2003). Recently, second generation OCT, termed optical frequency domain imaging (OFDI) (Vakoc, Lanning et al. 2009) has been very successful for the understanding of biological parameters of the tumor microenvironment *in vivo*.

Although substantially high-resolution at imaging depth up to 3 *mm* is readily achievable using OCT, its lack of molecular contrast especially incompatibility with fluorescence microscopy has restricted its applications for the study of many other biological processes.

3.4 Photo-acoustic tomography

Photo-acoustic tomography (PAT) (Wang, Xu et al. 2002; Wang, Ku et al. 2004), being one of the fastest-growing area of biomedical imaging technology over the last decade, offers high-resolution three-dimensional imaging with rich optical contrast *in vivo* at depths beyond the optical transport mean free path (i.e.$\sim 1\,mm$ in human skin) (Wang 2009). In the photoacoustic phenomenon, excitation light (short-pulsed laser is normally used for efficient ultrasound generation) is absorbed by a material and converted to heat, and the subsequent thermoelastic expansion generates an acoustic wave. This acoustic wave can then be detected by using an ultrasonic detector for the reconstruction of ultrasound image. In fluorescence mode, ultrasonic detection of pressure waves generated by the absorption of pulse light by fluorescence proteins in elastic media enable high-resolution visualization of fluorescent proteins few millimetres deep within highly light-scattering living organisms.

PAT combines the optical imaging and ultrasound imaging, enabling rich optical contrast and high ultrasonic resolution imaging modality. Typically, the ultrasonic scattering coefficient in biological tissue is $2 - 3$ orders of magnitude less than the optical equivalent. Hence, PAT can detect the ultrasonic waves even at a depth of multiple folds larger compared to existing high-resolution optical imaging techniques, such as confocal microscopy and two-photon microscopy, thus enabling deeply penetrating functional (Wang, Pang et al. 2003; Yang, Xing et al. 2007) and molecular (Li, Zemp et al. 2007; Li, Oh et al. 2008) imaging in biological samples. For instance, highly optimized PAT could enable visualization of fluorescent proteins few millimeters deep within highly light-scattering living organisms.

Nevertheless, the in-plane spatial resolution of the photo-acoustic images achievable is fundamentally limited by the effective bandwidth of the ultrasonic detector (20 MHz), leading to $\sim 38\,um$ diffraction limited resolution and even worse for axial resolution (Razansky, Distel et al. 2009). Recent higher lateral resolution around $5\,um$ has been reported but at a much shallower penetration depth of 0.7 *mm* (Wang 2009), which is not better than current techniques such as two-photon microscopy. Furthermore, very often the specimens have to be immersed in acoustic medium for better coupling of the propagation of acoustic wave to the ultrasonic detector, which might not be suitable for all types of living biological specimens.

3.5 Others recent developments

Another very promising technique, termed single plane illumination microscopy (SPIM) (Huisken, Swoger et al. 2004) or light-sheet-based fluorescence microscopy (Keller, Schmidt et al. 2010) in which a single plane in specimen is quickly scanned with a thin laser beam while a 2D camera-based detection arm records a fluorescence image at a right-angle to the illumination axis. Light-sheet-based microscopy could greatly enhance the image acquisition speed and the image contrast while limited the photobleaching and phototoxicity on the specimens (Keller, Schmidt et al. 2008; Keller and Stelzer 2008). However, this technique usually requires dedicated image post-processing to improve the spatial resolutions (for instance, deconvolution) (Verveer, Swoger et al. 2007; Keller, Schmidt et al. 2010) and no penetration depths over 100 μm have been reported up to date.

Other high-resolution optical imaging techniques such as 4-Pi (Hell, Stelzer et al. 1994) and I^5M (Gustafsson, Agard et al. 1999) microscopy based on coherent collection of fluorescence using a pair of diametrically opposed objectives which could enhance the axial resolution by a factor of 3-7 along the optical axis; far-field optical microscopy such as stimulated emission depletion (STED) microscopy (Dyba and Hell 2002) uses superlocalized depletion of the excited state by stimulated emission with few tens nanometers spatial resolution being demonstrated (probably the highest resolution using optical techniques for living cells) and total internal reflection fluorescence microscopy (TIRF) (Axelrod 2003) that uses decaying evanescent wave are all severely limited in penetration depth and thus not extensively reviewed here.

3.6 Summary

There is a considerable large gap in the development for optical microscopy techniques that can achieve high penetration depth with subcellular spatial resolution, for vast applications in biomedical researches. Table 1 summarizes the strengths and limitations of some of the imaging modalities for subcellular-resolution deep imaging being described in this book chapter. Therefore we developed Focal Modulation Microscopy (FMM) (Chen, Wong et al. 2008), a novel technique that aims for imaging depth greater than but not limited to 500 *um* with subcellular spatial resolution and molecular specificity. The principle of FMM will be further elaborated in the next section.

Embodiments	**Advantages**	**Limitations**
Confocal Fluorescence Microscopy	High-resolution with optical sectioning. Much cheaper laser source than two-photon imaging.	Shallow penetration depths due to multiple scattering effects.
Two-Photon Fluorescence Microscopy	Optical sectioning. Reduced photobleaching and photodamage with large penetration depths up to 1 *mm*.	High cost of ultrashort-pulsed laser and limited option of fluorescence probes.
Optical Coherence Tomography	Large penetration depth up to 3 *mm* and ease of implementation.	Lack of molecular contrast due to incompatibility with fluorescence imaging and high level of speckle noise.
Photoacoustic Tomography	Good penetration depths up to few mm and compatible with fluorescence imaging.	Poorer spatial resolutions than confocal and two-photon microscopy.
Focal Modulation Microscopy	Optical sectioning. Better penetration depths than confocal microscopy using cheaper continuous-wave laser. Can work in fluorescence and reflectance mode.	Photobleaching (same as confocal microscopy).

Table 1. A comparison of optical imaging modalities with good resolution and penetration depths.

4. Principle of focal modulation microscopy

Focal modulation microscopy (FMM) (Chen, Wong et al. 2008; Wong, Chong et al. 2009) is a novel optical microscopy technique based on single photon excited fluorescence. It can provide sub-micron spatial resolution at large penetration depth in living tissues mainly by preserving the SBR of the image. In FMM, a phase modulator is employed to sinusoidally phase modulate (or frequency shifting) half of the spatial extent of the excitation beam. As the beam being tightly focused by the objective lens, interference of the both half-beams generates an intensity modulation at the designated frequency around the focal volume. This modulated excitation focus thus results in a modulated fluorescence signal from the focal volume. Although both the ballistic and scattered photons could reach the focal plane, only the ballistic photons contribute to the oscillatory excitation, as they have well-defined phase and polarization. Therefore, in principle, "out-of-focus" fluorescence emission should not be modulated as they are originated from scattered excitation. Subsequently, a simple lock-in technique can be implemented to retrieve the fluorescence signal excited by ballistic light and to reject the contribution from diffusive-light-excited fluorescence.

4.1 Excitation beam modulation

Here we present the principle of FMM in mathematical model. As FMM is a technique that employs a spatiotemporal phase modulator to sinusoidally modulate a spatial fraction of the excitation beam, we can define the excitation field:

$$E_i(r_i) = h_{i1}(r_i) + h_{i2}(r_i)e^{i\varphi(t)} \tag{2}$$

in which r_i is the spatial coordinates and the $h_{i2}e^{i\varphi(t)}$ term describe the fraction of the excitation field being phase modulated with a periodic function $\varphi\,(t)$ (at the frequency f) in contrast to the unmodulated fraction h_{i1}. The corresponding excitation intensity around the focal spot is thus given by:

$$I_i(r_i) = |E_i(r_i)|^2 = E_i(r_i) \times E_i^*(r_i) = \left(h_{i1} + h_{i2}e^{i\varphi\,(t)}\right) \times \left(h_{i1} + h_{i2}e^{i\varphi\,(t)}\right)^* \tag{3}$$

Expanding the Eqn. 3, we obtained:

$$I_i(r_i) = h_{i1}[h_{i1}]^* + h_{i2}e^{i\varphi(t)}\left[h_{i2}e^{i\varphi\,(t)}\right]^* + h_{i1}\left[h_{i2}e^{i\varphi\,(t)}\right]^* + h_{i2}e^{i\varphi\,(t)}[h_{i1}]^* = |h_{i1}|^2 + |h_{i2}|^2 + 2Re\left(h_{i1}h_{i2}^*e^{i\varphi\,(t)}\right) = |h_{i1}|^2 + |h_{i2}|^2 + 2|h_{i1}h_{i2}^*|\cos(\varphi(t) + \arg(h_{i1}h_{i2}^*)) \tag{4}$$

We could observe from the last line of Eqn. 4 that the first two terms are the fraction of excitation intensity which is unchanged over time whereas the last term corresponds to oscillatory intensity at the modulation frequency f. In a FMM system, the unmodulated field $h_{i1}(r_i)$ and the modulated field $h_{i2}(r_i)$ are generally spatially separated, due to spatiotemporal phase modulation at the objective aperture. The excitation intensity is therefore a constant except at locations around the focal point, in which there is a significant overlapping between $h_{i1}(r_i)$ and $h_{i2}(r_i)$. At the focal point, $h_{i1}(r_i)$ and $h_{i2}(r_i)$ are usually in phase so that $\arg(h_{i1}h_{i2}^*) = 0$. The maximal excitation intensity is reached when $\cos(\varphi(t)) = 1$ (in phase),

$$I_{in-phase} = |h_{i1}|^2 + |h_{i2}|^2 + 2|h_{i1}h_{i2}^*| \tag{5}$$

The minimal excitation intensity is :

$$I_{off-phase} = |h_{i1}|^2 + |h_{i2}|^2 - 2|h_{i1}h_{i2}^*| \quad (6)$$

which corresponds to $\cos(\varphi(t)) = -1$. The difference between the in-phase and off-phase intensities provides the measure of peak-to-peak value of intensity modulation at the focal point.

4.2 Excitation point spread function of FMM

We can find the illumination intensity point spread function (PSF) of the FMM using the scalar diffraction theory. For an aberration-free lens of circular aperture, the illumination intensity distribution is given by (Gu 2000):

$$I_{illumination}(v,u) = \left|2\int_0^1 P(\rho)J_0(v\rho)e^{\frac{iu\rho^2}{2}}\rho d\rho\right|^2 \quad (7)$$

in which J_0 denotes the zero-order Bessel function and $v = k(NA)r$ and $u = 4k\left[\sin\frac{\alpha}{2}\right]^2 z$ are radial and axial normalized optical coordinates with the wavenumber $k = 2\pi/\lambda$. The excitation beam is split into two fractions. Let's consider an annular aperture as an example. The excitation beam passing through the outer ring of the annular aperture is subject to a phase-shift varying from $0\ to\ \pi$ with respect to the excitation beam passed through the inner circle. Hence, the pupil function $P(\rho)$ that describes the field distribution at the lens aperture can be described as:

$$P(\rho) = \begin{cases} 1, for\ 0 \ll \rho \ll \sqrt{2}/_2 \\ e^{i\varphi(t)}, for\ \sqrt{2}/_2 \ll \rho \ll 1 \end{cases} \quad (8)$$

where ρ is the normalized aperture diameter of the objective lens.

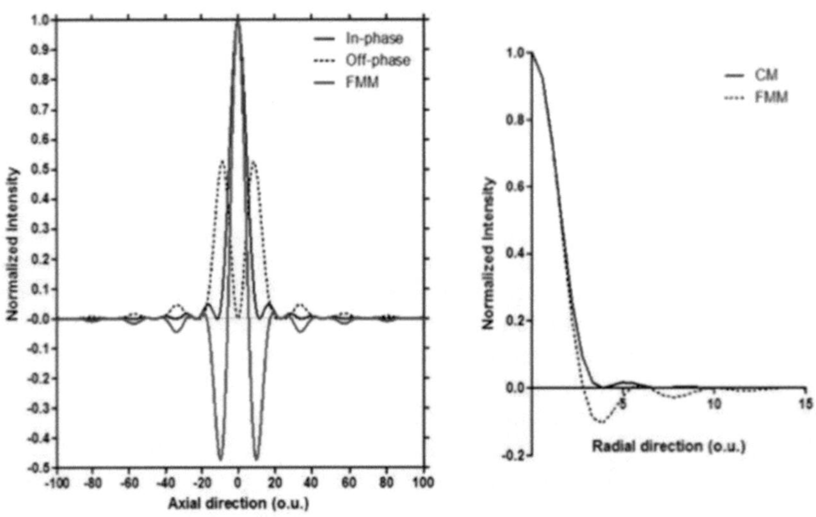

Fig. 5. (Left) Simulated excitation intensity profile along the axial direction of the in-phase, out-phase and FMM signals based on scalar diffraction theory. (Right) Simulated excitation intensity profile along lateral direction of the CM and FMM.

When the phase profile over the aperture is uniform (i.e. $\varphi(t) = 0$), the intensity distribution along the optical axis is identical to the illumination point spread function of CM; on the other hand, when $\varphi(t) = \pi$, there will be a strong destructive interference of the beams at the focal spot, leading to the off-phase intensity profile (dashed) as shown in Fig. 5 (Left). The difference between these two excitation intensity profiles is the effective illumination point spread function in FMM.

The excitation intensity distribution of the CM and FMM along the lateral direction is plot in Fig. 5 (Right). It is worth to mention that due to the differential mechanism of FMM, there are negative sidelobes in the excitation IPSF of the FMM, albeit with relatively smaller magnitude compared to that of lateral IPSF. In order to extract the FMM signal, an aperture pinhole of size slightly smaller that the central lobe is to be used, in order to exclude the negative side lobes being included in the retrieved signal. These negative side lobes, if being included in the detected signal, will dramatically reduce the FMM signal.

4.3 Signal-to-background ratio in FMM

While the basic principle of FMM is straightforward and its performance has been experimentally demonstrated (Chen, Wong et al. 2008), it is desirable to conduct theoretical studies to gain further insight into this technique. In this section, we present a theoretical model that combines the scalar diffraction theory (Gu 2000) with Monte Carlo simulation (Schmitt, Knuttel et al. 1994), in which the dependence of SBR on penetration depth are examined and compared for both FMM and CM.

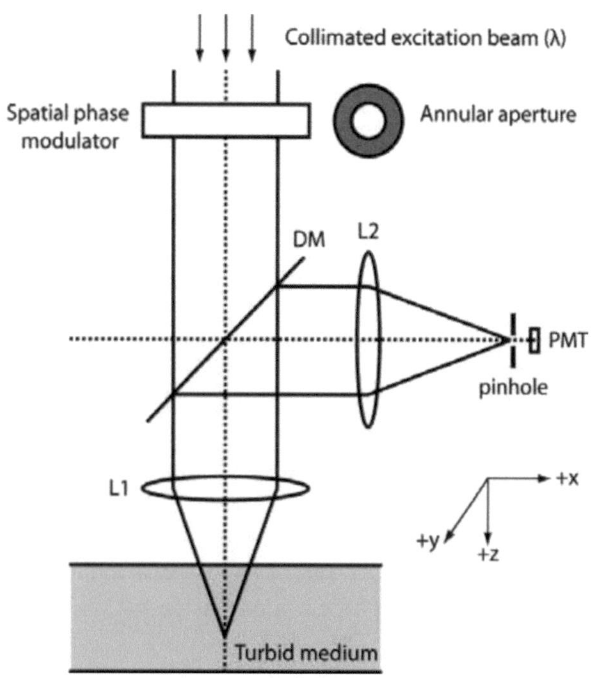

Fig. 6. Model geometry of a FMM/CM setup. Annular aperture with (shaded region) and without phase modulation is studied. L1 and L2 are lens with focal length **9 *mm***. DM is the dichroic mirror and PMT is the photomultiplier tube.

4.3.1 Model geometry

We consider a system geometry shown in Fig. 6. The collimated excitation laser beam is focused by the objective lens L1 to a point located in a slab of turbid medium. The refractive indices are assumed to be matched across the medium surface. The system includes lenses L1 and L2 (Diameter $D = 10\,mm$, focal length 9 mm), a dichroic mirror (DM), a pinhole 0.8 μm in diameter, a spatiotemporal phase modulator, and a PMT. The optical properties (absorption coefficient $\mu_a = 0.1\,cm^{-1}$, scattering coefficient $\mu_s = 100\,cm^{-1}$, anisotropy factor $g = 0.9$) of the turbid medium are typical for biological soft tissues. Fluorescent molecules are homogeneously distributed and are the only absorptive substance in the medium.

4.3.2 Excitation rate for confocal microscopy

The excitation light, once entering the turbid medium, is separated into a ballistic component and a scattered component due to scattering events. The fluorescence excitation rate for CM consists of ballistic (CMB) and scattered (CMS) components:

$$E_{CM}(r_F, r_M) = E_{CMB}(r_F, r_M) + E_{CMS}(r_F, r_M) \tag{9}$$

where $r_F = (x_F, y_F, z_F)$ and $r_M = (x_M, y_M, z_M)$ are the locations of the focal point and fluorescent molecules, respectively. The scalar diffraction theory is used to calculate the ballistic excitation rate (in polar coordinates):

$$E_{CMB}(r_F, r_M) = e^{-\mu_t z_M} \mu_a C \left| \int_0^1 J_0(v\rho) e^{iu\frac{\rho^2}{2}} \rho d\rho \right|^2 \tag{10}$$

Here J_o denotes the zero-order Bessel function. The normalized optical coordinates $v = kNA\rho$ and $u = 4k\Delta z \sin^2\left(\frac{\alpha}{2}\right)$ are related to the normalized radius $\rho = \sqrt{(x_F - x_M)^2 + (y_F - y_M)^2}$ and $\Delta z = z_M - z_F$, k is the wave number, and the numerical aperture $NA = \sin\alpha = \frac{a}{f'}$, with a being the radius of the diffraction aperture at the plane of the objective lens. The constant C is used to normalize the total excitation power to unity. Attenuation of the ballistic component depends on the extinction coefficient $\mu_t = \mu_a + \mu_s$ and the penetration depth z_M.

Monte Carlo simulation (Schmitt, Knuttel et al. 1994) is employed to obtain the scattered excitation rate $E_{CMS}(r_F, r_M)$. Given the focal point $(0, 0, z_F)$, photon packets with an initial weight of one are launched at the air-turbid medium interface ($z = 0$). Their initial position and direction are randomly assigned with the probability density function satisfying the following conditions: a) The excitation beam intensity is uniform over the aperture of L1, and b) the photon packets would converge to the focal point if there is no scattering. Then the trajectory of each photon packet is randomly generated following the standard propagation and interaction approach. The weight of a photon packet is adjusted after each interaction:

$$w_{new} = w_{old} - \left(\frac{\mu_a}{\mu_t}\right) w_{old} \tag{11}$$

At the same time, the 'lost' weight is deposited into that position grid as considered as being absorbed by the fluorescence molecules. A simulated trajectory ends when the photon escape from the slab surface or the weight drops below a preset threshold. A large number (10^7) of photons are traced to find the average excitation rate $E_{CMS}(r_F, r_M)$ for each focal depth. The contribution from the first interaction is attributed to ballistic light and thus excluded from $E_{CMS}(r_F, r_M)$.

4.3.3 Excitation rate for focal modulation microscopy

For FMM, the equivalent excitation rate is associated with the ballistic light only:

$$E_{FMM}(r_F, r_M) =$$
$$e^{-\mu_t z_M}\mu_a C\left\{\left|\int_0^1 J_0(v\rho)e^{iu\frac{\rho^2}{2}}\rho d\rho\right|^2 - \left|\int_0^{0.707} J_0(v\rho)e^{iu\frac{\rho^2}{2}}\rho d\rho - \int_{0.701}^1 J_0(v\rho)e^{iu\frac{\rho^2}{2}}\rho d\rho\right|^2\right\} \quad (12)$$

The first term in the above equation (i.e. enclosed in first modulus function) is the excitation intensity when $\varphi(t) = 0$ and the second term corresponds to excitation intensity when $\varphi(t) = \pi$.

In Fig. 7 , the excitation rates are compared for an imaging depth of 400 μm. Fig. 7 (a) shows FMM excitation rate (absolution value) as a function of the radial displacement and defocus, while Fig. 7 (b) is the ballistic excitation rate in the CM setup. They are highly concentrated around the focal point and decay rapidly outside of the focal volume. Such a behaviour is desirable for optimal optical sectioning and high-resolution imaging. On the contrary, the diffusive excitation rate for the CM setup (Fig. 7 (c)) is distributed in a rather large volume, although the peak value is about 2 orders of magnitude smaller than that of ballistic excitation rate.

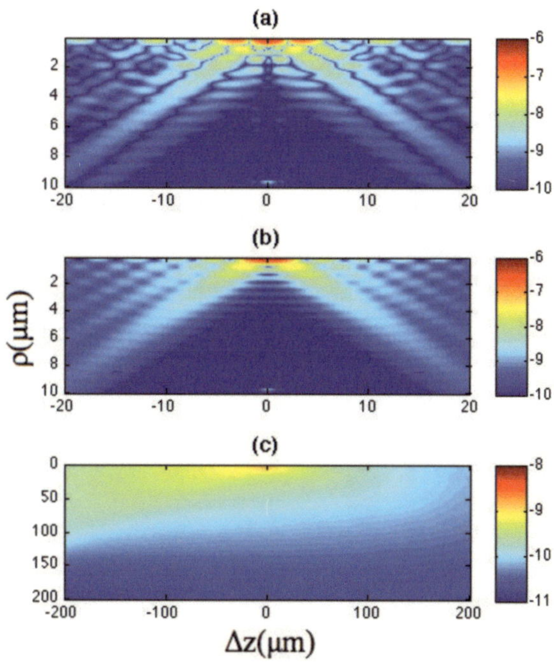

Fig. 7. Ballistic and diffusive excitation rates for an imaging depth of **400 μm**.

4.3.4 Detection point-spread-function

As CM and FMM have the same detection optics, their fluorescence detection efficiencies are identical. For the ballistic fluorescence light, the detection efficiency is given by:

$$D_B(r_F, r_M) = \frac{1-\cos\theta}{2} e^{-\mu_t z_M} C \iint_S dxdy \left| \int_0^1 J_0(v'\rho) e^{iu'\frac{\rho^2}{2}} \rho d\rho \right|^2 \quad (13)$$

where the two-dimensional integration is over S, the image of the pinhole in the medium and centered at r_F. The optical coordinates $v'$and u' are normalized radial and axial distances between r_M and the point (x, y, z_M) within S. The first term of Eqn. 13, $\frac{1-\cos\theta}{2}$ is the solid angles of the detection cone where θ is half of the angular aperture of L1.

Scattered fluorescence photons are again simulated by the use of Monte Carlo method. Photon packets are launched from a point $(0, 0, z_M)$ with the initial directions uniformly sampled. Trajectory of propagation and scattering steps for each photon is generated using the standard Monte Carlo approaches. Photons emerging from the surface without scattering are discarded. Scattered photons, once crossed the upper medium surface, are traced using geometric optics. In order to enhance the simulation efficiency by reusing the trajectories, we actually deploy an array of detectors after L2. The detector array consists of 101 planes along the optical axis, corresponding to focal depths sampled every 10 μm from 0 to 1000 μm in the medium. Each detection plane has a sensing area 1 mm in diameter and it is divided into a grid of 1 μm by 1 μm pixels. A photon captured by the pixel at r_{det} adds a normalized weight to the scattered detection efficiency:

$$D_S(r_F, r_M) = D_S(r_F, r_M) + \frac{S_P W}{N} \quad (14)$$

Here W is the weight of the photon packet, S_P is the pinhole area in $\mu m^2$and N is the total number of photons launched, and r_F is the conjugate point of r_{det} in the medium.

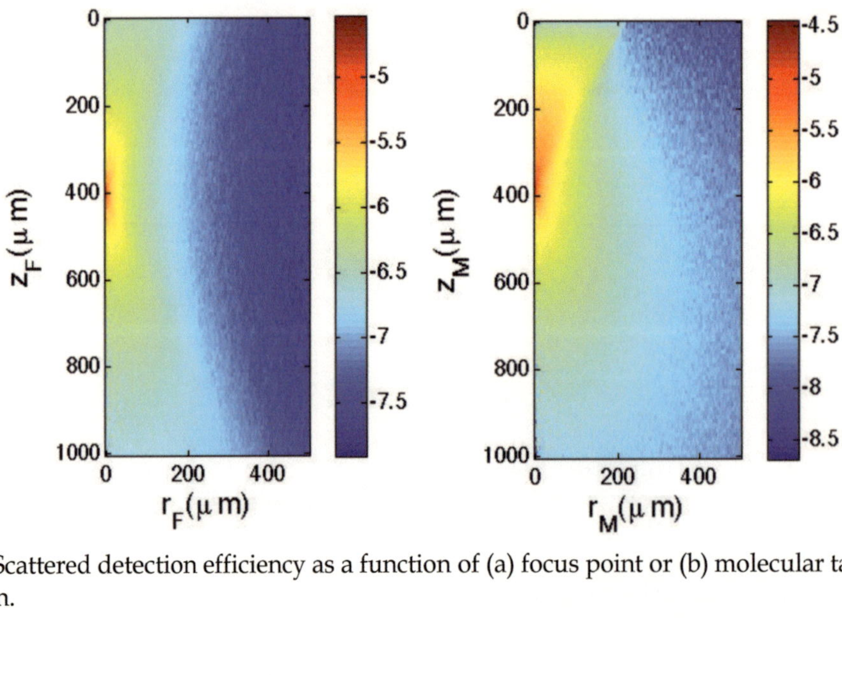

Fig. 8. Scattered detection efficiency as a function of (a) focus point or (b) molecular target position.

Shown in Fig. 8 (a) is $D_S(r_F, r_M = (0,0,400\mu m))$ as a function of r_F and z_F, obtained with 10^6 simulated photons. The simulation is repeated for the emitter depth range from 0 to 1 mm, at an incremental step of 10 μm. Then the results are combined to generate the spatial distribution as a function of r_M and z_M, for any given focal depth z_F. Shown in Fig 8 (b) is $D_S(r_F = (0,0,400\mu m), r_M)$, the scattered detection efficiency when the focal point is 400 μm deep.

4.3.5 Formulation for signal-to-background ratio

When the excitation and detection optics are focused at r_F, the total CM signal can be expressed as a sum of four terms:

$$I_{CM}(r_F) = \iiint dr_M\{E_{CMB}(r_F, r_M) + E_{CMS}(r_F, r_M)\} \times \{D_B(r_F, r_M) + D_S(r_F, r_M)\} = I_{CM}^{BB}(r_F) + I_{CM}^{SB}(r_F) + I_{CM}^{BS}(r_F) + I_{CM}^{SS}(r_F) \quad (15)$$

Here $I_{CM}^{BB}(r_F) = \iiint dr_M E_{CMB}(r_F, r_M) \times D_B(r_F, r_M)$ is related to ballistic excitation and ballistic fluorescence photons, and is the desired signal. All the three-dimensional integrals are over the entire volume of the turbid medium. The other three terms contribute to a background $I_{CM}^{BK} = I_{CM}^{SB} + I_{CM}^{BS} + I_{CM}^{SS}$, that is related to scattered photons. The signal to background ratio (SBR) is thus defined as:

$$SBR_{CM} = \frac{I_{CM}^{BB}}{I_{CM}^{BK}} \quad (16)$$

in which

$$I_{CM}^{BK} = \iiint dr_M\{E_{CMB}(r_F, r_M)D_S(r_F, r_M) + E_{CMS}(r_F, r_M)D_B(r_F, r_M) + E_{CMS}(r_F, r_M)D_S(r_F, r_M)\} = I_{CM}^{SB} + I_{CM}^{BS} + I_{CM}^{SS} \quad (17)$$

The total FMM signal is given by

$$I_{FMM}(r_F) = \iiint dr_M\{E_{FMM}(r_F, r_M)D_B(r_F, r_M) + E_{FMM}(r_F, r_M)D_S(r_F, r_M)\} = I_{FMM}^{BB}(r_F) + I_{FMM}^{BS}(r_F) \quad (18)$$

while the signal to background ratio is simply

$$SBR_{FMM} = \frac{I_{FMM}^{BB}}{I_{FMM}^{BS}} = \frac{\iiint dr_M E_{FMM}(r_F, r_M) D_B(r_F, r_M)}{\iiint dr_M E_{FMM}(r_F, r_M) D_S(r_F, r_M)} \quad (19)$$

4.3.6 Discussions and summary

Various CM and FMM signals are compared in Fig. 9 (a). I_{CM}^{BB} and I_{FMM}^{BB} decay exponentially with the focal depth as expected. I_{FMM}^{BB} is slightly weaker than I_{CM}^{BB} because the modulation depth is always less than one. The CM background is dominated by I_{CM}^{SS}, which is related to scattered excitation and scattered emission photons. It overwhelms I_{CM}^{BB} for imaging depths over 200 μm. In contrast, the FMM background I_{FMM}^{BS} is significantly lower than the FMM signal I_{FMM}^{BB}. The SBR ratios are plotted as functions of penetration depth in Fig. 9 (b). It is evident that FMM provides a much more superior SBR than CM even for small imaging depths. For a large imaging depth up to 1 mm, SBR_{FMM} is maintained at around 20 dB.

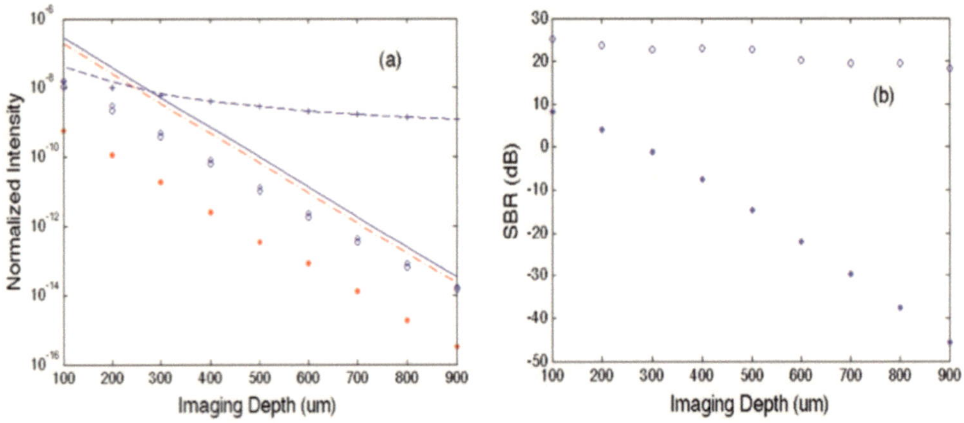

Fig. 9. Normalized intensity and signal-to-background ratio for various depths. (a) FMM signals I_{FMM}^{BB} (dashed-dotted) and I_{FMM}^{SB} (asterisks) compared with CM signals I_{CM}^{BB} (solid), I_{CM}^{BK} (dashed), I_{CM}^{SB} (diamonds), I_{CM}^{BS} (circles), and I_{CM}^{SS} (pluses); (b) SBR for FMM (circles) and CM (asterisks).

In this section, the advantage of FMM is well explained with the theoretical model combining the scalar diffraction theory and Monte Carlo methods. The SBR ratio of FMM is evaluated with such a model and is compared with that of CM. It is obvious that SBR is not a limiting factor for an imaging depth as large as $1\,mm$. Our model can also be used to analyse other performances such as spatial resolution and SBR ratio of FMM.

4.4 Effect of aperture configurations on the modulation depth of FMM

Another important parameter in FMM is the modulation depth, which can be defined as the ratio of the intensity of the modulated fluorescence signal (i.e. the ac component) to the average intensity (approximately the dc component) collected by the aperture pinhole. The modulation depth is crucial in designing illumination aperture for FMM because it determines the efficiency of FMM signal generation with respect to the total excitation power deposited on the sample. Principally, a larger modulation depth will give us enhanced FMM signal and therefore improved signal to noise ratio. In addition, a larger modulation depth allows us to reduce the threshold of excitation power for optical image quality when probing deep into thick living specimens, which is crucial in minimizing the probability of photobleaching and phototoxicity resulted from higher excitation power. In this section, we first define the modulation depth and an analytical expression for its calculation in FMM. In particular, various aperture designs are being considered to compare their effectiveness in generating high modulation depth. The spatial resolutions correspond to each aperture are also presented with some concluding remarks at the end.

4.4.1 Definition of modulation depth for FMM

The modulation depth of FMM can be defined as the ratio of the intensity of the modulated fluorescence signal (i.e. ac component) to the average intensity (i.e. dc component) collected by the aperture pinhole when exciting a fluorescence-stained sample:

$$M = \frac{\frac{1}{2}(I_{max}-I_{min})}{\frac{1}{2}(I_{max}+I_{min})} = \frac{I_{max}-I_{min}}{I_{max}+I_{min}} = \frac{I_{FMM}}{I_{CM}} \tag{20}$$

Here I denotes the signal intensity at the pinhole detector. In FMM, the illumination apertures consists of, non-modulated and modulated zones, as shown in Fig. 10, in which the green regions having a constant phase delay while the light passing through the blue regions is subject to a time-varying phase delay. The relative phase delay $\varphi(t)$ between the green and blue regions varies from 0 to π phase shift. All the apertures are designed such that the total area of the modulated regions equal to that of the unmodulated regions, in order to have the maximum modulation efficiency.

In previous section, we already described the 3D illumination point spread function (IPSF) after the objectives based on scalar diffraction theory. Assuming the wavefront of the illumination beams is uniform before spatial phase modulator, we can obtain the IPSF of CM and FMM using the following equation in Cartesian coordinates:

$$E(x,y,z,t) = \left| \iint_A P(x',y',t) e^{\left\{\frac{ik}{f}(x^2+y^2) - \frac{ik}{2z}[(x-x')^2+(y-y')^2]\right\}} dx'dy' \right|^2 \quad (21)$$

where A is the open area of the aperture and $P(x',y',t)$ is the instantaneous phase profile of the spatial phase modulator, which varies with time t according to designated modulation frequency. The lateral and axial coordinates x, y, and z are in the image space while x' and y' indicate the position in the aperture A. The wavenumber k is related to the wavelength of the illumination λ as $k = \frac{2\pi}{\lambda}$ and f is the focal length of the objective. Then, the intensity on the detector $I(t)$ can be expressed as:

$$I(t) = \iiint E(x,y,z,t) \times [|h_D(x,y,z)|^2 \otimes_2 D(x,y)] \, dxdydz \quad (22)$$

where $h_D(x,y,z)$is the amplitude point spread function of the detection optics, $D(x,y)$ is the sensitivity function for the detector and is related to the size of the aperture pinhole in front of the detector. Thus, when the phase over the apertures is uniform (i.e. $\varphi(t) = 0$), a strong constructive interference at the focal spot of the objectives is expected and the detected signal at the central focal spot will reach the maximum, which is also identical to that of CM. For CM, the phase profile is uniform (i.e. $P(x',y',t) = 1$) and thus the IPSF is simply:

$$E_{CM}(x,y,z) = \left| \iint_A P(x',y',t)|_{\varphi(t)=0} \, e^{\left\{\frac{ik}{f}(x^2+y^2) - \frac{ik}{2z}[(x-x')^2+(y-y')^2]\right\}} dx'dy' \right|^2 \quad (23)$$

Then, the detected signal of CM at the focal spot is:

$$I_{CM} = \iiint E_{CM}(x,y,z) \times [|h_D(x,y,z)|^2 \otimes_2 D(x,y)] \, dxdydz \quad (24)$$

On the other hand, when the relative phase delay of the modulated and unmodulated beams $\varphi(t)$ is equal to π, a strong destructive interference will occur at the central spot of the point spread function of the illumination beams (i.e. within the first zeroth of the IPSF of FMM) and the detected intensity approximately reach the minimum (i.e. I_{min}), with high-intensity side lobes appearing immediately outside the central focal spot. At such, we can define the effective FMM intensity point spread function as the difference of the intensity at the central focal spot for illumination with uniform phase (i.e. I_{max}) and that of modulated phase apertures (i.e. I_{min}); which can be easily shown to be proportionally equal to the FMM intensity detected using heterodyne detection in real implementation. Here, we outline the equations for the illumination PSF of FMM:

$$E_{FMM}(x,y,z) = E_{CM}(x,y,z) - \left| \iint_A P(x',y',t)|_{\varphi(t)=\pi}\, e^{\left\{\frac{ik}{f}(x^2+y^2) - \frac{ik}{2z}[(x-x')^2+(y-y')^2]\right\}} dx'dy' \right|^2 \quad (25)$$

Then, the FMM intensity is simply:

$$I_{FMM} = \iiint E_{FMM}(x,y,z) \times [|h_D(x,y,z)|^2 \otimes_2 D(x,y)]\, dxdydz \quad (26)$$

Finally, the modulation depth of FMM can be easily calculated using equations. It is important to understand that the total intensity loading on the focal plane inside the sample (as well as the whole sample) is always uniform regardless of the relative phase-delay of the patterned illumination beam, and the detection pinhole (as well as its size) is crucial in collecting only the intensity-modulated fluorescence emission from the focal volume. Else, the amplitude of FMM signal over the focal plane would drop significantly.

4.4.2 Simulation results

The simulation results based on analytical expressions described in the previous section are presented here. Typical system parameters are being used in our simulation. The laser wavelength is 633 nm. For simplicity, we assume the objective lens L_1 and the collection lens L_2 are identical and have the same numerical aperture of 0.55, and the excitation and emission lights have same wavelength as well. The pinhole diameter used is 0.8 μm, about $0.6d_{Airy}$ (d_{Airy} is the diameter of Airy disk). Eight apertures (see Fig. 10), which includes three annular apertures, three fan-shaped apertures and two stripe-shaped apertures, are investigated. These apertures are selected partly due to their ease of fabrication.

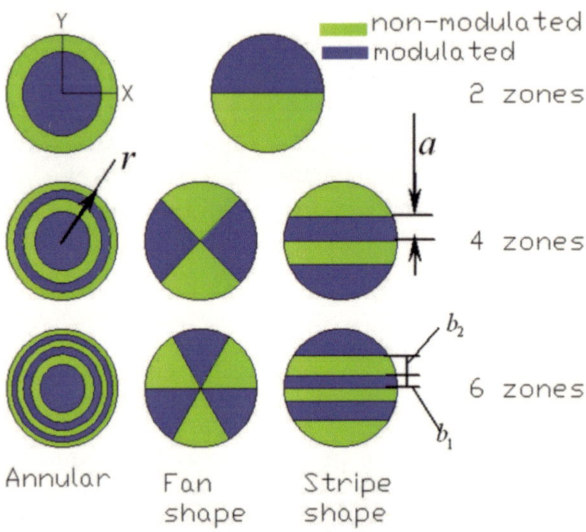

Fig. 10. Configurations of SPM apertures that are being investigated. The areas with green color are non-modulated, and those with blue are modulated. According to the first principle of aperture selection, the internal radii of annular apertures are $\frac{r}{\sqrt{2}}$ for 2-zone annular aperture, and $\frac{r}{2}, \frac{r}{\sqrt{2}}, \frac{\sqrt{3}r}{2}$ for 4-zone annular aperture, $\frac{r}{\sqrt{6}}, \frac{r}{\sqrt{3}}, \frac{r}{\sqrt{2}}, \frac{\sqrt{6}r}{3}, \frac{\sqrt{30}r}{6}$ for 6-zone annular aperture. Similarly, the widths for stripe apertures are $a \approx 0.404r$ for 4-zone stripe aperture and $b_1 \approx 0.215r$, $b_2 \approx 0.338r$ for 6-zone stripe aperture. r is the external radius of aperture.

The effective illumination IPSFs for different apertures calculated using equations described in section 4.4.1 are presented in Fig. 11. They are displayed as enface (upper row) and cross-sectional (lower row) 2D images of around the focal point. Fig. 11 (a) are the effective IPSFs for annular apertures of two zones (left column), four zones (middle column), and six zones (right column), respectively. The results for fan-shaped and stripe-shaped apertures are arranged in a similar way in Fig 11 (b) and (c). The coordinates of the Figs v_x, v_y and u are related to the practical coordinates x, y, and z by $v_x = kNAx$, $v_y = kNAy$ and $u = 4k\left[\sin\frac{\alpha}{2}\right]^2 z$ with NA the numerical aperture of objective lens, α the semi-angle aperture of the objective lens. The illumination IPSFs of FMM can be negative for some regions outside central focal volume due to differential excitation mechanism of FMM. If these negative side lobes are allowed to be included in the FMM image formation (i.e. by enlarging the detection pinhole), the FMM signals will diminish and become ineffective (Chen, Wong et al. 2008).

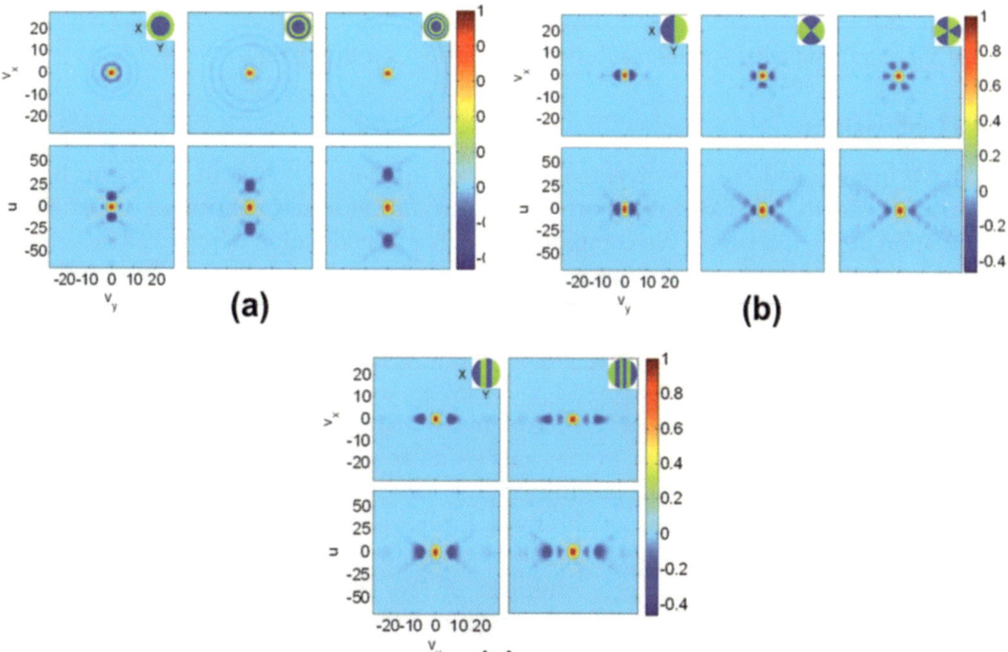

Fig. 11. IPSFs for (a) annular, (b) fan shape and (c) stripe shape apertures. In (a) and (b) the first, second and third columns are corresponding to two, four, and six zones. In (c) The result of two zones is omitted because it is the same as the two-zone fan-shape aperture. The icon on the top-right of each graph is the corresponding aperture shape.

From the IPSFs in Fig 11, we can calculate the modulation depth using the method described in previous section. The calculated modulation depth for the investigated apertures is shown in Table 2. Additionally, the lateral and axial spatial resolutions achievable are also expressed in term of full width half maximum (FWHM) of the simulated IPSFs (see Table 3), which is the diameter of the central spot where the intensity drops beyond half of the maximum. Basically, there are no significant differences between the achievable spatial resolutions in both lateral and axial directions.

Aperture pattern	Number of zones		
	2	4	6
Annular	0.446	0.757	0.865
Fan	0.361	0.602	0.762
Stripes	0.361	0.691	0.814

Table 2. Modulation depths for various aperture patterns.

	Lateral			Axial		
Aperture pattern	Number of zones					
	2	4	6	2	4	6
Annular	2.666	2.689	2.692	6.692	7.699	7.898
Fan	2.694	2.697	2.697	8.057	8.056	8.057
Stripes	2.694	2.696	2.696	8.057	8.060	8.059

Table 3. Lateral and axial spatial resolution for various aperture patterns.

4.4.3 Discussions

We have investigated the effectiveness of various aperture patterns in achieving higher modulation depth for FMM that are important for efficient generation of intensity modulation at the focal spot. We compare the resultant modulation depths and achievable spatial resolutions for these aperture patterns through analytical calculations, with several comments can be made.

First, with the number of zones increasing from 2 to 6, the modulation depths of the three types of apertures increase from 0.3~0.4 to 0.75~0.85, as shown in Table 2. As explained earlier, there are negative side lobes in the effective IPSFs as FMM is based on differential excitation mechanism (see Fig. 11). In the cases for an aperture with two zones, the negative side lobes appear very close to the positive central main lobe and their absolute peak values are greater than 0.4 (normalized to the main lobe peak value). Such behaviour lead to reduced FMM signal if these negative side lobes are included in FMM image formation when the pinhole size is too large. Alternatively, we can implement smaller detection pinhole to exclude these negative side lobes, which at the same time reduced FMM signals from central spot. By increasing the number of zones in the SPM aperture, however, we can disperse the negative side lobes, moving their peak positions slightly away from the focus and at the same time reducing their magnitudes. Thus, we have greater flexibility in selecting larger detection pinhole to capture maximum FMM signals from central focal spot. This is generally true for annular, fan-shape, and stripe-shape apertures.

Second, it is observed that there is slight degradation (from 6.7 to 7.9) for the axial resolution of annular aperture when the modulation depth is being increased by increasing the number of zones from 2 to 6, and almost no influence to the axial resolutions of other type of apertures, which is shown in Table 3. Previously, it has been shown that CM with an annular aperture and a point detector will result in improvement of lateral spatial resolution at the cost of degradation of optical sectioning strength (i.e. axial resolution) (Sheppard and Gu 1991). However, using a finite sized pinhole, annular aperture could give us improvement of axial resolution (Gu and Sheppard 1991). The effect of size of pinhole detector on the axial resolution of FMM with annular aperture as the number of zones increase is thus worth to be further investigated in future.

Last but not least, from the standpoint of modulation depth and axial resolution, the annular apertures are superior to the fan shape and stripe shape apertures, while the achievable lateral resolutions are approximately the same for all types of apertures. This is expected because neither the fan-shape nor the stripe-shape apertures have noticeable negative side lobes in the axial direction (Fig. 11 (b) and (c)), except the annular aperture that results in strong negative side lobes along the optical axis (Fig. 11 (a)), but has been taken care off by the pinhole. There are strong side lobes in the focal plane for the fan-shaped and stripe-shaped apertures due to their circular asymmetry and therefore better resolving power is expected in certain directions, such as, along y direction for fan shape and stripe shape apertures (see Fig. 11 (b) and (c)). Nevertheless, the poorest resolution along the lateral directions are being chosen as comparison. At such, we found no significant improvement of the lateral resolution for all apertures.

5. Implementations of focal modulation microscopy

Here, we describes on the implementations of two spatiotemporal phase modulation schemes for focal modulation microscope - double reflecting mirrors as well as FMM based on acousto-optical modulators that are significantly progressive in term of stability and image performance.

5.1 Double-reflecting mirror

5.1.1 System design

Shown in Fig. 12 is the schematic diagram of the first prototype FMM system developed at the Optical Bioimaging Lab, National University of Singapore. The light source is a 640 nm

solid state single frequency laser, whose 25 mW output beam is expanded to about 5 mm in diameter. When passing through the spatial phase modulator, the beam is split into two spatially separated half-beams, which are parallel and subject to different phase delays. The spatiotemporal phase modulation is implemented with two parallel mirrors (M1 and M2) inside the dashed box. M1 is mounted on a stationary base while M2 is mounted on a piezoelectric actuator. A sinusoidal voltage signal of a single frequency $f = 5\,kHz$ superimposed on an appropriate dc bias is applied to the actuator to induce a relative phase shift periodically between 0 and π. The spatiotemporal phase modulated excitation beam is reflected by a dichroic mirror and is then directed by a two-dimensional fast steering mirror to a 20X objective. Fluorescence emission is collected by the same objective and de-scanned is performed by the same fast steering mirror. A long pass emission filter is used to further reject the excitation light already suppressed by the DM. The cut-on wavelength for both the DM and the long pass filter is between 667 and 670 nm. Then the fluorescence light is focused by an achromat and coupled into a single mode (SM) optic fiber. A photomultiplier tube (R928, Hamamatsu Photonics Co.) converts the weak light signal to an electrical signal, which is digitized and sampled by a DAQ card in a personal computer (PC). The acquired photoelectrical signal contains a constant DC component and a time-varying AC component at 5 kHz due to modulated excitation. A Fast Fourier Transform (FFT) is performed on the PC to retrieve both FMM and CM signals respectively.

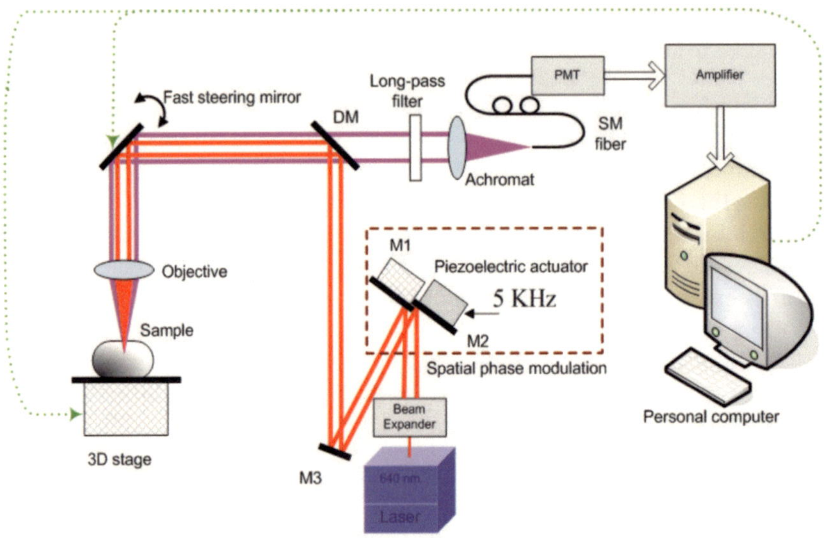

Fig. 12. Schematic diagram of the prototype focal modulation microscopy system. The spatial phase distribution of the 640 *nm* excitation beam (red) is modulated by the use of two parallel mirrors, M1 (stationary) and M2 (oscillating axially at **5** kHz). The fluorescence emission (purple) from the focal volume is collected by a fiber based confocal detection system, and then the oscillatory component at **5** kHz is retrieved for image formation. The personal computer is used for data acquisition and analysis, lateral scanning with the fast steering mirror, and axial scanning with the 3D stage.

5.1.2 Experiments and results

To demonstrate the capability of our method for *in vivo* imaging of cellular and sub-cellular structure and function, we used chicken cartilage as a sample tissue to evaluate the performance of FMM. Chondrocytes are the only cells found in cartilage. The cells are usually of a rounded or bluntly angular form, lying in groups of two or more in a glandular or almost homogeneous matrix. Chicken cartilage was cut into slices around **1** mm in thickness and stained with DiD (DiIC18 (5), Invitrogen Corp.), a lipophilic tracer for cell membrane labeling. The laser power was attenuated by 10 – 1000 times to avoid fast photobleaching. Fig. 13 (a) and 13 (b) are CM and FMM images acquired at a depth around 280 μm.

One can easily see that optical sectioning is not effective in the confocal image (Fig 13(a)). Fluorescence signals from layers other than the focal plane cast shadows in the image, resulting in overlapping structures and blurred cellular shapes. On the contrary, the FMM image (Fig. 13 (b)) shows uncompromised quality. The upper-central area was then scanned with a four times finer step (about 100 nm) and the high magnification images are displayed in Fig. 13 (c) and (d). The FMM image (Fig. 13 (d)) provides detailed information with sub-micron spatial resolution and excellent contrast, which are not available from the CM image (Fig. 13 (c)). We then pushed further to test the maximal penetration depth of our prototype FMM system. Shown in Fig 13. (e) and (f) are FMM images from 500 and 600 μm in depth. It is evident that resolution is still high enough to visualize cellular structures. Beyond 600 μm, the shot noise associated with the background will gradually overwhelm the FMM signal.

To the best of our knowledge, the penetration depth we report here has never been achieved by one photon fluorescence based microscopy when imaging optically dense biological tissues. However, there might be still room for further improvements. The tissue samples in our experiments were uniformly stained. As a result, the superficial layers strongly absorbed the excitation light and generated intense background emissions. For certain applications where only the deep region of interest is stained, an even larger penetration depth should be possible. More photostable and brighter fluorescent labels (e.g., quantum dots) can also help further increase the imaging depth.

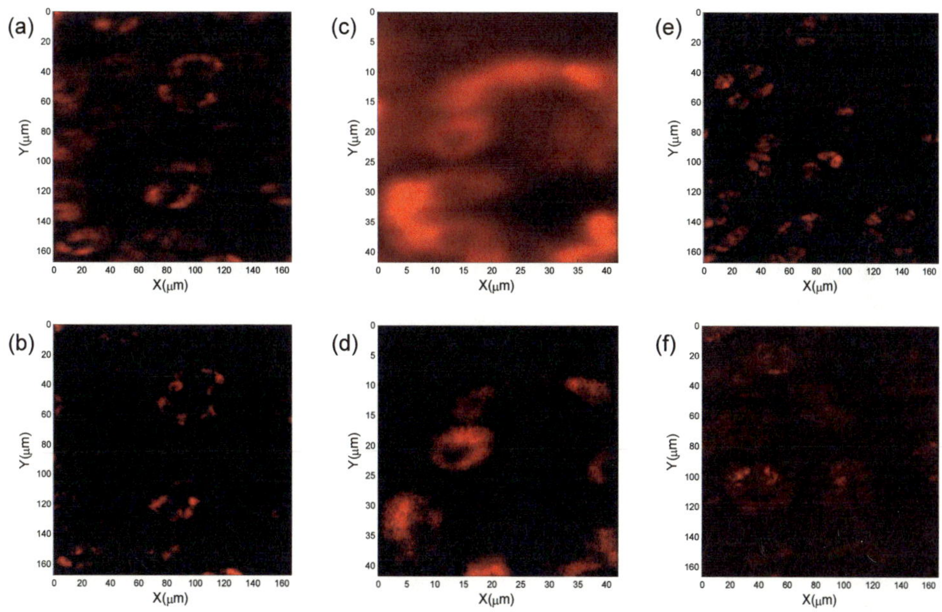

Fig. 13. Fluorescence images of chondrocytes obtained from chicken cartilage. Confocal images ((a) and (c)) were acquired simultaneously with the corresponding FMM images ((b) and (d)) at a depth of 280 μm. (e) and (f) are FMM images obtained from 500 and 600 μm in depth.

The imaging depth mentioned above was achieved with a relatively long excitation wavelength of 640 *nm*. For excitation light of shorter wavelength, such as UV or blue light, the achievable imaging depth is expected to be smaller due to stronger scattering. On the other hand, near infrared fluorescence dyes (Indocyanine Green, for example) would allow the use of an even longer excitation wavelength (780 *nm*) and deeper imaging. The imaging speed of this prototype FMM is limited by the spatiotemporal phase modulator consisting of two mirrors. The minimal dwelling time at each pixel is 0.2 ms, significantly longer than the typical 10 microsecond pixel dwelling time for commercial CM and MPM systems.

5.1.3 Discussions

The imaging depth demonstrated here is related to a relatively long excitation wavelength of 640 nm. Generally the scattering coefficient of biological tissue decreases with increasing wavelength, and in many situations the attenuation of ballistic light is dominated by scattering. For excitation light of shorter wavelength, such as UV or blue light, the achievable imaging depth should be smaller. On the other hand, near infrared fluorescence dyes (Indocyanine Green, for example) would allow the use of an even longer excitation wavelength (780 nm) and deeper imaging. In our future research, we will systematically study the dependence of imaging depth on excitation wavelength and fluorescence dye properties. The imaging speed of our prototype FMM is limited by the modulation frequency. The minimal dwelling time at each pixel is 0.2 ms, significantly longer than the typical 10 μs pixel dwelling time for commercial CM and MPM systems. We plan to develop electro-optical material based spatial phase modulators that can be modulated at a frequency more than a few MHz. Near-real-time FMM imaging (a few frames per second) would be possible with such a modulator.

5.2 FMM using acousto-optical modulators

We reported our FMM system implemented using tilting plate phase modulator (Wong, Chong et al. 2009) where a modulation frequency up to a few tens of kHz can been achieved. However, compared to most commercial laser scanning microscopes with microsecond pixel dwell time, that modulation frequency is still too low. In this section we describe a near-real-time FMM with AOMs and demonstrate the improved image acquisition speed and quality. Our FMM system is based on an Olympus FV300 confocal microscope

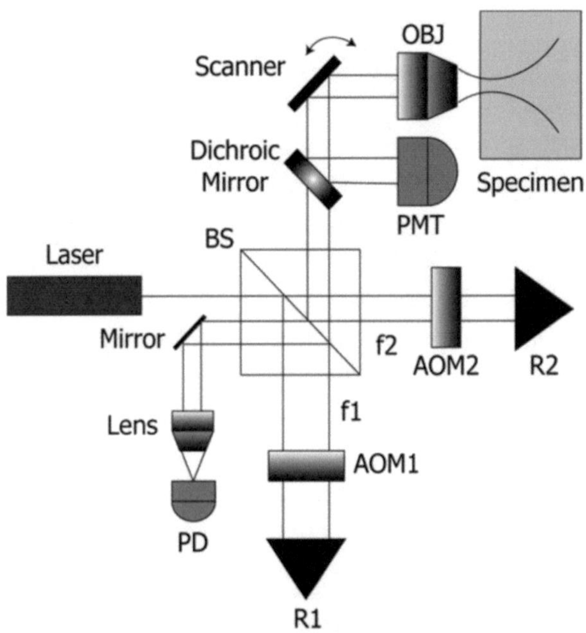

Fig. 14. Setup for a FMM implemented using acousto-optical modulators. Laser beam is split by a beam splitter (BS) in which light beam in each arm undergoing frequency shifting by two acoustic-optical modulators (AOM) with different resonance frequencies. Phase-shifted beams are reflected back to the BS by retroreflectors (R1 and R2). They are aligned in parallel non-overlapping manner when being split second times at BS in which one combined beam will be used to generate a reference signal while another combined beam is directed to the scanning unit of Olympus FV300 to excite the samples through the objective lens (OBJ). PD is a photodetector and M is a mirror.

5.2.1 Optical setup

The spatio-temporal phase modulator based on AOMs is shown schematically in see Fig. 14. The coherent laser beam is first split by a beam splitter into two beams which then passes through two AOMs with slightly different resonance frequencies (i.e. f_1 and f_2) where they undergo zeroth- and first-order diffractions. The first-order diffracted beams which are Doppler shifted at the f_1 and f_2 on each arm. They are reflected with slight lateral displacement using retroreflectors to return to the same AOMs and then are recombined at beam splitter. It is important to note that the two beams at the moment are Doppler shifted at twice the resonance frequencies of the AOMs respectively as they passed through the AOMs twice. Part of the combined beam is directed towards a fiber-optic photodetector, which generates a reference signal at the optical beating frequency of $2(f_1 - f_2)$. The remaining part of the modulated laser beam is directed to the scanning unit of a conventional CM (Olympus FV300) to excite the biological sample stained with fluorescence probes.

5.2.2 Detection of FMM signal

The fluorescence emissions are then detected by the built-in PMT detector (R3896, Hamamatsu Photonics Co.) behind a confocal pinhole. The PMT output is preamplified before feeding to an I/Q demodulator, where the oscillatory component at the beating frequency is picked up by mixing with the reference signal. The demodulated signal is further enhanced by the low-frequency amplifier and is then fed to the data acquisition device of the FV300 system (see Fig. 15 for the signal processing pathway).

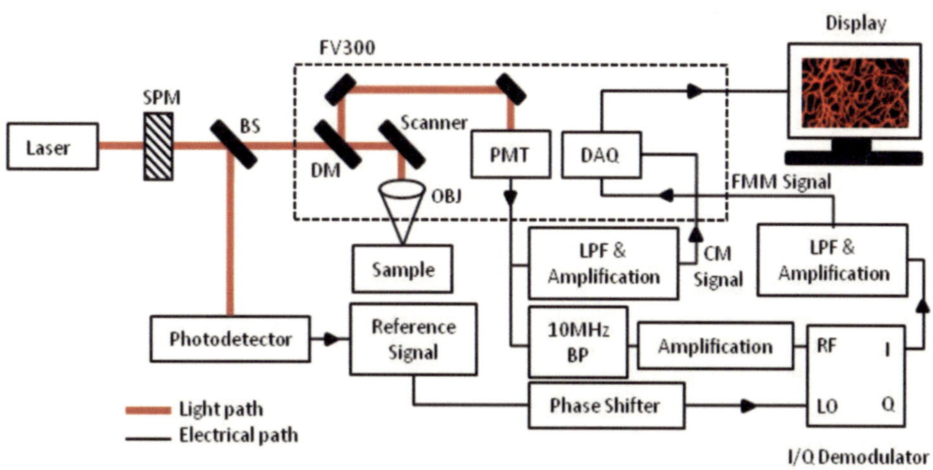

Fig. 15. Flow diagrams showing the signal-processing pathway.

The two AOMs we are using have resonant frequencies of 75 MHz and 80 MHz, respectively, resulting in a modulation frequency of 10 MHz. In principle, such a high modulation frequency allows a pixel dwell time as short as 0.1 microseconds. This instrument is a significant improvement in term of imaging speed, stability and noise level compared with the prototype setup we reported previously (Chen, Wong et al. 2008; Wong, Chong et al. 2009). CM and FMM images can be captured simultaneously with the same acquisition speed using our current system. The effectiveness of FMM in improving image quality is demonstrated by imaging blood vessels in mouse brain labeled with lipophilic carbocyanine dye DiI ('DiI'; DiIC18(3), Invitrogen), self-made tissue phantom as well as DiD stained chicken chondrocytes.

5.2.3 Experiments and results

The mouse brain samples were prepared using the established techniques described in the literature (Li, Song et al. 2008). A mouse was first sacrificed by overdose with CO_2 in a CO_2 chamber. A transverse incision was made to open the abdominal cavity. The diaphragm was exposed and cut. The chest was then cut on both sides up to the second rib. The anterior chest wall was turned toward the head of the mouse to expose the chest cavity. The butterfly needle of the perfusion device was inserted into the left ventricle, and the right atrium was punctured. $2ml$ of standard phosphate buffer solution (PBS) was injected from the perfusion device at the rate of $1 - 2ml/min$ for $5min$. Then, $5 - 10ml$ of the DiI solution was injected at a rate of $1 - 2ml/min$ for $5 - 10\ min$. Successful perfusion was monitored by observing color change in the ear, nose and palms of the mouse from pale while to purple. Lastly, the fixative (4% paraformaldehyde solution) was injected at a rate of $1 - 2ml/min$ for a total of 5min. It should be ensured that there are no air bubbles in the perfusion device as introduction of air into the circulatory system could block blood vessels, resulting in poor perfusion. The stained mouse brain was then extracted, and stored in 4% (wt/vol) paraformaldehyde solution. The whole fixed mouse brain is mounted by mounting medium (Polyvinyl alcohol mounting medium with DABCO®, antifading BioChemika, Sigma-Aldrich) in a coverslip bottom dish with cover (MatTek Corp) for imaging using our FMM.

Besides fluorescence imaging, we also apply our FMM system on imaging a cylindrical self-made tissue phantom slab mainly consisted of epoxy-resin, resin hardener, and titanium dioxide (TiO_2). The TiO_2 powder acts as scattering components and the main contrast agent inside the tissue phantom. This tissue phantom was made based on the procedures reported in literature (Firbank, Oda et al. 1995) and is commonly used for calibration in diffuse optical tomography (DOT) (Mo and Chen 2008). The chicken cartilage sample is prepared in the similar way described in section 5.1.2.

A. Mouse brain vasculatures imaging

The mouse brain samples were imaged using our FMM system with either objectives UPLSAPO 10x/0.40 numerical aperture (NA) or LUCPLANFLN 20x/0.45 NA to evaluate our FMM system in term of image quality improvement. Here we show the images captured using CM and FMM simultaneously to demonstrate the robustness of FMM in rejecting out-of-focus fluorescence background and retaining high-resolution features even imaging deep inside tissues (depicted by Fig. 16).

A blood vessel bifurcation imaged using CM (Fig. 16 (a)) and FMM (Fig. 16. (b)) shows that much finer features can be visualized by FMM clearly at the penetration depth around $200um$. Fig. 16 (c) and (d) shows the digital magnification near the bifurcation of the main blood vessel (indicated by white boxes in Fig. 16 (a) and (b)) which also reveals better contrast on the fine structures of the blood vessels by the image captured by FMM as compared to CM. From the intensity profiles spanning the both white lines (top-down) in the Fig. 16 (c) and (d), we can also observe that the peaks are more clearly visible and distinctive from each other's in the FMM image with sharper valleys, and significant reduction in background as well. This indicates that our FMM system can provide better image contrast and more structural information of the tissue being studied.

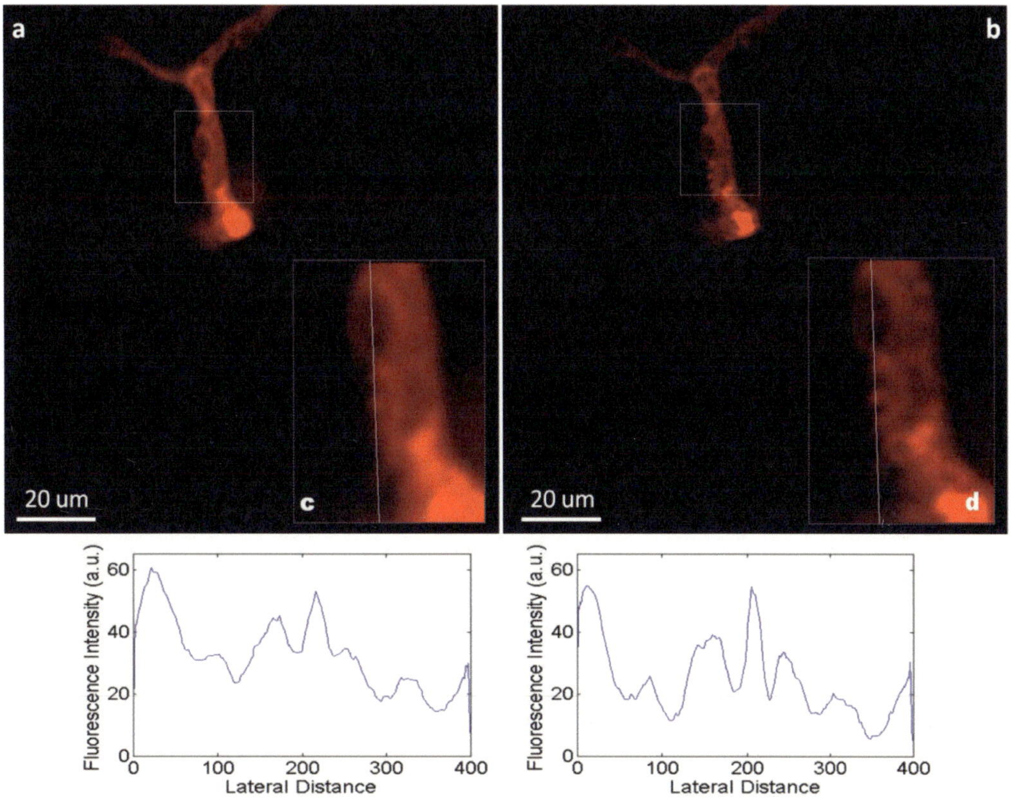

Fig. 16. Demonstration of FMM in retaining high-resolution features by rejecting out-of-focus fluorescence background. A blood vessel bifurcation image acquired with Olympus LUCPLANFLN 20x/0.45 NA using (a) CM and (b) FMM shows much finer features can be revealed by FMM even at penetration depth up 200um. Fig. 16 (c) and (d) shows the digital magnification near the bifurcation of the main blood vessel which reveals much richer features on the image captured by FMM. The plot at the bottom of the images shows the intensity profiles of the white lines (top-down) in the images.

B. Tissue phantom imaging

We also performed imaging in the tissue phantom over the depths of $300 - 400\ \mu m$ with $0.5\ \mu m$ increments. A single frame image of a cluster of TiO_2 powder (see Fig. 17) embedded at $320\ \mu m$ inside the self-made tissue phantom captured using CM and FMM operated in reflectance mode.

Similarly, FMM (see Fig. 17 (b)) could significantly improve the image quality by providing superior contrast and sharp edges as compared to CM which are blurred mainly by multiple scattering effects. The peaks are also more clearly distinguished from each other in FMM despite the TiO_2 granules are in close proximity, as shown by the intensity profile spanning the white line (left-right), with higher SBR ratio due to lower background intensity.

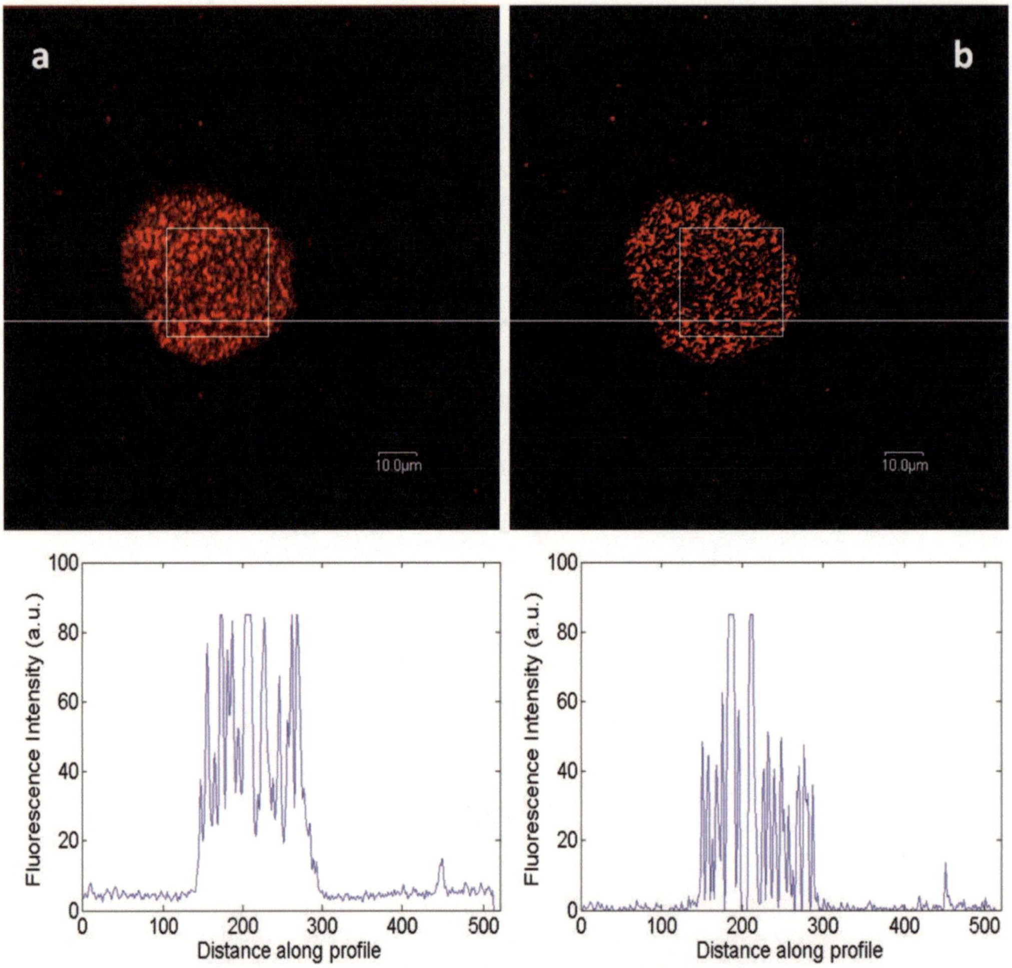

Fig. 17. Image of cluster of TiO_2 embedded 320um inside tissue phantom captured with Olympus LUCPLANFLN 20x/0.45 NA using (a) CM and (b) FMM. Better image quality is achieved using FMM, with less blurring and structures are more clearly distinguishable due to sharp boundaries. The plot at the bottom of the images shows the intensity profile of the white lines in the images. Peaks are more distinct with better contrast can be observed.

To perform more quantitative analysis of image quality improvement by FMM, we selected a pair of identical region of interest (ROI) from Fig. 17 (a) and (b) respectively and compare their normalized spectra (with respect to the dc values). From Fig. 18, we can observe that the high frequency components (>1 cycle/μm) in the FMM image are about 13 dB stronger than those in the CM image. This can be translated to a 13 dB improvement in the SBR ratio provided by FMM. However, our previous theoretical model (Chong, Wong et al. 2010) predicted a 20 dB enhancement by FMM at a similar imaging depth of 2 scattering mean free paths (the scattering coefficient of our tissue phantom is around 6 cm^{-1} (Mo and Chen 2008) . This discrepancy could be due to slight overlapping of the two excitation beams and the resultant residual intensity modulation which can be minimized by improved modulator designs.

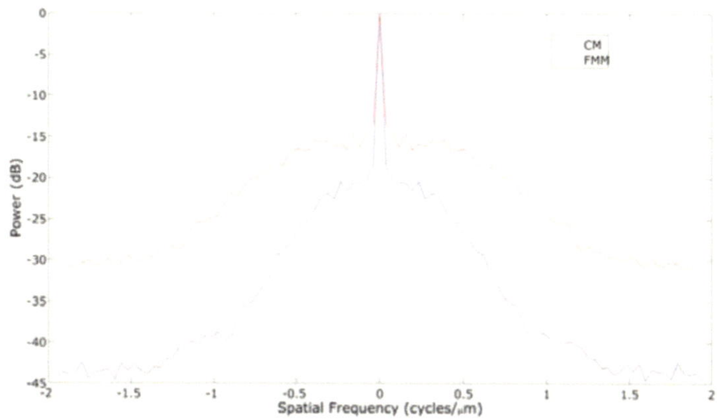

Fig. 18. Normalized spatial spectra (with respect to dc values) of the region of interests labeled by square boxes in Fig. 17 (a) and (b) showing the spatial frequency components of CM and FMM respectively.

C. Chicken chondrocytes samples

We also imaged chondrocytes of the chicken cartilage samples labelled with lipophilic carbocyanine dye DiD (DiD′ solid; DiIC18 (5) solid, Invitrogen) using objectives UPLSAPO 10x/0.40 numerical aperture (NA).

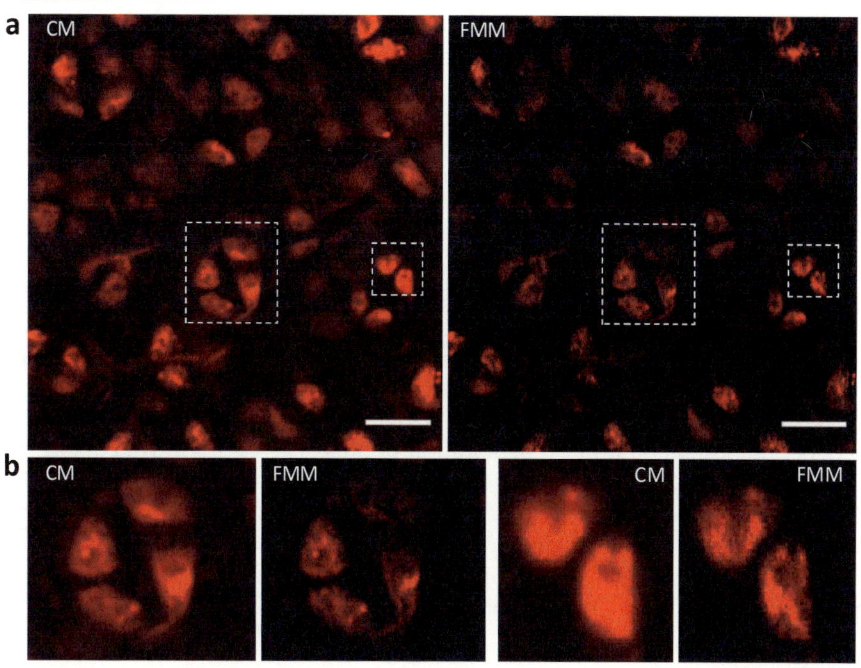

Fig. 19. Comparison of FMM and confocal fluorescence microscopy of chondrocytes of chicken cartilages at penetration depth around **350** μm. (a) The chondrocytes were labeled with DiD (red). (b) Magnifications of the indicated regions. Scale bars **20** μm.

Generally, it is evident that the FMM image gives us less background than raw confocal fluorescence microscopy image (Fig. 19 (a)). The optical contrast of FMM image is also greatly improved, whereas the confocal data are blurred as a result of light scattering. The removal of scattered light also translated directly into enrichment in information quality, revealing features inside the cellular compartments that were obscured in confocal images (Fig. 19 b), indicating that FMM can preserve the optical contrast for large penetration depth in which the fluorescence background dominates the collected signals. The advantages of FMM in terms preserving optical contrast and providing richer subcellular information will be important for imaging of subcellular studies of thick specimens such as characterizing the morphological changes of nuclei in cancers cells (Yao, Maslov et al. 2010).

5.2.4 Discussions and summary

We have validated the capability of FMM in improving image quality at large penetration depth by visualizing various specimens. All the images were taken at 512x512 pixels, with a pixel dwell times of around 10 μs, resulting image acquisition time of around 2.7s. We emphasized that as the mouse brain samples are specifically stained in which only blood vessels void of blood (one of the major absorbers and scatterers inside biological tissues) are labeled with DiD, generally less background will be observed while larger penetration depth is expected compared to uniformly stained samples. Nevertheless, CM still suffers from poor image quality especially in observation of finer features; while FMM can work robustly in detecting fluorescence by ballistic photons and rejecting out-of-focus fluorescence background even at the large depth. This is an important feature for investigations and characterizations of thick tissue with sub-micron spatial resolution when confocal pinhole fails to reject majority of the out-of-focus fluorescence background. Better characterization of microvasculatures in animal model over large observation volume using FMM can be potentially useful especially for quantification of angiogenesis in term of density/diameter of blood vessels in live animal cancer model (Lunt, Gray et al. 2010). We also highlight that though FMM can reject most of the background, it cannot increase the signal level and thus if the FMM signal falls below the shot noise floor at extreme depths, other strategies (i.e. denoise image processing and/or extended image acquisition time) may be needed to improve the image quality.

A modulation frequency of 160 MHz can be achieved if only a single AOM is used. However, a too high modulation frequency could cause significant attenuation of the FMM signals as the signal intensity is proportional to $e^{-2\pi f\tau}$ in which f is the modulation frequency and τ is the lifetime of fluorescent probes. As most of the fluorescent molecules have a typical lifetime of a few nanoseconds, deterioration of the signal-to-noise ratio will thus be a serious problem at large penetration depths. The 10 MHz we choose falls in the optimal frequency range for fast image acquisition and negligible signal attenuation, and it is compatible with available demodulation components. In future, the issues of inherent Poisson statistical noise that gradually becoming significant in the case of low intensity signal related to deep imaging of biological tissues and further improvement of the image quality with the inclusion of Poisson noise removal will be studied.

6. Conclusions

It is a seemingly endless endeavour as microscopists seek to push ever deeper into biological specimens, while resolving micro-structural details and observing specific molecular events. This book chapter describes the development of high-speed focal modulation microscopy and the corresponding technological advancement, in which the aim is to extend the penetration depth limit in thick specimens, without the necessity of the usage of long wavelength excitation or non-linear effect, i.e. currently two main approaches for achieving large penetration depth in biological specimens. FMM has thus far proved to be a significant improvement over the conventional confocal microscopy in term of SBR ratio at large penetration depths and potentially useful for cellular and molecular *in vivo* imaging. Its overall low-cost implementation also means its potential to be widely adopted as a basic research tool in biomedical and clinical applications.

In summary, the principles of FMM is elaborated and two implementations of FMM which varies in term of phase modulation schemes - double-mirrors phase modulator and FMM based on acousto-optical modulator that are significantly progressive in term of stability and image performance as compared to first FMM prototype based on double mirror spatial phase modulator (Chen, Wong et al. 2008) are being demonstrated. It is worth to mention that the modulation frequency is greatly enhanced from kHz range to MHz range, and the accompanied benefits include higher image acquisition speed and possible adaptation to fluorescence lifetime imaging. We also demonstrated the capability of FMM in improving the imaging contrast of various types of samples over a large penetration depth. We also highlight that FMM can operate in both fluorescence and back-scattered/reflectance mode. This is contrasted to the non-linear methods such as two-photon microscopy which only improve the imaging depth in fluorescence mode. FMM can switch between fluorescence and back-scattered/reflectance mode by enabling/disabling the phase modulation components in the illumination arm, thus allowing observation of surface topology and tissue morphology based on the back-scattered/reflectance mode as well as rich functional and molecular-specific information through the fluorescence mode.

6.1 Future directions

We believe FMM technique will be useful for many biological applications, which large penetration depth is required. Future works to combine the technique of FMM with multi-photon microscopy and microendoscopy are underway to further improve the penetration depth achievable by optical techniques through better rejection of background fluorescence; and for clinical usage to help in early disease detection and diagnosis. On top of that, the application of adaptive optics in FMM to pre-conditioning the beam profile of the excitation beam will further improve the modulation efficiency of FMM, which currently hampered by optical aberrations due to biological samples inhomogeneity. Much stronger FMM signal can be obtained if these optical aberration effects can be dampened which allows better focusing at the focal region and more efficient generation of intensity modulation. The development of FMM microendoscopy, thanks to the technological advancement in miniature fiber-optics and micro-mechanical scanning mechanism, will be invaluable for *in vivo* cellular-level imaging of tissues in regions that are otherwise inaccessible by bench-top microscope, such as the lung, bladder, cervix, uterus, colon, and peritoneum (Sabharwal, Rouse et al. 1999; Flusberg, Cocker et al. 2005). This ability enables determination of abnormalities localized on the surface or those being more aggressive (i.e. invading below the surface) which will be crucial for early cancer detection.

In addition, the high modulation frequency of FMM based on acousto-optical modulators can also be further developed for fluorescence lifetime imaging. Fluorescence lifetime measurements are independent of fluorophores concentrations and thus insensitive to wavelength-dependent light scattering, making it attractive especially in certain scenario such as when uniform illumination for visualization of fluorescent probes deep in tissues cannot be easily achieved over the area of interest owing to its irregular surface (Sun, Phipps et al. 2009).

6.2 Take home message

It is always a trade-off between the penetration depths limit and spatial resolutions when adopting an optical microscopy technique in visualization of thick biological specimens. Depending on the applications, it is important to balance the overall cost and imaging qualities to maximize the research outputs. With the advancement of optical engineering, faster scanning mechanisms and higher–performance photodetector, it is expected that biomedical imaging will be benefited with higher-throughput and larger penetration depths.

7. References

Axelrod, D. (2003). "Total internal reflection fluorescence microscopy in cell biology." Biophotonics, Pt B 361: 1-33.

Chen, N., C. H. Wong, et al. (2008). "Focal modulation microscopy." Opt Express 16(23): 18764-18769.

Chen, N., C. H. Wong, et al. (2008). "Focal modulation microscopy." Optics Express 16(23): 18764-18769.

Chong, S. P., C. H. Wong, et al. (2010). "Focal modulation microscopy: a theoretical study." Optics letters 35(11): 1804-1806.

Conchello, J. A. and J. W. Lichtman (2005). "Optical sectioning microscopy." Nature methods 2(12): 920-931.

Deng, X. and M. Gu (2003). "Penetration depth of single-, two-, and three-photon fluorescence microscopic imaging through human cortex structures: Monte Carlo simulation." Applied Optics 42(16): 3321-3329.

Denk, W., J. H. Strickler, et al. (1990). "Two-photon laser scanning fluorescence microscopy." Science 248(4951): 73-76.

Detrich, H. W., 3rd, M. Westerfield, et al. (2010). "The zebrafish: cellular and developmental biology, part A. Preface." Methods Cell Biol 100: xiii.

Dittrich, P. S. and P. Schwille (2001). "Photobleaching and stabilization of fluorophores used for single-molecule analysis with one- and two-photon excitation." Applied Physics B-Lasers and Optics 73(8): 829-837.

Dunn, A. K., C. Smithpeter, et al. (1996). "Sources of contrast in confocal reflectance imaging." Applied Optics 35(19): 3441-3446.

Dyba, M. and S. W. Hell (2002). "Focal spots of size lambda/23 open up far-field fluorescence microscopy at 33 nm axial resolution." Physical review letters 88(16): 163901.

Fercher, A. F. (2010). "Optical coherence tomography - development, principles, applications." Zeitschrift Fur Medizinische Physik 20(4): 251-276.

Fercher, A. F., W. Drexler, et al. (2003). "Optical coherence tomography - principles and applications." Reports on Progress in Physics 66(2): 239-303.

Firbank, M., M. Oda, et al. (1995). "An improved design for a stable and reproducible phantom material for use in near-infrared spectroscopy and imaging." Physics in Medicine and Biology 40(5): 955-961.

Flusberg, B. A., E. D. Cocker, et al. (2005). "Fiber-optic fluorescence imaging." Nat Methods 2(12): 941-950.

Fujimoto, J. G. (2003). "Optical coherence tomography for ultrahigh resolution in vivo imaging." Nature biotechnology 21(11): 1361-1367.

Fujimoto, J. G., M. E. Brezinski, et al. (1995). "Optical Biopsy and Imaging Using Optical Coherence Tomography." Nature Medicine 1(9): 970-972.

Gan, X., S. Schilders, et al. (1997). "Combination of annular aperture and polarization gating methods for efficient microscopic imaging through a turbid medium: Theoretical analysis." Microscopy and Microanalysis 3(6): 495-503.

Gu, M. (1996). Principles of three dimensional imaging in confocal microscopes. Singapore ; River Edge, NJ, World Scientific.

Gu, M. (2000). Advanced optical imaging theory. Berlin ; New York, Springer.

Gu, M. and C. J. R. Sheppard (1991). "3-Dimensional Imaging in Confocal Fluorescent Microscopy with Annular Lenses." Journal of Modern Optics 38(11): 2247-2263.

Gustafsson, M. G., D. A. Agard, et al. (1999). "I5M: 3D widefield light microscopy with better than 100 nm axial resolution." Journal of microscopy 195(Pt 1): 10-16.

Hell, S. W., E. H. K. Stelzer, et al. (1994). "Confocal Microscopy with an Increased Detection Aperture - Type-B 4pi Confocal Microscopy." Optics Letters 19(3): 222-224.

Helmchen, F. and W. Denk (2005). "Deep tissue two-photon microscopy." Nature methods 2(12): 932-940.

Huang, D., E. A. Swanson, et al. (1991). "Optical coherence tomography." Science 254(5035): 1178-1181.

Huisken, J., J. Swoger, et al. (2004). "Optical sectioning deep inside live embryos by selective plane illumination microscopy." Science 305(5686): 1007-1009.

Izatt, J. A., M. R. Hee, et al. (1994). "Optical coherence microscopy in scattering media." Optics letters 19(8): 590-592.

Jain, R. K., L. L. Munn, et al. (2002). "Dissecting tumour pathophysiology using intravital microscopy." Nature Reviews Cancer 2(4): 266-276.

Keller, P. J., A. D. Schmidt, et al. (2010). "Fast, high-contrast imaging of animal development with scanned light sheet-based structured-illumination microscopy." Nature methods 7(8): 637-U655.

Keller, P. J., A. D. Schmidt, et al. (2008). "Reconstruction of Zebrafish Early Embryonic Development by Scanned Light Sheet Microscopy." Science 322(5904): 1065-1069.

Keller, P. J. and E. H. Stelzer (2008). "Quantitative in vivo imaging of entire embryos with Digital Scanned Laser Light Sheet Fluorescence Microscopy." Current opinion in neurobiology 18(6): 624-632.

Kempe, M., W. Rudolph, et al. (1996). "Comparative study of confocal and heterodyne microscopy for imaging through scattering media." Journal of the Optical Society of America a-Optics Image Science and Vision 13(1): 46-52.

Kempe, M., A. Thon, et al. (1994). "Resolution Limits of Microscopy through Scattering Layers." Optics Communications 110(5-6): 492-496.

Kleinfeld, D., P. P. Mitra, et al. (1998). "Fluctuations and stimulus-induced changes in blood flow observed in individual capillaries in layers 2 through 4 of rat neocortex." Proc Natl Acad Sci U S A 95(26): 15741-15746.

Kobat, D., M. E. Durst, et al. (2009). "Deep tissue multiphoton microscopy using longer wavelength excitation." Optics Express 17(16): 13354-13364.

Li, L., R. J. Zemp, et al. (2007). "Photoacoustic imaging of lacZ gene expression in vivo." Journal of Biomedical Optics 12(2): 020504.

Li, M. L., J. T. Oh, et al. (2008). "Simultaneous molecular and hypoxia imaging of brain tumors in vivo using spectroscopic photoacoustic tomography." Proceedings of the Ieee 96(3): 481-489.

Li, Y., Y. Song, et al. (2008). "Direct labeling and visualization of blood vessels with lipophilic carbocyanine dye DiI." Nature protocols 3(11): 1703-1708.

Lunt, S. J., C. Gray, et al. (2010). "Application of intravital microscopy in studies of tumor microcirculation." Journal of Biomedical Optics 15(1): 011113.

Minsky, M. (1961). Microscopy Apparatus. US.

Minsky, M. (1988). "Memoir on Inventing the Confocal Scanning Microscope." Scanning 10(4): 128-138.

Misgeld, T. and M. Kerschensteiner (2006). "In vivo imaging of the diseased nervous system." Nature reviews. Neuroscience 7(6): 449-463.

Mo, W. and N. Chen (2008). "Fast time-domain diffuse optical tomography using pseudorandom bit sequences." Opt. Express 16(18): 13643-13650.

Oheim, M., E. Beaurepaire, et al. (2001). "Two-photon microscopy in brain tissue: parameters influencing the imaging depth." J Neurosci Methods 111(1): 29-37.

Patterson, G. H. and D. W. Piston (2000). "Photobleaching in two-photon excitation microscopy." Biophysical journal 78(4): 2159-2162.

Pavlova, I., M. Williams, et al. (2008). "Understanding the biological basis of autofluorescence imaging for oral cancer detection: high-resolution fluorescence microscopy in viable tissue." Clinical cancer research : an official journal of the American Association for Cancer Research 14(8): 2396-2404.

Pawley, J. B. (2006). Handbook of biological confocal microscopy. New York, NY, Springer.

Prati, F., E. Regar, et al. (2010). "Expert review document on methodology, terminology, and clinical applications of optical coherence tomography: physical principles, methodology of image acquisition, and clinical application for assessment of coronary arteries and atherosclerosis." European Heart Journal 31(4): 401-415.

Razansky, D., M. Distel, et al. (2009). "Multispectral opto-acoustic tomography of deep-seated fluorescent proteins in vivo." Nat Photon 3(7): 412-417.

Sabharwal, Y. S., A. R. Rouse, et al. (1999). "Slit-scanning confocal microendoscope for high-resolution in vivo imaging." Applied Optics 38(34): 7133-7144.

Sandison, D. R., D. W. Piston, et al. (1995). "Quantitative Comparison of Background Rejection, Signal-to-Noise Ratio, and Resolution in Confocal and Full-Field Laser-Scanning Microscopes." Applied Optics 34(19): 3576-3588.

Schmitt, J. M., A. Knuttel, et al. (1994). "Confocal Microscopy in Turbid Media." Journal of the Optical Society of America a-Optics Image Science and Vision 11(8): 2226-2235.

Schmitt, J. M., A. Knuttel, et al. (1994). "Confocal microscopy in turbid media." Journal of the Optical Society of America. A, Optics, image science, and vision 11(8): 2226-2235.

Sheppard, C. J. R. and M. Gu (1991). "3-Dimensional Optical Transfer-Function for an Annular Lens." Optics Communications 81(5): 276-280.

Sheppard, C. J. R. and T. Wilson (1980). "Image-Formation in Confocal Scanning Microscopes." Optik 55(4): 331-342.

Smithpeter, C. L., A. K. Dunn, et al. (1998). "Penetration depth limits of in vivo confocal reflectance imaging." Applied Optics 37(13): 2749-2754.

Sun, Y., J. Phipps, et al. (2009). "Fluorescence lifetime imaging microscopy: in vivo application to diagnosis of oral carcinoma." Opt Lett 34(13): 2081-2083.

Svoboda, K., F. Helmchen, et al. (1999). "Spread of dendritic excitation in layer 2/3 pyramidal neurons in rat barrel cortex in vivo." Nat Neurosci 2(1): 65-73.

Svoboda, K. and R. Yasuda (2006). "Principles of two-photon excitation microscopy and its applications to neuroscience." Neuron 50(6): 823-839.

Theer, P. and W. Denk (2006). "On the fundamental imaging-depth limit in two-photon microscopy." Journal of the Optical Society of America. A, Optics, image science, and vision 23(12): 3139-3149.

Theer, P., M. T. Hasan, et al. (2003). "Two-photon imaging to a depth of 1000 microm in living brains by use of a Ti:Al2O3 regenerative amplifier." Opt Lett 28(12): 1022-1024.

Theer, P., M. T. Hasan, et al. (2003). "Two-photon imaging to a depth of 1000 mu m in living brains by use of a Ti : Al2O3 regenerative amplifier." Optics Letters 28(12): 1022-1024.

Vakoc, B. J., R. M. Lanning, et al. (2009). "Three-dimensional microscopy of the tumor microenvironment in vivo using optical frequency domain imaging." Nat Med 15(10): 1219-1223.

Verveer, P. J., J. Swoger, et al. (2007). "High-resolution three-dimensional imaging of large specimens with light sheet-based microscopy." Nature methods 4(4): 311-313.

Wang, L. V. (2009). "Multiscale photoacoustic microscopy and computed tomography." Nature photonics 3(9): 503-509.

Wang, X., Y. Pang, et al. (2003). "Noninvasive laser-induced photoacoustic tomography for structural and functional in vivo imaging of the brain." Nature biotechnology 21(7): 803-806.

Wang, X., Y. Xu, et al. (2002). "Photoacoustic tomography of biological tissues with high cross-section resolution: reconstruction and experiment." Medical Physics 29(12): 2799-2805.

Wang, X. D., G. Ku, et al. (2004). "Non-invasive functional photoacoustic tomography of blood oxygen saturation in the brain." Photons Plus Ultrasound: Imaging and Sensing 5320: 69-76.

Wong, C. H., S. P. Chong, et al. (2009). "Simple spatial phase modulator for focal modulation microscopy." Applied Optics 48(17): 3237-3242.

Yang, S., D. Xing, et al. (2007). "Functional imaging of cerebrovascular activities in small animals using high-resolution photoacoustic tomography." Medical Physics 34(8): 3294-3301.

Yao, D. K., K. Maslov, et al. (2010). "In vivo label-free photoacoustic microscopy of cell nuclei by excitation of DNA and RNA." Opt Lett 35(24): 4139-4141.

Ying, J., F. Liu, et al. (1999). "Spatial distribution of two-photon-excited fluorescence in scattering media." Appl Opt 38(1): 224-229.

Zeng, C., S. Vangveravong, et al. (2007). "Subcellular localization of sigma-2 receptors in breast cancer cells using two-photon and confocal microscopy." Cancer research 67(14): 6708-6716.

8

Automated Segmentation and Morphometry of Cell and Tissue Structures. Selected Algorithms in ImageJ

Dimiter Prodanov and Kris Verstreken
Bioelectronic systems group, BIONE, Imec
Belgium

1. Introduction

This chapter covers selected aspects of the segmentation and measurements of spatial or temporal features (i.e. morphometry) of biological objects in biomedical (non-optical)[1] and microscopic images. The term *measurement* refers to a succinct quantitative representation of image features over space and time. This implies the application of the act of geometric measurement to the raw imaging data, i.e. "morphometry". Measurements arise in a defined experimental context.

1.1 Information complexity aspects

The life science experimentation strives to answer defined research questions via quantitative analysis of multiple experimental trials. This process can be described by a workflow[2] which starts by defining the research hypotheses or questions (Fig. 1). During the last stage the images are transformed into measurements, which are finally interpreted in the light of the original research question (Fig. 1).

A substantial decrease of the volume of output data occurs at each step of the so-described processing workflow. In contrast, this decrease is translated into an increase of the complexity of generated information (e.g. derived data). For example, if one takes a microscopic image representing a cell and measures its shape, then the raster image data (supposedly a matrix of *width* x *height*) transforms into a set of shape parameters, each one having a different semantic context (for example, neurite length, orientation, cell size). While in the raster data set the biological object is only implicitly present, in the derived data the representation of at least one attribute of the object under study is explicitly constructed (for example, the cell size). At this stage, the explicit information contained in the raw image about the illumination and staining distribution is lost. Therefore, the process of object (i.e. pattern) recognition and reconstruction is accompanied by irreversible reduction of the input information. At each step of the workflow the information in the previous step is transformed into contextual data,

[1] The bioluminescence imaging methods will not be discussed here.
[2] A workflow provides an abstracted view over the experiment being performed. It describes what procedures need to be enacted, but not necessarily all the details of how they will be executed.

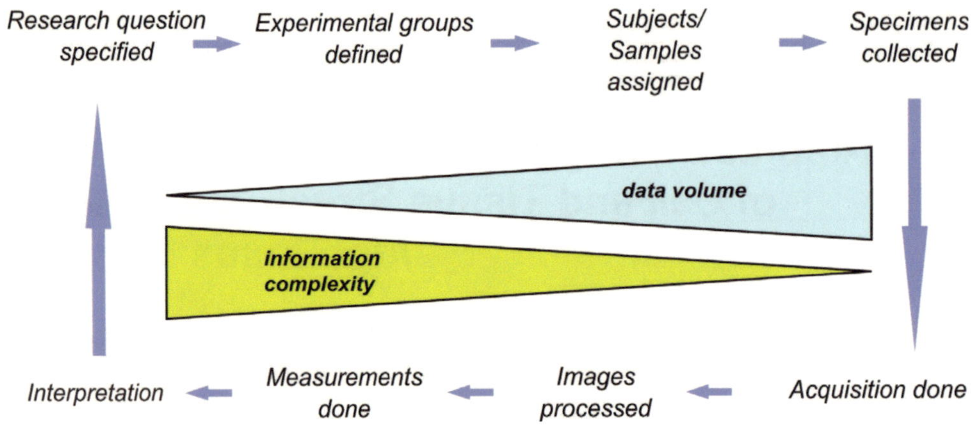

Fig. 1. The experimental workflow in life science imaging

The experimental workflow in life sciences aims at answering the initially- posed research question via quantitative analysis of multiple experimental trials. It starts with definition of experimental design and assignment of subjects (samples) to the experimental groups. Upon completion of the manipulations, the final specimens are collected and the raw data are acquired. Subsequent process of analysis leads to a decrease of the volume of the input data and an increase in their structural complexity.

called *meta data*. In such manner, the information complexity increase is also mapped to an increase of the complexity of the data structure.

Measurements, therefore, are reduced representations of the image features of interest, which have higher information complexity compared to the raw data. Due to the irreversible information loss introduced by the process of measurement, in order to be able to replicate the measurements given the original data, one needs an instance of the applied algorithm. Therefore, measurements are only implicitly "present" in images.

1.2 Biomedical imaging modalities

Processing and extraction of information from images have become indispensable aspects of the experimental workflow in life science research. Two major branches of imaging methods in life sciences can be discerned: microscopic imaging and biomedical imaging [3].

Biomedical imaging integrates aspects of medicine, medical physics, biomedical engineering, and computer science. Notably, pre-clinical imaging comprises an assembly of techniques exploiting different physical modalities[4]: (i) **micro-ultrasound**, (ii) micro Photoacoustic tomography μ**PAT**, (iii) micro Magnetic Resonance Imaging μ**MRI**, (iv) micro Computed Tomography μ**CT**, (v) micro Positron Emission Tomography μ**PET** and (vi) micro Single Photon Emission Computed Tomography μ**SPECT**.

[3] The biomedical imaging can be narrowly defined as an assembly of imaging methods developed for the study of human disorders and diseases for the purposes of mechanism characterization and development of treatments in model organisms, i.e. **pre-clinical imaging**.

[4] Since most of the work with animal models is done in rodent species the mirco aspect of the techniques is emphasized.

1.3 Drivers for biomedical imaging software development

The continuous improvement of biomedical imaging hardware enables development of novel imaging methods for acquisition and visualization. Novel imaging techniques progress in 3 main aspects: improvement of the signal-to-noise ratio, improvement of the spatial resolution, or adding new physical modalities to images. In microscopy, examples of the former can be given in laser scanning confocal (van Meer et al., 1987; White et al., 1987), spinning disc confocal (Nakano, 2002), wide-field deconvolution (Hiraoka et al., 1987) and multiphoton microscopes (Denk et al., 1990) ubiquitously used in cell and developmental biology. In non-optical imaging for example, the resolution in μMRI reached the order of 150 um, while different super-resolution microscopic approaches brought up the spatial resolution of microscopes to the order of 100 nm. Images having more than 3 dimensions (i.e. 3 spatial plus time, wavelength, orientation, decay times, etc) have become ubiquitous in biomedical imaging and life science microscopy.

Some examples can be also given in time-lapse microscopy, confocal microscopy (Canaria & Lansford, 2010), hyperspectral imaging (Marcsisin et al., 2010) and non-invasive imaging, such as MRI and PET. For example, contemporary tract reconstruction techniques in MRI require computations on 5D image datasets, representing position and orientation (Jonasson et al., 2005). As a result, developing novel image processing, data mining and database tools gained an increasing focus in the scientific community (Peng, 2008).

2. Biomedical imaging software

Each step of the experimental workflow typically requires the use of different hardware and software tools. Ideally, obtained raw data should be directly available for use in other applications either by remote instrument read-out or by transfer of the data upon application request. However, such ideal situation is far from reality and is inherently restricted by the heterogeneity of meta data describing different experiments. Other impeding factors are the limited interoperability between equipment vendor applications and the frequent incompatibility between proprietary data storage formats. As a result, the field of biomedical imaging suffers from considerable segmentation. There are numerous proprietary and open-source software products.

2.1 Proprietary software

Proprietary software for **pre-clinical imaging** is usually distributed with the specialized data acquisition hardware, such as MRI or PET scanners. Without being exhaustive, we could give several examples:

The Paravision® package of Bruker is used to operate the Biospin™ MR scanner. The software performs image reconstruction, 3D visualization of the reconstructed images, computation of parametric image maps and morphometry.

The IMALYTICS® package of Philips is used to analyze ultrasound, PET, CT, SPECT and MRI images (Fischer & Paulus, 2010). The package is targeted at the pharmaceutical industry and provides project-based workflows, rigid registration, segmentation and visualization. Advanced options are non-rigid registration, pharmacokinetic modeling and analysis of SPECT data.

Amira is a general purpose package for imaging data rendering and 3D modeling and analysis. Among its processing capabilities can be included image filtering, segmentation, registration and morphing, deconvolution and tensor computation. Among its measurement capabilities can be included spatial measurements, densitometry, co-localization and statistics. Its functionality to an extent matches the one offered by the Fiji distribution of *ImageJ*.

Pre-clinical imaging systems usually do not comply with any specific standard regarding raw data storage. In contrast, each manufacturer usually develops a proprietary storage format, which makes it difficult to share data and distribute data processing efforts.

In the field of **imaging for microscopy** there are also several powerful commercial systems distributed by the microscopic equipment manufacturers; for example the AxioVision™ and ZEN™ systems of Carl Zeiss (Germany) or the Cell-R™ system of Olympus (Japan). They all provide image processing and measurement features to a varying extent. The most-popular specialized morphometry software packages are listed in the paragraphs below:

Huygens is a package specialized in deconvolution, rendering and visualization developed by Scientific Volume Imaging, The Netherlands. Its advanced characteristics include estimation of the 3D point spread function from images and simulation of microscopic image formation.

Image-Pro Plus is a package specialized in 2D and 3D image processing, enhancement, and analysis developed by Media Cybernetics, USA. Among its advanced capabilities can be counted image fusion, extended depth of view, object tracking, thresholding of color images and morphological segmentation. Its functionality closely matches the one developed in *ImageJ*.

Imaris is a package for image rendering and visualization of 3D and 4D microscopy datasets of Bitplane Scientific Software, Switzerland. Its advanced capabilities include object fusion, illumination, segmentation and volume rendering. Its functionality to an extent matches the one offered by the Fiji distribution of *ImageJ*.

MetaMorph is an advanced system for image processing and morphometry developed by Molecular Devices, USA. The advantages of the system include different filtering and segmentation algorithms and the integration between measurements and display of results. Its functionality closely matches the one developed in *ImageJ*.

Volocity is a package of PerkinElmer (USA) for microscopic image rendering, interactive exploration, and analysis. Among the analysis options can be included colocalization, ratioed images, Fluorescence Recovery After Photobleaching (FRAP) and Fluorescence Resonance Energy Transfer (FRET). Its functionality closely matches the one offered by the McMaster's distribution of *ImageJ*.

In addition, general purpose data-processing languages, such as IDL® (ITT Visual Information Solutions, USA) and Matlab® (The Mathworks Inc, USA) computational environments are also used by the community.

A substantial and usual shortcoming of proprietary software is that the researcher is forced to use the offered package as a black box. In contrast, open-source implementations allow the researcher to critically examine the used approaches and the correctness of the implementation. Due to this, open-source solutions typically have faster development cycles including faster bug fixing. Consequently, to the authors' understanding they are preferable for development of new image processing and morphometric algorithms.

2.2 Open source software

There are numerous open-source programs for biomedical image processing. This can be attributed in part to the fact that in the past every imaging center developed its own analysis tools. Traditionally, many image processing algorithms were developed in C or C++. Attempts to overcome the fragmentation of the field of C/C++ programs were funded in 1990s by NIH in USA, which lead to the development of the general-purpose platforms for image visualization – *VTK* (Visualization Toolkit), and image registration and filtering – *ITK* (Insight Toolkit) which are currently supported by Kitware Inc (Ibanez et al., 2005). Both sets of libraries are implemented in C++ and require sophisticated building systems. However, their use in life-science microscopy is very limited.

While C/C++ platforms dominated the field before the year 2000, the evolution of *Java* and the continuous improvement of its performance in the last 10 years made it a language of choice for scientific software. Among the advantages of *Java* can be counted its portability across platforms; the richness of the available functionality; the extended user base including academic, commercial and community end-users and developers; its automated multi-threading and its object-oriented architecture.

The analysis packages having more extensive functionality are listed in Table 1 (Ciliberti, 2009). For didactic purposes, the open-source packages can be classified into **analysis suites**, which are suitable for comprehensive analytical tasks, and **specialized toolsets**, which focus into a limited number of processing and analysis tasks.

name	web site	platform	language
Mango	`http://ric.uthscsa.edu/mango/`	JAMA	Java
Seg3D	`http://www.sci.utah.edu/SCIRunDocs/index.php/CIBC:Seg3D`	ITK/VTK	C++
MedINRIA	`http://www-sop.inria.fr/asclepios/software/MedINRIA/`	ITK/VTK	C++
BioImage Suite	`http://www.bioimagesuite.org/`	ITK/VTK	C++
3D Slicer	`http://www.slicer.org/`	ITK/VTK	Tcl/Tk
FSL	`http://www.fmrib.ox.ac.uk/fsl/fsl/list.html`	FMRIB	C++
FreeSurfer	`http://surfer.nmr.mgh.harvard.edu/`	FMRIB	C++

Table 1. Some popular open source biomedical imaging programs

2.2.1 Analysis suites

BioImage Suite provides image editing, voxel classification, deformable user-interactive segmentation, rigid and non-rigid registration, modules for Diffusion Tensor Imaging (DTI) analysis and General Linear Model (GLM) functionality for fMRI analysis (Papademetris et al., 2008).

Seg3D is a volume segmentation and processing tool, which is distributed under the MIT License and is developed by the NIH Center for Integrative Biomedical Computing at the University of Utah. The data are organized in multiple layered volumes supporting either manual or filter-based segmentation and annotation.

3D Slicer is a software package for visualization and image annotation (Pieper et al., 2004). Present versions of 3D Slicer provide a workflow engine, command-line and GUI interfaces and scripting. The packages is distributed under BSD-style license.

Mango is a Java 3D-based program which supports image registration, surface rendering and analysis (statistics and profiling) (Lancaster & Martinez, 2007). It also provides extensibility via plugins and high level API.

FSL is a set of command line and GUI image analysis and statistical tools for fMRI, structural MRI and DTI analysis (Smith et al., 2004). FSL is written mainly by members of the Analysis Group, FMRIB, Oxford University, UK. It is distributed under non for profit use license.

2.2.2 Specialized tool-sets

Among the specialized tools, two main application areas can be discerned: DTI analysis and fMRI.

Diffusion Tensor Imaging – MedINRIA is a program based on VTK and ITK, which is developed by INRIA in France (Fillard et al., 2009). It is specialized in DTI and fiber tracking, tensor visualization and image registration.

fMRI – **SPM** is a software package designed for the analysis of brain imaging data sequences. The sequences can be a series of images from different cohorts, or time-series from the same subject. The current release is designed for the analysis of fMRI, PET and SPECT data. SPM is developed by the Functional Imaging Laboratory at University College London, UK (Ashburner et al., 2010). It is based on the proprietary MATLAB® (The MathWorks, Inc) environment. The **FreeSurfer** program provides reconstruction of the brain cortical surface from structural MRI data, and overlay of functional MRI maps. **CARET** is a software program for the structural and functional analysis of the cerebral and cerebellar cortex. The name is an abbreviation from Computerized Anatomical Reconstruction Toolkit. **AFNI** is an environment for processing and displaying functional MRI data[5].

3. *ImageJ* in the big picture

ImageJ is a public domain image processing program written in Java. Since its inception in 1997 *ImageJ* has evolved to become a standard analytical tool in life science imaging. It has an open architecture providing extensibility via 3rd party Java modules (called plugins) and scripting macros. It is developed by Wayne Raspband since 1997 and expanded via contributed software code by an international group of contributors (Abramoff et al., 2004; Collins, 2007). Plugins are distributed together with their source code under various licences determined by the pluing authors. Occasionally, some plugins are included in the main body of the program.

ImageJ supports a large number of file formats either natively or through the plugin extensions, for example using the Bio-Formats library [6].

There are several popular plugin distributions and collections. The most popular distributions are listed in the next paragraphs:

NIH's plugin collection is historically the 1st plugin collection. It is hosted on the *ImageJ* web site itself [7]. Main categories include acquisition, analysis, color processing, filters, segmentation, graphics, input/output, stacks, utilities and links to developers's sites.

Fiji is a plugin distribution aimed at microscopic applications in Neuroscience. It is developed and maintained since 2008 with the support of the Max Planck Institute of

[5] `http://afni.nimh.nih.gov/afni/about/summary`
[6] `http://www.openmicroscopy.org/site/products/bio-formats`
[7] `http://rsbweb.nih.gov/ij/plugins/`

Molecular Cell Biology and Genetics (MPI-CBG), Dresden, Germany. The collection includes plugins and libraries for neurite tracing (Longair et al., 2011), 3D reconstructions, trainable interactive segmentation (Schindelin, 2008) and mathematical morphology (Prodanov et al., 2006). It also comes with several additional scripting engines such as Jython and JRuby and *Java* enhancements like *Java* 3D. Every plugin included in the collection has a user manual.

The McMaster's University plugin collection[8] is aimed at fluorescent microscopy applications. There are specialized plugins for collocalization analysis, spectral and iterative deconvolution for image denoising (Dougherty, 2005) including parallel implmentations[9]. The distribution includes a user manual.

The CRP Tudor's plugin collection is structured around the documentation Wiki web site[10] and is hosted and maintained with the support of the Public Research Centre Henri Tudor, Luxembourg. It is a general purpose collection. Different categories include: filtering, color processing, morphometry and processing, segmentation and others. Every plugin included in the collection has a user manual and a history page.

It should be noted that some of the contributed plugins are present in all plugin distributions; while others are only distribution-specific.

While developed more for microscopic analysis *ImageJ* can be also used as a tool for visualization and measurements of pre-clinical imaging data. Key features of *ImageJ* are its support of (i) different modes of segmentation, (ii) the advanced image editing, (iii) the advanced filtering and processing capabilities and (iv) the well-established user and developer communities.

ImageJ can also produce derived results plots. Supported modalities are linear and surface plots. The basic measurement types in *ImageJ* are: areas, diameters, perimeters, angles, circularity, coordinates in 2D and 3D, intensities, and calibrated pixel values. Finally, *ImageJ* can also produce image and measurement statistics. A complete user guide of *ImageJ* is maintained by T. Ferreira and W. Rasband since 2010 (Ferreira & Rasband, 2010). What makes *ImageJ* superior to most of the specialized biomedical imaging programs are its capabilities:

- to support add-on functionality via plugins;
- to implement several scripting languages, such as its native macro script and JavaScript;
- to provide extensive measurement functions (e.g. morphometry and statistics).
- to run without modification on multiple operation systems.

4. Applications of *ImageJ* in MRI

Although historically analysis of non-optical biomedical images was one of the first applications of *ImageJ* there are still not so many algorithms for such types of images. Recently, however, with the spread of common non-optical biomedical imaging modalities the demand to use *ImageJ* for processing of such data has grown (Prodanov et al., 2010).

---

[8] `http://www.macbiophotonics.ca/imagej`

[9] `http://sites.google.com/site/piotrwendykier/software/deconvolution/paralleliterativedeconvolution`

[10] `http://imagejdocu.tudor.lu/`

The most common MRI techniques map the distribution of hydrogen atoms in different tissues. The primary contrast mechanisms exploit relaxation of the atomic magnetization: *spin-lattice relaxation*, characterized by the relaxation time T1, i.e T1-contrast, and *spin-spin relaxation*, characterized by the relaxation time T2, i.e. T2-contrast. MRI can be used for non-invasive monitoring of models of human diseases, such as traumatic brain edema, stroke or spinal cord injury. Such monitoring requires development of differential contrasting techniques either for T1 or for T2.

Parametric mapping functionality for *ImageJ* 3D and 4D datasets is provided by the *MRI Processor* plugin made available from the *ImageJ* documentation Wiki website (Prodanov et al., 2010). The plugin calculates parametric maps based on reconstructed MR images. Such parametric maps are derived images where each pixel value represents a parametric fit to time varying data sequence. Parametric maps are, for example, T1, T2 and proton density maps. Data fitting is available using either the Levenberg-Marquardt or the Simplex algorithm. Currently supported types are T2 and T1 maps. Unique features of the plugin are (i) the possibility to fit multicomponent exponential models, (ii) the support of 4D data sets and (iii) the support of arbitrary closed *Regions of Interest* (ROIs). The T2-map functionality has been already validated against the Paravision 4.0 software.

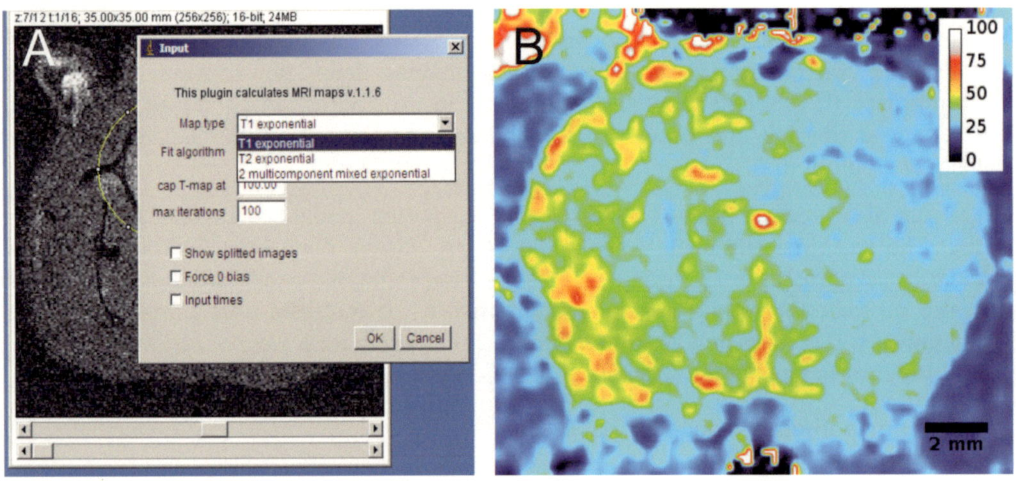

Fig. 2. Operation of the MRI Processor plugin
A – UI of the MRI Processor. The user can select different types of maps and fitting algorithms.
B – Computed T2 map. The image was colorized using the *royal* LUT. The calibration is given in *ms*. Scale bar – 2 mm.

The T2 maps are computed by fitting of the MRI dataset to the equation:

$$M_{xy}(t) = M_{xy}(0)e^{-t/T_2} + \epsilon \tag{4.1}$$

where M_{xy} is the transverse field magnetization component and ϵ is the offset term introduced by the unsigned pixel representation. The T1 maps are computed by fitting of the dataset to the equation:

$$M_z(t) = M_{z,eq}(0)(1 - 2e^{-t/T_1}) + \epsilon \tag{4.2}$$

where M_z is the longitudinal field magnetization component and ϵ is the offset term introduced by the unsigned pixel representation.

5. Selected Morphometric algorithms

Cell and tissue structures can be segmented in a variety of ways. For a successful image segmentation it is important to have prior knowledge of the image composition, i.e. the texture properties of the background and the objects of interest. In general, a typical algorithm includes the following stages:

- preprocessing steps, which decrease the spatial variation of the image
- thresholding, which produces one or more binary masks
- masking or Region of interest (ROI) selection
- postprocessing steps, for example including second thresholding or parametric fitting
- final measurement of volume, area, angles, etc.

Image processing algorithms can be classified based on the spatial (temporal) transformations which they introduce into the image. **Point operations** transform an input pixel into an output value. An example for such an operation can be given by histogramming or contrast adjustment. **Zonal operations** transform all the pixels in a certain spatially- or temporally-connected neighborhood into some output. Such neighborhoods are, for example, defined by structuring elements or convolution kernels. **Map operations** compute output image based on 2 or more input images. For example masking, addition and subtraction of images are such operations.

In the next sections we describe protocols based on granulometric filtering (a class of morphological filters), differential contrast enhancement, area thresholding, or distance map transforms.

5.1 Thresholding

Thresholding is performed using a labeling operator *Tr*. By definition, *Tr* labels a pixel in the image only if its intensity g exceeds certain value T_{min}:

$$Tr_{\alpha}\left[g(\mathbf{x}) \geq T_{\mathrm{min}}\right] : g(\mathbf{x}) \rightarrow 1(\mathbf{x})$$

where *1* is the binary pixel label denoting the foreground value and g – the pixel intensity at the co-ordinates vector **x**. There are different ways to propose a T_{min} value based on zonal or regional statistical variables. Some of the most popular methods include Otsu, maximal entropy and percentile thresholding. A good review on thresholding techniques can be found in Sezgin & Sankur (2004).

5.2 Local area thresholding

The local area thresholding is a regional image operation depending on the parameter α. If it is assumed that this ROI represents predominantly the image texture, α acts as a sensitivity parameter that determines the overall proportion of the "noise" pixels in the ROI. If so determined threshold level is extended to the overall image then a signal to noise ratio, SNR can be calculated as

$$SNR = \frac{T_{min}}{\bar{g}} \tag{5.3}$$

where $\bar{g}$ is the mean intensity of the image.

The action of a parametric thresholding operator Tr_α is conditioned on the ratio between the area of the labeled pixels and the total ROI area:

$$Tr_\alpha \left[\mathbf{x} \in ROI | \ \frac{H_{ROI}(T_{min})}{A_{ROI}} \geq 1 - \alpha \right] : g(\mathbf{x}) \rightarrow 1(\mathbf{x}) \tag{5.4}$$

where A_{ROI} denotes the ROI area, T_{min} is the locally-computed threshold level and $H()$ the cumulative histogram of the ROI (Prodanov & Feirabend, 2008).

5.3 Granulometric filtering

The algorithm is implemented as an *ImageJ* plugin. Particles of different sizes can be extracted from an image if two images from a granulometric image sequence are subtracted (see Appendix 12). Accordingly, the *granulometric filtering* is defined as:

$$D = I \circ SE[d_{low}] - I \circ SE[d_{high}]$$

where $\circ$ denotes *morphological opening* and SE is a structuring element defining the neighborhood around a pixel.

5.4 Differential Contrast Enhancement

The algorithm assumes that one of the images samples only background $I_{background}$ while the other samples background and objects of interest $I_{objects}$. Further, it is assumed that the histograms of the background and the objects overlap to an extent so that it is not-possible to separate them by thresholding. The contrast of the image (channel) of interest is rescaled with a coefficient assuring that $0 \notin Confidence_{95}[I_{background} - I_{objects}]$. This condition is achieved if the original image is contrast-rescaled by a factor

$$k_b = \frac{E[I_{objects}]}{P_{95}[I_{background}]} \tag{5.5}$$

where P_{95} denotes the 95th percentile of the empirical pixel intensity distribution and $E[]$ denotes the expectation. Next, to obtain the objects, the contrast-rescaled image is subtracted from the objects image in order to produce an output image R.

$$R = I_{objects} - k_b \cdot I_{background} \tag{5.6}$$

5.5 Distance map transformations

Distance map are produced from binary images. The map is an image derived from the original image where every pixel in the background is assigned the shortest possible distance to a foreground pixel given a certain metrics. The most popular distance maps are derived from the city-block (e.g. having diamond equidistant contours), the chessboard (e.g. having square equidistant contours) or the euclidean (e.g. having circular equidistant contours) metrics. In mathematical terms:

$$D(\mathbf{x}) = min_p\{dist(\mathbf{x}, p) \mid g(p) = 1\}$$

where 1 denotes the foreground label, **x** and **p** denote pixel coordinates, and g denotes intensity. From this equation a naive implementation can be derived directly. However, its execution time scales very badly with the image size and is of little practical use. *ImageJ* implements an approximate Euclidean distance map algorithm as part of its EDM plugin. The EDM algorithm is similar to the 8SSEDT in Leymarie & Levine (1992). The algorithm provides a fast approximation of the EDM, with the deviation from a full calculation being between -0.09 and 0.

6. Spatial distribution of labeled cells around a lesion site

Distance distribution of cell structures around an object can be used to demonstrate spatially-distributed effects or interactions. The distance from an arbitrary pixel set (for example a connected ROI representing the objects of interest) can be computed using the (approximate) Euclidean distance map transformation. In such case, the quantity of the effect (e.g. the amount of immuno-reactivity) can be given by the support volume. Since the area of a ring enclosed by two equidistant levels in the distance map increases monotonously with distance, to allow for comparison one needs to normalize the integral intensity by the ring area. Such normalization produces so called *support volume density*, having the same mathematical expression as the mean intensity inside the ring formed between 2 concentric contours:

$$\overline{G} = \frac{1}{A_r} \sum_{g=0}^{255} h(g) \cdot g \tag{6.7}$$

where A_r denotes the are of the ring.

The algorithm is demonstrated on images produced from transversal cortical histological slices stained for ED1 (microglial cell marker) and GFAP (astrocytic cell marker). The principle of the algorithm is similar to the previous work of Blacher et al. (2001), which employed distance maps to determine the effects of small molecules (Blacher et al., 2001) or enzymes (Chabottaux et al., 2006) on vascularization. In contrast to the works of Blacher et al., we did not attempt segmenting individual glial cells, since their processi form an overlapping mesh.

The application, which is presented here, is the measurement of the amount and distribution of glial cells in a histological section encompassing an implanted microelectrode. Following chronic implantation, the brain matter around the electrode forms glial scar spanning about 500 um from the electrode (review in Polikov et al. (2005)). Shortly after implantation, the astroglial and microglial cells undergo activation and hypertrophy and invade the region of primary injury. The distribution of glial cells around a lesion in the brain can be used to measure the extent of reactive gliosis and compare effects of treatments with anitinflammatory agents after such an implantation. In particular, such distributions can be used to study the brain tissue response to chronically implanted silicon microelectrode arrays (Welkenhuysen, 2011).

6.1 Imaging protocol

Tissue slices were stained using the following protocol: preincubation - 4h in 10 % normal goat serum, containing 0.1 % Triton-X 100; incubation - rabbit GFAP antibody (1:500, Dakocytomation) + mouse ED1 (1:200, Abcam) overnight at room temperature. Following secondary incubation with antibodies for 4h with a cocktail of anti-mouse Alexa-444 and Alexa-568 (1:500, Molecular Probes) in blocking buffer, the sections were cover-slipped with Vectashield-DAPI (Vector Labs) mounting medium.

Confocal images were acquired on LSM5 Pascal confocal microscope (Carl Zeiss Microimaging GmbH, Germany) using Plan Apochromat 5x/0.16 objective. The images were composed of 2 acquisition channels (having 8-bit dynamic range each) for demonstration of Alexa-444 (green LUT) and Alexa-568 emission (red LUT), respectively. The implant side was centered in the field of view (Fig. 3A). Exposure times were optimized to provide best compromise between cell contrast and saturation fraction. Images were imported in *ImageJ* using the LSM Reader plugin.

6.2 Outline of the algorithm

The following algorithm was used for computation of the binary mask from the ED1 image:

1. Perform Gaussian filtering, kernel diameter 5 pixels;
2. Perform morphological erosion with SE of d=5 pixels;
3. Perform morphological dilation with SE of d=10 pixels;
4. Do median thresholding (Doyle, 1962) (Fig. 3B).
5. Do magic wand selection from a point in the lesion site.
6. Clear the non selected area.
7. This mask is then transformed by Euclidean distance mapping and serially thresholded at increasing distances.

The resulting ring-like images are then overlaid in turn onto the GFAP image (Fig. 3D).

Proposed approach can be used to investigate the factors which contribute to the loss of signal in chronic microelectrode recordings. From the side of the brain this phenomenon can be caused by (i) spatial shift caused by the formation of the glial scar, (ii) neuronal cell death around the implanted probe or (iii) silencing of the surrounding neurons (review in Braeken & Prodanov (2010)). Activation of microglial cells results in a substantial increase in their phagocytic capacity. So-described process could lead to changes of the neuronal activity of the remaining neurons and may lead to atrophy or cell death of the neuronal cell bodies and axons, respectively. This in turn increases the variability of recorded bioelectrical signals and impedes the interpretation of the acquired physiological data. Moreover, the glial scar in the brain has growth-inhibitory properties for the regenerating axons, which could additionally impede the signal readout.

7. Morphometry of cultured neurons

To establish the dose- or time- dependence of a specific pharmacological effect often a large number of different experimental groups are needed. This rapidly increases the number of individual samples to be evaluated. Because of the high variability of the localizations of synapses on dendrites and the clustering of boutons, the stereological assumption of homogeneity of spatial distribution is violated. Therefore, complete dendritic trees are counted. To facilitate counting in cell cultures we have developed a reproducible and robust method for automatic identification and morphometry of synaptic boutons (Prodanov et al., 2006). The method is further illustrated with identification of synaptic boutons marked for *synapsin I* immuno-fluoresecence from micro-island cultures of neocortical neurons.

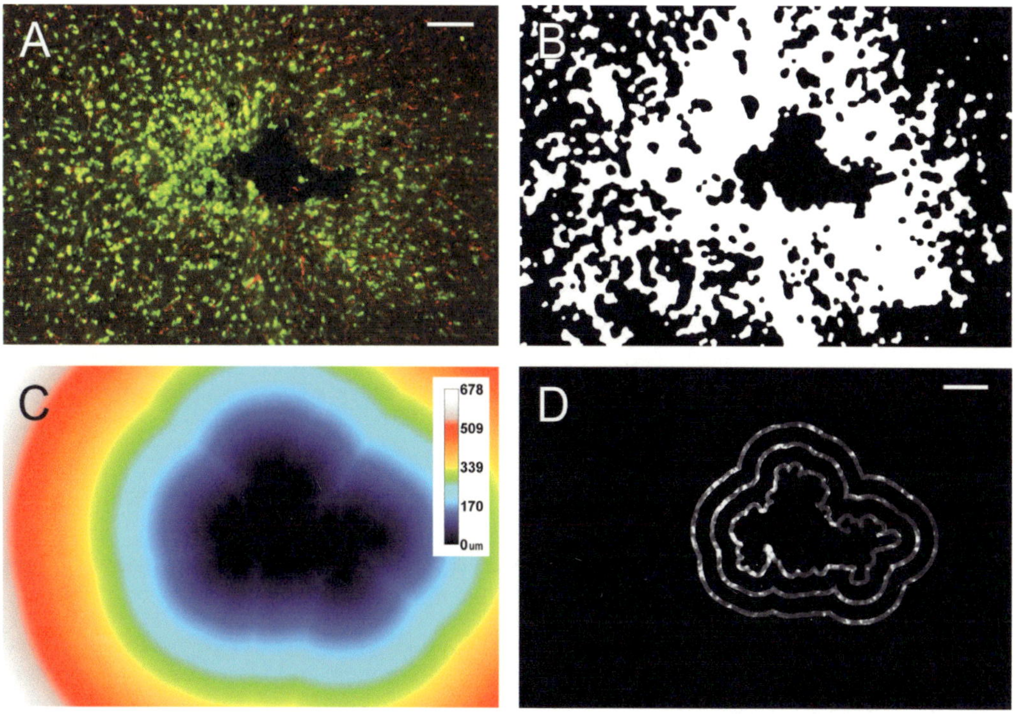

Fig. 3. Spatial distribution of GFAP immunoreactivity around an electrode insertion track

A – ED1-labeled neuronal cell bodies (red) overlaid on GFAP-positive glial cells (green). The electrode insertion track can be recognized as the tissue defect in the center of the image.
B – mask of the insertion track segmented as a background object in the center of the image;
C – Euclidean distance map of the insertion track. The closest distance to a point on the track border is represented by the intensity value of the pixel. D – concentric equidistant regions overlaid on the GFAP-image. Original image resolution 1.217 pixels/μm; scale bar – 100 μm.

7.1 Imaging protocol

Micro island cortical cultures were prepared from embryonic day 18 murine embryos. Cultures were stained with antibodies against a marker for dendrites, *microtubule-associated protein 2* (MAP-2), and a marker for synaptic vesicles, *synapsin I*. Cultures were fixed by 4% paraformaldehyde, washed with 0.1M Phosphate buffered saline (PBS) and incubated in 0.1% Triton X-100 followed by 4% fetal calf serum for 20 minutes. After washing with PBS, cultures were incubated for 1 hour at room temperature in a mixture containing 0.1% Triton X-100, mouse monoclonal anti-MAP-2, 1:200 (Boehringer, Alkmaar, The Netherlands) and rabbit polyclonal anti-synapsin I, 1:1000 antibodies diluted in PBS. After washing with PBS, the cells were incubated for 1 hour at room temperature in secondary antibodies conjugated to anti-rabbit-Cy5 or anti-mouse-Alexa546 (Molecular Probes, Oregon, USA). Finally, the slides were washed in PBS and cover-slipped with Dabco-Mowiol (Prodanov et al., 2006).

Samples were analyzed on a Zeiss 510 Meta confocal microscope (Carl Zeiss, Heidelberg, Germany). A set of high-resolution digital images of different cultures was recorded at a resolution of 4.45 pixels per μm. Images were acquired on 2 channels - *cyan*, comprising anti-synapsin staining and *red*, comprising anti-MAP-2 staining.

7.2 Outline of the algorithm

The algorithm employed in the study can be outlined in the following main steps:

1. Perform granulometry of the image and compute its granulometric size density *G(d)* (Appendix 12).
2. Identify the scale of interest by the pattern of the peaks in *G(d)*; select low bound $I_{low} = S \circ E_{low}$ and high bound images $I_{high} = S \circ E_{high}$ and subtract the images.
3. Construct the binary "mask" using the *k-means clustering* segmentation algorithm.
4. Delete irrelevant structures by superimposing the mask on the original image using bit-plane logical AND operation (masking).
5. Threshold the resulting image using the area thresholding (Sec. 5.2).
6. Construct disjoint grains from the pixels that are above the threshold based on their 8-connected neighborhoods.
7. Enumerate and measure the grains constructed in this way. Produce derivative images where the identification numbers of the positive fibers are visible.

The algorithm was applied to the synapsin channel of every image. The identified boutons were numbered and their areas, equivalent diameters, and planar co-ordinates were automatically measured and recorded. The final measurements were uploaded in the *LabIS* system using the SQL Results plugin (see Sec. 10.3).

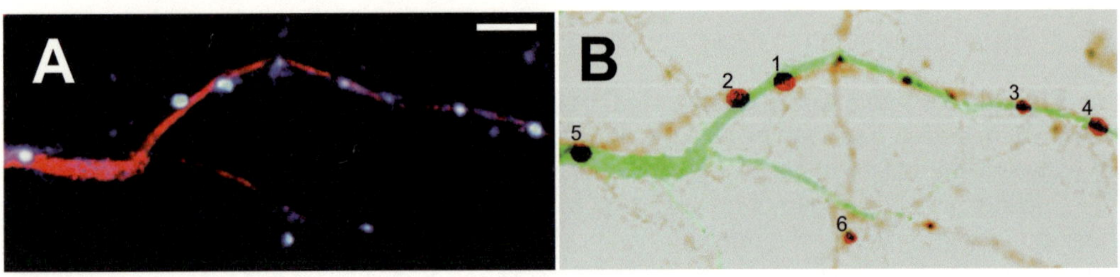

Fig. 4. Illustration of the granulometric filtering technique on a real image. A - Co-localization of synapsin I (cyan) and MAP-2 (red); B - co-localization of the detected synaptic boutons (red outline) with the inverted image from A. Scale bar - 5 μm.

As the fluorescent patches in the real images were round, granulometry was performed with a family of flat disk-shaped SEs ranging from d=1 to d=25 (0.2 μm - 5.6 μm). For the construction of I_{low} values of either d_{low}=3 or d_{low}=5 were selected depending on the amount of debris in an image; d_{high}=11 was selected as a parameter for I_{high}. Based on the discrimination of dark background, auto-fluorescing cell mass, and synapsin positive grains *three* brightness classes were used during k-means clustering. During the area thresholding, sufficient overlap of the thresholded particles with the actual synapsin grains was typically achieved for $\alpha = 0.8$. The brightest class was selected for the construction of the mask. A typical result of the detection procedure is presented in Fig. 4B.

An advantage of the proposed automated approach is that, apart from the number of synaptic boutons in a light microscopic image, it also allows to be measured morphological characteristics such as area, circularity, and maximal diameter.

8. Spatial mapping of tracer-filled axons

Specific populations of myelinated nerve fibers can be investigated by retrograde tracing from a muscle followed by morphometric assessment of the labeled fibers at different anatomical levels. Transversal sections of so-labeled nerves would then represent spatial maps of the specific muscle representations (Fig. 5). To facilitate such mapping studies we have developed a reproducible approach for image segmentation and morphometry (Prodanov & Feirabend, 2008).

Gastrocnemius muscles of adult rats were injected under anesthesia with the retrograde tracer Fluoro-Gold. After a survival period of 3 days, the sciatic nerves and spinal roots were harvested and fixed in 4% paraformaldehyde.

8.1 Imaging protocol

The samples were sectioned at 14 μm, mounted on glass slides and inspected on an Axioplan (Carl Zeiss Microimaging GmmbH, Germany) fluorescence microscopes. The fluorescent signal from the specimens was recorded on 2 channels. Fluoro-Gold signal was recorded using a standard filter set for DAPI (4′,6-Diamidino-2-phenylindole) detection (excitation 320 - 370 nm), see Fig. 5/Fluoro-Gold. The signal from the myelin sheaths (comprising autofluorescence) was recorded using a standard filter set for FITC (Fluorescein) detection (excitation 450 - 490 nm), see Fig. 5/FITC. Tracer-positive axonal profiles were isolated from the resulting images by means of Differential Contrast Enhancement and Granulometric filtering.

The following procedure was employed to identify the Fluoro-Gold-positive fibers. Due to the excitation characteristics of Fluoro-Gold its signal was absent from the FITC channel (Fig. 5/FITC). Therefore, it was possible to isolate the Fluoro-Gold using the DCE implemented as the *Channel Filter* plugin. For the optimal differential brightness enhancement a thin rectangle ROI was drawn across the image and the intensities of the pixels were averaged in the direction perpendicular to the larger side of the rectangle and the input images were transformed according to Eq. 5.6.

8.2 Outline of the algorithm

The algorithm employed in the study can be outlined in the following main steps:

1. Perform DCE (Sec. 5.4).
2. Perform granulometry on the resulting image and compute *G(d)*.
3. Identify the scale of interest by the pattern of the peaks in G(d); select $I_{low} = S \circ E_{low}$ and $I_{high} = S \circ E_{high}$ and subtract the images.
4. Interactively threshold the resulting image.
5. Construct disjoint grains from the pixels that are above the threshold based on their 8-connected neighborhoods.
6. Enumerate and measure the grains constructed in this way. Produce derivative images where the identification numbers of the positive fibers are visible.

Spatial maps obtained in this way were uploaded to *LabIS* using the SQL Results plugin. The data were imported to Matlab and the spatial distribution of the Fluoro-Gold-positive axons was further studied on demand using custom code (Prodanov & Feirabend, 2008; Prodanov et al., 2007).

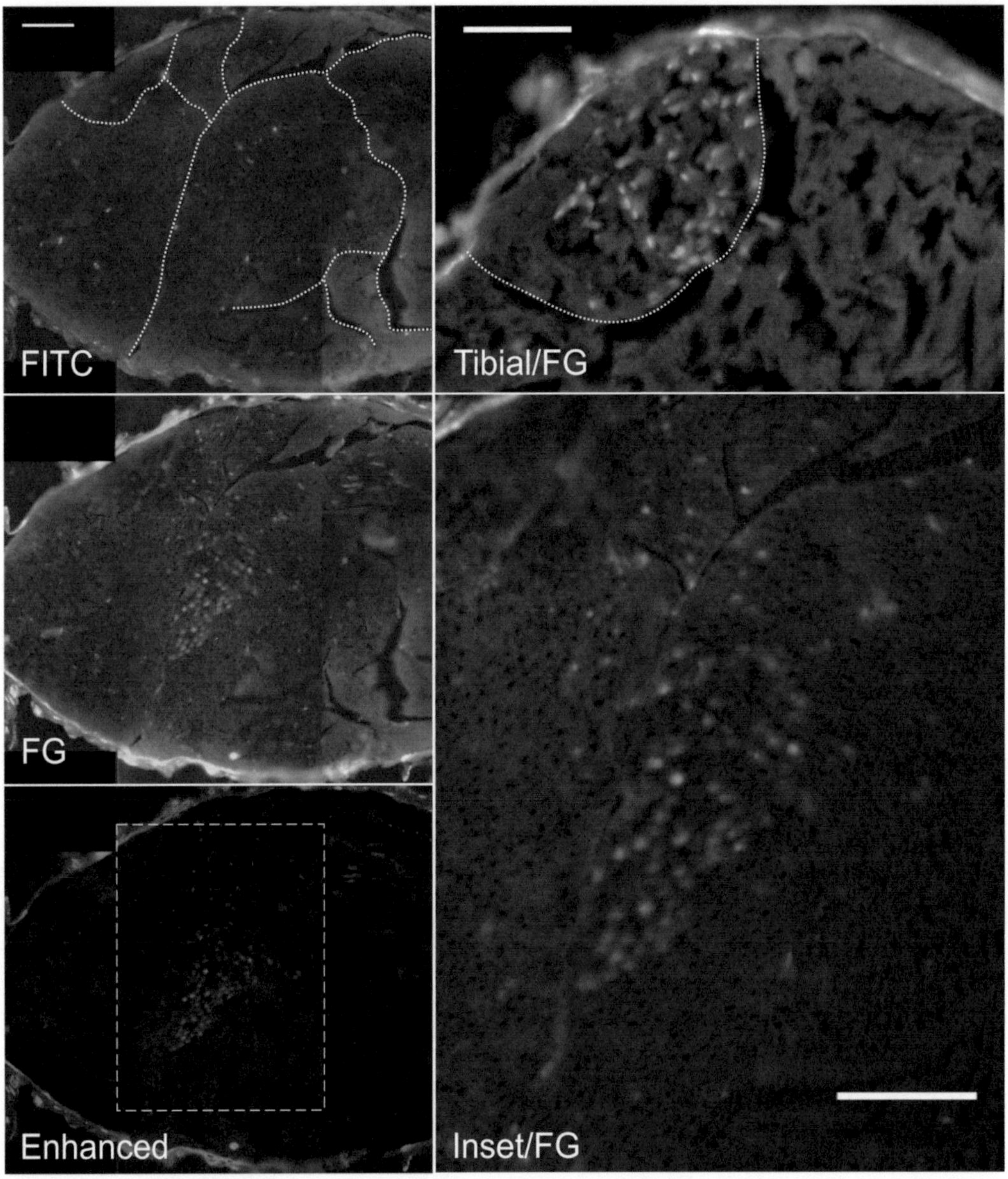

Fig. 5. Gastrocnemius topography in the sciatic and tibial nerves revealed by the Differential Contrast Enhancement algorithm (Prodanov & Feirabend, 2008)

Left pane: **FITC** – showing the myelin sheath auto-fluorescence; FG – showing **Fluoro-Gold** fluorescence and **Enhanced** – showing the subtraction of the other two. Images are composed of several "stitched" complete microscopical fields. Stitching was performed semi-automatically using the the 2D stitching plugin (Preibisch et al., 2009). Fascicle borders are enhanced by dotted lines. **Enhanced** image was generated by the *Channel Filter* plugin. Right pane: *Gastrocnemius* axons inside a fascicle of the tibial nerve (top - **Tibial/FG**) and a microscopic field in the sciatic nerve (bottom - **Inset/FG**). The corresponding inset is outlined in the Enhanced image. **Tibial/FG** – the *Gastrocnemius* fascicle borders are outlined by a dotted line. Scale bars – 100 μm.

9. Outlook

Presented algorithms can be developed further in two directions.

Parallelization: As the sizes of available images increase and the parallel computer architectures become increasingly available a logical step would be the development of parallel implementations. Such parallelizations can be especially useful in zonal and map algorithms where the same elementary operations are repeated multiple times on different pixels. Notably we expect substantial speedups for image convolutions and morphology operations. Parallelization can be implemented either using general purpose semi-automatic parallelization libraries, or optimized at a low level for the specific algorithms.

Multidimensionality: Another direction for future development is the support of multidimensional kernels and structuring elements in zonal operations. Multidimensional imaging data are increasingly used in life sciences but at present they are not well supported by the data model in *ImageJ*, which assumes at best a collection of loosely-coupled 2D images. Such support can be achieved by development of a multidimensional data model in combination with generic zonal image transform algorithms.

It is expected that the development and support of *ImageJ* will continue in the future as the user and developer base of the program is growing and there are structured institutional efforts to sustain and support this trend. Therefore, both directions will be pursued further in the context of *ImageJ* and the developed plugins and libraries will be made available to the user community.

10. Management of the information flow

Until recently, management of the data produced along the life science workflow (Fig. 1) was not perceived as a pressing issue in the academic environments. Traditionally, the scientific publications were considered as the *only* sufficient reports of the experimental findings. However, the scale of current imaging experiments and the volumes of data generated by them would also require persistent data management and collaboration solutions. This is a situation already recognized in brain mapping studies (Bjaalie, 2002). On the second place, sharing of raw data and code gains momentum in Neuroscience. The exchange of raw imaging data between groups offers the opportunity to differently re-analyze previously collected data and encourage new interpretations (Eckersley et al., 2003). While something new for Neurosciences such practices are common in other fields like Physics and to some extend in Bioinformatics, i.e. in Proteomics. With the increase of experimental complexity and the article size restrictions imposed by the scientific publishers, frequently essential experimental details are omitted from the final peer reviewed publications. This eventually impedes the reproduction of the original experiments and could eventually lead to unnecessary reproduction of experiments and waste of time and resources. In contrast, data sharing can reduce the experimental and analytical errors. However, both high-level data archiving and the raw data sharing will have limited utility if they are not backed by information system solutions on the research laboratory level.

In the following sections we present an integrated information system for image measurements, *LabIS*. The system was publicly demonstrated for the first time at the 6th FENS Forum of European Neuroscicence, although developmental versions existed since

2004. Previous versions of the system supported data analyzed in publications about: motor endplate distributions in (Prodanov, 2006; Prodanov et al., 2005); synaptic boutons morphometry in (Prodanov, 2006; Prodanov et al., 2006); peripheral axon spatial distributions in (Prodanov, 2006; Prodanov & Feirabend, 2008; Prodanov et al., 2007). Development of *LabIS* has the objectives to automate (i) the process of storage, annotation and querying of image measurements and (ii) to provide means for data sharing with 3rd party applications utilizing measurement data (Prodanov, 2008). A developmental snapshot of the system is available through the website Sourceforge.net at `http://labinfsyst.sourceforge.net/`.

10.1 System realization

LabIS realizes 3-tier architecture with a relational database back-end and an application logic middle tier realizing web-based user interface for reporting and annotation and a web service communication layer. *LabIS* is a distributed Internet and intranet application. It can be accessed (i) through the web user interface by a web browser, (ii) through web-service or (iii) database clients (Fig. 6). *LabIS* is based on commonly-accepted open-source software technologies and open communication and data storage protocols. In order to enforce data organization in a structured manner, *LabIS* realizes a centralized data storage model. *LabIS* is designed and developed in a modular manner and the data model for communication with 3rd party applications is also extendable.

Interaction with users is executed via dynamically-generated web pages. All user-interface modules are organized in a similar manner: users can generate reports, enter data or annotate already present database records. The *Project planning* module is used for management of the records of research projects. The users can perform tasks, such as deployment of new and/or changing the state or the attributes of ongoing projects. Groups of results can be organized in *results collections*. The *Subject management* module manages the records for experimental animals. The users can perform tasks, such as registration of new subjects/animals, editing of records, introduction of new species etc. The subjects can be assigned to projects and to experimental groups. Dynamic reports can be generated for arbitrary periods. The *Manipulation management* module manages the records for performed manipulations. The users can perform tasks, such as registration and editing of manipulations. Dynamic reports can be generated for arbitrary periods. The *Image Measurements and Morphometry* module manages uploaded measurement records. Uploaded measurements can be associated to a project, an experimental subject, experimental group, sample, result collection, or paired to other measurements. The measurements can be queried by the name of the measured image, by the internal ID or simply browsed. There are possibilities for flexible reporting of the performed measurements. The *Administration* module manages the user roles, the maintenance of the database, and the system configuration. The users can also define custom ontologies.

It should be noted that *LabIS* is not a raw image database. The raw images are let to reside in remote repositories, such as on a local client file system or 3rd party file server, while only references to them are stored centrally. In contrast, the imaging meta data and the produced measurements are stored centrally in the relational database. Such an approach provides a definite advantage for the integration of 3rd party imaging data, such as large scale digital atlases. It also increases the portability of the system since its entire database can be easily copied from one host to another. Most notable characteristics of *LabIS* are the possibilities to annotate and collate measurements and its interoperability with 3rd party software. In this

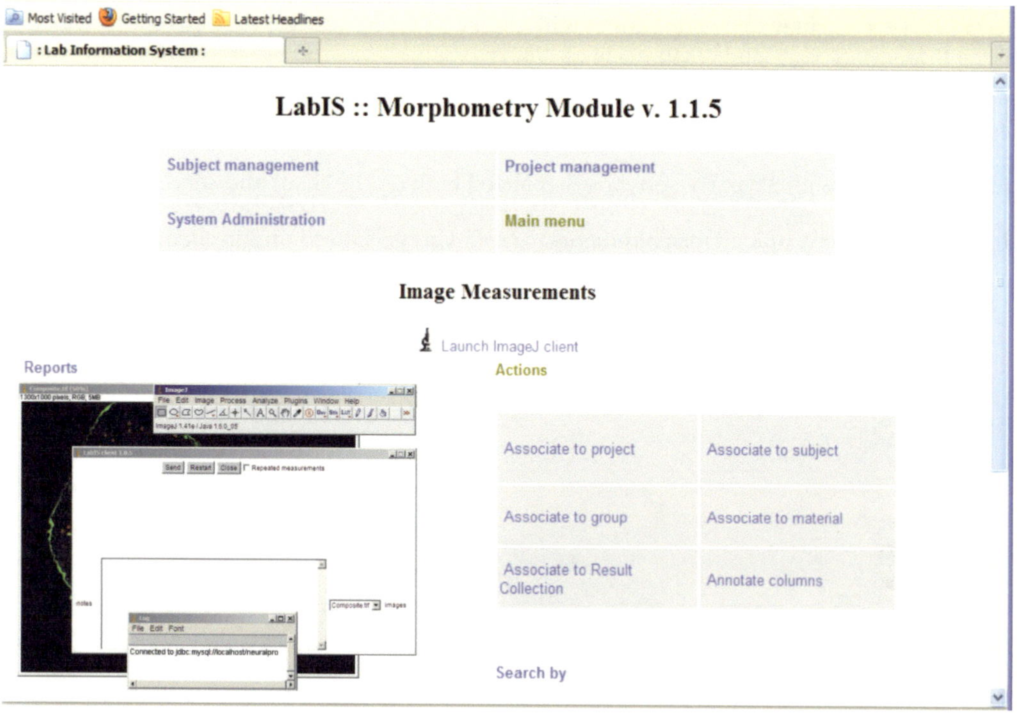

Fig. 6. *LabIS* user interface and data upload clients

The information system can be accessed through the web user interface by a web browser. The user interface of the *ImageJ* SQL access plugin for measurement upload and annotation is overlaid onto a web browser window displaying the Morphometry module.

context, interactions with *LabIS* are executed either by exchange of structured messages over the web or by database queries in an intranet.

10.2 Annotations of measurements

Measurement type annotations Uploaded measurements can be annotated by ontology entries. Support of 3rd party ontologies is provided using the publicly available Ontology Lookup Service (OLS) registry web site [11]. This support is realized on 2 levels: (i) individual measurement types can be annotated with ontology keys, for example using the Unit Ontology; (ii) the complex measurement objects can be annotated using terms of any of the ontologies supported by OLS. The integration with OLS is transparent for the user and is realized using a cascade of client and 3rd party server calls. This is an example of mixed client-server interoperability.

Spatial annotations *LabIS* provides also atlas mapping and registration functionality. Major features include the possibility to associate a *Results collection* to an atlas and to map individual measurement entries of the collection to the atlas imaging space. An example is demonstrated in Fig. 7 where some measurements are mapped to a rat coronal histological

[11] http://www.ebi.ac.uk/ontology-lookup/

atlas. This is achieved by integration with public atlas datasets, for example those available at Brain Maps web site[12] (Mikula et al., 2007) .

10.3 Interoperability

Interoperability with 3rd party software is realized both on the client and server sides.

ImageJ can directly upload measurements to *LabIS* via specialized plugin clients. In such way, the entire image processing functionality of *ImageJ* can be made available to the end user. The user can perform arbitrary measurements using any type of built-in or customized

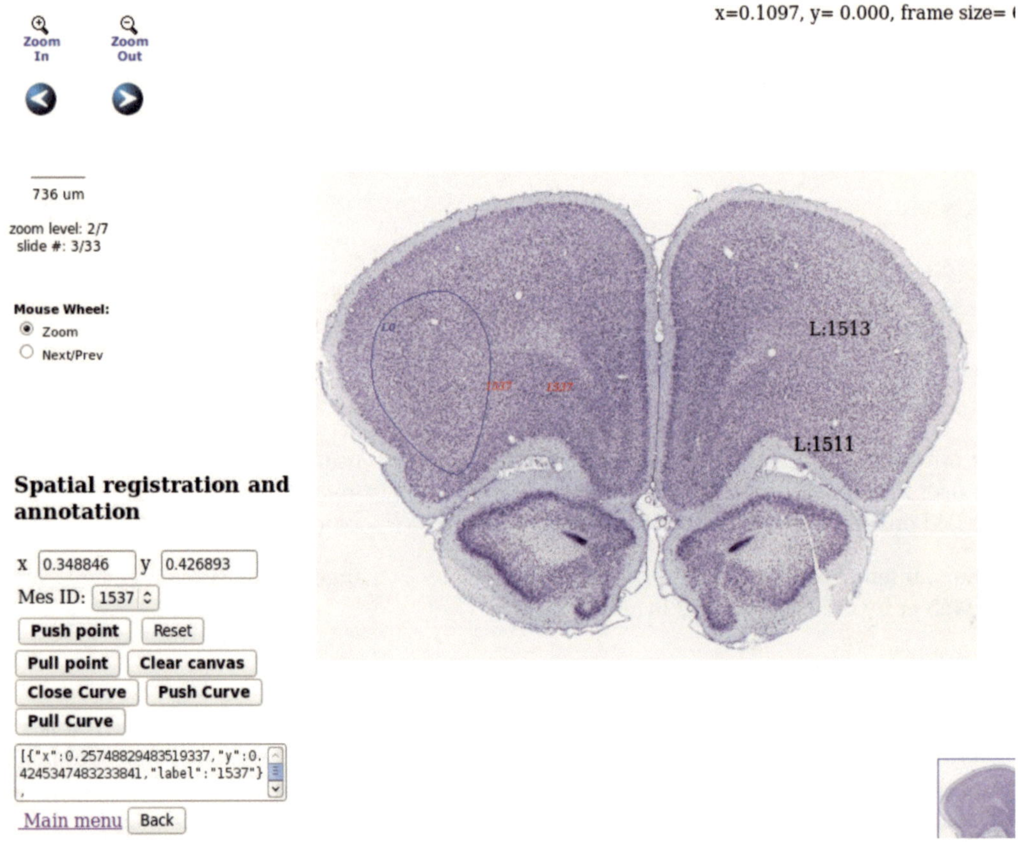

Fig. 7. Spatial annotation and atlas registration

Three types of atlas annotations are demonstrated in the figure. A ROI annotation delineating a region in the frontal cortex is displayed in *solid blue*, Nissl stating, source Brain Maps, contributed by Edward Jones, 2007. In *red* are demonstrated provisional annotations produced by mouse clicks on the client side. In *black* are demonstrated measurements already stored on the server. Spatial annotation storage and retrieval can be done using the user interface in the bottom left part of the web page. Spatial navigation in the atlas dataset can be done using the icons in the top left part of the web page.

[12] `http://brainmaps.org/`

ImageJ plugins. After the end of the measurement session this object together with a JPEG-encoded thumbnail view of the active image are upload either using the SQL client or using the web service client. Known measurement unit types are associated automatically to terms in 3rd party ontologies, i.e. the Unit Ontology. If a new measurement type is encountered it is also automatically included in the database. Such a new type can be later annotated using the web UI and the ontology terms lookup service. The GUI front-end clients were implemented as a set of plugins: the SQL Results plugin and web-service plugins SOAP Results and JSON Results plugins. The SQL-plugin implements a MySQL client that interacts directly with the database server. It is intended for use in intranet environments. The web-service plugins interact with the *Object Server* interfaces of *LabIS* (Fig. 6). This functionality is an example of interoperability on the client side.

Matlab® can directly query *LabIS* via its web-service interface. Since its R2007 version, Matlab® provides client functionality for web services. The generation of client scripts is fully automated and transparent to the end-user by the service discovery mechanisms.

On the application level, advantages of the system are the use of open communication standards and the integration of server and client technologies, which are transparent for the end-user. On the system level, advantages of *LabIS* are the extendable data model, the independence of a particular programming language and the scalability of the component technologies. On the level of exploitation and deployment, advantages of the system are the use of open-source platforms, which are available as standard hosting options in the most web hosting services.

11. Summary

This chapter presents several techniques for morphometry of microscopic and non-optical images. The main focus of the manuscript is the automation of image processing and measurement steps along the experimental workflow. Main algorithms are implemented as either plugins or macros for the public domain image processing program *ImageJ*. We present several generic processing and segmentation techniques, which can be used in a variety of applications.

Notably, the utility of mathematical morphology was demonstrated in several image filtering and segmentation algorithmic steps. Morphology-based Granulometric filtering was used to facilitate segmentation of globular structures, such as synaptic boutons or cross sections of axons. In the first application, morphological granulometry was used to estimate size of synaptic boutons, which are then segmented by means of granulometric filtering followed by thresholding. Using this approach quantitative effects of different treatments of cell cultures can be measured. In the second application, Differential Contrast Enhancement and granulometry were used to segment images of fluorescent tracer filled axons. An additional application of the morphological image simplification were the preprocessing steps in the analysis of astroglial distribution.

The computation of spatial parametric maps was demonstrated in the context of MRI data sets. Such maps are produced by parametric fitting to time-varying spatial measurements.

The utility of the Local Area Thresholding was demonstrated in the context of segmentation of histological images. The Differential Contrast Enhancement algorithm can be used to reduce bleed-through artifacts from a background channel to a signal channel. Presented algorithm was used in the context of image enhancement in fluorescent tracer studies.

The utility of distance transform for analysis of spatial distribution of objects was demonstrated in the context of estimation of radial distributions of the glial fraction of the neuropil.

In addition, we also present an information system, which is capable of managing the measurements uploaded from *ImageJ*. The system provides a structured information context for querying and retrieval of primary morphometric information, which goes beyond acquisition metadata. In such way, the increase of the information complexity along the experimental workflow is supported. The system is a step towards providing the link between the raw image, the performed measurements and their meaning in the context of the experiment.

12. Appendix

A. Mathematical morphology

Mathematical morphology is a branch of mathematics applicable to image processing. Morphology operators are a class of zonal operations where the pixels of a certain neighborhood (Structure Element) are combined to produce a single output value. Principal operations in mathematical morphology are *erosion*, *dilation*, *opening* and *closing* (Matheron, 1975; Serra, 1982).

Grey level images can be represented by 3D geometric bodies (called umbras) where the elevation conventionally signifies intensity. Morphology operations of gray level images can be constructed from ordering and ranking of the pixels. If $S(x)$ is the umbra of the image S and $E(x)$ is a *Structuring Elements* (SEs) set, *erosion* ($\ominus$) and *dilation* ($\oplus$) are defined by:

$$S \ominus E = \left\{ \min_{b \in \hat{E}} \left[S(\mathbf{x} + \mathbf{b}) + \hat{E}(\mathbf{b}) \right] \right\} \tag{12.8}$$

$$S \oplus E = \left\{ \max_{b \in \hat{E}} \left[S(\mathbf{x} - \mathbf{b}) - \hat{E}(\mathbf{b}) \right] \right\} \tag{12.9}$$

where $\hat{E}$ is the complement of the structure element and $\mathbf{x}$ or $\mathbf{b}$ denote vector coordinates.

Opening is defined as $I \circ E = (I \ominus E) \oplus E$ and *closing* as $I \bullet E = (I \ominus E) \oplus E$.

An example of the four major morphological operations is given in Fig. 8.

As seen from their definition, erosion and closing increase the number of dark pixels and decrease image brightness, while dilation and opening do the opposite.

Sizes of different objects present in an image can be collectively studied by the operation of granulometry, introduced by Matheron (1975).

In a way similar to sieving grains, pixels comprising an image are "sieved" according to their connectivity imposed by a certain SE. Granulometry is formally defined as a set of openings by a family of SEs, characterized by certain scale parameter d. In the case of closings, the set

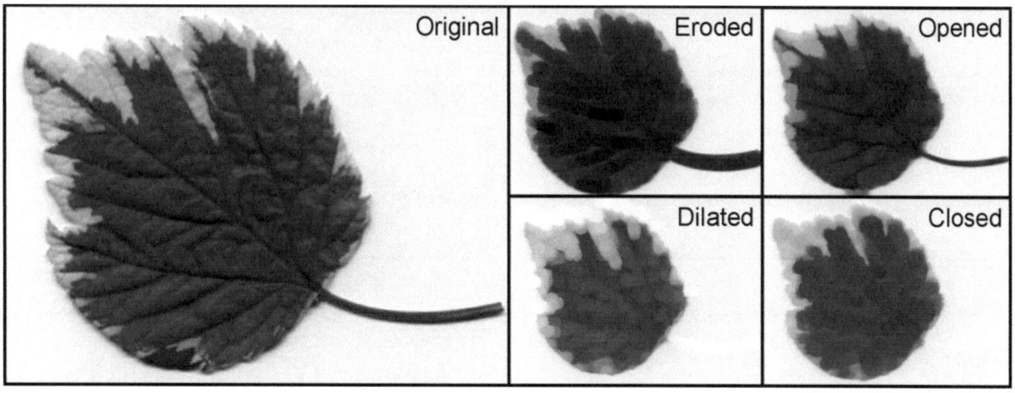

Fig. 8. Prinicipal morphological operations

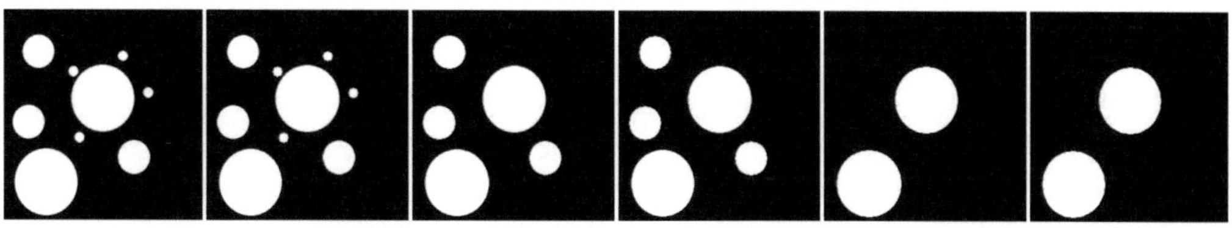

Fig. 9. Granulometry of a synthetic image

Granulometric image sequence; from left to right: original image, d=5; d=10, d=15, d=20, d=25

is termed antigranulometry. If the SEs are homothetic, that is $E[d] = d \cdot E$, the granulometry is calculated as

$$G_d(I) = \bigcup_d I \circ (d \cdot E) \tag{12.10}$$

where d denotes the proportionality parameter of the homothety. By convention $G_0(S) = S$ and for negative *d opening* is replaced by *closing*.

For greyscale images, the measure of the interaction with SE is the support volume removed after opening. This can be expressed by the granulometric (size) density distribution:

$$GSD\,(d) = \frac{V[I \circ dE] - V[I \circ (d-1)E]}{V[I]} \tag{12.11}$$

where g is the intensity. The support volume is estimated from the image histogram $H = \{h(g)\}$. In particular, for unsigned 8-bit images $g \in [0,\ 255]$ and

$$V[I] = \sum_{g=0}^{255} h(g) \cdot g$$

Gray-level morphological operations erosion, dilation, opening and closing are implemented as a plugins for *ImageJ*.

B. Resources

Grayscale Morphology	http://rsbweb.nih.gov/ij/plugins/gray-morphology.html
Granulometric filtering	http://rsbweb.nih.gov/ij/plugins/gran-filter.html
Color Histogram	http://rsbweb.nih.gov/ij/plugins/color-histogram.html
MRI Processor	http://imagejdocu.tudor.lu/doku.php?id=plugin:filter:mri_processor:start
DCE	http://imagejdocu.tudor.lu/doku.php?id=plugin:filter:differential_contrast_enhancement:start

Table 2. Lsit of Plugins

13. References

Abramoff, M., Magalhaes, P. & Ram, S. (2004). Image processing with ImageJ, *Biophotonics International* 11(7): 36 – 42.

Ashburner, J., Barnes, G., Chen, C.-C., Daunizeau, J., Flandin, G., Friston, K., Gitelman, D., Kiebel, S., Kilner, J., Litvak, V., Moran, R., Penny, W., Stephan, K., Gitelman, D., Henson, R., Hutton, C., Glauche, V., Mattout, J. & Phillips, C. (2010). *SMP8 Manual*, Functional Imaging Laboratory.

Bjaalie, J. G. (2002). Opinion: Localization in the brain: new solutions emerging., *Nat Rev Neurosci* 3(4): 322–325.
URL: http://dx.doi.org/10.1038/nrn790

Blacher, S., Devy, L., Burbridge, M. F., Roland, G., Tucker, G., Noël, A. & Foidart, J. M. (2001). Improved quantification of angiogenesis in the rat aortic ring assay., *Angiogenesis* 4(2): 133–142.

Braeken, D. & Prodanov, D. (2010). *New Developments in Biomedical Engineering*, In-Teh, Vukovar, chapter New trends and challenges in the development of microfabricated probes for recording and stimulation of excitable cells, pp. 311 – 339.

Canaria, C. A. & Lansford, R. (2010). Advanced optical imaging in living embryos., *Cell Mol Life Sci* 67(20): 3489–3497.
URL: http://dx.doi.org/10.1007/s00018-010-0440-5

Chabottaux, V., Sounni, N. E., Pennington, C., English, W. R., van den Brûle, F., Blacher, S., Gilles, C., Munaut, C., Maquoi, E., Lopez-Otin, C., Murphy, G., Edwards, D. R., Foidart, J.-M. & Noël, A. (2006). Membrane-type 4 matrix metalloproteinase promotes breast cancer growth and metastases., *Cancer Res* 66(10): 5165–5172.
URL: http://dx.doi.org/10.1158/0008-5472.CAN-05-3012

Ciliberti, C. (2009). *MRI-evaluation of implantable neural probes: Software tools and data analysis*, Master's thesis, University of Calabria.

Collins, T. J. (2007). ImageJ for microscopy., *Biotechniques* 43(1 Suppl): 25–30.

Denk, W., Strickler, J. H. & Webb, W. W. (1990). Two-photon laser scanning fluorescence microscopy., *Science* 248(4951): 73–76.

Dougherty, P. (2005). Extensions of DAMAS and benefits and limitations of deconvolution in beamforming, 11th AIAA/CEAS Aeroacoustics Conference, pp. Dougherty, R.P., "Extensions of DAMAS and benefits and limitations of deconvolution in beamforming", 2961.

Doyle, W. (1962). Operation useful for similarity-invariant pattern recognition, *J. ACM* 9: 259 – 267.

Eckersley, P., Egan, G. F., Amari, S., Beltrame, F., Bennett, R., Bjaalie, J. G., Dalkara, T., Schutter, E. D., Gonzalez, C., Grillner, S., Herz, A., Hoffmann, K. P., Jaaskelainen, I. P., Koslow, S. H., Lee, S.-Y., Matthiessen, L., Miller, P. L., da Silva, F. M., Novak, M., Ravindranath, V., Ritz, R., Ruotsalainen, U., Subramaniam, S., Toga, A. W., Usui, S., van Pelt, J., Verschure, P., Willshaw, D., Wrobel, A., Tang, Y. & on Neuroinformatics,

O. E. C. D. W. G. (2003). Neuroscience data and tool sharing: a legal and policy framework for neuroinformatics., *Neuroinformatics* 1(2): 149–165.

Ferreira, T. & Rasband, W. (2010). *ImageJ User Guide*, NIH.
URL: `http://rsbweb.nih.gov/ij/docs/guide/index.html`

Fillard, P., Souplet, J.-C. & Toussaint, N. (2009). *Medical Image Navigation and Research Tool by INRIA (MedINRIA 1.9) Tutorial*, 2 edn, INRIA Sophia Antipolis.

Fischer, A. & Paulus, T. (2010). IMALYTICS 1.3: Translational research workstation.

Hiraoka, Y., Sedat, J. W. & Agard, D. A. (1987). The use of a charge-coupled device for quantitative optical microscopy of biological structures., *Science* 238(4823): 36–41.

Ibanez, L., Schroeder, W., Ng, L. & Cates, J. (2005). *The ITK Software Guide: ITK version 2.4*, 2 edn, Insight Software Consortium.

Jonasson, L., Hagmann, P., Bresson, X., Thiran, J.-P. & Wedeen, J. V. (2005). Representing diffusion MRI in 5D for segmentation of white matter tracts with a level set method., *Inf Process Med Imaging* 19: 311–320.

Lancaster, J. & Martinez, M. (2007). Mango – Multi-image analysis GUI, http://ric.uthscsa.edu/mango/index.html.
URL: `http://ric.uthscsa.edu/mango/index.html`

Leymarie, F. & Levine, M. (1992). Fast raster scan distance propagation on the discrete rectangular lattice, *CVGIP: Image Understanding* 55: 84 –94.

Longair, M., Baker, D. & Armstrong, J. (2011). Simple neurite tracer: open source software for reconstruction, visualization and analysis of neuronal processes., *Bioinformatics* 27(17): 2453–2454.
URL: `http://dx.doi.org/10.1093/bioinformatics/btr390`

Marcsisin, E. J. S., Uttero, C. M., Miljković, M. & Diem, M. (2010). Infrared microspectroscopy of live cells in aqueous media., *Analyst* 135(12): 3227–3232.
URL: `http://dx.doi.org/10.1039/c0an00548g`

Matheron, G. (1975). *Random Sets and Integral Geometry*, Wiley series in probability and mathematical statistics, 2 edn, Wiley, New York.

Mikula, S., Trotts, I., Stone, J. M. & Jones, E. G. (2007). Internet-enabled high-resolution brain mapping and virtual microscopy., *Neuroimage* 35(1): 9–15.
URL: `http://dx.doi.org/10.1016/j.neuroimage.2006.11.053`

Nakano, A. (2002). Spinning-disk confocal microscopy – a cutting-edge tool for imaging of membrane traffic., *Cell Struct Funct* 27(5): 349–355.

Papademetris, X., Jackowski, M., Rajeevan, N., Constable, R. & Staib, L. (2008). *BioImage Suite User's Manual*, Yale School of Medicine.

Peng, H. (2008). Bioimage informatics: a new area of engineering biology., *Bioinformatics* 24(17): 1827–1836.
URL: `http://dx.doi.org/10.1093/bioinformatics/btn346`

Pieper, S., Halle, M. & Kikinis, R. (2004). 3D slicer, Vol. 1, IEEE International Symposium on Biomedical Imaging, ISBI 2004, pp. 632–635.

Polikov, V. S., Tresco, P. A. & Reichert, W. M. (2005). Response of brain tissue to chronically implanted neural electrodes., *J Neurosci Methods* 148(1): 1–18.
URL: `http://dx.doi.org/10.1016/j.jneumeth.2005.08.015`

Preibisch, S., Saalfeld, S. & Tomancak, P. (2009). Globally optimal stitching of tiled 3D microscopic image acquisitions., *Bioinformatics* 25(11): 1463–1465.
URL: `http://dx.doi.org/10.1093/bioinformatics/btp184`

Prodanov, D. (2006). *Morphometric analysis of the rat lower limb nerves. Anatomical data forneural prosthesis design*, PhD thesis, Twente University, Enschede, The Netherlands.

Prodanov, D. (2008). Bidirectional communication of imaging data over the internet using ImageJ, *in* A. Jahnen & C. Moll (eds), *Proceedings of the 2nd ImageJ User and Developer Conference*, pp. 76 – 84.

Prodanov, D. & Feirabend, H. K. P. (2008). Automated characterization of nerve fibers labeled fluorescently: determination of size, class and spatial distribution., *Brain Res* 1233: 35–50.
URL: http://dx.doi.org/10.1016/j.brainres.2008.07.049

Prodanov, D., Heeroma, J. H. & Marani, E. (2006). Automatic morphometry of synaptic boutons of cultured cells using granulometric analysis of digital images, *J. Neurosci. Methods* 151 (2): 168 – 177.

Prodanov, D., Nagelkerke, N. & Marani, E. (2007). Spatial clustering analysis in neuroanatomy: applications of different approaches to motor nerve fiber distribution., *J Neurosci Methods* 160(1): 93–108.

Prodanov, D., Roussel, S., Trekker, J., Dresselaers, T. & Himmelreich, U. (2010). ImageJ in biomedical imaging applications, *in* A. Jahnen & C. Moll (eds), *Proceedings of the 3rd ImageJ User and Developer Conference*, pp. 20 – 27.

Prodanov, D., Thil, M.-A., Marani, E., Delbeke, J. & Holsheimer, J. (2005). Three-dimensional topography of the motor endplates of the rat gastrocnemius muscle., *Muscle Nerve* 32(3): 292–302.
URL: http://dx.doi.org/10.1002/mus.20378

Schindelin, J. (2008). Fiji is just ImageJ – batteries included, *in* A. Jahnen & C. Moll (eds), *Proceedings of the 2nd ImageJ User and Developer Conference*, Luxembourg.

Serra, J. (1982). *Image Analysis and Mathematical Morphology*, Academic Press Ltd, London.

Sezgin, S. & Sankur, B. (2004). Survey over image thresholding techniques and quantitative performance evaluation, *J. Electron. Imaging* 13(1): 146–165.

Smith, S., Jenkinson, M., Woolrich, W., Beckmann, C., Behrens, T., Johansen-Berg, H., Bannister, P., Luca, M. D., Drobnjak, I., Flitney, D., Niazy, R., Saunders, J., Vickers, J., Zhang, Y., Stefano, N. D., Brady, J. M. & Matthews, P. (2004). Advances in functional and structural MR image analysis and implementation as FSL., *Neuroimage* 23 Suppl 1: S208–S219.
URL: http://dx.doi.org/10.1016/j.neuroimage.2004.07.051

van Meer, G., Stelzer, E. H., van Resandt, R. W. W. & Simons, K. (1987). Sorting of sphingolipids in epithelial (madin-darby canine kidney) cells., *J Cell Biol* 105(4): 1623–1635.

Welkenhuysen, M. (2011). *Electrical brain stimulation and microrecording: Research in animal models of psychiatric disorders and in vivo evaluation of a neural probe*, PhD thesis, Catholic university of Leuven, KU Leuven, Leuven.

White, J. G., Amos, W. B. & Fordham, M. (1987). An evaluation of confocal versus conventional imaging of biological structures by fluorescence light microscopy., *J Cell Biol* 105(1): 41–48.

Part 2

Specific Applications with Clinical Examples

9

Molecular Imaging of Stem Cells: A New Area for Neuroscience

Nora Sandu[1,2], Fatemeh Momen-Heravi[3], Pooyan Sadr-Eshkevari[4], Ali Arvantaj[5] and Bernhard Schaller[2]
[1]*Department of Neurosurgery, University of Lausanne, Lausanne,*
[2]*Department of Neurosurgery, University of Paris 7, Paris,*
[3]*Craniomaxillofacial Research Center, Shariati Hospital, Tehran University of Medical Sciences*
[4]*Dental Section, Farzan Clinical Research Institute, Tehran,*
[5]*Department of Neurology, Baylor College of Medicine, Houston,*
[1]*Switzerland*
[2]*France*
[3,4]*Iran*
[5]*USA*

1. Introduction

Nowadays, new imaging modalities such as molecular imaging have enabled both practitioners and researchers to visualize, trace and measure biological processes at the level of cells or even single molecules. Instruments of nuclear medicine, like Positron Emission Tomography (PET), Single-Photon Emission Computed Tomography (SPECT) and gamma scintigraphy have largely contributed to the evolving and promising era of personalized medicine. Such recently introduced molecular imaging techniques take advantage of an additional potential for broad application in imaging molecular or cellular events in vivo: gene/protein function and regulation, signal transduction, transcriptional regulation and characterization of transgenic animals (Jacobs et al., 2003). Most importantly, molecular imaging will render possible the identification of potential molecular therapeutic targets, in the development of new treatment strategies, and in their successful implementation into clinical application (Jacobs et al., 2003). As a description, molecular imaging is a process of getting signals originating from live organisms after the administration of specific agents that target specific markers found at tissue or cellular level. Such nuclear imaging is the most well-known instrument of all molecular imaging methods and has been set as the gold standard.

In this chapter, the authors will discuss PET and other more recent molecular imaging techniques such as near infrared fluorescence (NIRF). Moreover, we will put emphasis on the application of molecular imaging in visualization of stem cell transplantation as a ground breaking treatment modality for neurodegenerative and other neurological diseases. The authors stand among the very first who has implemented recently introduced molecular imaging techniques into experimental research and clinical practice.

2. Cell therapy

Cell therapy, as a promising method using live components of human tissue for treatment of neurological diseases, is one of the mainstays of the wide field of regenerative medicine.. Among stem cell sources available up to date, mesenchymal stem cells (MSCs) have generated a great deal of interest because of their potency in terms of regeneration and tissue engineering (Wislet-Gendebien et al., 2012).

Neurodegenerative disease is a term which encompasses a wide range of acute and chronic neurological diseases such as Parkinson's disease, Huntington's disease, amyotrophic lateral sclerosis (ALS), Alzheimer's disease, multiple sclerosis (MS), stroke, and spinal cord injury. Because of the fact that central nervous system reveals limited capacity of regeneration and tissue replacement, cell therapy and tissue regeneration of injured or degenerated tissue, as a potential new therapeutic modality, draws lots of attention (Wislet-Gendebien et al., 2012). Stem cells have the potential to differentiate into many different cell types. Recent research has concerned an exciting opportunity to apply MSCs especially in the management of neurodegenerative diseases, because of their potential to differentiate into neurons (Lee et al., 2010).

It has been shown that the injection of MSCs could be profitable in the treatment of neurodegenerative diseases such as Parkinson’s disease (Levy et al.), Spinal Stroke and cerebral ischemia (Sieber-Blum, 2010), Alzheimer's disease (Lee et al., 2010), Multiple Sclerosis (Grigoriadis et al., 2011), Huntington's Disease (Snyder et al., 2010). The advantages of using stem cells for regenerative medicine are not only the eases of harvesting from bone marrow or other donor sites but also the minimal risk of tissue rejection because of the application of autologous cells.

Interestingly, recent data suggest that intravenously injected MSCs could migrate into the brain and pass blood-brain barrier (BBB), which is basically formed by brain microvascular endothelial cells (BMECs), and restrict the passage of immune cells and different molecules into the brain. The exact mechanism of this phenomenon, whether it is based on Integrin-mediated adhesion or is matrix metalloproteinase dependent extracellular matrix degradation, is yet not clear (Krampera et al., 2007, Matsushita et al., 2011).

One of the main clinical problems of stem cell transplantation is the difficulty of detection, localization, and examination of the stem cells in vivo at both cellular and molecular levels (Sandu et al.). State-of-the-art molecular imaging techniques provide new superior means of noninvasive, repeated, and quantitative tracking of stem cell implants or transplants (Sandu et al.). From initial deposition to the survival, migration, and differentiation of the transplant/implanted stem cells, current molecular imaging methods allow monitoring of the infused cells in the same live recipient bed over time (Sandu et al.).

3. Positron Emission Tomography (PET)

Over the past two decades, PET has been introduced and applied widly in the milieu of diagnosis including head and neck diseases. Along with a growing interest to use PET in tracing different types of molecules such as amino acids, receptor ligands, glucose and other metabolic substrates which follow specific metabolic pathways have been utilized to assess different tissue functions, especially in neoplasms (Cornelius et al., 2011). The main substances for radio-labeling are fluorine-18 (F), gadolinium-68 (Ga) and Carbon-11 (C). The advantages that they confer upon other positron emitting isotopes such as O, N and C are their longer half-life time which results in superior tissue distribution and consequently a dynamic imaging of higher accuracy (de Langen et al., 2008, Keiding et al., 2010, Floeth et al., 2011, Henze et al., 2005).

Among metabolic substrates, F-fluorodeoxyglucose is the most renowned molecular tracer in oncology. It has been shown that F-FDG uptake may increase in neoplasmic cells which are believed to be indicative of an increased glycolysis and a subsided respiratory rate of tumoral tissues (Di Chiro et al., 1987). It has been demonstrated that amino acid synthesis is up regulated in tumor cells in comparison to normal tissues. Until now, F-Tyrosine and C-Methionine uptakes are studied at different grades of oncologic tumors such as meningimoma (Cremerius et al., 1997).

C-colin, another marker which represents phospholipid synthesis, is hiked in malignant tumors. It has been shown that the metabolism and proliferation of C-colin are strongly correlated with breast and prostate cancers, indicating high uptake as a measurement of cellular proliferation (Cornelius et al., 2011). Other markers, with a better theoretical profile, have also been introduced in neuroscience but are mostly used only in a limited number of experiments, so that no knowledge is about their potential for imaging stem cell transplantation.

4. Near-InfRared Fluorescence (NIRF) imaging

NIRF confers similar capability for tracing of imaging agents as PET. NIRF dyes are chemically conjugated on targeting molecule such as antibodies, carbohydrates and peptides. After administration into tissues, the dye molecules are excited by the radiation of tissue penetrating NIR excitation light (750-900nm).

Considering radioactive decay, a photon of lower energy which has a higher wavelength is emitted and the fluorescent dye relaxes back to its basic state, ready to repeat the same process. Each fluorescent dye absorb excitation light and afterward, just in a nanosecond, produce fluorescent light. Accordingly, each fluorescent dye molecule provides about 100,000,000 photons per second for collection and image formation. As a consequence, low-energy fluorescent photons are slightly absorbed and maximally scattered, reduced by the tissues between the targeted tissue and the tissue surface before being collected by detectors in a few milliseconds. In contrast with radionuclides, a fluorescent dye has no physical half-life. Moreover, this methodology is not clinically approved yet and no devices is available for human imaging with NIRF contrast agents, and NIRF contrast imaging agents do not posses approval for human study as well. Interestingly, some investigators utilized NIRF imaging for human applications such as functional lymphatic imaging, sentinel lymph node mapping, activated probes, and promising advances in 3D imaging (Sevick-Muraca EM, 2012).

5. Potential clinical applications of molecular imaging

Many surgical techniques are mainly based on histological grading of the tumor. Molecular imaging enables surgeons to have the gross picture of these tumors. Pre-surgical molecular imaging of neurological tumors enables us to establish better surgical procedure and strategy. Also, it would allow physicians to have a better pre-assessment of prognosis and risk benefit ratio. Moreover, PET might be helpful in the early discovery of molecular-level changes, which are undetectable in CT and MRI. Also, within a specific tumor, the most metabolically active and aggressive tumor areas could be mapped.

Intriguingly, emerging data suggest that molecular imaging could be used as an outcome assessment tool for different treatment modalities. For instance, a recent study compared MRI response assessment with metabolic O-(2-(18)F-fluoroethyl)-L-tyrosine ((18)F-FET) PET response assessment during antiangiogenic treatment in patients with recurrent high-grade glioma (see table 1). Good results are already known for (18)FDG-PET, but results revealed that (18)F-FET PET, on the other hand, seems also to be predictive of treatment failure in that it contributes important information to response assessment based only on MRI and response assessment in neurooncology (RANO) criteria (Hutterer et al., 2011).

Gold Standard	FDG-PET diagnosis		FDG-PET diagnosis in brain metastasis patients only		FDG-PET diagnosis in primary tumor patients only		Magnetic resonance imaging diagnosis	
	Tumor (%)	Necrosis (%)	Tumor (%)	Necrosis (%)	Tumor (%)	Necrosis (%)	Tumor (%)	Necrosis (%)
Tumor	47	16	42	17	75	13		
Necrosis	7	3	8	33	0	13	36	9
Sensitivity	75	0	71	0	86	0	94	0
Specificity	81	0	80	0	100	0	50	0

Legend: FDG: ^{8}F-fluoro-2-deoxy-D-glucose; PET: positron emission tomography.

Table 1. (18)F-FDG Positron Emission Tomography with a Gold Standard of Biopsy or Radiography Follow-up (Schaller et al., 2008)

6. Stem cell imaging at neurodegenerative pathways and pathologies

Regenerative medicine is a developing era that seeks to restore or replace damaged tissue and organs via natural or bioengineered tools. Regenerative medicine via stem cells is considered as one of the most promising means to repair tissues. Stem cells could be isolated from both adult human and embryonic tissues. There is a great body of evidence demonstrating successful cases of expanded stem cell in vitro and then grafted in vivo for regenerative purposes at different tissues such as bone, cartilage, and myocardium.

It seems that inflammation and degeneration are the two main aspects of CNS pathogenesis. It seems that there is an intrinsic connection between these two phenomena because in several cases inflammation trigger degeneration. Also, endogenous neural stem cells, which have the capacity of renewing cells of CNS, may migrate to the affected area and robust the process of repair. This scenario drives scientists to seek a natural healing framework based on Trans stem cell therapy. In fact, it may improve the efficacy and decrease the toxicity of treatment modalities which are the main concepts of personalized medicine.

7. Molecular imaging in Alzheimer's disease

Alzheimer's disease (AD) is describes as a chronic and complex progressive neurodegenerative disorder, and is the most common cause of dementia among the elderly. A great body of evidences indicates that neuronal degeneration in AD progresses in a certain way while the pathology advances over several decades. Establishing an accurate dynamic map of this sequence is vital for the understanding and mapping the complex endophenotype of AD, providing a basis for successful treatments designed to resist or prevent disease progression.

PET scanning has long been used to trace alterations in cerebral blood flow and metabolism in AD, and is useful for the differential diagnosis of dementia in individual patients. For instance, hypometabolism of the posterior cingulate cortex could be observed early in AD using fluoro-deoxyglucose (FDG) PET scanning, even while MRI results are normal (Ewers et al., 2011, Mosconi et al., 2004). As disease progresses, there is diminished cerebral metabolism and perfusion in posterior cingulate and association cortices, but the basal ganglia and thalamus, cerebellum, and primary sensorimotor cortices are largely spared until later stages of the disease. Some studies have tracked AD with PET, using new molecular probes sensitive to amyloid-beta (Aβ) or neurofibrillary tangle pathology, or both types of pathology (Braskie et al., 2010, Klunk et al., 2004, Mintun et al., 2006, Small et al., 2006).

8. Stem cell in Multiple Sclerosis (MS)

Multiple sclerosis appears to result from defective innate and adaptive immune system actions in the CNS, likely begins with a kind of autoimmune response that leads to demyelination and neuronal degeneration. It seems that auto activity of immune system followed by neuroinflamation gradually causes death of oligodendrocytes. Increasing body of evidence represents that the brain's inability to repair is one of the main factors that make this disease irreversible and causes permanent damages. This claim is in accordance with the fact that the progression of disease and state of remyelination is different in every patient. Consistently, Patrikios et al. (Patrikios et al.), recently performed 51 autopsies of MS patients with different clinical courses and disease durations and traced variable extents of remyelination. In 20% of patients - both relapsing and progressive patients - the extent of remyelination was extensive with 60–96% of the global lesion area remyelinated.

Several attempts have been made since about four decades to replace demieylinated cells with myelin forming cells; however, as neural cells are highly differentiated and have limited ability for growth and expansion, these efforts have been mostly abortive in vivo. With the advent of stem cell regenerative medicine, scientists further discovered the functional and special characteristics of adult stem cells and attempted to utilize them for the treatment of neurodegenerative multiple sclerosis.

Adult stem cells have not only provided us with a readily available cell source for cell therapy but also with much safer and far less toxic tumor treatment measures. There are two basic routes for cell administration including in-site cell transplantation or blood injection (circulation). Tangible examples for the former include Parkinson's disease, acute spinal cord injury and brain trauma. For multifocal diseases such as MS and epilepsy, the model of in-site injection is not effective; rather blood circulation or cerebrospinal fluid circulation should be used. There are several studies demonstrating successful results with the transplantation of hematopietic, mesenchymal and neural stem cells into the CNS injured areas in MS, SCI, epilepsy, and stroke cases (Pluchino et al., 2009).

9. Mechanisms of Stem Cell Repairing

A great amount of data demonstrates that HSCs have a great capacity to differentiate into different cell types including muscle, skin, neural tissue and lung (Pluchino et al., 2009). Several studies used HSCs injection as a treatment modality for hematological malignancies and shows that HSCs have the capability of entering the brain and as well as differentiating and producing new neural cells including neurons and microglia; these findings were in concordance by the detection of Y chromosome- positive Purkinje cells in the cerebellum of female rats who have undergone bone marrow transplantation from male donors (Koshizuka et al., 2004 2005). In addition, in an animal studies on rats suffering from a demyelinated lesion of the spinal cord, intravenous or intraparenchimal HSCs therapy lead to different degrees of remyelination which was proportional to the number of injected stem cells (Akiyama et al., 2002a 2002, Inoue et al, 2003, Akiyama et al., 2002b 2002, Inoue et al, 2003).

Several studies have challenged the idea of cell replacement in stem cell regeneration theories. Despite the fact that MSCs can exert various therapeutic effects, some data suggest that they protect immune system from demyelination via alternative mechanism to cell replacement.

The suggested therapeutic effect is based on the intrinsic capacities of such cells to secret a large number of cytokines and chemokines. It has been shown that the pattern of secretion changes as early as transplanted stem cell encounter new (micro) environment in vivo. Some studies have shown that mesenchymal stem cells mainly act by suppressing inflammation, via cell-to-cell contact as well as through the activation of anti-inflammatory pathways; and consequently the proliferation, migration and differentiation of endogenous progenitor cells are enhanced.

Utilizing fluorescent dyes and imaging modalities in humans is not possible due to limited depth of tissue penetration. On the other hand, magnetic resonance imaging (MRI) and positron emission tomography (PET) have shown promising value and also great feasibility for treatment via stem cell. As well as above PET scan imaging, stem cells could be tagged with ferromagnetic material or with gadolinium rhodamine dextran and then detect via MRI (Brekke et al., 2007) (Carney and Shah, 2011). These imaging modalities along with alteration of genes via genetic engineering and consequent labeling methods, enabled scientists to monitor different phase of repair and stem cell therapy. This allows not only the imaging in real time of stem cell migration, but also its integration, and therapeutic effects at the single cell level. Also, the above-mentioned capacities for tracing and monitoring of grafted stem cell behavior, enable us to assess both quantitatively and qualitatively the interaction between stem cell and its environment.

10. View to the future

Molecular imaging will gain more and more importance in neurosciences. PET is currently the gold standard and that will not change very soon. However, the different methods have different advantages and disadvantages, but it is not only for the researcher but also for the physician important to know this differences. In the near future, imaging on the molecular but also on the cellular level will not be an exception, as it is still now, but rather the rule. Such improvements open widely the door to a personalized medicine, a fact that has special importance in neurosciences.

11. Take-home-message

Molecular imaging has gained step-by-step importance in neuroscience. To know this method in detail is demanding but important in the area of personalized medicine.

12. References

Akiyama, Y., Radtke, C., Honmou, O. & Kocsis, J. D. 2002a. Remyelination of the spinal cord following intravenous delivery of bone marrow cells. *Glia,* 39, 229-36.

Akiyama, Y., Radtke, C. & Kocsis, J. D. 2002b. Remyelination of the rat spinal cord by transplantation of identified bone marrow stromal cells. *The Journal of neuroscience : the official journal of the Society for Neuroscience,* 22, 6623-30.

Braskie, M. N., Klunder, A. D., Hayashi, K. M., Protas, H., Kepe, V., Miller, K. J., Huang, S. C., Barrio, J. R., Ercoli, L. M., Siddarth, P., Satyamurthy, N., Liu, J., Toga, A. W., Bookheimer, S. Y., Small, G. W. & Thompson, P. M. 2010. Plaque and tangle imaging and cognition in normal aging and Alzheimer's disease. *Neurobiology of aging,* 31, 1669-78.

Brekke, C., Williams, S. C., Price, J., Thorsen, F. & Modo, M. 2007. Cellular multiparametric MRI of neural stem cell therapy in a rat glioma model. *NeuroImage,* 37, 769-82.

Carney, B. J. & Shah, K. 2011. Migration and fate of therapeutic stem cells in different brain disease models. *Neuroscience,* 197, 37-47.

Cornelius, J. F., Langen, K. J., Stoffels, G., Hanggi, D., Sabel, M. & Steiger, H. J. 2011. Pet Imaging Of Meningioma In Clinical Practice: Review of literature and future directions. *Neurosurgery.*

Cremerius, U., Bares, R., Weis, J., Sabri, O., Mull, M., Schroder, J. M., Gilsbach, J. M. & Buell, U. 1997. Fasting improves discrimination of grade 1 and atypical or malignant meningioma in FDG-PET. *Journal of nuclear medicine : official publication, Society of Nuclear Medicine,* 38, 26-30.

De Langen, A. J., Van Den Boogaart, V. E., Marcus, J. T. & Lubberink, M. 2008. Use of H2(15)O-PET and DCE-MRI to measure tumor blood flow. *The oncologist,* 13, 631-44.

Di Chiro, G., Hatazawa, J., Katz, D. A., Rizzoli, H. V. & De Michele, D. J. 1987. Glucose utilization by intracranial meningiomas as an index of tumor aggressivity and probability of recurrence: a PET study. *Radiology,* 164, 521-6.

Ewers, M., Frisoni, G. B., Teipel, S. J., Grinberg, L. T., Amaro, E., Jr., Heinsen, H., Thompson, P. M. & Hampel, H. 2011. Staging Alzheimer's disease progression with multimodality neuroimaging. *Progress in neurobiology,* 95, 535-46.

Floeth, F. W., Sabel, M., Ewelt, C., Stummer, W., Felsberg, J., Reifenberger, G., Steiger, H. J., Stoffels, G., Coenen, H. H. & Langen, K. J. 2011. Comparison of (18)F-FET PET and 5-ALA fluorescence in cerebral gliomas. *European journal of nuclear medicine and molecular imaging,* 38, 731-41.

Grigoriadis, N., Lourbopoulos, A., Lagoudaki, R., Frischer, J. M., Polyzoidou, E., Touloumi, O., Simeonidou, C., Deretzi, G., Kountouras, J., Spandou, E., Kotta, K., Karkavelas, G., Tascos, N. & Lassmann, H. 2011. Variable behavior and complications of autologous bone marrow mesenchymal stem cells transplanted in experimental autoimmune encephalomyelitis. *Experimental neurology,* 230, 78-89.

Henze, M., Dimitrakopoulou-Strauss, A., Milker-Zabel, S., Schuhmacher, J., Strauss, L. G., Doll, J., Macke, H. R., Eisenhut, M., Debus, J. & Haberkorn, U. 2005. Characterization of 68Ga-DOTA-D-Phe1-Tyr3-octreotide kinetics in patients with meningiomas. *Journal of nuclear medicine : official publication, Society of Nuclear Medicine,* 46, 763-9.

Hutterer, M., Nowosielski, M., Putzer, D., Waitz, D., Tinkhauser, G., Kostron, H., Muigg, A., Virgolini, I. J., Staffen, W., Trinka, E., Gotwald, T., Jacobs, A. H. & Stockhammer, G. 2011. O-(2-18F-fluoroethyl)-L-tyrosine PET predicts failure of antiangiogenic treatment in patients with recurrent high-grade glioma. *Journal of nuclear medicine : official publication, Society of Nuclear Medicine,* 52, 856-64.

Jacobs, A. H., Li, H., Winkeler, A., Hilker, R., Knoess, C., Ruger, A., Galldiks, N., Schaller, B., Sobesky, J., Kracht, L., Monfared, P., Klein, M., Vollmar, S., Bauer, B., Wagner, R., Graf, R., Wienhard, K., Herholz, K. & Heiss, W. D. 2003. PET-based molecular imaging in neuroscience. *European journal of nuclear medicine and molecular imaging,* 30, 1051-65.

Keiding, S., Sorensen, M., Munk, O. L. & Bender, D. 2010. Human (13)N-ammonia PET studies: the importance of measuring (13)N-ammonia metabolites in blood. *Metabolic brain disease,* 25, 49-56.

Klunk, W. E., Engler, H., Nordberg, A., Wang, Y., Blomqvist, G., Holt, D. P., Bergstrom, M., Savitcheva, I., Huang, G. F., Estrada, S., Ausen, B., Debnath, M. L., Barletta, J., Price, J. C., Sandell, J., Lopresti, B. J., Wall, A., Koivisto, P., Antoni, G., Mathis, C. A. & Langstrom, B. 2004. Imaging brain amyloid in Alzheimer's disease with Pittsburgh Compound-B. *Annals of neurology,* 55, 306-19.

Koshizuka, S., Okada, S., Okawa, A., Koda, M., Murasawa, M., Hashimoto, M., Kamada, T., Yoshinaga, K., Murakami, M., Moriya, H. & Yamazaki, M. 2004. Transplanted Hematopoietic Stem Cells from Bone Marrow Differentiate into Neural Lineage

Cells and Promote Functional Recovery after Spinal Cord Injury in Mice. *Journal of Neuropathology & Experimental Neurology,* 63, 64-72.

Krampera, M., Franchini, M., Pizzolo, G. & Aprili, G. 2007. Mesenchymal stem cells: from biology to clinical use. *Blood transfusion = Trasfusione del sangue,* 5, 120-9.

Lee, J. K., Jin, H. K., Endo, S., Schuchman, E. H., Carter, J. E. & Bae, J. S. 2010. Intracerebral transplantation of bone marrow-derived mesenchymal stem cells reduces amyloid-beta deposition and rescues memory deficits in Alzheimer's disease mice by modulation of immune responses. *Stem cells,* 28, 329-43.

Levy, Y. S., Bahat-Stroomza, M., Barzilay, R., Burshtein, A., Bulvik, S., Barhum, Y., Panet, H., Melamed, E. & Offen, D. 2008. Regenerative effect of neural-induced human mesenchymal stromal cells in rat models of Parkinson's disease. *Cytotherapy,* 10, 340-52.

Matsushita, T., Kibayashi, T., Katayama, T., Yamashita, Y., Suzuki, S., Kawamata, J., Honmou, O., Minami, M. & Shimohama, S. 2011. Mesenchymal stem cells transmigrate across brain microvascular endothelial cell monolayers through transiently formed inter-endothelial gaps. *Neuroscience letters,* 502, 41-5.

Mintun, M. A., Larossa, G. N., Sheline, Y. I., Dence, C. S., Lee, S. Y., Mach, R. H., Klunk, W. E., Mathis, C. A., Dekosky, S. T. & Morris, J. C. 2006. [11C]PIB in a nondemented population: potential antecedent marker of Alzheimer disease. *Neurology,* 67, 446-52.

Mosconi, L., Pupi, A., De Cristofaro, M. T., Fayyaz, M., Sorbi, S. & Herholz, K. 2004. Functional interactions of the entorhinal cortex: an 18F-FDG PET study on normal aging and Alzheimer's disease. *Journal of nuclear medicine : official publication, Society of Nuclear Medicine,* 45, 382-92.

Patrikios, P., Stadelmann, C., Kutzelnigg, A., Rauschka, H., Schmidbauer, M., Laursen, H., Sorensen, P. S., Bruck, W., Lucchinetti, C. & Lassmann, H. 2006. Remyelination is extensive in a subset of multiple sclerosis patients. *Brain : a journal of neurology,* 129, 3165-72.

Pluchino, S., Zanotti, L., Brini, E., Ferrari, S. & Martino, G. 2009. Regeneration and repair in multiple sclerosis: the role of cell transplantation. *Neuroscience letters,* 456, 101-6.

Sandu, N., Momen-Heravi, F., Sadr-Eshkevari, P. & Schaller, B. 2012. Molecular imaging for stem cell transplantation in neuroregenerative medicine. *Neuro-degenerative diseases,* 9, 60-7.

Schaller, B. J., Cornelius, J. F., Sandu, N. & Buchfelder, M. 2008. Molecular imaging of brain tumors personal experience and review of the literature. *Current molecular medicine,* 8, 711-26.

Sieber-Blum, M. 2010. Epidermal neural crest stem cells and their use in mouse models of spinal cord injury. *Brain research bulletin,* 83, 189-93.

Small, G. W., Kepe, V., Ercoli, L. M., Siddarth, P., Bookheimer, S. Y., Miller, K. J., Lavretsky, H., Burggren, A. C., Cole, G. M., Vinters, H. V., Thompson, P. M., Huang, S. C., Satyamurthy, N., Phelps, M. E. & Barrio, J. R. 2006. PET of brain amyloid and tau in mild cognitive impairment. *The New England journal of medicine,* 355, 2652-63.

Snyder, B. R., Chiu, A. M., Prockop, D. J. & Chan, A. W. 2010. Human multipotent stromal cells (MSCs) increase neurogenesis and decrease atrophy of the striatum in a transgenic mouse model for Huntington's disease. *PloS one,* 5, e9347.

Wislet-Gendebien, S., Laudet, E., Neirinckx, V. & Rogister, B. 2012. Adult bone marrow: which stem cells for cellular therapy protocols in neurodegenerative disorders? *Journal of biomedicine & biotechnology,* 2012, 601560.

10

Molecular MRI of Atherosclerosis

B.C. Te Boekhorst and K. Nicolay
Department of Biomedical Engineering, Eindhoven University of Technology, The Netherlands

1. Introduction

Atherosclerosis and its consequences contribute to more than 50% of mortality in Europe, the United States of America and many developed or developing countries (Schafers et al., 2010). The main pathologic substrate in atherosclerosis is the atherosclerotic lesion. The classical high-risk plaque is characterized by a large lipid core, a thin fibrous cap and many macrophages in the shoulder regions of the plaque (Falk et al., 1995; Stary et al., 1995). Rupture of the fibrous cap or, more subtle, erosion leads to exposure of the thrombogenic sub-endothelial matrix to blood leading to thrombus formation. Recurrent thrombosis or major atherothrombosis may lead to an acute cardiovascular event via sub(total) occlusion of the vessel of interest. Macrophages are the key mediators of plaque inflammation and progression (Lusis, 2000; Ross, 1999). Inflammatory activity can be evaluated at the cellular (macrophages and neutrophils) or sub-cellular (secreted enzymes, membrane-bound proteins) level. Sensitive and specific biomarkers of plaque inflammation and instability are highly desired for more accurate definition of high-risk plaques in high risk patient populations. At present, serologic markers do not accomplish this need sufficiently. Therefore, there is a need for noninvasive imaging techniques for identification and quantification of local plaque biomarkers, which can direct interventional cardiologists and vascular surgeons to diseased sites and can monitor therapeutic response.

2. Atherosclerosis

Atherosclerosis is characterized by various more or less orderly processes taking place during the development from a fatty streak to a rupture-prone or ruptured plaque (Ross, 1999). Several morphological stages of plaque development related to risk of rupture were described by the American Heart Association (Stary et al., 1995). However, recently other plaques than the classical vulnerable plaque with a large lipid core and thin fibrous cap were also recognized as high-risk plaque, like highly calcified and obstructive plaques (Naghavi et al., 2003a, 2003b). During the process of atherogenesis, inflammation aggravates endothelial dysfunction and *vice versa*. First, low density lipoproteins are deposited in the subintima, where rare neutrophils and macrophages produce myeloperoxidase. This leads to generation of tyrosyl radicals and aldehydes resulting in oxidation of LDL. Oxidized LDL (ox-LDL) irritates endothelial cells which become dysfunctional, leading to inflammatory cell migration and activation. Macrophage activation leads to release of matrix metalloproteinases, cathepsins and other matrix degrading enzymes. Activated macrophages also release factors that eventually cause apoptosis of smooth muscle cells, endothelial cells and macrophages themselves. Fibrous cap thinning, lipid core growth, formation of fragile intra-plaque neovasculature, intra-plaque hemorrhage and finally fibrous cap rupture may be the result of these processes. Fibrous cap rupture leads to exposure of the tissue under the broken endothelial barrier to the blood stream which activates coagulation. Subsequent formation of a thrombus may cause an acute thrombotic event (Libby, 2002; Lusis, 2000; Ross, 1999) .

All these processes can serve as the target of molecular imaging techniques, at the cellular or subcellular/molecular level. The next section describes an overview of the available methods for in vivo molecular imaging of atherosclerosis.

3. Molecular imaging techniques for atherosclerosis

Various noninvasive imaging techniques are available for evaluation of the levels of the above inflammation-related cells, proteins or enzymes. Fluorescence imaging (FI), ultrasound (US), computed tomography (CT), positron emission tomography (PET), single-photon-emission computed tomography (SPECT) and magnetic resonance imaging (MRI) are all imaging modalities with in vivo applicability that could play a role in molecular imaging of plaque inflammation (I.Y. Chen & Wu, 2011).

Because light attenuation by tissue is wavelength dependent, fluorescent proteins with more red-shifted emission wavelength have been developed to maximize FI sensitivity and specificity. The advent of quantum dot technology alleviates the problems associated with protein-based optical reporters, e.g. photobleaching, low quantum yield, low absorbance and broad emission band. However, because of the limited imaging depth an intravascular catheter is needed for clinical application (Calfon et al., 2010). Further, cytotoxicity of quantum dots needs to be addressed and a second imaging modality (MRI or CT) is needed for anatomic colocalization before FI with quantum dots may be clinically implemented (Iga et al., 2007).

Ultrasound with targeted micro-bubbles is restricted to the endothelial molecular targets, because the size of the bubbles (~1-10 μm) precludes their extravasation (I.Y. Chen & Wu, 2011). Other disadvantages of US include the high degree of operator dependency, low micro-bubble adhesion efficiency and poor ability to image past bony structures.

Recently, an iodinated CT contrast agent was used for imaging of macrophage activity in atherosclerotic plaques (Hyafil et al., 2007). The unknown toxicity of the high concentrations of organometallics needed for effective imaging, limited differentiation between diverse soft plaque constituents and the high radiation exposure limit clinical application of molecular CT.

After intravenous administration of the PET-tracer F-18-fluorodeoxyglucose, metabolically active cells may take up this tracer. This has been shown useful for PET/CT imaging of atherosclerotic plaque inflammation in carotid, iliac and femoral arteries of patients (Rudd et al., 2007). PET and SPECT are techniques allowing imaging of disease processes in vivo with nanomolar/picomolar sensitivity (Massoud & Ghambir, 2003). SPECT was applied for imaging of plaque apoptosis in an atherosclerotic rabbit model (Kolodgie et al., 2003), and lipid-rich lesions of mice and rabbits via an epitope on ox-LDL (Tsimikas et al., 2000). PET and SPECT lack definition of anatomical structure and have limited spatial resolution, and therefore need to be combined with an imaging modality (CT or MRI), which can define anatomic structure.

In terms of broad clinical applicability and availability, MRI is the most versatile technique. MRI does not involve ionizing radiation, has a high penetration depth, is safe and non-invasive, suitable as a screening tool, which can be repeated at will and provides both anatomical and physiological information. Disadvantages of MRI are relatively long acquisition times and poor suitability for patients, who are claustrophobic. Molecular MRI of coronary artery plaque is difficult due to motion caused by respiration and cardiac contractions. These motions pose an upper limit to the time window of MRI signal acquisition during the cardiac cycle. However, development of more efficient pulse sequence protocols may reduce these problems in future.

Molecular MRI employs contrast agent carriers to which antibodies, peptides or receptor (ant)agonists with affinity for the target of interest are conjugated (Mulder et al., 2007a). Larger carriers can harbor a higher payload of MR contrast generating Gd or iron oxides and can therefore have higher relaxivity. However, carriers which are very large may not enter the plaque due to the limited size of endothelial cell fenestrations. In atherosclerosis these fenestrations may exceed the regular size of 5 nm by far. In the apoE-/- mouse model neo-intimal thickening of the carotid artery induced by a constrictive collar could be visualized with paramagnetic liposomes which could pass the endothelial barrier despite a mean diameter of 90 nm (Mulder et al., 2006). In another study the effect of size of the contrast agent on plaque permeation was investigated (Van Bochove et al., 2011). This effect was tested in apoE-/- mice in which a tapered cast around the right carotid artery generated thin cap fibroatheromas and non-thin cap fibroatheromas as published previously (Cheng et al. 2006). Low molecular weight Gd-chelates (Gd-HP-DO3A) and micelles led to plaque enhancement which was highest with the longest retention in the non-thin cap fibroatheromas, whereas liposomes did not accumulate in any of the plaques (Van Bochove et al., 2011). These results implicate that targeted liposomes are most suitable for the imaging of plaque-associated endothelial markers, whereas micelles, which accumulate extravascularly on a long timescale, are suited for imaging of less abundant markers inside plaques. Low molecular weight compounds may be employed for target-specific imaging of highly abundant extravascular plaque-associated targets.

4. Molecular MRI of atherosclerosis

4.1 Extracellular matrix proteins

The potential for *in vivo* molecular imaging of plaque collagen using a liposome functionalized with a collagen adhesion protein, CNA35, has been suggested after a series of in vitro tests (Sanders et al., 2009). Indirectly, quantification of collagen using this method could provide information about plaque phenotype, in particular plaque stability.

Another extracellular matrix protein of plaque, which has potential for noninvasive assessment of plaque burden by molecular MRI *in vivo* is elastin. Changes in elastin content and the high abundance of elastin during plaque development make it a good quantitative marker of plaque burden, which was recently confirmed in a mouse model of atherosclerosis with an elastin-specific MR contrast agent (Makowski et al., 2011). The strong MRI signal change provided by this agent allowed for imaging with high spatial resolution, not only resulting in accurate assessment of plaque burden, but also plaque characterization by quantification of intra-plaque elastin content using signal intensity measurements (Makowski et al., 2011).

Gadofluorine M is an amphiphile with perfluorinated side chains, which forms micelles with a diameter of 5 to 6 nm in aqueous solution. Accumulation of Gadofluorine M micelles in atherosclerotic plaque has been attributed to the enhanced vessel-wall permeability and also to its affinity for both extracellular matrix proteins (Meding et al. 2007) and plaque lipids (Barkhausen et al., 2003).

4.2 Cholesterol deposition

Antibody-conjugated paramagnetic micelles have been used for targeted MRI of specific epitopes of ox-LDL in atherosclerotic plaque. At 72 and 96 hours after intravenous injection of ox-LDL-targeted micelles in apoE-/- mice, specific MRI signal enhancement of aortic plaque was observed. MRI signal enhancement was significantly lower after injection of control non-conjugated micelles and nonspecific IgG-conjugated micelles (Briley-Saebo et al., 2008). Despite this success in the preclinical setting, clinical application of the ox-LDL targeted micelles may be hampered by the long blood circulation times (>14 hours) and high liver uptake (20% of the injected dose). Cell apoptosis (Hak et al., 2009; Ide et al. 2005) and nephrogenic systemic fibrosis in patients with renal dysfunction (Pedersen, 2007) have been implied to be caused by gadolinium (Gd) released from paramagnetic MRI contrast agents. Therefore, excessive and prolonged retention of Gd-chelates in organs needs to be avoided.

Ox-LDL in the plaque of apoE-/- mice has also been targeted with functionalized lipid-coated ultra-small superparamagnetic iron particles (LUSPIOs) (<20 nm) (Briley-Saebo et al., 2011). The aortic wall was enhanced on gradient echo images after injection in apoE-/- mice using a positive contrast method (GRASP). In contrast, no enhancement was observed after injection of control non-targeted LUSPIOs and larger (~40 nm) LSPIOs. *In vivo* specificity of the particles to ox-LDL increased after coating of the particles with lipids which prevented ingestion by macrophages.

Another targeted imaging approach which features interaction with plaque cholesterol is the use of HDL-like particles. These particles have the advantages of being endogenous and biodegradable, do not trigger immune reactions and are not recognized by the RES (Cormode et al., 2008, 2009; Frias et al., 2006; Skajaa et al., 2010). Other attractive biological properties of HDL-like particles are that HDL enables reverse cholesterol transport from the plaque, has anti-atherothrombotic properties, and reduces oxidation and plaque inflammation (Skajaa et al., 2010). Various versions of HDL-mimicking nanoparticles have been designed for plaque imaging: reconstituted HDL-like spherical or discoid particles, fully synthetic HDL-like particles and fully synthetic nanocrystal HDL (Cormode et al., 2009a; Skajaa et al., 2010). Spherical HDL-like particles were made up by apoA-I, extracted from human plasma, and reconstituted with commercially available phospholipids and Gd-conjugated lipids (Frias et al., 2004). The signal intensity of the aortic wall of mice was highest at 24 hours after injection of the above particles and returned to baseline levels at 48 hours after injection (Frias et al., 2004). Cheaper and easier manufacturing procedures would facilitate the use of HDL-like particles. Two different methods of preparation of reconstituted HDL discs were compared for their in vivo efficacy of imaging aortic wall in apoE-/- mice (Frias et al., 2006). Both types of discs showed highest signal intensity of macrophage-rich plaques at 24 hours after injection, while advanced plaques containing more cholesterol crystals and less macrophages revealed most enhancement at 72 hours after injection (Frias et al., 2006). Two fully synthetic HDL-like disks based on two synthetic lipid-binding apo A-I mimicking peptides, 37pA and the cheaper and easier synthesized 18A, were compared for their potential for *in vivo* MR enhancement. At 24 hours after injection both HDL disks provided similar plaque enhancement in the aorta of atherosclerotic mice (Cormode et al., 2008). In nanocrystal HDL the natural HDL core is replaced by inorganic nanocrystals while retaining the phospholipid coating. Via modification of both their core and their corona, these particles can be made suitable for multimodality imaging. In one study Gd-chelates were incorporated in the corona while the nanocrystal core was chosen to be based on gold for CT detection, quantum dots for optical imaging or iron oxide (FeO) for MRI visualization (Cormode et al., 2008). In vivo MRI showed positive enhancement of plaque when the core consisted of gold or quantum dot, whereas a significant decrease in signal was observed when the core contained FeO. Histology revealed at least partial colocalization with plaque macrophages (Cormode et al., 2008). Additionally, all mentioned MRI-visible HDL-like nanoparticles might be useful to study the role of HDL in plaque progression (Skajaa et al., 2010).

As mentioned earlier, Gadofluorine M is supposed to have affinity for plaque lipids (Barkhausen et al., 2003) and extracellular matrix proteins. In a rabbit model of atherosclerosis injection of Gadofluorine M led to a high contrast-to-background ratio on T_1-weighted MR images of aortic plaque (Barkhausen et al., 2003). The contrast-enhanced regions corresponded with Sudan-positive lipid-rich aortic wall segments on histological slices (Barkhausen et al., 2003).

4.3 Endothelial cells

Endothelial cells respond to several stimuli with increased expression of cell adhesion molecules. The inflammatory mediators, IL-1 and TNFα, are among these stimuli and lead to increased expression of ICAM-1, VCAM-1 and P-selectin by endothelial cells (Libby, 2002). Oxidized low-density lipoproteins, accumulating in plaque during atherogenesis, represent a stimulus for enhanced expression of VCAM-1 by endothelial cells (Libby, 2002; Lusis, 2000; Ross, 1999). Leukocytes extravasate after interaction of VCAM-1 with very late antigen-4 (VLA-4) on the leukocyte membrane surface (Libby, 2002).

The binding capacity of microparticles of iron oxide conjugated with antibodies directed against VCAM-1 (diameter ~4.5 μm) to TNFα-stimulated mouse endothelial cells was demonstrated *in vitro* (McAteer et al., 2010). These VCAM-1-targeted microparticles were applied for *in vivo* imaging of inflammation in peritubular capillaries in murine kidneys after ischemia reperfusion injury (Akhtar, 2010). VCAM-1 expression on dysfunctional endothelial cells of cholesterol-fed apoE-/- mouse aorta was targeted with a cross-linked iron oxide (CLIO) fluorescent nanoparticle conjugated to a peptide sequence with homology to the a-chain of VLA-4 for both MRI and fluorescence imaging (Kelly et al., 2005). Higher signal amplification of atherosclerotic mouse aorta was anticipated and found by this group using newly developed second-generation VCAM-1-targeted magnetic nanoparticles that undergo internalization and trapping in endothelial cells and macrophages that express VCAM-1 (Nahrendorf et al., 2006).

P-selectin expression by endothelial cells has been imaged with a slow-clearing blood-pool MRI contrast agent functionalized with sulfate groups with homology to the P-selectin binding region of P-selectin glycoprotein ligand-1 (Alsaid et al., 2009). Application of this P-selectin-targeted paramagnetic agent led to specific plaque enhancement in apoE-/- mice between 10 and 30 minutes after intravenous injection. *Ex vivo* fluorescence microscopy confirmed specific binding of the agent to P-selectin (Alsaid et al., 2009).

4.4 Neovascularization

The reason for the development of neovasculature in atherosclerotic plaques is uncertain. One theory emphasizes the hypoxia in the thickened intimal layer (>500 μm) as a stimulant for neoangiogenesis (Sluimer & Daemen, 2009). Another theory however states that neovascularization may exist early on during atherogenesis and promotes plaque inflammation and progression by facilitating extravasation of inflammatory cells (Dunmore et al., 2007). Intraplaque hemorrhage of the fragile neovasculature has also been related to rapid carotid atherosclerotic plaque growth (Takaya et al., 2005).

Dynamic contrast enhanced (DCE) MRI was applied first for quantitative assessment of neovasculature in tumors, but has been exploited more recently for quantification of human carotid plaque neovasculature (Yuan et al., 2002). DCE-MRI uses serial MRI acquisitions with high temporal resolution enclosing a time window around the injection of a low molecular weight Gd-containing contrast agent. Differentiation between fibrous tissue (enhancement ~80%) and lipid core (enhancement ~30%) by virtue of the neovessel density in fibrous tissue has been demonstrated (Yuan et al., 2002). Quantitative information on plaque uptake kinetics of contrast agent, amount of neovascularization and vessel permeability may be provided by appropriate modeling of the signal intensity time course in the plaque (Calcagno et al., 2010).

Recently, Gadofluorine M uptake in the balloon-injured aorta of New Zealand White rabbits has been found to correlate with plaque neovessel and macrophage density (Sirol et al., 2009). Histological evaluation showed that plaque neovessels, lipid-rich regions and Gadofluorine M co-localized. However, non-specificity of Gadofluorine M, which also has affinity for other plaque constituents like extracellular matrix proteins and lipids, will complicate mathematical modeling of quantitative parameters.

Also targeted approaches have been used for the molecular MR imaging of plaque neovascularization. The $\alpha_v\beta_3$ integrin is expressed amongst others by endothelial cells on angiogenic vessels in plaque. A low molecular weight peptidomimetic of Arg-Gly-Asp conjugated to Gd-DTPA led to enhancement of aortic plaque in apoE-/- mice which was diminished after "presaturation" with the MRI-silent, Europium-chelated analogue of the Gd-conjugated compound (Burtea et al., 2008).

Targeting of proteins expressed on the outer endothelial cell membrane indicative for neovascularization has the distinct advantage that the contrast agent does not need to enter the plaque. This approach allows for the use of large, very potent, nanoparticulate MR contrast agents, like Gd-containing perfluorocarbon emulsion nanoparticles with a size of about 250 nm (Anderson et al., 2000). Transgenic rats with a mutation in the leptin receptor represent a model for metabolic syndrome, resulting in abdominal obesity, atherosclerosis and myocardial lesions. The Gd-containing perfluorocarbon emulsion targeted towards the $\alpha_v\beta_3$ integrin was used for imaging neovessels in aortic plaques of these rats (Cai et al., 2010). Additionally, the effect of treatment with the anorectic and hypolipidemic drug benfluorex on plaque neovascularization was studied. Treated animals displayed an overall lower and patchy plaque enhancement in comparison to non-treated ones, indicative for a decreased angiogenic vessel density in the plaque (Cai et al., 2010). So, modulation of neovascularization by therapeutics could be studied using this molecular MRI approach. The same $\alpha_v\beta_3$-targeted perfluorocarbon emulsion was used to monitor collateral formation after treatment with angiogenic L-arginine in a rabbit femoral artery ligation model (Winter et al., 2010). The results achieved in these diverse studies argue against a straightforward interpretation of MR imaging results in atherosclerosis using $\alpha_v\beta_3$-targeted nanoparticles. Molecular MRI of neovascularization with these nanoparticles may not discriminate between adverse plaque neovascularization and beneficial sprouting of collaterals. At the time, pharmacokinetic profiling information on $\alpha_v\beta_3$-targeted and non-targeted perfluorocarbon nanoparticles has been obtained in rabbits with *in vivo* MRI and blood samples (Neubauer et al., 2008).

4.5 Macrophages

Macrophages play a key role in the inflammatory process of atherosclerosis. Therefore, they are most extensively studied using molecular MRI. Previously, superparamagnetic particles of iron oxide were used for lymph node imaging in the context of tumor staging and detection of focal liver lesions (Schmitz, 2003). During a phase III trial which investigated the use of the ultra-small dextran-coated counterparts of these particles (USPIOs, diameter 18-30 nm) for discrimination between healthy lymph nodes and lymph node metastases, these USPIOs were found by co-incidence to be ingested by aortic plaque macrophages (Schmitz et al., 2001). Since then these USPIOs have been extensively studied for their potential to monitor inflammation in atherosclerosis in patients and regression after treatment with aggressive lipid-lowering therapy (Tang et al., 2009).

The versatility of these USPIOs for imaging of both lymph nodes and atherosclerotic plaque constitutes an important drawback of these USPIOs. Lymph nodes often develop in close proximity to the inflamed plaque lesion. We have shown that differentiation between peri-vascular lymph nodes and aortic wall in atherosclerotic mouse models may be difficult using USPIOs (Te Boekhorst et al., 2010a). Successful visualization will depend on spatial resolution and the imaging sequence (Te Boekhorst et al., 2010a). Recently, a newly developed positive contrast technique for (U)SPIOs, "GRASP", has been shown capable to differentiate between peri-vascular lymph nodes and atherosclerotic vessel wall (Briley-Saebo et al., 2011).

Apart from this cellular MRI approach, also specific macrophage membrane proteins have been targeted. Among others targeting of the macrophage scavenger receptor-A (MSR-A) has been achieved in a mouse model of atherosclerosis with paramagnetic Gd-containing micelles (Amirbekian et al., 2007). Plaques in the aortic wall of apoE-/- mice displayed a 79% increase in signal intensity upon injection of the MSR-A-targeted micelles, whereas control micelles resulted in 34% signal increase (Amirbekian et al., 2007). MSR-A together with MSR-B is responsible for 75-90% of ox-LDL uptake by macrophages. *Ex vivo* targeting of MSR-B in dissected human aortic atherosclerotic plaque has been achieved with 125-nm-diameter lipid-based nanoparticles (Lipinski et al., 2009). However, the potential of these MSR-B-targeted nanoparticles for *in vivo* targeting has still to be demonstrated. Bimodal micelles for MSR (A and B) containing both Gd and an optical label (rhodamine-conjugated lipid or a quantum dot) led to a signal increase of aortic wall in apoE-/- up to 200% (Mulder et al., 2007b). MSR-targeted rhodamine micelles could be detected with fluorescence microscopy and were found to be associated with macrophages. Quantum dots allowed *ex vivo* detection of aortic macrophage-rich regions with UV illumination (Mulder et al., 2007b).

Plaque macrophages express the ox-LDL receptor LOX-1 and binding of ox-LDL induces apoptosis, expression of adhesion molecules and release of MMPs (Ross, 1999; Li et al., 2010). Paramagnetic liposomes conjugated to anti-LOX-1 antibodies were injected in LDL-R-/- mice. Aortic plaques were specifically enhanced on T1 weighted MR images, while no enhancement was observed on MR images from double knockout LDL-R-/- LOX-1-/- mice or from LDL-R-/- mice injected with nonspecific IgG-conjugated liposomes (Li et al., 2010). Histological analyses revealed that most LOX-1 co-localized with macrophages, apoptotic cells and MMP-9 and only a small proportion with proliferated smooth muscle cells.

The use of antibodies for making contrast agents target specific has important disadvantages: the high costs of antibodies, their immunogenicity and difficulty in handling and preparation. Application of other specific targeting moieties of non-antibody origin is therefore attractive. An example is the use of phosphatidylserine (PS) incorporated in self-assembled lipid-based contrast agents. PS is expressed on apoptotic cells and is specifically recognized by macrophages. PS-containing paramagnetic liposomes showed *in vitro* specificity for RAW cells (mouse macrophages) and significant MR enhancement of aortic plaques during the first 4 hours after injection in apoE-/- mice (Maiseyeu et al., 2009).

Another targeted approach avoiding the use of antibodies employs a potent synthetic agonist (HU-308) of the peripheral cannabinoid receptor (CB2-R) (Te Boekhorst et al., 2010b). T-lymphocytes and macrophages in advanced mouse and human atherosclerotic plaque CB2-R have been shown to express this CB2-R (Steffens et al., 2005). Activation of CB2-R by HU-308 results in amelioration of plaque phenotype in atherosclerotic mice (Steffens et al., 2005). The suggested mechanism is an immune system modulating effect through CB2-R, which involves a regulatory negative feedback effect dampening the inflammatory process in advanced plaques (Steffens et al., 2005). Self-assembly of polymeric micelles was easily achieved by mixing HU-308, which has a 7-carbon tail and a hydrophilic head group, with Gd-containing and PEG-ylated lipids (Te Boekhorst et al., 2010b). T_1-weighted inversion recovery fast spin echo MR images revealed *in vivo* plaque enhancement in the aortas of double knockout apoE-/-, eNOS-/- mice between 36 and 48 hours after injection of CB2-R-targeted micelles (Te Boekhorst et al., 2010c).

The earlier mentioned flexible HDL platform could be easily functionalized for more specific retention into plaques. A third example of targeted approach avoiding the application of antibodies concerns incorporation of an apoE-derived lipopeptide into HDL particles enriched with Gd-based lipids (W. Chen et al., 2008). Application of this material led to both higher association with mouse macrophages *in vitro* and more pronounced *in vivo* enhancement of aortic plaque in mice relative to reconstituted HDL without incorporation of the apoE-derived lipopeptide (W. Chen et al., 2008).

Furthermore, hyaluronic acid, which targets the CD44 receptor on activated macrophages, has been conjugated to a lipid coating enclosing iron oxide nanoparticles (Kamat et al., 2010). In vitro experiments have revealed ingestion by activated THP-1 macrophages, suggesting potential for *in vivo* imaging of plaque inflammation (Kamat et al., 2010). Transient cellular location of the HDL particles was suggested by a series of Prussian blue stainings for iron. Despite these promising findings, the *in vivo* potential of these macrophage-targeted iron oxides for MRI of plaque inflammation has still to be confirmed.

Apart from direct targeting of macrophages, one can also address released macrophage products. An example of an extracellular released enzyme in atherosclerotic plaque is represented by the matrix metalloproteinases (MMPs). Increased activity of MMPs produced by smooth muscle cells and macrophages has been reported to be related to plaque rupture (Vink & Pasterkamp, 2002; Schafers et al., 2010). A small peptide with affinity for MMPs was conjugated to Gd-DOTA and employed for *in vivo* MR imaging of plaque (Lancelot et al., 2008). The plasma half-life of this small peptide was only 30 minutes and the concentrations in artery specimens were 3 times as high as those after injection of Gd-DOTA, with prolonged retention at least until 22 hours after injection (Lancelot et al., 2008). The mentioned peptide has affinity for various MMPs. However, the MMP family is large and the role of each MMP member is not entirely known. It has been shown, that expression of MMP-2 and MMP-9 is upregulated in shoulder regions of human vulnerable plaques (Galis & Khatri, 2002). The advent of specific inhibitors of MMP-9 and -2 and their application in small paramagnetic peptides may improve specificity for unstable plaque.

Another protein that has been linked to adverse cardiovascular events in patients after carotid endarterectomy surgery is neutrophil gelatinase-associated lipocalin-2 (NGAL) (Te Boekhorst et al., 2011). NGAL is produced and released particularly by macrophages, although first discovered in neutrophils (Hemdahl et al., 2006). MMP-9 activity is prolonged and degradation prevented after binding to NGAL. Apart from forming a stable and biologically active complex with MMP-9, NGAL mediates inflammatory activity through binding to formyl-methionyl-leucyl-phenylalanine (fMLP; a chemotactic peptide), leukotriene B4, and platelet-activating factor (Hemdahl et al., 2006). *In vivo* MRI of severely advanced atherosclerotic plaques of the double knockout apoE-/-, eNOS-/- mouse was performed at 24 and 72 hours after injection of 24p3(mouse homologue of NGAL)-targeted micelles and IgG isotype antibody-conjugated micelles (Te Boekhorst et al., 2011). Both 24p3-targeted and control micelles led to an increased average Normalized Enhancement Ratio (NER) at 24 hours after injection (~1.45 versus ~1.30 respectively), while at 72 hours after injection of 24p3-targeted micelles average NER further increased and after injection of control micelles average NER had decreased (~1.70 versus ~1.20) (Te Boekhorst et al., 2011). Histology revealed that micelles co-localized with 24p3 and partially with macrophages. The results of this study are summarized in Figure 1A-H.

Targeting of extracellular located molecules such as MMPs and NGAL has the advantage over intracellular targets that the target is readily available. On the other hand, it may carry the drawback that the contrast agent is easily washed out from the plaque, together with the target, into the blood. Nevertheless, imaging of intact excreted proteins and particularly their activity could provide important insights in the inflammatory state of the plaque. For

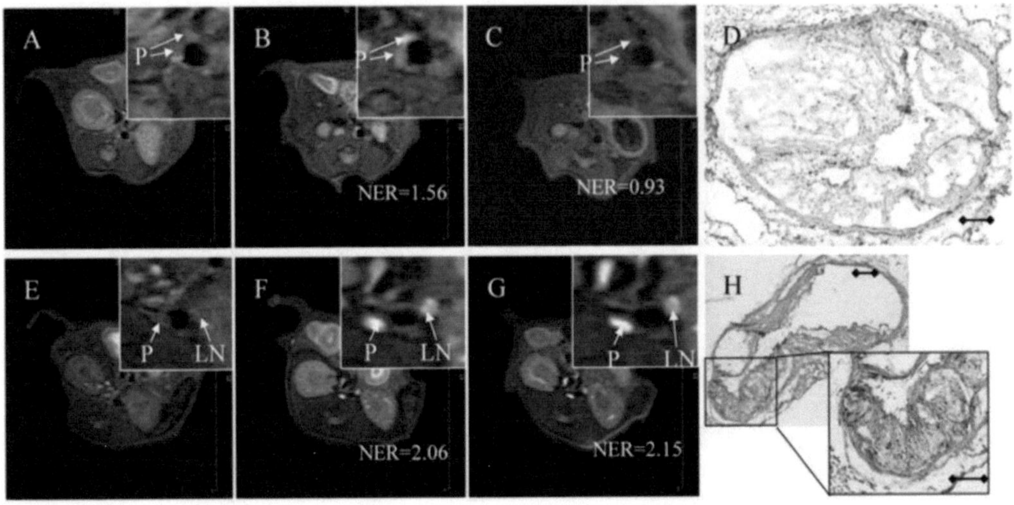

Fig. 1. MR images and histological stainings of atherosclerotic plaque after intravenous injection of NGAL/24p3-targeted micelles. Pre- and post-injection (0, 24 and 72 h) MR images of aortic wall in apoE-/-/eNOS-/- mice injected with control (A-C) and NGAL/24p3-targeted (E-G) micelles and immunohistochemistry at 72 hours for micelle-conjugated rat antibodies in control micelles (D) and NGAL/24p3-targeted micelles (H). P=plaque, LN=lymph node. NER= Normalized Enhancement Ratio. The post-injection MR images show increased signal intensity at 24 hours for both NGAL/24p3-targeted micelles and control micelles, while signal intensity at 72 hours stays at the higher level for NGAL/24p3-targeted micelles but returned to baseline for control micelles. Note that the signal intensity of the peri-aortic lymph node, which was removed during harvesting of the aorta, is also increased after injection. Histology of the mouse aorta at 72 hours after injection revealed no staining of micelles for injections with control micelles and extensive red staining for injections with NGAL/24p3-targeted micelles.. H: scale bar = 100μm (original magnification: 100x) (Te Boekhorst et al., 2011).

example, peroxidase-based hematologic profiling has been shown to predict adverse cardiac events during a follow-up of 1 year (Brennan et al., 2010). In order to prevent washout of the agent, Bogdanov and coworkers have designed an activatable (smart) low-molecular weight Gd-containing probe for imaging of myeloperoxidase, an enzyme released by macrophages that is responsible for oxidation of LDL via the formation of reactive oxygen species (J.W. Chen et al., 2004). Activation of the probe by myeloperoxidase leads to polymerization, increasing its size and relaxivity, and prolonging its retention in the target region - hence providing an indirect readout of enzyme activity. This probe enabled MR imaging of increased myeloperoxidase activity in plaques in the aorta of rabbits, as is summarized in Figure 2A-G (Ronald et al., 2009).

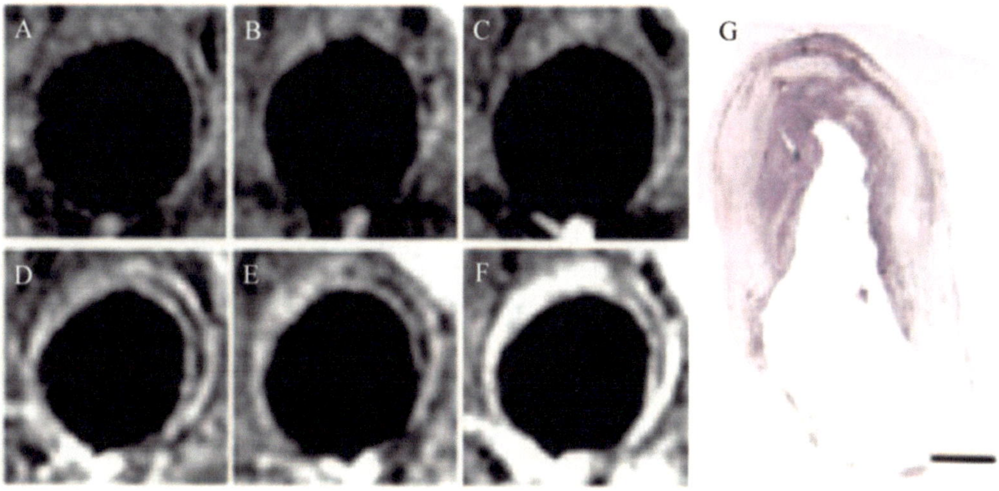

Fig. 2. Imaging of diseased aortas of cholesterol-fed rabbits before and after injection of an activatable MPO sensor.

Imaging before and 2 hours after injection of DTPA-Gd (A,D), before and 2 hours after injection of bis-tyr-DTPA-Gd (B,E) which is a nonactivatable analog of MPO-Gd, and before and 2 hours after injection of the functional agent MPO-Gd (C,F). Histology of the rabbit aorta after injection of MPO-Gd revealed focal MPO presence in the plaque and confirmed the MR findings (G). Printed with permission from (Ronald et al., 2009).

4.6 Apoptotic cells

When cells become apoptotic, phosphatidylserine (PS), initially mainly found in the inner leaflet of the viable cell membrane, is also expressed on the outer leaflet of the cell. The expression of PS can be detected with molecular MRI using the protein annexin A5 as a targeting ligand. Annexin A5 binds specifically to PS in the presence of calcium (Gerke et al., 2002). Apoptosis in atherosclerotic plaques in the aorta of apoE-/- mice was studied using Gd-containing micelles conjugated to annexin A5. T_1-weighted MR images showed at 24 hours after injection a slight, but significant, increase of plaque intensity relative to control non-conjugated micelles (Van Tilborg et al., 2010).

Phage display may identify small peptides with specific affinity to selected targets. One study employed a PS-specific peptide, identified by phage display and conjugated to Gd-DTPA, for detection of apoptotic cells in aortic plaques of apoE-/- mice at 30 minutes after injection (Burtea et al., 2009). The use of such small peptides has certain advantages above proteins or antibodies in terms of reduced immunogenicity and a cheaper and easier production process.

However, studies with apoptosis-directed agents in a number of apoptosis-associated pathologies have also revealed the limitation of apoptosis-targeted contrast agents. The publication of a SPECT study reporting visualization of apoptosis of cardiomyocytes in patients with acute myocardial infarction (Hofstra et al., 2000) may serve as an example. Apoptosis may not be useful for targeted imaging of vulnerable plaque in the coronary arteries, due to the possibly overwhelming background signal of enhanced cardiac muscle in a compromised patient group.

4.7 Activated platelets and thrombus

Activated platelets play a crucial role in the formation of repetitive micro-thrombi, which suddenly may result in a major thrombus, followed by an acute cardiovascular event (Naghavi et al., 2003a, 2003b; Stary et al., 1995). Therefore, early recognition of a high incidence of micro-thrombi by molecular imaging of activated platelets has important prognostic value.

Activated platelets express αIIbβ3 integrin, which has been targeted with cyclic arginine–glycine–aspartic acid (RGD) peptides, which are specific for the αIIβ3 integrin among others, and are conjugated to ultra-small particles of iron oxide for T2* weighted MRI (Johansson et al., 2001). Unfortunately, the resolution, which was achieved with RGD-USPIO-enhanced MRI, was too low to detect thrombus *in vivo* (Johansson et al., 2001). Chemical conjugation to nanoparticles typically results in the loss of antibody functionality. A biochemically robust, highly reproducible and site-specific coupling method using the Staphylococcus aureus sortase A enzyme for the conjugation of single-chain antibodies (scFv) to amine-coated superparamagnetic iron oxide nanoparticles was developed (Ta et al., 2011). Conjugation efficiency ranged between 50 and 70% and the bioactivity of the scFv with specific affinity to activated platelets was preserved after conjugation. In vivo MRI showed that these scFv-conjugated SPIOs effectively bound to activated platelets on $FeCl_3$ induced thrombus in carotid arteries of mice (Ta et al., 2011).

Fibrin-targeted small peptides conjugated to Gd-DTPA have been employed successfully in pigs, showing the feasibility of MRI to differentiate between acute and subacute (1-3 days old) coronary thrombus (Botnar, 2004a, 2004b). More recently, MR enhancement of thrombus has been achieved in a phase II trial using these peptides in patients, with a diagnosed symptomatic thrombus in vessel territories potentially associated with stroke (Spuentrup et al., 2008).

Gd-perfluorocarbon nanoparticles functionalized with fibrin-targeted peptides were also applied for MR imaging of *in vitro* human thrombus (Winter et al., 2003). These perfluorocarbon nanoparticles can be used for T_1-weighted proton MRI as well as for ^{19}F hot-spot MR imaging. The advantage of the latter feature is the natural absence of background signal precluding the necessity of a baseline scan, which is attractive for clinical application from a logistical point of view.

Also contrast agents based on the paramagnetic chemical exchange saturation transfer (PARACEST) mechanism have been employed for MR imaging of fibrin. This technique has been pioneered by the group of Balaban et al. (Ward et al., 2000). PARACEST agents have exchangeable protons (-NH, -OH, etc.) that resonate at a chemical shift position that is distinguishable from the bulk water signal. When an RF pulse is applied at the resonance frequency of the exchangeable protons, these protons will be saturated. Transfer into the bulk water pool will lead to reduced equilibrium magnetization. This so-called saturation transfer effect can be switched "on" and "off" by simply changing the pulse sequence. The PARACEST agents are potentially attractive for *in vivo* use, because contrast can be switched on and off by selective RF pulse saturation, avoiding the need for baseline imaging and spatial registration of images acquired hours or days apart. The main disadvantage of PARACEST agents, however, is low sensitivity, which hampers the ability to image molecular targets. One method of increasing the sensitivity of paraCEST agents is to incorporate multiple metal chelates into a macromolecular scaffold. Proof of concept CEST imaging of fibrin was provided *in vitro* for fibrin clots, using a fibrin-specific perfluorocarbon nanoparticle containing multiple PARACEST units (Winter et al., 2006). This first generation PARACEST nanoparticle agent, however, introduced a large cationic charge on the particle surface. Cationic particles can cause significant in vivo toxicity and are not suitable for biomedical applications. In a recent study, a neutral lipid conjugated PARACEST chelate was incorporated onto the surface of PFC nanoparticles leading to a negative surface charge. PARACEST and ^{19}F MRI showed a linear increase in both PARACEST contrast to noise ratio and the 19F signal with increasing nanoparticle concentration. Artificial fibrin clots were efficiently targeted using these nanoparticles and imaged using PARACEST and ^{19}F MRI (see Figure 3) with detection limits of 2.30 nM and 4.60 nM respectively (Cai et al., 2011).

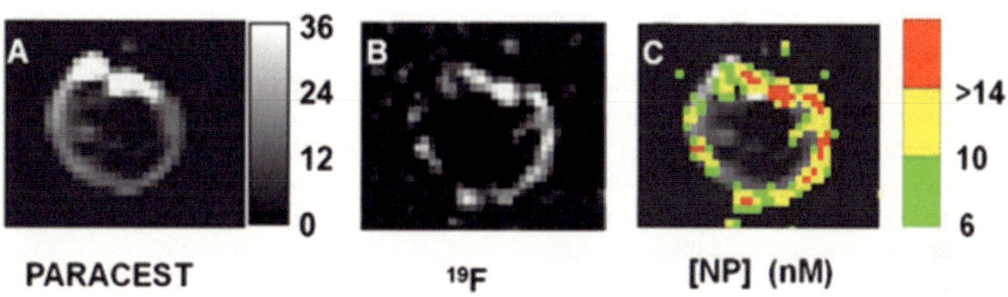

Fig. 3. Dual PARACEST and ^{19}F MR imaging of a clot treated with fibrin-targeted PARACEST nanoparticles.
PARACEST contrast to noise ratio map (A) and ^{19}F image (B) collaboratively show nanoparticles bound to the surface of the clot. The grayscale color bar represents the PARACEST CNR depicted in (A). (C) The nanoparticle concentration (nM) is color-coded and overlaid onto the PARACEST subtraction image to demonstrate colocalization of these two definitive signals. Printed with permission from (Cai et al., 2011).

Various products of the coagulation cascade may serve as targets for molecular MRI as well. Very recently, a thrombin inhibitor was conjugated to perfluorocarbon nanoparticles for localized *in vivo* control of thrombus in the common carotid artery of a mouse after acute photochemical injury (Myerson et al., 2011). The modified nanoparticles outperformed heparin and the free thrombin inhibitor according to the activated partial thromboplastin time.

The earlier mentioned fibrin-targeted small-peptide MR contrast agents have low sensitivity for the estimation of thrombus age. Specific targeting of earlier phases of thrombus formation could help into this respect. Activated factor XIII cross-links fibrin chains and covalently cross-links α2-antiplasmin to fibrin, with a rapid decline in catalytic activity. Therefore, the potential of an α2-antiplasmin-based peptide labeled with rhodamine and Gd for specific detection of early thrombus was investigated both *in vitro* and *in vivo* (Miserus et al., 2009). Thrombus was induced via application of $FeCl_3$ to the carotid artery of mice. In one group the contrast agent was injected seconds after thrombus formation, while in another group injection was postponed 24 to 48 hours after thrombus formation. Only early thrombus was enhanced using this contrast agent while thrombus with an age of 24 -48 hours was not enhanced (Miserus et al., 2009).

5. View-to-future

As described above, MRI is capable of providing detailed cellular and molecular imaging information, which combined with the wealth of anatomical and functional MRI readouts, makes MR imaging of atherosclerosis a very powerful asset to study plaque vulnerability, progression and to evaluate effects of treatment. A potential limitation of MRI, however, is the limited sensitivity of the technique in the detection of low concentrations of targeted contrast agent.

Development of improved MR techniques may enhance the sensitivity of detection. Hyperpolarization of nuclear spins through dynamic nuclear polarization (DNP) has recently attracted considerable attention for increasing the signal-to-noise ratio in an NMR experiment by several orders of magnitude (Ragavan et al., 2011). However, application of this technique to larger molecules has so far proven challenging. Recently, a full length protein was hyperpolarized at low temperature and dissolved for NMR signal acquisition in the liquid state in mixtures of organic solvent and water. Signal enhancements of 300-2000 are obtained in partially deuterated polypeptide when hyperpolarized on 13C and of 30-180 when hyperpolarized on 1H (Ragavan et al., 2011). Additionally, low-field (1 T) compact benchtop MRI systems (ASPECT, IconBruker) are ideally suited to take advantage of the higher relaxivity of Gd-based contrast agents at low magnetic fields.

Although MRI-based single cell detection with the use of iron oxides has been reported, in general, much higher doses are needed as compared to for example the nuclear imaging techniques (Leuschner et al., 2011). Moreover the effect of covalent binding of peptides/lipids to Gd on the pharmacokinetics and biodistribution of the various contrast agent ingredients is uncertain. This complicates rapid approval of Gd-based MR contrast agents and its carriers for human application by the Food and Drug Administration (FDA (USA)) and European Medicines Agency (EMEA (Europe)), because of the concerns about retention in the body and toxicity. Issues are, amongst others, the unknown metabolic fate of the carrier material in the body, transmetallation of Gd^{3+} with native metal-ions in the body (Hak et al., 2009), and worries about Gd-induced nephrogenic systemic fibrosis (Pedersen, 2007). In this respect, nanocrystal HDL-like particles with iron oxide cores (Cormode et al., 2008; Mulder Acc Chem Res 2009; Skajaa et al., 2011) are very promising MR contrast agent candidates for clinical application because they seem to avoid most of these toxicity concerns. Figure 4 shows a schematic depiction of a nanocrystal HDL-like nanoparticle and summarizes some results achieved with it (Skajaa et al., 2011).

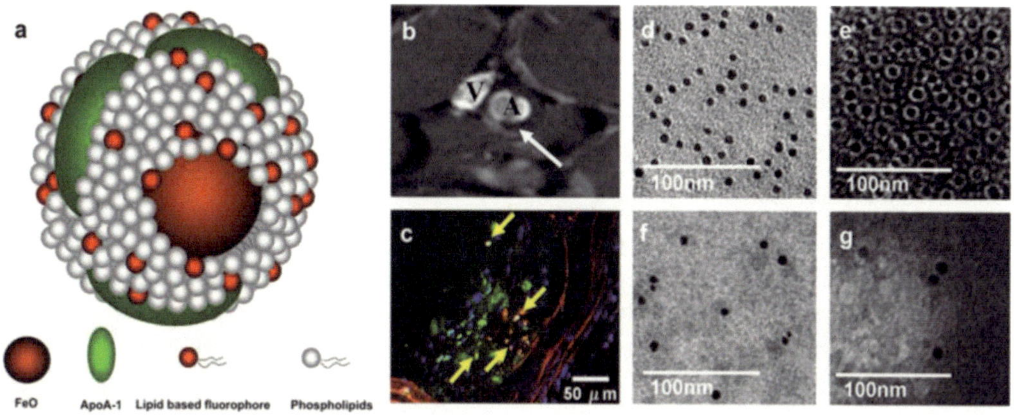

Fig. 4. Nanocrystal HDL with FeO core. Schematic depiction of FeO-HDL (a). (b) *In vivo* T2*-weighted (TR = 10 ms, TE = 4 ms) MR image of abdominal region of an apoE-/- mouse, 24 h post-injection of FeO-HDL. The white arrow denotes the black rim (black spot) in the aortic wall observed after FeO-HDL administration. (A, aorta, V, inferior cava vein). (c) *Ex vivo* confocal laser microscopy of excised aorta section. Nuclei are shown in blue via DAPI staining, FeO-HDL in red (rhodamine), green color marks macrophages, stained with Alexa 647-CD68 and yellow marks co-localization of FeO-HDL and macrophages. (d) *In vitro* TEM images of FeO-HDL in buffer. (e) *In vitro* negative staining TEM image of FeO-HDL, showing that each iron oxide (IO) particle is coated with a single monolayer of phospholipids. (f, g) TEM and negative staining TEM of blood samples 5 min after the administration of FeO-HDL revealed individually dispersed particles, i.e. no aggregation and that the lipid coating is intact. Printed with permission from (Skajaa et al., 2011).

The use of frequency-selective paraCEST agents or perfluorocarbon nanoparticles in principle permits imaging of various target species simultaneously. Although *in vitro* proof of principle has been provided, *in vivo* application has been limited so far. Problems for paraCEST agents are related to low sensitivity and susceptibility artifacts, whereas ^{19}F imaging also suffers from relatively low sensitivity. Concerning clinical translation, the iron oxides are most promising, since they enable the most sensitive detection with MRI while toxicity is low. The larger iron oxides provide sensitive hypointense contrast on T_2-weighted images, whereas small iron oxides (~5 nm) can also be used for T_1-weighted imaging with hyperintense contrast (Taboada et al., 2007).

The application of both diagnostic and therapeutic MR agents for monitoring of drug delivery and therapeutic responses is very promising. Gd-containing liposome-encapsulated prednisolone phosphate was injected in atherosclerotic rabbits and delivery at the balloon-injured aorta was imaged with MRI (Lobatto et al., 2010). The therapeutic anti-inflammatory and anti-angiogenic effects of the glucocorticoid were monitored with DCE MRI (Lobatto et al., 2010). Another study employed paramagnetic αvβ3-targeted fumagillin-loaded perfluorocarbon nanoparticles, releasing fumagillin via "contact facilitated drug delivery" (only upon ligand-directed binding) (Winter et al., 2006). These nanoparticles resulted after 1 week in a significant reduction in degree and spatial distribution of MR enhancement. This effect was not observed when no drug or non-targeted fumagillin-loaded nanoparticles were administered (Winter et al., 2006), thus providing evidence for the specific therapeutic effect of the targeted, drug-loaded nanoparticles.

6. Clinical application

In patient studies iron oxide particles and Gadofluorine M have already been successfully applied for MRI of inflammation. The use of MRI with these particles combined with MRI assessment of cardiovascular function and myocardial tagging in selected patient populations with specific co-morbidity that increases risk for atherosclerotic disease may further stratify cardiovascular risk groups. Clinical application of self-assembling Gd-based molecular contrast agents is difficult due to the large amounts needed for detection and toxicity issues, especially in patients with kidney disease. Molecular targeted iron oxide nanoparticles conjugated to small peptides, recognized by phage display have lower immunogenicity when compared to full antibodies but toxicity may still hamper clinical application. Into this respect, the use of synthetic (ant)agonists or peptidomimetics for conjugation to MR visible nanoparticles combined with MRI of plaque targets in selected patient groups is anticipated to be more successful. Clinical application of perfluorocarbon nanoparticles for imaging of intravascular targets (endothelial cell markers and thrombus/activated platelets) employing the zero-background ^{19}F signal is attractive. The safety of fluorine and the high payload of ^{19}F which counterbalances low sensitivity of ^{19}F MRI, make these perfluorocarbon nanoparticles (without Gd) useful contrast agents with clinical potential for targeted imaging of intravascular targets. However, first the pharmokinetic profiling information obtained in rabbits (Neubauer et al., 2008) needs to be expanded and should be obtained in patients. Activatable Gd- or iron oxide-based contrast agents sensing plaque enzyme activity may be used for detection of enzymes available at nM concentrations owing to enhanced relaxivity related to oligomerization of substrates or coupling of them to proteins (Tu et al., 2011). This approach is interesting in the scope of clinical application because it measures activity instead of presence of enzymes and lower toxicity is anticipated because lower Gd (or iron oxide) concentrations are needed for a certain degree of enhancement. The endogenous nature of the lipid coat of FeO-HDL-like nanoparticles, the easy incorporation of natural or synthetic lipids for increased accumulation in plaque macrophages, and the low toxicity of FeO makes these nanoparticles an attractive contrast agent for clinical MRI of atherosclerotic plaque. Clinical application of a specific molecular MRI method will also depend on costs of the contrast agent for a specific target of interest, the versatility of that agent and the contribution of this MRI approach to clinical decision making.

7. Conclusion

A number of strategies for cellular and molecular MRI of atherosclerosis were successfully developed. Proof of concept clinical application was already established for imaging of macrophages using non-targeted iron oxides and at a more immature stage for the fibrin-targeted small-molecule peptides conjugated to Gd-DTPA. Future studies will have to clarify whether the targeted contrast agents have diagnostic or prognostic added value in the evaluation of atherosclerotic plaque progression/rupture in humans. Promising new developments include activatable contrast agents, which are able to report on enzyme activity, perfluorocarbon nanoparticles exploiting the zero-background ^{19}F signal, as well as the use of modified MRI-visible endogenous nanoparticles, such as HDL and LDL, for imaging of atherosclerosis and specific plaque components.

8. Acknowledgements

This work was supported by the European Network of Excellence Diagnostic Molecular Imaging (DIMI, LSHB-CT-2005-512146), the Integrated European Union Project Targeted Delivery of Nanomedicine (MEDITRANS, FP6-2004-NMP-NI-4/IP 026668-2), and the Netherlands Heart Foundation Grant (NHF, 2006T106 and 2003B249).

9. References

Akhtar, A., Schneider, J., Chapman, S., Jefferson, A., Digby, J., Mankia, K., Chen, Y., McAteer, M., Wood, K., & Choudhury, R. (2010). In vivo quantification of VCAM-1 expression in renal ischemia reperfusion injury using non-invasive magnetic resonance molecular imaging. *PLoS One,* Vol.5, No.9, (September 2010), pp. e12800, ISSN 1932-6203

Alsaid, H., De Souza, G., Bourdillon, M., Chaubet, F., Sulaiman, A., Desbleds-Mansard, C., Chaabane, L., Zahir, C., Lancelot, E., Rousseaux, O., Corot, C., Douek, P., Briguet, A., Letourneur, D., & Canet-Soulas E. (2009). Biomimetic MRI contrast agent for imaging of inflammation in atherosclerotic plaque of ApoE-/- mice: a pilot study. *Investigative Radiology,* Vol.44, No.3, (March 2009), pp. 151-158, ISSN 1536-0210

Amirbekian, V., Lipinski, M., Briley-Saebo, K., Amirbekian, S., Aguinaldo, J., Weinreb, D., Vucic, E., Frias, J., Hyafil, F., Mani, V., Fisher, E., & Fayad, Z. (2007). Detecting and assessing macrophages in vivo to evaluate atherosclerosis noninvasively using molecular MRI. *Proceedings of the National Academy of Sciences of the United States of America,* Vol.104, No.3, (January 2007), pp. 961-966, ISSN 0027-8424

Anderson, S., Rader, R., Westlin, W., Null, C., Jackson, D., Lanza, G., Wickline, S., & Kotyk, J. (2000). Magnetic resonance contrast enhancement of neovasculature with alpha(v)beta(3)-targeted nanoparticles. *Magnetic Resonance in Medicine,* Vol.44, No.3, (September 2000), pp. 433–439, ISSN 0740-3194

Barkhausen, J., Ebert, W., Heyer, C., Debatin, F., & Weinmann H. (2003). Detection of atherosclerotic plaque with Gadofluorine-enhanced magnetic resonance imaging. Circulation, Vol.108, No.5, (August 2003), pp. 605-609, ISSN 1524-4539

Brennan, M., Reddy, A., Tang, W., Wu, Y., Brennan, D., Hsu, A., Mann, S., Hammer, P., & Hazen, S. (2010). Comprehensive peroxidase-based hematologic profiling for the prediction of 1-year myocardial infarction and death. Circulation, Vol.122, No.1, (July 2010), pp. 70-79, ISSN 1524-4539

Briley-Saebo, K., Shaw, P., Mulder, W., Choi, S., Vucic, E., Aguinaldo, J., Witztum, J., Fuster, V., Tsimikas, S., & Fayad, Z. (2008). Targeted molecular probes for imaging atherosclerotic lesions with magnetic resonance using antibodies that recognize oxidation-specific epitopes. *Circulation,* Vol.117, No.25, (June 2008), pp. 3206-3215, ISSN 1524-4539

Briley-Saebo, K., Cho, Y., Shaw, P., Ryu, S., Mani, V., Dickson, S., Izadmehr, E., Green, S., Fayad, Z., & Tsimikas, S. (2011). Targeted iron oxide particles for in vivo magnetic resonance detection of atherosclerotic lesions with antibodies directed to oxidation-specific epitopes. *Journal of the American College of Cardiology*, Vol.57, No.3, (January 2011), pp. 337-347, ISNN 1558-3597

Burtea, C., Laurent, S., Lancelot, E., Ballet, S., Murariu, O., Rousseaux, O., Port, M., Vander Elst, L., Corot, C., & Muller, R. (2009). Peptidic targeting of phosphatidylserine for the MRI detection of apoptosis in atherosclerotic plaques. *Molecular Pharmaceutics*, Vol.6, No.6, (November-December 2009), pp. 1903-1919, ISSN 1543-8392

Cai, K., Caruthers, S., Huang, W., Williams, T., Zhang, H., Wickline, S., Lanza, G., & Winter, P. (2010). MR molecular imaging of aortic angiogenesis. *Journal of the American College of Cardiology. Cardiovascular Imaging*, Vol.3, No.8, (August 2010), pp. 824-832, ISSN 1876-7591

Cai, K., Kiefer, G., Caruthers, S., Wickline, S., Lanza, G., & Winter, P. (2011). Quantification of water exchange kinetics for targeted PARACEST perfluorocarbon nanoparticles. *NMR in Biomedicine*, Epub ahead of print (July 2011), ISSN 1099-1492

Calcagno, C., Mani, V., Ramachandran, S., & Fayad, Z. (2010). Dynamic contrast enhanced (DCE) magnetic resonance imaging (MRI) of atherosclerotic plaque angiogenesis. *Angiogenesis*, Vol.13, No.2, (June 2010), pp. 87-99, ISSN 1573-7209

Calfon, M., Vinegoni, C., Ntziachristos, V., & Jaffer, F. (2010). Intravascular near-infrared fluorescence molecular imaging of atherosclerosis: toward coronary arterial visualization of biologically high-risk plaques. *Journal of Biomedical Optics*, Vol.15, No.1. (January-February 2010), pp. 011107, ISSN 1560-2281

Chen, I., & Wu, J. (2011). Cardiovascular molecular imaging: focus on clinical translation. *Circulation*, Vol.123, No.4, (February 2011), pp. 425-443, ISSN 1524-4539

Chen, J., Pham, W., Weissleder, R., & Bogdanov, A. (2004). Human myeloperoxidase: a potential target for molecular MR imaging in atherosclerosis. *Magnetic Resonance in Medicine*, Vol.52, No.5, (November 2004), pp. 1021–1028, ISSN 0740-3194

Chen, W., Vucic, E., Leupold, E., Mulder, W., Cormode, D., Briley-Saebo, K., Barazza, A., Fisher, E., Dathe, M., & Fayad Z. (2008). Incorporation of an apoE-derived lipopeptide in high-density lipoprotein MRI contrast agents for enhanced imaging of macrophages in atherosclerosis. Contrast Media & Molecular Imaging, Vol.3, No.6, (November-December 2008), pp. 233-242, ISSN 1555-4317

Cheng, C., Tempel, D., Van Haperen, R., Van der Baan, A., Grosveld, F., Daemen, M., Krams, R., & De Crom, R. (2006). Atherosclerotic lesion size and vulnerability are determined by patterns of fluid shear stress. *Circulation*, Vol.113, No.23, (June 2006), pp. 2744-2753, ISSN 1524-4539

Cormode, D., Briley-Saebo, K., Mulder, W., Aguinaldo, J., Barazza, A., Ma, Y., Fisher, E., & Fayad, Z. (2008). An ApoA-I mimetic peptide high-density-lipoprotein-based MRI contrast agent for atherosclerotic plaque composition detection. *Small*, Vol.4, No.9, (September 2008), pp. 1437-1444, ISSN 1613-6829

Cormode, D., Skajaa, T., Van Schooneveld, M., Koole, R., Jarzyna, P., Lobatto, M., Calcagno, C., Barazza, A., Gordon, R., Zanzonico, P., Fisher, E., Fayad, Z., & Mulder W. (November 2008). Nanocrystal core high-density lipoproteins: a multimodality contrast agent platform. *Nano Letters*, Vol.8, No.11, (November 2008), pp. 3715-23, ISSN 1530-6984

Cormode, D., Chandrasekar, R., Delshad, A., Briley-Saebo, K., Calcagno, C., Barazza, A., Mulder, W., Fisher, E., Fayad, Z. (2009). Comparison of synthetic high density lipoprotein (HDL) contrast agents for MR imaging of atherosclerosis. *Bioconjugate Chemistry,* Vol.20, No. 5, (May 2009), pp. 937–943, ISSN 1520-4812

Dunmore, B., McCarthy, M., Naylor, A., & Brindle, N. (2007). Carotid plaque instability and ischemic symptoms are linked to immaturity of microvessels within plaques. *Journal of Vascular Surgery,* Vol.45, No.1, (January 2007), pp. 155-159, ISSN 0741-5214

Falk, E., Shah, P., & Fuster, V. (1995). Coronary plaque disruption. *Circulation,* Vol.92, No.3, (August 1995), pp. 657-671, ISSN 0009-7322

Frias, J., Williams, K., Fisher, E., & Fayad, Z. (2004). Recombinant HDL-like nanoparticles: a specific contrast agent for MRI of atherosclerotic plaques. *Journal of the American Chemical Society,* Vol.126, No.50, (December 2004), pp. 16316-16317, ISSN 0002-7863

Frias, J., Ma, Y., Williams, K., Fayad, Z., & Fisher, E. (2006). Properties of a versatile nanoparticle platform contrast agent to image and characterize atherosclerotic plaques by magnetic resonance imaging. Nano Letters, Vol.6, No.10, (October 2006), pp. 2220–2224, ISSN 1530-6984

Galis, Z., & Khatri, J. (2002). Matrix metalloproteinases in vascular remodeling and atherogenesis: the good, the bad, and the ugly. Circulation Research, Vol.90, No.3, (February 2002), pp. 251–262, ISSN 1524-4571

Gerke, V., & Moss, S. (2002). Annexins: from structure to function. *Physiological Reviews,* Vol.82, No.2, (April 2002), pp. 331-371, ISSN 0031-9333

Hak, S., Sanders, H., Agrawal, P., Langereis, S., Grüll, H., Keizer, H., Arena, F., Terreno, E., Strijkers, G., & Nicolay, K. (2009). A high relaxivity Gd(III)DOTA-DSPE-based liposomal contrast agent for magnetic resonance imaging. *European Journal of Pharmaceuticsand Biopharmaceutics,* Vol.72, No.2, (June 2009), pp. 397-404, ISSN 1873-3441

Hemdahl, A., Gabrielsen, A., Zhu, C., Eriksson, P., Hedin, U., Kastrup, J., Thorén, P., & Hansson, G. (2006). Expression of neutrophil gelatinase-associated lipocalin in atherosclerosis and myocardial infarction. *Arteriosclerosis, Thrombosis, and Vascular Biology,* Vol.26, No.1, (January 2006), pp. 136-142, ISSN 1524-4636

Hofstra, L., Liem, I., Dumont, E., Boersma, H., van Heerde, W., Doevendans, P., De Muinck, E., Wellens, H., Kemerink, G., Reutelingsperger, C., & Heidendal, G. (2000). Visualisation of cell death in vivo in patients with acute myocardial infarction. *Lancet,* Vol.356, No.9225, (July 2000), pp. 209–212, ISSN 0140-6736

Hyafil, F., Cornily, J., Feig, J., Gordon, R., Vucic E., Amirbekian, V., Fisher, E., Fuster, V., Feldman, L., & Fayad, Z. (2007). Noninvasive detection of macrophages using a nanoparticulate contrast agent for computed tomography. *Nature Medicine,* Vol.13, No.5, (May 2007), pp. 636-641, ISSN 1078-8956

Ide, M., Kuwamura, M., Kotani, T., Sawamoto, O., & Yamate, J. (2005). Effects of gadolinium chloride (GdCl(3)) on the appearance of macrophage populations and fibrogenesis in thioacetamide-induced rat hepatic lesions. *Journal of Comparative Pathology,* Vol.133, No.2-3, (August-October 2005), pp. 92-102, ISSN 0021-9975

Iga, A., Robertson, J., Winslet, M., & Seifalian, A. (2007). Clinical potential of quantum dots. *Journal of Biomedicine & Biotechnology*, Vol.2007, No.10, (2007), pp. 1-10, ISSN 1110-7243

Johansson, L., Bjornerud, A., Ahlstrom, H., Ladd, D., & Fujii, D. (2001). A targeted contrast agent for magnetic resonance imaging of thrombus: implications of spatial resolution. *Journal of Magnetic Resonance Imaging*, Vol.13, No.4, (April 2001), pp. 615-618, ISSN 1053-1807

Kamat, M., El-Boubbou, K., Zhu, D., Lansdell, T., Lu, X., Li, W., & Huang, X. (2010). Hyaluronic acid immobilized magnetic nanoparticles for active targeting and imaging of macrophages. *Bioconjugate Chemistry*, Vol.21, No.11, (November 2010), pp. 2128-2135, ISSN 1520-4812

Kelly, K., Allport, J., Tsourkas, A., Shinde-Patil, V., Josephson, L., Weissleder, R. (2005). Detection of vascular adhesion molecule-1 expression using a novel multimodal nanoparticle. *Circulation Research*, Vol.96, No.3, (February 2005), pp. 327-336, ISSN 1524-4571

Kolodgie, F., Petrov, A., Virmani, R., Narula, N., Verjans, J., Weber, D., Hartung, D., Steinmetz, N., Vanderheyden, J., Vannan, M., Gold, H., Reutelingsperger, C., Hofstra, L., & Narula, J. (2003). Targeting of apoptotic macrophages and experimental atheroma with radiolabeled annexin V: a technique with potential for noninvasive imaging of vulnerable plaque. *Circulation*, Vol.108, No.25, (December 2003), pp. 3134–3139, ISSN 1524-4539

Lancelot, E., Amirbekian, V., Brigger, I., Raynaud, J., Ballet, S., David, C., Rousseaux, O., Le Greneur, S., Port, M., Lijnen, H., Bruneval, P., Michel, J., Ouimet, T., Roques, B., Amirbekian, S., Hyafil, F., Vucic, E., Aguinaldo, J., Corot, C., & Fayad, Z. (2008). Evaluation of matrix metalloproteinases in atherosclerosis using a novel noninvasive imaging approach. *Arteriosclerosis, Thrombosis, and Vascular Biology*, Vol.28, No.3, (March 2008), pp. 425-432, ISSN 1524-4636

Leuschner, F., & Nahrendorf, M. (2011). Molecular imaging of coronary atherosclerosis and myocardial infarction: considerations for the bench and perspectives for the clinic. *Circulation Research*, Vol.108, No.5, (March 2011), pp. 593-606, ISSN 1524-4571

Li, D., Patel, A., Klibanov, A., Kramer, C., Ruiz, M., Kang, B., Mehta, J., Beller, G., Glover, D., & Meyer C. (2010). Molecular imaging of atherosclerotic plaques targeted to oxidized LDL receptor LOX-1 by SPECT/CT and magnetic resonance. Circulation. Cardiovascular Imaging, Vol.3, No.4, (July 2010), pp. 464-472, ISSN 1942-0080

Libby, P. (2002). Inflammtion in atherosclerosis. *Nature*, Vol.420, No.6917, (December 2002), pp. 868-874, ISSN 0028-0836

Lipinski, M., Frias, J., Amirbekian, V., Briley-Saebo, K., Mani, V., Samber, D., Abbate, A., Aguinaldo, J., Massey, D., Fuster, V., Vetrovec, G., & Fayad, Z. (2009). Macrophage-specific lipid-based nanoparticles improve cardiac magnetic resonance detection and characterization of human atherosclerosis. *Journal of the American College of Cardiology. Cardiovascular Imaging*, Vol.2, No.5, (May 2009), pp. 637-647, ISSN 1876-7591

Lobatto, M., Fayad, Z., Silvera, S., Vucic, E., Calcagno, C., Mani, V., Dickson, S., Nicolay, K., Banciu, M., Schiffelers, R., Metselaar, J., Van Bloois, L., Wu, H., Fallon, J., Rudd, J., Fuster, V., Fisher, E., Storm, G., & Mulder, W. (2010). Multimodal clinical imaging to longitudinally assess a nanomedical anti-inflammatory treatment in experimental atherosclerosis. *Molecular Pharmaceutics,* Vol.7, No.6, (December 2010), pp. 2020-2029, ISSN 1543-8392

Maiseyeu, A., Mihai, G., Kampfrath, T., Simonetti, O., Sen, C., Roy, S., Rajagopalan, S., & Parthasarathy, S. (2009). Gadolinium-containing phosphatidylserine liposomes for molecular imaging of atherosclerosis. Journal of Lipid Research, Vol.50, No.11, (November 2009), pp. 2157-2163, ISSN 0022-2275

Makowski, M., Wiethoff, A., Blume, U., Cuello, F., Warley, A., Jansen, C., Nagel, E., Razavi, R., Onthank, D., Cesati, R., Marber, M., Schaeffter, T., Smith, A., Robinson, S., & Botnar, R. (2011). Assessment of atherosclerotic plaque burden with an elastin-specific magnetic resonance contrast agent. *Nature Medicine,* Vol.17, No.3, (March 2011), pp. 383-388, ISSN 1546-170X

Massoud, T., & Gambhir, S. (2003). Molecular imaging in living subjects: seeing fundamental biological processes in a new light. *Genes & Development,* Vol.17, No.5, (March 2003), pp. 545–580, ISSN 0890-9369Lusis, A. (2000). Atherosclerosis. *Nature,* Vol.407, No.6801, (September 2000), pp. 233–241, ISSN 0028-0836

McAteer, M., Akhtar, A., Von zur Muhlen, C., & Choudhury, R. (2010). An approach to molecular imaging of atherosclerosis, thrombosis, and vascular inflammation using microparticles of iron oxide. *Atherosclerosis,* Vol.209, No.1, (March 2010), pp. 18-27, ISSN 1879-1484.

Meding, J., Urich, M., Licha, K., Reinhardt, M., Misselwitz, B., Fayad, Z., & Weinmann H. (2007). Magnetic resonance imaging of atherosclerosis by targeting extracellular matrix deposition with Gadofluorine M. *Contrast Media & Molecular Imaging,* Vol.2, No.3, (May-June 2007), pp. 120-129, ISSN 1555-4317

Miserus, R., Herias, M., Prinzen, L., Lobbes, M., Van Suylen, R., Dirksen, A., Hackeng, T., Heemskerk, J.,Van Engelshoven, J., Daemen, M., Van Zandvoort, M., Heeneman, S., & Kooi, M. (2009). Molecular MRI of early thrombus formation using a bimodal alpha2-antiplasmin-based contrast agent. *Journal of the American College of Cardiology. Cardiovascular Imaging,* Vol.2, No.8, (August 2009), pp. 987-996, ISSN 1876-7591

Morawski, A., Winter, P., Yu, X., Fuhrhop, R., Scott, M., Hockett, F., Robertson, J., Gaffney, P., Lanza, G., Wickline, S. (2004). Quantitative "magnetic resonance immunohistochemistry" with ligand-targeted (19)F nanoparticles. *Magnetic Resonance in Medicine,* Vol.52, No.6, (December 2004), pp. 1255-1262, ISSN 0740-3194

Mulder, W., Douma, K., Koning, G., Van Zandvoort, M., Lutgens, E., Daemen, M., Nicolay, K., & Strijkers, G. (2006). Liposome-enhanced MRI of neointimal lesions in the ApoE-KO mouse. *Magnetic Resonance in Medicine,* Vol.55, No.5, (May 2006), pp. 1170-1174, ISSN 0740-3194

Mulder, W., Strijkers, G., Vucic, E., Cormode, D., Nicolay, K., & Fayad, Z. (2007). Magnetic resonance molecular imaging contrast agents and their application in atherosclerosis. *Topics in Magnetic Resonance Imaging,* Vol.18, No.5, (October 2007a), pp. 409-417, ISSN 0899-3459

Mulder W., Strijkers, G., Briley-Saebo, K., Frias, J., Aguinaldo, J., Vucic, E., Amirbekian, V., Tang, C., Chin, P., Nicolay, K., & Fayad, Z. (2007b). Molecular imaging of macrophages in atherosclerotic plaques using bimodal PEG-micelles. *Magnetic Resonance in Medicine,* Vol.58, No.6, (December 2007), pp. 1164-1170, ISSN 0740-3194

Mulder W., Strijkers, G., Van Tilborg, G., Cormode, D., Fayad, Z., & Nicolay K. (2009). Nanoparticulate assemblies of amphiphiles and diagnostically active materials for multimodality imaging. *Accounts of Chemical Research,* Vol.42, No.7, (July 2009), pp. 904-914, ISSN 1520-4898

Naghavi, M., Libby, P., Falk, E., Casscells, S., Litovsky, S., Rumberger, J., Badimon, J., Stefanadis, C., Moreno, P., Pasterkamp, G., Fayad, Z., Stone, P., Waxman, S., Raggi, P., Madjid, M., Zarrabi, A., Burke, A., Yuan, C., Fitzgerald, P., Siscovick, D., de Korte, C., Aikawa, M., Airaksinen, K., Assmann, G., Becker, C., Chesebro, J., Farb, A., Galis, Z., Jackson, C., Jang, I., Koenig, W., Lodder, R., March, K., Demirovic, J., Navab, M., Priori, S., Rekhter, M., Bahr, R., Grundy, S., Mehran, R., Colombo, A., Boerwinkle, E., Ballantyne, C., Insull, W. Jr, Schwartz, R., Vogel, R., Serruys, P., Hansson, G., Faxon, D., Kaul, S., Drexler, H., Greenland, P., Muller, J., Virmani, R., Ridker, P., Zipes, D., Shah, P., & Willerson, J. (2003a). From vulnerable plaque to vulnerable patient: a call for new definitions and risk assessment strategies: Part I. *Circulation,* Vol.108, No.14, (October 2003), pp. 1664-1672, ISSN 1524-4539

Naghavi, M., Libby, P., Falk, E., Casscells, S., Litovsky, S., Rumberger, J., Badimon, J., Stefanadis, C., Moreno, P., Pasterkamp, G., Fayad, Z., Stone, P., Waxman, S., Raggi, P., Madjid, M., Zarrabi, A., Burke, A., Yuan, C., Fitzgerald, P., Siscovick, D., de Korte, C., Aikawa, M., Airaksinen, K., Assmann, G., Becker, C., Chesebro, J., Farb, A., Galis, Z., Jackson, C., Jang, I., Koenig, W., Lodder, R., March, K., Demirovic, J., Navab, M., Priori, S., Rekhter, M., Bahr, R., Grundy, S., Mehran, R., Colombo, A., Boerwinkle, E., Ballantyne, C., Insull, W. Jr, Schwartz, R., Vogel, R., Serruys, P., Hansson, G., Faxon, D., Kaul, S., Drexler, H., Greenland, P., Muller, J., Virmani, R., Ridker, P., Zipes, D., Shah, P., & Willerson, J. (2003b). From vulnerable plaque to vulnerable patient: a call for new definitions and risk assessment strategies: Part II. *Circulation,* Vol.108, No.15, (October 2003), pp. 1772-1778, ISSN 1524-4539

Nahrendorf, M., Jaffer, F., Kelly, K., Sosnovik, D., Aikawa, E., Libby, P., & Weissleder, R. (2006). Noninvasive vascular cell adhesion molecule-1 imaging identifies inflammatory activation of cells in atherosclerosis. *Circulation,* Vol.114, No.14, (October 2006), pp. 1504-1511, ISSN 1524-4539

Neubauer, A., Sim, H.,Winter, P., Caruthers, S., Williams, T., Robertson, J., Sept, D., Lanza, G., & Wickline, S. (2008). Nanoparticle pharmacokinetic profiling in vivo using magnetic resonance imaging. *Magnetic Resonance in Medicine,* Vol.60, No.6, (December 2008), pp. 1353-1361, ISSN 1522-2594

Pedersen, M. (2007). Safety update on the possible causal relationship between gadolinium-containing MRI agents and nephrogenic systemic fibrosis. *Journal of Magnetic Resonance Imaging,* Vol.25, No.5, (May 2007), pp. 881-883, ISSN 1053-1807

Ragavan, M., Chen, H., Sekar, G., & Hilty, C. (2011). Solution NMR of polypeptides hyperpolarized by dynamic nuclear polarization. *Analytical Chemistry,* Vol.83, No.15, (August 2011), pp. 6054-6059, ISSN 1520-6882

Ronald, J., Chen, J., Chen, Y., Hamilton, A., Rodriguez, E., Reynolds, F., Hegele, R., Rogers, K., Querol, M., Bogdanov, A., Weissleder, R., & Rutt, B. (2009). Enzyme-sensitive magnetic resonance imaging targeting myeloperoxidase identifies active inflammation in experimental rabbit atherosclerotic plaques. *Circulation,* Vol.120, No.7, (August 2009), pp. 592-599, ISSN 1524-4539

Ross, R. (1999). Atherosclerosis—an inflammatory disease. *New England Journal of Medicine,* Vol.340, No.2, (January 1999), pp. 115-126, ISSN 0028-4793

Rudd, J., Myers, K., Bansilal, S., Machac, J., Rafique, A., Farkouh, M., Fuster, V., & Fayad, Z. (2007). (18)Fluorodeoxyglucose positron emission tomography imaging of atherosclerotic plaque inflammation is highly reproducible: implications for atherosclerosis therapy trials. *Journal of the American College of Cardiology,* Vol.50, No.9, August 2007), pp. 892-896, ISSN 1558-3597

Sanders, H., Strijkers, G., Mulder, W., Huinink, H., Erich, S., Adan, O., Sommerdijk, N., Merkx, M., & Nicolay, K. (2009). Morphology, binding behavior and MR-properties of paramagnetic collagen-binding liposomes. *Contrast Media & Molecular Imaging,* Vol.4, No.2, (March-April 2009), pp. 81-88, ISSN 1555-4317

Schafers, M., Schober, O., & Hermann, S. (2010). Matrix-metalloproteinases as imaging targets for inflammatory activity in atherosclerotic plaques. *Journal of Nuclear Medicine,* Vol.51, No.5, (May 2010), pp. 663-666, ISSN 1535-5667

Schmitz, S., Taupitz, M., Wagner, S., Wolf, K., Beyersdorff, D., & Hamm, B. (2001). Magnetic resonance imaging of atherosclerotic plaques using superparamagnetic iron oxide particles. *Journal of Magnetic Resonance Imaging,* Vol.14, No.4, (October 2001), pp. 355–361, ISSN 1053-1807

Schmitz, S. (2003). [Iron-oxide-enhanced MR imaging of inflammatory atherosclerotic lesions: overview of experimental and initial clinical results]. *Rofo,* Vol.175, No.4, (April 2003), pp. 469-476, ISSN 1438-9029

Sirol, M., Moreno, P., Purushothaman, K., Vucic, E., Amirbekian, V., Weinmann, H., Muntner, P., Fuster, V., & Fayad, Z. (2009). Increased neovascularization in advanced lipid-rich atherosclerotic lesions detected by gadofluorine-M-enhanced MRI: implications for plaque vulnerability. *Circulation. Cardiovascular Imaging,* Vol.2, No.5, (September 2009), pp. 391-396, ISSN 1942-0080

Skajaa, T., Cormode, D., Falk, E., Mulder, W., Fisher, E., & Fayad, Z. (2010). High-density lipoprotein-based contrast agents for multimodal imaging of atherosclerosis. *Arteriosclerosis, Thrombosis, and Vascular Biology,* Vol.30, No.2, (February 2010), pp. 169-176, ISSN 1524-4636

Skajaa, T., Cormode, D., Jarzyna, P., Delshad, A., Blachford, C., Barazza, A., Fisher, E., Gordon, R., Fayad, Z., & Mulder, W. (2011). The biological properties of iron oxide core high-density lipoprotein in experimental atherosclerosis. *Biomaterials,* Vol.32, No.1, (January 2011), pp. 206-213, ISSN 1878-5905

Sluimer, J., & Daemen, M. (2009). Novel concepts in atherogenesis: angiogenesis and hypoxia in atherosclerosis. *Journal of Pathology,* Vol.218, No.1, (May 2009), pp. 7-29, ISSN 1096-9896

Spuentrup, E., Botnar, R., Wiethoff, A., Ibrahim, T., Kelle, S., Katoh, M., Ozgun, M., Nagel, E., Vymazal, J., Graham, P., Günther, R., & Maintz, D. (2008). MR imaging of thrombi using EP-2104R, a fibrin-specific contrast agent: initial results in patients. *European Radiology,* Vol.18, No.9, (September 2008), pp. 1995-2005, ISSN 0938-7994

Stary, H., Chandler, A., Dinsmore, R., Fuster, V., Glagov, S., Insull, W. Jr, Rosenfeld, M., Schwartz, C., Wagner, W., & Wissler, R. (1995). A definition of advanced types of atherosclerotic lesions and a histological classification of atherosclerosis. A report from the Committee on Vascular Lesions of the Council on Arteriosclerosis, American Heart Association. *Arteriosclerosis, Thrombosis, and Vascular Biology,* Vol.15, No.9, (September 1995), pp. 1512-1531, ISSN 1079-5642

Steffens, S., Veillard, N., Arnaud, C., Pelli, G., Burger, F., Staub, C., Karsak, M., Zimmer, A., Frossard, J., & Mach, F. (2005). Low dose oral cannabinoid therapy reduces progression of atherosclerosis in mice. Nature, Vol.434, No.7034, (April 2005), pp. 782-786, ISSN 1476-4687

Ta, H., Prabhu, S., Leitner, E., Jia, F., Von Elverfeldt, D., Jackson, K., Heidt, T., Nair, A., Pearce, H., Von Zur Muhlen, C., Wang, X., Peter, K., & Hagemeyer, C. (2011). Enzymatic Single-Chain Antibody Tagging: A Universal Approach to Targeted Molecular Imaging and Cell Homing in Cardiovascular Disease. *Circulation Research,* Vol.109, No.4, (August 2011), pp. 365-373, ISSN 1524-4571

Taboada, E., Rodriguez, E., Roig, A., Oró, J., Roch, A., Muller, R. (2007). Relaxometric and magnetic characterization of ultrasmall iron oxide nanoparticles with high magnetization. Evaluation as potential T1 magnetic resonance imaging contrast agents for molecular imaging. Langmuir, Vol.23, No.8, (April 2007), pp. 4583-4588, ISSN 0743-7463

Takaya, N., Yuan, C., Chu, B., Saam, T., Polissar, N., Jarvik, G., Isaac, C., McDonough, J., Natiello, C., Small, R., Ferguson, M., & Hatsukami, T. (2005). Presence of intraplaque hemorrhage stimulates progression of carotid atherosclerotic plaques: a high-resolution magnetic resonance imaging study. Circulation, Vol.111, No.21, (May 2005), pp. 2768-2775, ISSN 1524-4539

Tang, T., Howarth, S., Miller, S., Graves, M., Patterson, A., U-King-Im, J., Li, Z., Walsh, S., Brown, A., Kirkpatrick, P., Warburton, E., Hayes, P., Varty, K., Boyle, J., Gaunt, M., Zalewski, A., & Gillard, J. (2009). The ATHEROMA (Atorvastatin Therapy: Effects on Reduction of Macrophage Activity) Study. Evaluation using ultrasmall superparamagnetic iron oxide-enhanced magnetic resonance imaging in carotid disease. *Journal of the American College of Cardiology,* Vol.53, No.22, (June 2009), pp. 2039-2050, ISSN 1558-3597

Te Boekhorst, B., Bovens, S., Nederhoff, M., Van de Kolk, K., Cramer, M., Van Oosterhout, M., Ten Hove, M., Doevendans, P., Pasterkamp, G., & Van Echteld, C. (2010a). Negative MR contrast caused by USPIO uptake in lymph nodes may lead to false positive observations with in vivo visualization of murine atherosclerotic plaque. *Atherosclerosis,* Vol.210, No.1, (May 2010), pp. 122-129, ISSN 1879-1484

Te Boekhorst, B., Bovens, S., Van de Kolk, C., Cramer, M., Doevendans, P., Ten Hove, M., Van der Weerd, L., Poelmann, R., Strijkers, G., Pasterkamp, G., & Van Echteld, C. (2010b). The time window of MRI of murine atherosclerotic plaques after administration of CB2 receptor targeted micelles: inter-scan variability and relation between plaque signal intensity increase and gadolinium content of inversion recovery prepared versus non-prepared fast spin echo. NMR in Biomedicine, Vol.23, No.8, (October 2010), pp. 939-951, ISSN 1099-1492

Te Boekhorst, B., Bovens, S., Rodrigues-Feo, J., Sanders, H., Van de Kolk, C., De Kroon, A., Cramer, M., Doevendans, P., Ten Hove, M., Pasterkamp, G., & Van Echteld, C. (2010c). Characterization and in vitro and in vivo testing of CB2-receptor- and

NGAL-targeted paramagnetic micelles for molecular MRI of vulnerable atherosclerotic plaque. *Molecular Imaging and Biology,* Vol.12, No.6, (December 2010), pp. 635-651, ISSN 1860-2002

Te Boekhorst, B., Bovens, S., Hellings, W., Van der Kraak, P., Van de Kolk, K., Vink, A., Moll, F., Van Oosterhout, M., De Vries, J., Doevendans, P., Goumans, M., De Kleijn, D., Van Echteld, C., Pasterkamp, G., & Sluijter, J. (2011). Molecular MRI of murine atherosclerotic plaque targeting NGAL: a protein associated with unstable human plaque characteristics. *Cardiovascular Research,* Vol.89, No.3, (February 2011), pp. 680-688, ISSN 1755-3245

Tsimikas, S., Shortal, B., Witztum, J., & Palinski, W. (2000). In vivo uptake of radiolabeled MDA2, an oxidation-specific monoclonal antibody, provides an accurate measure of atherosclerotic lesions rich in oxidized LDL and is highly sensitive to their regression. Arteriosclerosis, Thrombosis, and Vascular Biology, Vol.20, No.3, (March 2000), pp. 689–697, ISSN 1079-5642

Tu, C., Osborne, E., & Louie, A. (2011). Activatable T_1 and T_2 magnetic resonance imaging contrast agents. *Annals of Biomedical Engineering,* Vol.39, No.4, (April 2011), pp. 1335-1348, ISSN 1521-6047

Van Bochove, G., Paulis, L., Segers, D., Mulder, W., Krams, R., Nicolay, K., & Strijkers, G. (2011). Contrast enhancement by differently sized paramagnetic MRI contrast agents in mice with two phenotypes of atherosclerotic plaque. *Contrast Media & Molecular Imaging,* Vol.6, No.1, (January-February 2011), pp. 35-45, ISSN 1555-4317

Van Tilborg, G., Vucic, E., Strijkers, G., Cormode, D., Mani, V., Skajaa, T., Reutelingsperger, C., Fayad, Z., Mulder, W., & Nicolay, K. (2010). Annexin A5-functionalized bimodal nanoparticles for MRI and fluorescence imaging of atherosclerotic plaques. *Bioconjugate Chemistry,* Vol.21, No.10, (October 2010), pp. 1794-1803, ISSN 1520-4812

Vink, A., & Pasterkamp, G. (2002). Atherosclerotic plaque burden, plaque vulnerability and arterial remodeling: the role of inflammation. Minerva Cardioangiologica, Vol.50, No.2, (April 2002), pp. 75–83, ISSN 0026-4725

Ward, K., Aletras, A., & Balaban, R. (2000). A new class of contrast agents for MRI based on proton chemical exchange dependent saturation transfer (CEST). *Journal of Magnetic Resonance,* Vol.143, No.1, (March 2000), pp. 79-87, ISSN 1090-7807

Winter, P., Caruthers, S., Yu, X., Song, S., Chen, J., Miller, B., Bulte, J., Robertson, D., Gaffney, P., Wickline, S., & Lanza G. (2003). Improved molecular imaging contrast agent for detection of human thrombus. Magnetic Resonance in Medicine, Vol.50, No.2, (August 2003), pp. 411–416, ISSN 0740-3194

Winter, P., Cai, K., Chen, J., Adair, C., Kiefer, G., Athey, P., Gaffney, P., Buff, C., Robertson, J., Caruthers, S., Wickline, S., & Lanza, G. (2006). Targeted PARACEST nanoparticle contrast agent for the detection of fibrin. *Magnetic Resonance in Medicine,* Vol.56, No.6, (December 2006), pp. 1384-1388, ISSN 0740-3194

Winter, P., Caruthers, S., Allen, J., Cai, K., Williams, T., Lanza, G., & Wickline, S. (2010). Molecular imaging of angiogenic therapy in peripheral vascular disease with alphanubeta3-integrin-targeted nanoparticles. *Magnetic Resonance in Medicine,* Vol.64, No.2, (August 2010), pp. 369-376, ISSN 1522-2594

Yuan, C., Kerwin, W., Ferguson, M., Polissar, N., Zhang, S., Cai, J., & Hatsukami, T. (2002). Contrast-enhanced high resolution MRI for atherosclerotic carotid artery tissue characterization. Journal of Magnetic Resonance Imaging, Vol.15, No.1, (January 2002), pp. 62-67, ISSN 1053-1807

11

Molecular Imaging of Atherosclerotic Coronary Plaques by Fluorescent Angioscopy

Yasumi Uchida[1] and Yuko Maezawa[2]
[1]*Japan Foundation for Cardiovascular Research, Funabashi,*
[2]*Sick Children's Hospital, Toronto,*
[1]*Japan*
[2]*Canada*

1. Introduction

It is generally believed that the coronary plaques with lipid-laden thin fibrous cap and a large lipid core beneath are vulnerable and imaging methods such as intravascular ultrasonography[1], optical coherence tomography[2], and angioscopy[3-5] are clinically employed to detect this type of plaques. However, the coronary plaques that have a thin cap composed of tight calcium layers are frequently observed during post-mortem examinations[3]. Moreover, plaques wherein the deposition of lipids and macrophages is confined to just the superficial layers and in which a lipid core is not present also exist[3,6]. These evidences indicate the necessity of detailed molecular characterization for the detection of vulnerable plaques.

Oxidized low-density lipoprotein (ox-LDL) plays an important role in the initiation, progression and destabilization of atherosclerotic plaques by inducing the proliferation and elongation of survival of macrophages[7,8].

Normal collagen fibers (CFs) that contain collagen-I in abundance protect the coronary plaques against mechanical stress. During plaque growth, collagen-I is replaced by collagen-III, -IV and/or -V[9-11], and CFs are degenerated, disrupted, and finally destroyed by matrix metalloproteinases released by macrophages[12]. During this process, macrophages accumulate lipids such as cholesteryl esters (CEs) and ox-LDL[13,14] and become foam cells while simultaneously producing ceramide within themselves[15]; their death results in formation of the lipid core. Therefore, demonstrating the lack of collagen-I which is mainly contained in normal CFs, deposition of lipids and existence of ox-LDL and the substances that comprising ox-LDL is an essential requisite for the detection of vulnerable plaques, but *in-vivo* clinical tools to visualize them in the coronary plaques are lacking.

Structurally, ox-LDL is composed of cortex and core. The cortex is composed of lysophosphatidylcholine (LPC), free cholesterol (C) and Shiff base derived by oxidation from apolipoprotein B (apoB), and the core is composed of triglyceride (TG), cholesteryl esters (CEs), and proteins (Figure 1).

High-density lipoprotein (HDL) is composed of the same substances except Apo B, and plays a key role in reverse cholesterol transport but also stimulates prostacyclin release, enhances endothelial repair, inhibits monocyte recruitment into the arterial wall, and inhibits progression of and enhances regression of atherosclerosis[16, 17].

LPC itself is a pro-inflammatory substance, and plays a critical role in the atherogenic activity of ox-LDL. This substance is generated by lipoprotein-associated phospholipase A_2 [18]; induces vascular endothelial cell dysfunction[19]; causes endothelial cell apoptosis by DNA fragmentation[20]; stimulates adhesion and activation of lymphocytes and initiates chemotaxis of macrophages[21]; causes transformation of vascular smooth muscle cells that is characteristic of atherosclerosis.

Apolipoprotein B-100 (apo B-100) is a major protein of low density lipoprotein (LDL)[22]. Serum Apo B-100 is elevated in patients with type 2 diabetes mellitus[23] as well as in those with coronary artery disease[24]. Apo B-100 and apo B-100/apo A-1 ratio predict not only coronary artery disease[25] but also other cardiovascular disease[26], and metabolic syndrome[27]. Medical treatments have been directed to lower Apo B-100[28].

TG is also considered an important risk of cardiovascular disease, but lowering TG levels remains difficult to achieve[29, 30].

Although these substances in serum are measureable, measurement of these substances in the atherosclerotic plaques is difficult. If they become visible in patients *in-vivo*, initiation, progression and destabilization, and the effects of medical and interventional therapies on atherosclerotic plaques can be objectively evaluated.

Based upon the knowledge about the pathophysiology of atherosclerosis, *in-vitro* and *in-vivo* animal studies and clinical trials have been performed using different tracers for plaque imaging studies, including radioactive-labelled lipoproteins, components of the coagulation system, cytokines, mediators of the metalloproteinase system, cell adhesion receptors, and even whole cells, or antibodies of the substances composing atherosclerotic plaques. However the majority of them are still not applicable clinically.

Spectroscopy has been attempted intensively for molecular imaging of lipids within the atherosclerotic lesions *in-vitro*[31,32]. However, its clinical application started only recently[33]. Also, magnetic resonance imaging or computed tomography has been attempted for lipid imaging, however their clinical application is yet not established[34,35].

Although invasive, angioscopy is a clinically established high resolution technique, which enables direct, colored and three-dimensional imaging of the coronary arterial wall. Recently, fluorescent angioscopy, both color and near-infrared, was developed and is used for molecular imaging of the substances within the human coronary plaques not only *in-vitro*[36-39] but also in patients *in-vivo*[36,37].

The present article reviews recent advances in molecular imaging of the substances comprising atherosclerotic coronary plaques by fluorescent angioscopy.

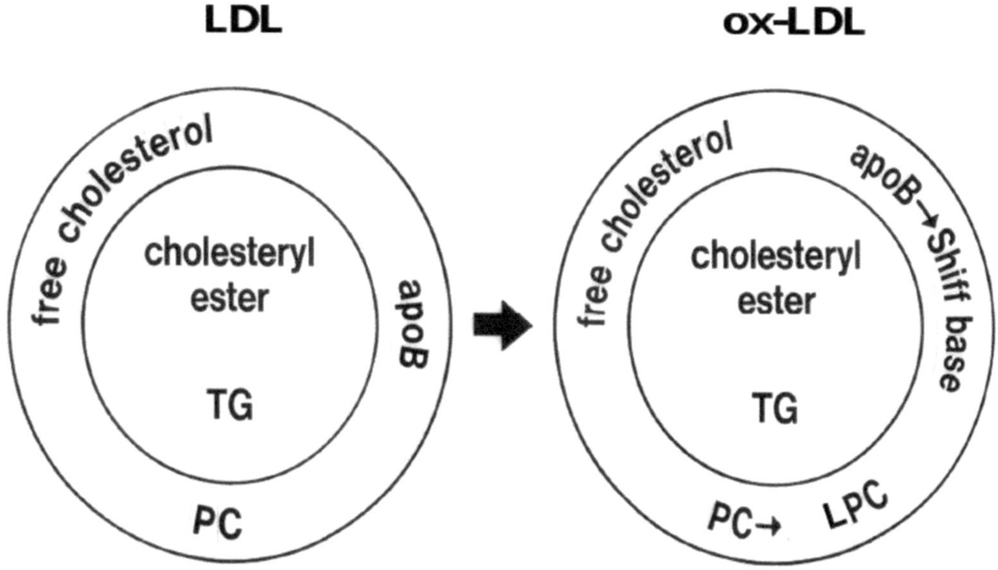

TG: triglyceride. apo B: apolipoprotein B . PC: phosphatidylcholine. LPC: lysophosphatidylcholine.

Fig 1. Schematic Representation of Structure of Low-density Lipoprotein (LDL) and Oxidized Low-density Lipoprotein (Ox-LDL).

2. Fluorescent angioscopy system

a. Color fluorescent angioscopy

The color fluorescent angioscopy (CFA) system is composed of a fluorescence-excitation unit, an angioscope, a fluorescence-emission unit and a camera. The fluorescence-excitation unit is composed of a mercury-xenon lamp and seven sets of band-pass filter (BPF) discs, exchangeable by rotation for selection of the desired wave length of light ranging from 320- to 760-nm. The remaining single disc, which did not have any filter, was used to irradiate white light for carrying out conventional angioscopy. The angioscope (modified VecMover, Clinical Supply Co, Gifu, Japan) was composed of a 2.5-F fiberscope which contained 6000 quartz fibers for the image guide and 300 quartz fibers for the light guide. This fiberscope was incorporated in a 5-F guiding balloon catheter and was steerable along a 0.014-inch guide wire; it also enabled observation of a coronary segment up to 7 cm in length by a single saline flush. This angioscope was approved for clinical use by the Japanese Ministry of Health and Labor and Welfare, and is widely used clinically in Japan.

The fluorescence-emission unit is composed of seven sets of dichroic membrane (DM) and 7 sets of band-absorption filter (BAF) discs which receive light ranging from 360- to 880-nm and is connected to a 3CCD digital camera (C7780, Hamamatsu Photonics, Hamamatsu). The obtained images are displayed on a computer screen through a camera controller (C7780, Hamamatsu Photonics, Hamamatsu).

To observe the vascular lumen, the light and image guides are connected to the excitation and emission units, respectively. After selecting the desired BPF and BAF, the light is irradiated through the BPF and the light guide toward the target. A pair of BPF of 345±15 nm and BAF of 420 nm ("A" imaging), and another pair of 470±20 nm BPF and BAF of 515 nm ("B" imaging) are usually used for imaging The evoked fluorescence is received by the digital camera through the DM and BAF for successive three-dimensional imaging at an adequate time-interval from 0.01 to 1 s. The details of this CFA system are described elsewhere.[41]

The intensity of the fluorescence images is arbitrarily defined as strong, weak and absent when the exposure-time required for imaging is within 0.5, more than 0.5 and within 1 and more than 1 s, respectively (Figure 2).

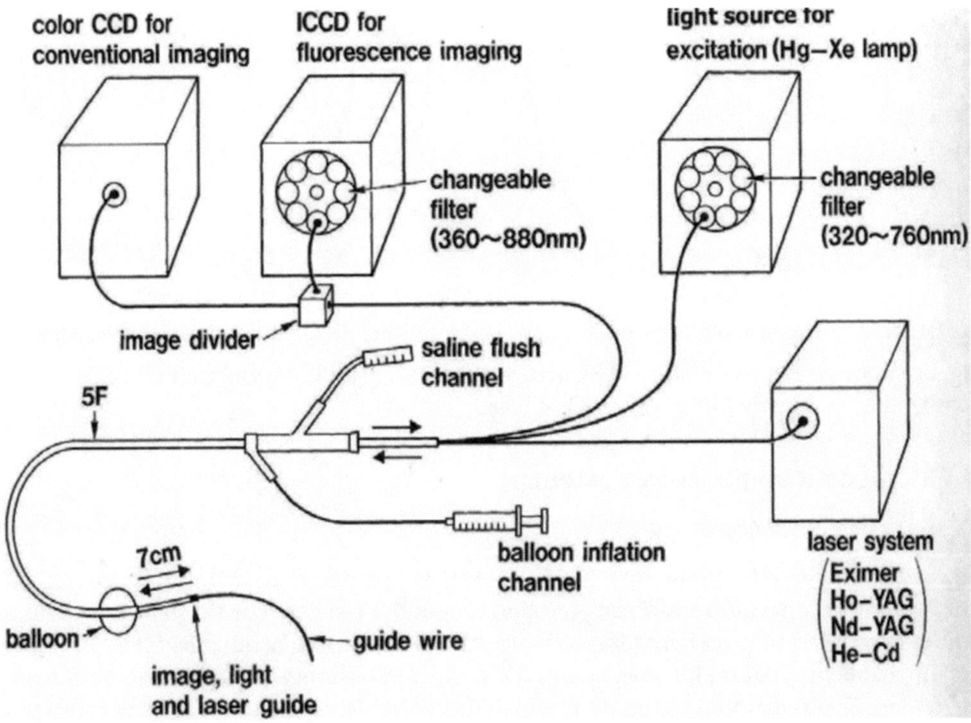

Cited from Ref. 41, with permission.

Fig. 2. Schematic Representation of A Fluorescent Angioscopy System

b. Near-infrared fluorescent angioscopy (NIRFA)

For NIRFA, the BPF and BAF of the angioscopy system used for color fluorescent angioscopy system are replaced by a 710±25 nm BPF disc and 780-nm BAF disc by rotation, respectively, and color CCD camera is replaced by an intensified CCD camera (C3505, Hamamatsu Photonics)[37].

3. Color fluorescence of major substances that comprising atherosclerotic plaques examined by fluorescent microscopy

a. Autofluorescence at "A"-imaging

Among the major substances that constitute atherosclerotic plaques, collagen-I and -IV exhibit blue and light blue autofluorescence, respectively whereas collagen-III and -V did not. Blue or light blue auto-fluorescence was not exhibited by other substances. Calcium phosphate, ceramide, and β-carotene which co-exists with lipid in the vascular wall, exhibited white, purple and orange auto-fluorescence, respectively (Figure. 3; Table 1)

In the presence of β-carotene, collagen-I and -IV exhibited green fluorescence, collagen-III and -V showed white fluorescence, cholesterol (C) exhibited yellow fluorescence and cholesteryl esters (CEs) showed orange fluorescence (Figure 3; Table 1).

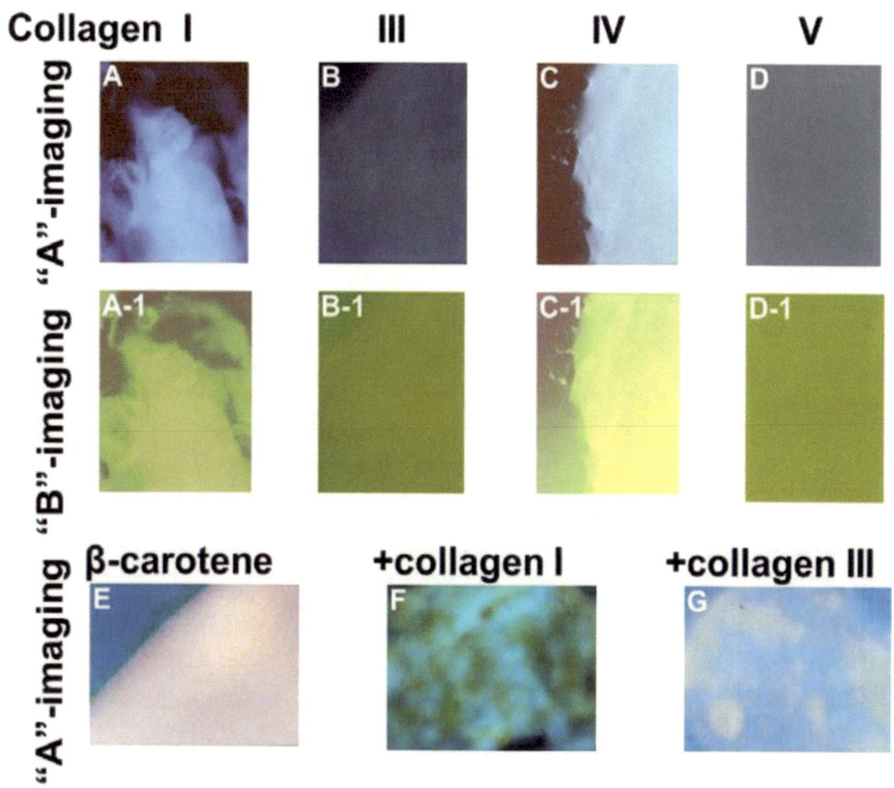

From A to D: "A"-imaging of and E to H: "B"-imaging of collagens-I, -III, -IV and -V, respectively. By "A"-imaging, blue fluorescence was seen in collagen-I, no fluorescence in collagen-III, light blue fluorescence in collagen-IV and no fluorescence in collagen-V. I: β-carotene (10^{-5} M) showing orange in fluorescence color by "A"-imaging. J: mixture of collagen-I and β-carotene showing green in fluorescent color by "A"-imaging. K: mixture of collagen-III and β-carotene showing white-to-light blue in fluorescence by "A"-imaging. Horizontal bar of each panel: 100 μ m. cited from Ref. 36, with permission.

Fig. 3. Fluorescence of Collagen Subtypes Visualized by "A"- and "B"-Imagings of Color Fluorescent Microscopy (CFM) Before and After Mixing with β-Carotene.

	Color fluorescent microscopy									
	Fluorescence evoked by dyes									
	AF		EB		TB		NB		Ho+TB	
	"A"	"B"	"A"	"B"	"A"	"B"	"A"	"B"	"A"	"B"
LDL	-	-	-	-	V	O	-	**Br**	R	**Go**
Ox-LDL	-	-	**V**	**RBr**	V	O	-	-	V	**Go**
VLDL	-	-	-	R	V	O	-	-	P	O
HDL	-	-	R	R	P	R	SB	G	-	P
LPC	-	-	R	R	**R**	**R**	P	**R**	V	**R**
PC	-	-	-	O	P	O	-	-	P	O
TG	-	-	-	-	-	-	P	Br	-	-
Apo B-100	-	-	-	R	P	O	-	**Go**	P	**R**
Apo A-1	-	-	-	-	-	-	-	-	-	-
Apo E-2	-	-	-	-	-	-	-	-	-	-
MMP-9	-	-	-	-	-	-	-	-	-	-
Cholesterol	W	Y	-	O	-	-	-	-	W	G
Chole oleate	-	-	-	-	-	-	-	-	-	-
Chole linoleate	-	-	-	-	-	-	-	-	-	-
7-Keto chol	-	-	-	-	-	-	-	-	-	-
5-Cholesten-3 β -ol	-	-	-	-	-	-	V	Br	-	-
Oleic acid	-	-	-	-	-	-	-	-	-	-
Linoelic acid	-	-	-	-	-	-	-	-	-	-
Collagen I	**B**	**G**	-	-	-	-	B	G	-	-
Collagen IV	**LB**	**G**	-	-	-	-	LB	G	-	-
Collagen III, V	-	-	-	-	-	-	-	-	-	-
Heparan sulfate	-	-	-	-	-	-	-	-	-	-
Hyaluronic acid	-	-	-	-	-	-	-	-	-	-
Albumin	-	-	-	-	-	-	-	-	-	-
Globulins	-	-	-	-	-	-	-	-	-	-
Amino acids	-	-	-	-	-	-	-	-	-	-
Ceramide	P	G	-	-	-	-	**R**	**R**	-	-
Calcium phosphate	W	Y	B	Y	-	-	-	-	-	-
β -Carotene	**O**	**O**	O	O	-	-	-	-	P	O

AF: autofluorescence. EB: Evans blue. TB: Trypan blue. NB: Nile blue. Ho: Homidium chloride.
"A" : "A"-imaging.
"B" : "B"-imaging.
LDL: low-density lipoprotein. Ox-LDL: oxidized low-density lipoprotein. VLDL: very low-density

lipoprotein. HDL: high-density lipoprotein. LPC: lysophosphatidylcholine. PC: phosphatidylcholine. TG: triglyceride. Apo: apolipoprotein. MMP: matrix metalloproteinase. Chole: cholesteryl. 7-Keto chol: 7-ketocholesterol.
B: blue. **Br**: brown. **G**: green. **Go**: gold. **LB**: light blue. **LY**: light yellow. **O**: orange. **P**: purple. **R**: red. **RBr**: reddish brown. **SB**: sky blue. **V**: violet. **W**: white. **Y**: yellow. - : no significant fluorescence.
Underlined colors are characteristic for the corresponding substances.

Table 1. Fluorescence Color of the Major Substances That Comprising Atherosclerotic Plaques

b. Autofluorescence at "B"-imaging

Collagen I and IV exhibit green autofluorescence whereas collagen III and V not. Calcium phosphate, ceramide and β-carotene exhibit yellow, yellow and orange autofluorescence, respectively. Other major subtances comprising atherosclerotic plaques do not exhibit autofluorescence (Table 1).

c. Color fluorescence of major substances that comprising atherosclerotic plaques evoked by markers

Evans blue dye (EB) has been clinically used for intravascular imaging[41-43], and its beneficial effects proved[44].

Oxidized low-density lipoprotein (ox-LDL) does not show autofluorescence, but presents a violet and a reddish brown fluorescence in the presence of EB by "A"- and "B"-imaging, respectively (Figure 4). This combination of fluorescent colors is not exhibited by any other major substances in the atherosclerotic plaques, indicating that this combination of fluorescent colors is due to ox-LDL (Table 1).

TB has been clinically applied for treatment of Tripanosoma parasitemia many years ago[45,46]. Although LPC and TB do not exhibit autofluorescence independently, a red fluorescence is evoked at both "A"- and "B"-imaging when they are mixed together. PC exhibits a pink and an orange fluorescence by "A"- and "B"-imaging, respectively[38] (Figure 4).

Nile blue dye (NB), which has been used as a electromechanical biosensor of DNA[47]. Apolipoprotein B-100 (apo B-100) exhibits no fluorescence at "A"-imaging but exhibits a golden fluorescence in the presence of NB at "B"-imaging (Figure 4, Table 1).

In the presence of a mixture of homidium chloride (Ho) and TB, ox-LDL and LDL exhibit a golden fluorescence whereas LPC and apo B-100 a red fluorescence at "B"-imaging (Table 1).

Since not exhibited by other major substances comprising atherosclerotic plaques, these fluorescent colors can be used for identification of the substances mentioned above.

4. Near-infrared fluorescence (NIRF) of major substances that comprising atherosclerotic plaques

Cholesterol, cholesteryl esters and calcium phosphate (Ca) individually do not exhibit NIRF but exhibit NIRF in the presence of β-carotene which is known to coexists with lipids in the vascular wall. The other substances that are contained in atherosclerotic plaques did not[37] (Figure 5; Table 2).

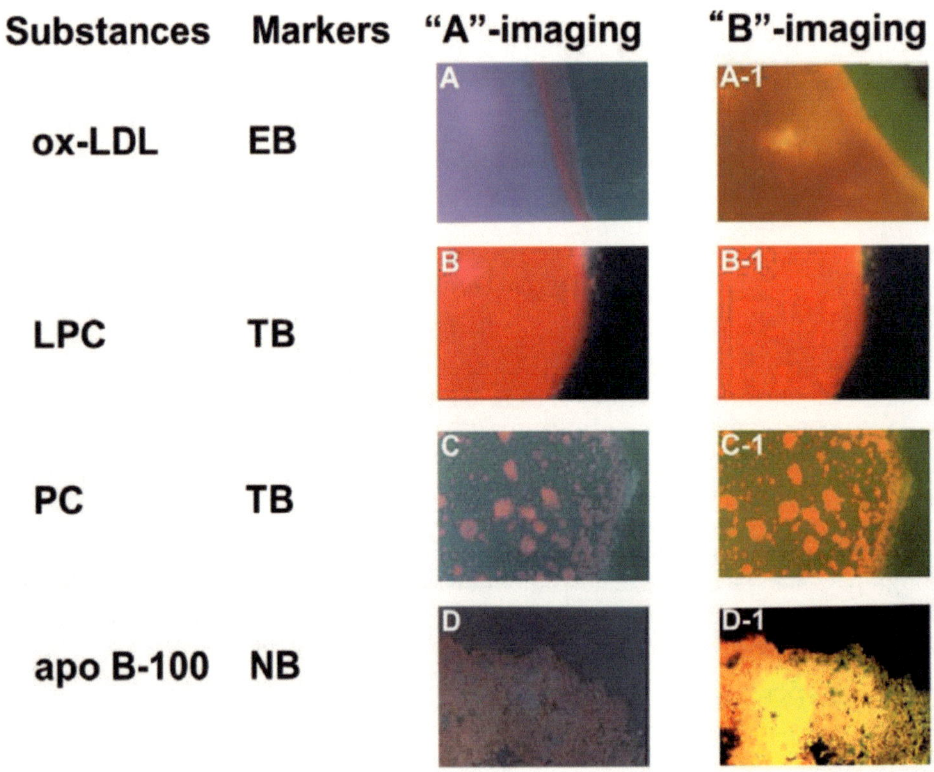

EB: Evans blue. TB: Trypan blue. NB: Nile blue. Ho+TB: Homidium chloride and Trypan blue.

Fig. 4. Fluorescent Colors of Major Lipid Components Evoked by Biocompartible Markers Examined by Microscopy

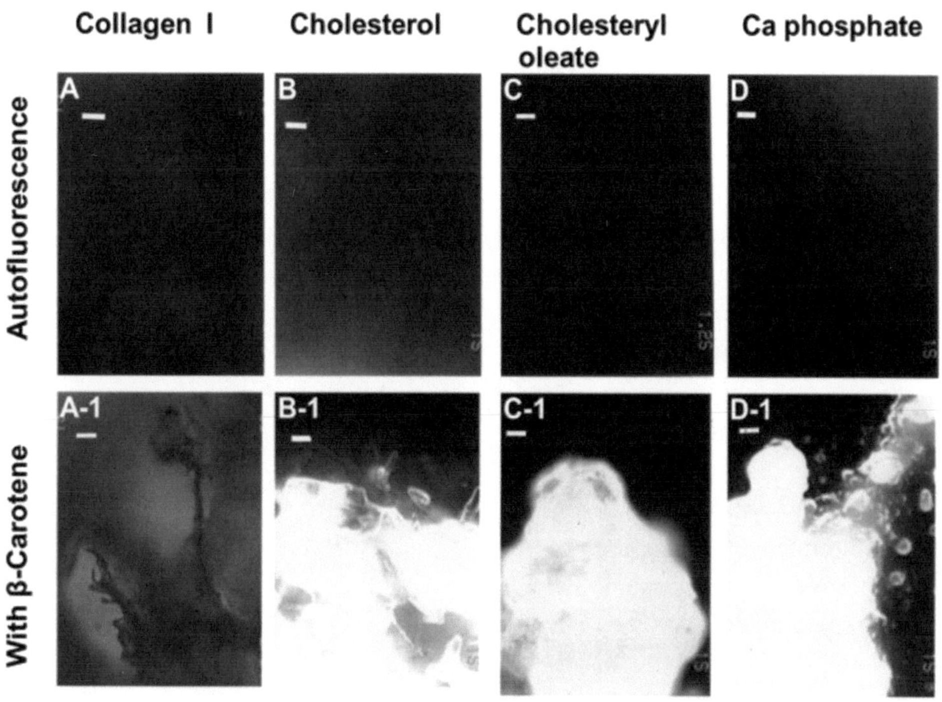

Images before (upper panels) and after mixing with β-carotene (lower panels); From A to D: collagen I, free cholesterol, cholesteryl oleate, calcium phosphate, respectively; From A-1 to D-1: corresponding NIRFM images evoked after mixing with β-carotene (10^{-5}M). Horizontal bar in each panel: 100µm. Cited from Ref. 37, with permission.

Fig. 5. Near-infrared Fluorescent Microscopy (NIRFM) Images of Collagen I, Cholesterol, Choresteryl Oleate and Calcium Phosphate.

Substances		NIRF	
		Autofluorescence	with β-Carotene
Cholesterol	(c)	-	+
Chole oleate	(c)	-	+
Chole linoleate	(c)	-	+
5-Cholesten- 3β-ol	(l)	-	+
7-Ketochol	(c)	-	-
Oleic acid	(c)	-	-
Linoleic acid	(c)	-	-
Ox-LDL	(l)	-	-
LDL	(l)	-	-
VLDL	(l)	-	-
HDL	(l)	-	-
Apo B-100	(c)	-	-
Apo A-1	(c)	-	-
Apo E-2	(c)	-	-
Matrix metalloproteinase-9	(c)	-	-
PC	(c)	-	-
LPC	(c)	-	-
TG	(l)	-	-
Collagens I, III, IV, V	(c)	-	-
Hyaluronic acid	(c)	-	-
Ceramide	(c)	-	±
Heparan sulfate	(c)	-	-
Albumin	(c)	-	-
Globulins	(c)	-	-
Calcium phosphate	(c)	-	+
β-Carotene	(l)	-	

(c): crystal. (l): liquid. - : NIRF absent. ±= NIRF weak. += NIRF strong.

Table 2. Near-infrared Fluorescence (NIRF) of the Major Substances That Comprising Atherosclerotic Plaques

5. Color fluorescent angioscopy of excised human coronary plaques

a. Detection of vulnerable coronary plaques based on collagen subtype imaging

Excised human coronary plaques exhibit blue, green, white-to-light blue, or yellow-to-orange fluorescence. Fluorescent microscopic studies revealed that collagen subtypes, cholesterol, cholesteryl esters, calcium and β-carotene determine the fluorescent color of the plaques[36]. Histological examinations revealed abundant CFs without lipids in blue plaques;

CFs and lipids in green plaques; meager CFs and abundant lipids in white-to-light blue plaques; and the absence of CFs and deposition of lipids, calcium and macrophage foam cells in the thin fibrous cap in yellow-to-orange plaques, indicating that the yellow-to-orange plaques were most vulnerable[36] (Figures 6, 7).

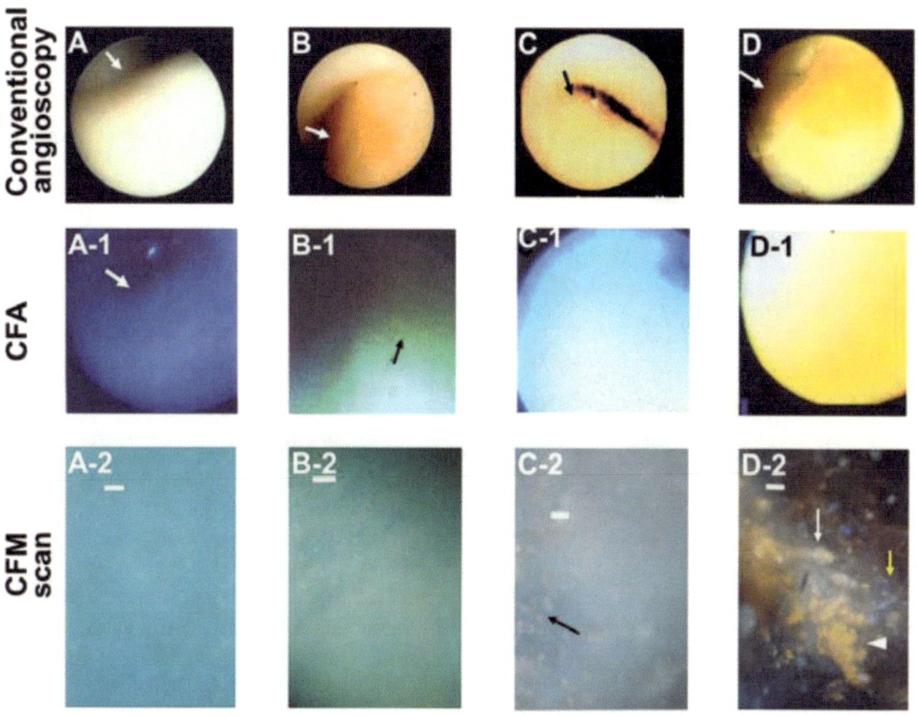

From A to D: conventional angioscopic images of coronary plaques. From A-1 to D-1: corresponding CFA images using "A" imaging. From A-2 to D-2: corresponding CFM scanned images using "A" imaging. Horizontal bar:100 μ m. A: a white plaque observed during conventional angioscopy (arrow) exhibited blue fluorescence by CFA (arrow in A-1) and CFM scan (A-2). B: a yellow plaque observed during conventional angioscopy (arrow) exhibited green fluorescence seen during CFA (arrow in B-1) and CFM scan (arrow in b-2). C: a yellow plaque observed during conventional angioscopy (arrow) exhibited white-to-light blue fluorescence seen during CFA (C-1) and deposition of yellow substances in the white-to-light blue area (arrow in C-2). D: a yellow plaque observed during conventional angioscopy (arrow) exhibited yellow fluorescence observed during CFA (D-2) and deposition of orange (white arrowhead), white (white arrow) and blue (yellow arrow) substances in the area of no fluorescence by CFM scanning. Cited from Ref. 36, with permission.

Fig. 6. Relationships between Images of Coronary Plaques Produced by Conventional Angioscopy, Color Fluorescent Angioscopy (CFA) and Color Fluorescent Microscopy (CFM) Scanning

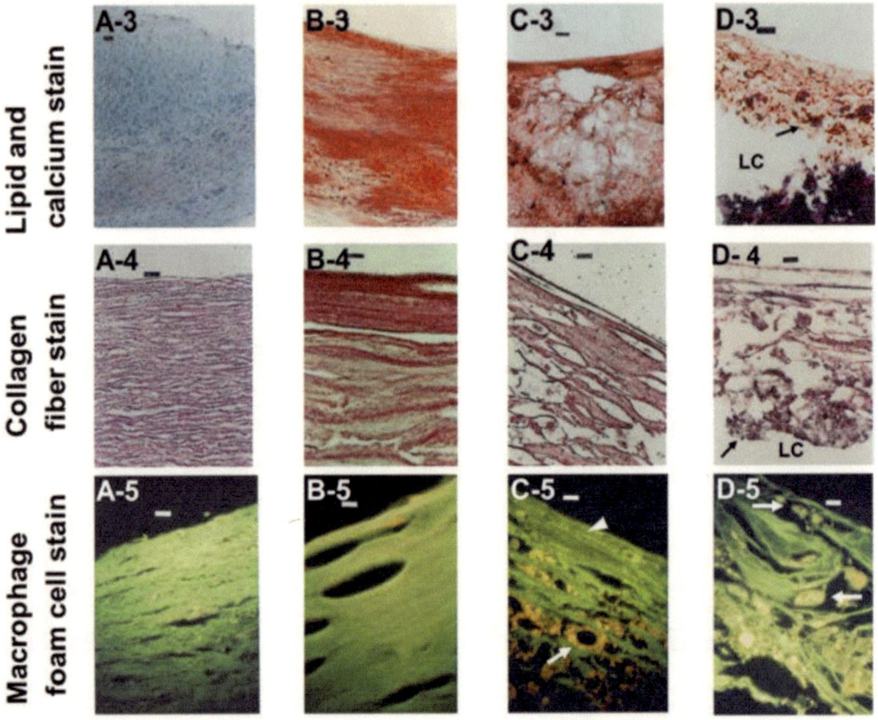

From A-3 to D-3: microscopic images after Oil-red O and methylene blue staining obtained from the same plaques in A, B, C and D as shown in Figure. 6, respectively. Red: lipids. Black: calcium. LC: lipid core. Horizontal bar: 100 μ m. From A-4 to D-4: CFs stained by silver staining. No normal CFs in D-4. Arrow in D-4: plaque debris. Horizontal bar: 20 μ m. From A-5 to D-5: images of ceramide in macrophage foam cells obtained by "B" imaging of CFM after Ziel-Neelsen staining. Orange fluorescence (arrows): ceramide. Arrowhead in C-5: residual CFs. Horizontal bar: 20 μ m. A-3: a plaque without lipids, with abundant normal CFs (A-4) and without macrophage foam cells (A-5). B-3: a plaque with lipids, with thick CFs (B-4) but without macrophage foam cells (b-5). C-3: a plaque with lipid deposition and cavity formation, meager CFs (C-4) and disseminated macrophage foam cells (arrow inC-5). D-3: a plaque with a thin fibrous cap with lipids and calcium (arrow in D-3), without CFs (D-4) and with multiple macrophage foam cells (arrows inD-5). Cited from Ref. 36, with permission.

Fig. 7. Lipids, Calcium Compounds, Collagen Fibers (CFs), and Macrophage Foam Cells in the Same Plaques as Those Shown in Figure. 6.

b. Oxidized low-density lipoprotein (Ox-LDL) imaging

After the administration of EB in an *ex-vivo* study, not only the yellow plaques but also the white plaques studied by conventional angioscopy frequently presented a violet fluorescence by "A"-imaging and a reddish brown fluorescence by "B" imaging, indicating the existence of ox-LDL (Figure 8). The distribution of this fluorescence appeared in a patchy or diffuse manner. There was a tendency for this fluorescent color to appear more frequently in yellow plaques rather than the white plaques classified by conventional angioscopy[36]. By scanning microscopy, a violet and a reddish brown fluorescence distributed diffusely or in web-like configuration, indicating plaque to plaque differences in deposition pattern of ox-LDL[36].

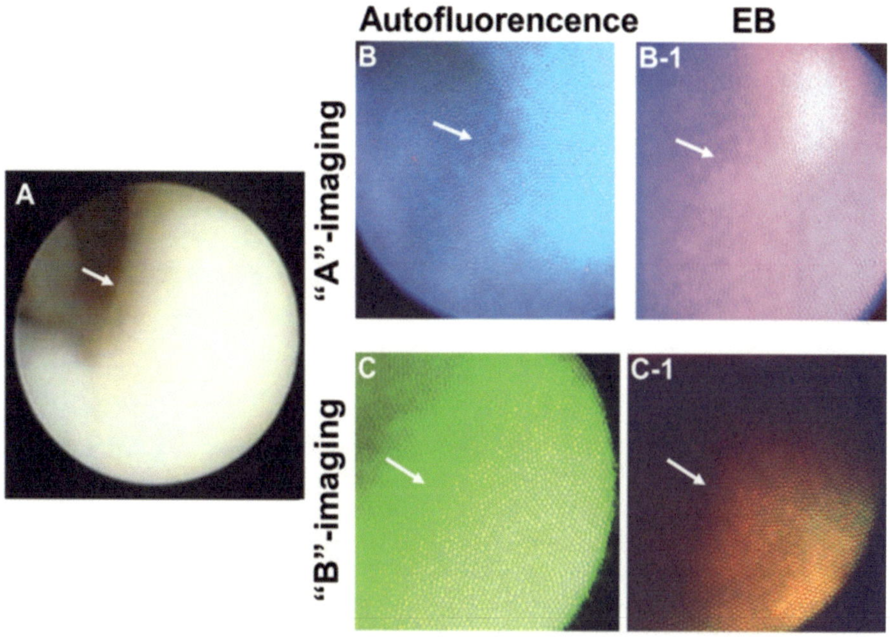

A: a white plaque imaged by conventional angioscopy. Arrow: the portion observed by CFA. B: "A"-image of the same plaque before administration of EB. The plaque showed green autofluorescence, indicating existence of collagens-I and/or -IV (Table 1). B-1: CFA image after administration of EB. The plaque showed diffuse and violet fluorescence. C: "B"-image of the same plaque, showing green autofluorescence. C-1: "B"-image after administration of EB, showing reddish brown fluorescence. This combination of EB-evoked fluorescent color indicates the existence of ox-LDL. Cited from Ref. 36, with permission.
Blue fluorescence (arrowhead in A-1) and green fluorescence(arrowhead in B-1) indicate collagen I and/or IV.

Fig. 8. Ox-LDL in An Excised Coronary Plaque Imaged by Color Fluorescent Angioscopy (CFA)

c. *Lysophosphatidylcholine (LPC) imaging*

The red fluorescence of LPC was investigated by color fluorescent angioscopy in the excised human coronary plaques. This fluorescent color both at "A"-and "B"-imaging was detected frequently by color fluorescent angioscopy in both white and yellow plaques that were classified by conventional angioscopy using white light (Figure 9). As in case of ox-LDL, this fluorescent color was found to be distributed in web-like or diffuse configuration by color fluorescent microscopic scanning[38] (Figure 10).

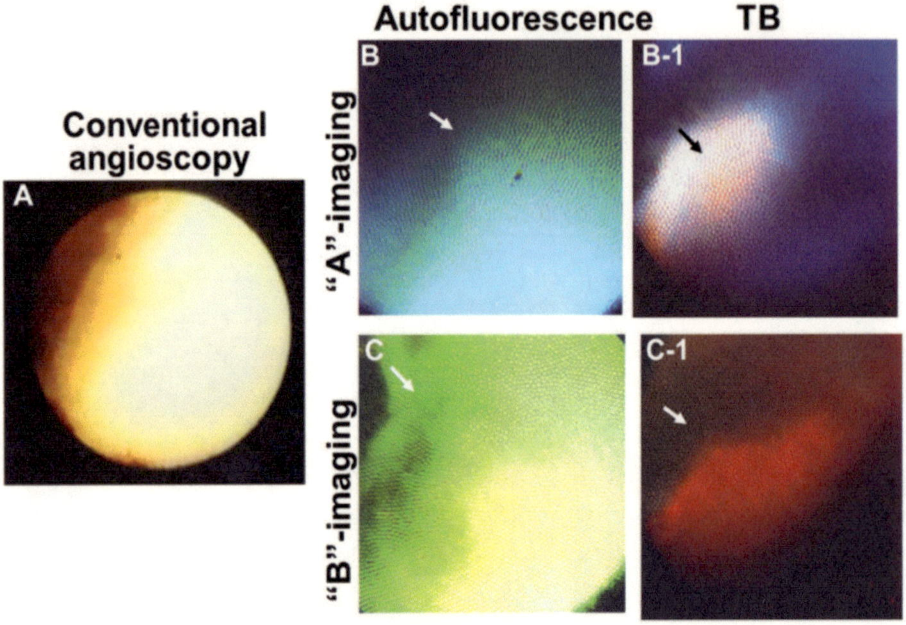

A: a yellow plaque imaged by conventional angioscopy. Arrow: the portion observed by CFA. B and C: CFA images of the same plaque before administration of TB. The plaque showed green and blue fluorescence in mosaic pattern by "A" imaging, and green and yellow fluorescence in mosaic pattern by "B" imaging, indicating the co-existence of collagen I and/or IV and lipids. B-1 and C-1: CFA images after administration of TB. The plaque showed red fluorescence by both" A"-and "B"-imaging, indicating the existence of LPC. Cited from Ref. 38, with permission.

Fig. 9. Lysophosphatidylcholine (LPC) in A Coronary Plaque Imaged by Color Fluorescent Angioscopy (CFA)

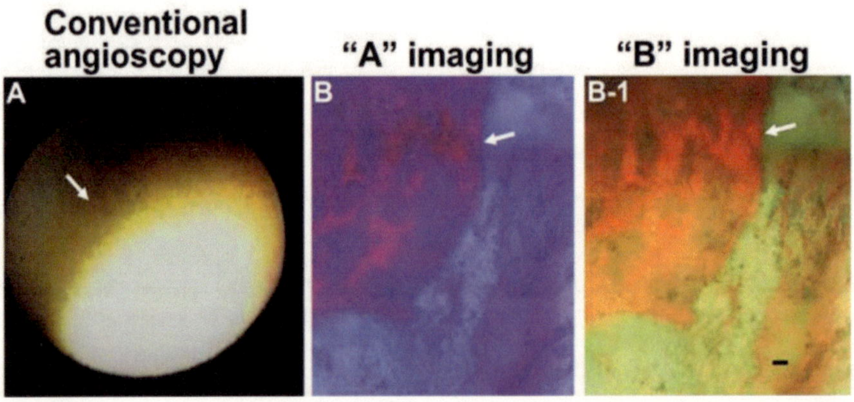

A: yellow plaque imaged by conventional angioscopy. B and B-1: CFM scanned luminal surface of the same plaque after the application of TB, showing wed-like distribution of red fluorescence and therefore web-like deposition of LPC (arrows). Horizontal bar in B-1: 100 μ m. This bar is also applicable to B. Cited from Ref. 38, with permission.

Fig. 10. Distribution Patterns of Lysophosphatidylcholine (LPC) in A Coronary Plaque by Color Fluorescent Microscopy (CFM) Scanning

d. Apo B-100 imaging

In the presence of NB, golden fluorescence, diffuse, spotty or web-like configuration, was observed in excised human coronary arteries by "B"-imaging, indicating deposition of apo B-100. However, the relationship between deposition patterns of this substance and plaque structure by histology is not clarified.

e. Triglyceride (TG) imaging

Imaging of TG, a major component of the core of ox-LDL, by CFA is yet not successful because of a lack in appropriate biocompartible markers.

f. HDL and LDL imaging

Selective imaging of HDL and LDL by fluorescent angioscopy is yet not successful as in case of TG.

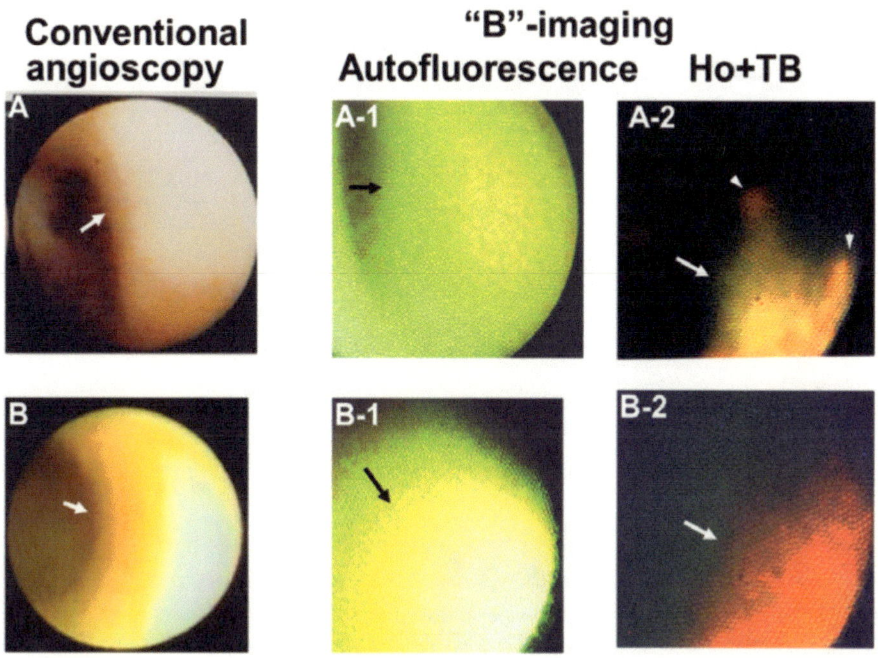

A: Yellow plaque imaged by conventional angioscopy. Arrow: the portion observed by CFA A-1 and A-2: CFA images of the same plaque before and after administration of Ho and TB solution (Ho+TB), respectively. The plaque showed greenish yellow autofluorescence before (arrow in A-1) and red (arrowheads in A-2) and golden fluorescence (arrow in A-2) in a mosaic pattern after the administration of Ho and TB, indicating co-existence of ox-LDL and/or LDL, and LPC and /or apo B-100. B: Yellow plaque by conventional angioscopy (arrow). B-1 and B-2: CFA images before and after administration of Ho and TB solution (Ho+TB), respectively. The plaque showed yellow autofluorescence (arrow in B-1) before and red fluorescence (arrow in B-2) after the administration of Ho and TB solution, indicating deposition of LPC and/or apo B-100.
Cited from Ref. 39, with permission.

Fig. 11. Oxidized Low-density Lipoprotein (Ox-LDL), LDL, Lysophosphatidylcholine (LPC), and Apolipoprotein (ApoB) in Coronary Plaques Imaged by Color Fluorescent Angioscopy (CFA)

g. *Simultaneous imaging of oxidized low-density lipoprotein (Ox-LDL), low-density lipoprotein (LDL), lysophosphatidylcholine (LPC) and apolipoprotein B-100 (apo B-100)*

By "B"-imaging, ox-LDL and LDL (group A) exhibit golden fluorescence, while LPC and apo B-100 (group B) exhibit red fluorescence. By color fluorescent angioscopy, coronary plaques frequently exhibited red and golden fluorescence in a mosaic pattern, indicating co-deposition of A and B. Red fluorescence was also observed in a small number of plaques, indicating solitary deposition of B[39] (Figure 11).

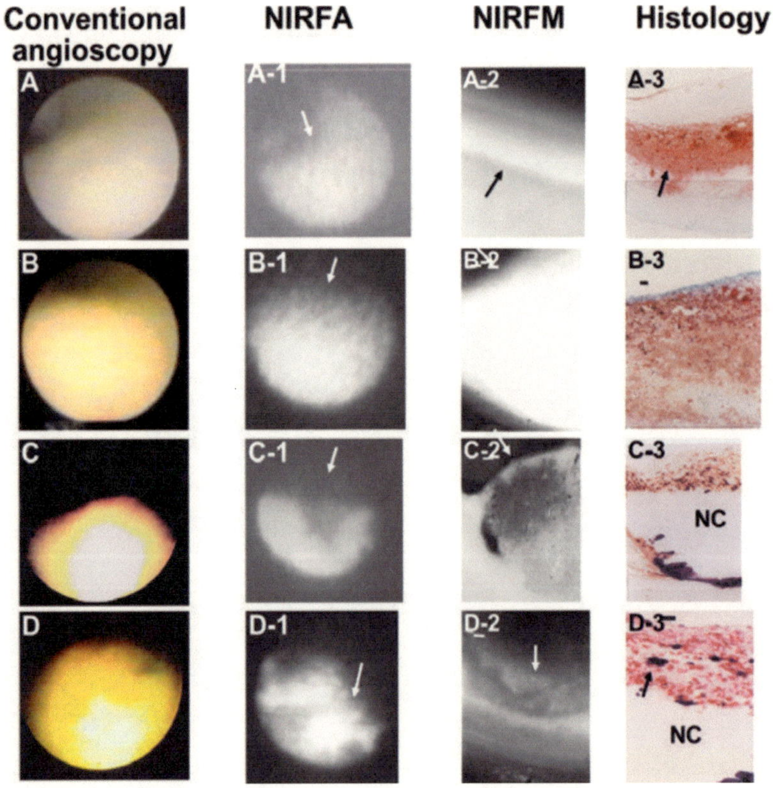

From A to D: the images of coronary plaques by conventional angioscopy.
From A-1 to D-1: corresponding NIRFA images of the same plaques. From A-2 to D-2 : corresponding NIRFM scanned images of the cut wall surface of the same specimens . From A-3 to D-3: corresponding histological images after staining with Oil Red-O and methylene blue. Red and black portions indicate lipids and calcium, respectively. Horizontal bar at the left upper corner of each panel: 100 µm.
A: a white plaque. From B to D: yellow plaques. A-1 and B-1: homogenous type. Arrows: homogenous NIRF; C-1: doughnut-shaped type. Arrow: NIRF absent portion surrounded by strong NIRF region; D-1: spotty type. Arrow: spots. A-2 and B-2: homogenous NIRF (arrows); C-2 : necrotic core lacking NIRF (arrow) surrounded by strong NIRF region; D-2: fibrous cap with strong NIRF spots (arrow). A-3: homogenous deposition of lipids deep in the plaque (arrow); B-3: lipid deposition in entire plaque. C-3: lipid-deposited fibrous cap with a necrotic core (NC) belowD-3: calcium particles distributed within a lipid-laden fibrous cap. Red: lipids. Black: calcium compounds (arrow).
Horizontal bar: 100µm. Cited from Ref. 37, with permission.

Fig. 12. Relationships Among Conventional Angioscopic, Near-infrared Fluorescent Angioscopic (NIRFA), and Near-infrared Fluorescent Microscopic (NIRFM) Scanned Images and Histological Changes in Excised Human Coronary Plaques.

6. Near-infrared fluorescent angioscopy of excised human coronary plaques

a. Cholesterol (C) and cholesteryl ester (CE) imaging

In an ***ex-vivo*** study, excised human coronary plaques were classified as those with NIRF and those without. The former plaques were classified into homogenous, doughnut-shaped and spotty types[37].

Histological examinations revealed that these image patterns were determined by the differences in the locations of cholesterol, cholesteryl esters and Ca, and that those deposited within 700 μm in depth from plaque surface were imaged by NIRFA[37] (Figure 12).

7. Clinical application of fluorescent angioscopy

a. Oxidized low-density lipoprotein (ox-LDL)

In our catheterization laboratory, CFA was performed during routine coronary angioscopy in patients with coronary artery disease.

After selective injection of the EB solution into the coronary artery, not only the plaques but also the apparently normal coronary segments frequently exhibited a reddish brown fluorescence by "B"-imaging, indicating the existence of ox-LDL[36] (Figure 13).

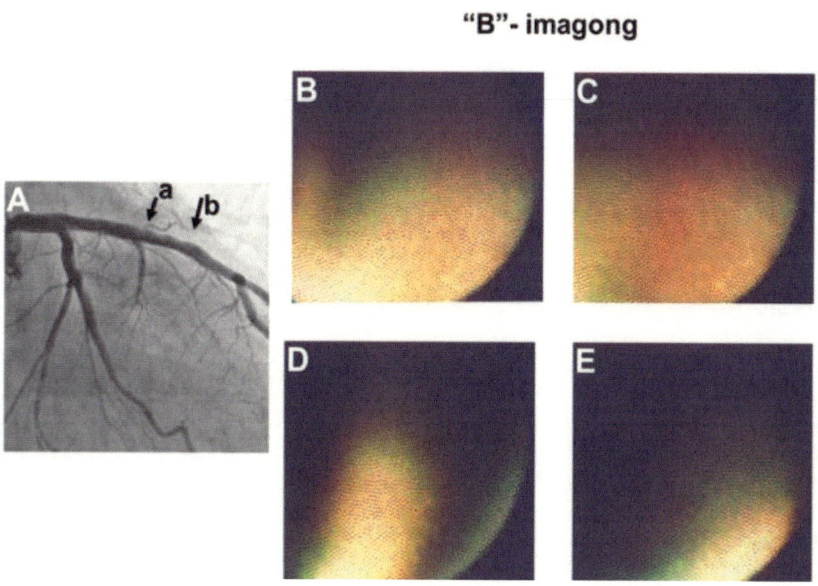

Reddish brown fluorescence observed in a non-stenotic proximal segment of the left anterior descending coronary artery after the intracoronary injection of EB in a patient with stable angina pectoris.
A: an angiogram of the left coronary artery. Arrows a to b: the proximal segment observed by CFA. The wall of the segment was uneven but significant stenosis was not found.
From .B to E: CFA images of the same segment obtained after injecting EB, by advancing the angioscope distally from a to b of panel A. Reddish brown portions indicate ox-LDL. The luminal surface was uneven, indicating early stage of atherosclerosis. Cited from Ref. 36, with permission.

Fig. 13. Ox-LDL Imaged by "B"-imaging of Color Fluorescent Angioscopy (CFA) in the Coronary Artery in A Patient with Angina Pectoris

b) Cholesterol and cholesteryl esters

The present authors examined coronary plaques by NIRFA during coronary angiography in 25 patients with coronary artery disease. Figure 14 shows a yellow plaque by conventional angioscopy. This plaque exhibited homogenous NIRF, indicating homogenous deposition of cholesterol and/ or choresteryl esters. Homogenous, doughnut-shaped or spotty NIRFA images were also observed in patients[37].

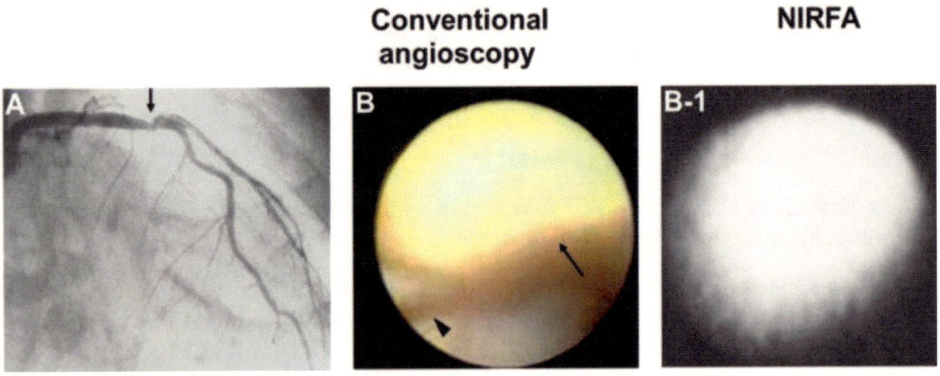

From A to C: angiogram, conventional angioscopic image and NIRFA image of a plaque in the proximal segment of the left anterior descending coronary artery (arrow in A). The yellow plaque (arrow in B) presented a homogenous type NIRF image (B-1). Arrowhead: guide wire.
Cited from Ref. 37, with permission.

Fig. 14. Near-infrared Fluorescent Angioscopy (NIRFA) Study in a 61-year-old Male with Stable Angina.

8. Discussion

The use of an antibody of individual components that comprising vessel wall is a more specific indicator for their imaging *in-vivo*. However, there are many limitations to its clinical application. Therefore, the use of a low molecular weight substance that selectively binds to individual components and presents specific fluorescence color is another option that can be used for the imaging of individual lipid components.

In the present study, low molecular weight dyes with, EB, TB, NB, Ho+TB were found to evoke fluorescence specific to ox-LDL and its components except TG and Schiff base. Thus, visualization of ox-LDL and its major components in a given plaque was achieved, enabling analysis of the differences in their deposition patterns in human coronary plaques. The mechanisms by which these dyes evoked fluorescence are not known. One possibility is that dyes became conjugated to the target substances to form an adduct to provoke a fluorescent color specific to individual substances.

Ox-LDL, which plays an important role in the initiation, progression and destabilization of atherosclerotic plaques, became visible for the first time by CFA in patients. Furthermore, the substances that comprising ox-LDL became visible by CFA or NIRFA in excised human coronary arteries.

However, CFA and NIRFA have been limited to collagen subtypes, ox-LDL, cholesterol and cholesteryl esters in clinical situations. Imaging of other substances by CFA or NIRFA in patients is yet not performed because clinical applicability of biocompartible markers other than EB is not established.

Fluorescent angioscopy faced some shortcomings; (1) The visualization by CFA is limited only to the substances deposited within 200μm from the vascular luminal surface and by NIRFA within 700 μm (Table 3). Therefore deposits in the deeper layers can not be analyzed by this system of CFA and NIRFA. (2) Differing in function to antibodies, biomarkers employed in CFA do not selectively bind to the target substance, and therefore, there may be other unknown substances which exhibit the same fluorescent color in the presence of the markers used. (3) Because a lens is used, the pictures obtained by CFA and NIRFA are fish-eye images and therefore quantitative assessment of the target substance is difficult (Table 3).

	Conventional angioscopy	CFA	NIRFA
1. Simultaneous visualization of two or more substances[39]	yes	yes	no
2. Determination of substance	no	yes	yes
3. Quantitative measurement of substances[41]			
Size	no	no	no
Density	no	no	no
Distance from luminal surface	no	no	no
4. Depth from luminal surface to the substances which can be visualized[37]	100-200 μm	200 μm	700 μm
5. Two-dimensional imaging	yes	yes	yes

CFA: color fluorescent angioscopy. NIRFA: near-infrared fluorescent angioscopy.

Table 3. Advantages and Disadvantages of Angioscopy

At present, imaging by fluorescent angioscopy is limited to several substances that comprise coronary plaques. By selecting adequate biomarkers, the substances other than those mentioned above may become visible.

Fluorescent angioscopy was established only recently and therefore its clinical application is limited to a few laboratories. As in spectroscopy, this technique will become prevalent when clinically applicable biomarkers for the substances comprising atherosclerotic lesions become complete.

9. Conclusion

LDL has cortex and core. The cortex is composed of PC, free cholesterol and apo B-100, and the core is composed of TG and cholesteryl esters. Ox-LDL is derived from LDL by oxidation of its component PC into LPC and apo B-100 into Shiff base, and plays an important role in the initiation, progression and destabilization of atherosclerotic plaques by inducing the proliferation and elongation of survival of macrophages.

We succeeded in molecular imaging of ox-LDL not only in the excised human coronary plaques but also in coronary arteries in patients ***in-vivo*** by CFA using EB as a biomarker. Also, LPC, apo B-100, free cholesterol, and cholesteryl esters in human coronary plaques became visible by either CFA or NIRFA. These imaging techniques will give us much information which is otherwise not obtainable on the mechanisms of atherosclerosis in clinical situation.

10. References

[1] Ge J, Baumgart D, Hauda M, et al. Role of intravascular ultrasound imaging in identifying vulnerable plaques. Herz. 1999; 24: 32-41.

[2] Jang IK, Tearney GJ, MacNeil B, et al. In vivo characterization of coronary atherosclerotic plaque by use of optical coherence tomography. Circulation. 2005; 111: 1551-1555.

[3] Uchida Y. Coronary Angioscopy. Futura Publishing Co, NY, 2001: 11-81

[4] Uchida Y, Prediction of acute coronary syndromes by percutaneous angioscopy in patients with stable angina. Am Heart J 1995, 130: 195-203.

[5] Thieme T, Wernecke KD, Meyer R, et al. Angioscopic evaluation of atherosclerotic plaques: validation by histomorphologic analysis and association with stable and unstable coronary syndromes. J Am Coll Cardiol 1996; 28: 1-6.

[6] Uchida Y, Uchida Y, Hiruta N. Histological characteristics of glistening yellow coronary plaques seen on angioscopy: with special reference to vulnerable plaques. Circ J. 2011; 75: 1913-1919.

[7] Matsuura E, Hughes GR, Khamashta MA. Oxidation of LDL and its clinical implication. Autoimmun Rev. 2008; 7: 558-566.

[8] Chen JH, Riazzy, Smith EM, Proud CG, Steinbrecher UP, Duronio V. Oxidized LDL-mediated macrophage survival involves elongation of factor-2 kinase. Arterioscler Thromb Vasc Biol 2009; 29: 92-98.

[9] Katsuda S, Okada Y, Minamoto T, Matsui Y, Nakanishi I. Collagens in human atherosclerosis: Immunohistochemical analysis using collagen type-specific antibodies. Atheroscler Thromb. 1992; 12:494-502.

[10] Murata K, Motoyama T. Collagen species in various sized arteries, their changes with intimal proliferation. Artery. 1990; 17: 96-106.

[11] Murata K, Kotake C, Motoyama T: Collagen species in human aorta: with special reference to basement membrane-associated collagens in the intima and media and their alteration with atherosclerosis. Artery. 1987; 14: 229-247.

[12] Shah PK, Falk E, Badimon JJ, et al. Human monocyte-derived macrophages induce breakdown in fibrous caps of atherosclerotic plaques. Potential role of matrix-metalloproteinases and implication for plaque rupture. Circulation 1995; 92: 1565-1569.

[13] Takano T, Itabe H, Mori M, et al. Molecular pathology in atherosclerosis: the mechanisms by which cholesteryl ester accumulates in atherosclerotic aorta. Yakugaku Zasshi. 2008; 128: 1383-1401.

[14] Li W, Yuan XM, Olsson AG, Brunk UT. Uptake of oxidized LDL by macrophages results in partial lysosomal enzyme inactivation and relocation. Arterioscler Thromb Vasc Biol. 1998; 18: 177-184.

[15] Grandl M, Bared SM, Liebisch G, Werner T, Barlage S, Schmitz G. E-LDL and ox-LDL differentially regulate ceramide and cholesterol raft microdomains in human macrophages. Cytometry A. 2006; 69: 189-191.

[16] Tardif JC. Emerging high-density lipoprotein infusion therapies: fulfilling the promise of epidemiology? J Clin Lipidol. 2010; 4: 399-404.

[17] Negi S, Ballantyne CM. Insights from recent meta-analysis: role of high-density lipoprotein cholesterol in reducing cardiovascular events and rates of atherosclerotic disease progression. J Clin Lipidol. 2010; 4: 365-370.

[18] Vilani SS, Nambi V. The role of lipoprotein-associated phospholipase A_2 as a marker of atherosclerosis. Curr Atheroscler Rep 2007; 9: 97-103.

[19] Erdogan A, Schaefer MB, Kulmann CR, Most A, Hartmann M, Mayer K, Renner FC, Schaefer C, Abdallah Y, Hoelschermann H, Schaefer CA. Activation of Ca2+-induced potassium channels is involved in lysophosphatidylcholine-induced monocyte adhesion to endothelial cells. Atherosclerosis. 2007; 190: 100-105.

[20] Matsubara M, Hasegawa K. Benipine, a dihydopyridine-calcium channel blocker, prevents lysophosphatidylcholine-induced injury and reactive oxygen species production in human aortic endothelial cells. Atherosclerosis. 2005; 178: 57-66.

[21] Matsumoto T, Kobayashi T, Kamata K. Role of lysophosphadidylcholine (LPC) in atherosclerosis. Curr Med Chem. 2007; 14: 3209-3220.

[22] Stollenberk MM, Svensson O, Schiopu A, Jansson B, Arnebrant T, Fredrikson GN. A desorption of low-density lipoprotein, its oxidation, and subsequent binding of specific recombinant antibodies: an in situ ellipsometric study. Biochim Acta. 2011; 1810: 211-217.

[23] Kanani FH, Alam JM. Apolipoprotein B in type 2 diabetes—a cross sectional study in a tertiary care set-up. J Pak Med Assoc. 2010; 60: 653-656.

[24] Holewijn S, den Heijer M, Swinkels DW, Stalenhoef AF, de Graaf J. Apolipoprotein B, non-HDL cholesterol and LDL cholesterol for identifying individuals at increased cardiovascular risk. J Intern Med. 2010; 68: 567-677.

[25] Enkhmaa B, Annurad E, Zhang Z, Pearson TA, Berglund L. Usefulness of apolipoprotein B/ apolipoprotein A-1 ration to predict coronary artery disease independent of the metabolic syndrome in African Americans. Am J Cardiol. 20210; 106: 1264-1269.

[26] Kappelle PJ, Gansevoort RT, Hillege JL, Wolffenbultel BH, Dullaart RP. Apolipoprotein B/A-1 and total cholesterol/high-density lipoprotein cholesterol rations both predict cardiovascular events in the general population independently of nonlipid risk factors, albuminuria and C-reactive protein. J Interm Med. 2011; 269: 232-242

[27] Lee YH, Choi SH, Lee KW, Kim DJ. Apolipoprotein B/A1 ratio is associated with free androgen index and visceral adiposity and may be an indicator of metabolic syndrome in male children and adolescence. Clin Endoclinol. 2011; 74: 579-588

[28] Rosenson RS, Carlson DM, Kelly MT, Setze CM, Hirshberg B, Stolzenbach JC, Williams LA. Achievement of lipid targets with combination of rosuvastatin and fenofibric acid in patients with type 2 diabetes mellitus. Cardiovasc Drugs Ther. 2011; 25: 47-57

[29] Labreuche J, Touboul PJ, Amarenco P. Plasma triglyceride levels and risk of stroke and carotid atherosclerosis: a systematic review of the epidemiological studies. Atherosclerosis. 2009; 203: 331-345.

[30] Gandotra P, Miller M. The role of triglycerides in cardiovascular risk. Curr Cardiol Rep. 2008; 10: 505-511.

[31] Colley CS, Kazarian SG, Weinberg PD, Lever MJ. Spectroscopic imaging of arteries and atherosclerotic plaques. Biopolymers. 2004; 74: 328-335.
[32] Krisko A, Stjepanoic G, Pifat G, Ruysechaert JM, Goormaghtigh E. Detection of apolipoprotein B 100 early conformatical changes during oxidation. Biochim Biophys Acta. 2007; 1768: 2923-2930.
[33] Garg S, Serruys PW, van der Ent M, Schultz C, Mastik F, van Soest G, van der Steen AF, Wilder JE, Regar E. First use in patients of a combined infra-red spectroscopy and intra-vascular ultrasound catheter to identify composition and structure of coronary plaque. Eurointervention. 2010; 5: 755-756.
[34] Li D, Patel AR, Klibanov AL, Kramer CM, Ruiz M, Kang BY, Mehta JL, Beller GA, Glover DK, Meyer CH. Molecular imaging of atherosclerotic plaques targeted to oxidized LDL receptor LOX-1 by SPECT/CT and magnetic resonance. Circ Cardiovasc Imaging. 2010; 3: 464-472.
[35] Briley-Saebo KC, Shaw PX, Mulder WJ, Choi SH, Vucic E, Aguinaldo JG, Wiltztum JL, Fuster V, Tsimikas S, Fayad ZA. Targeted molecular probes for imaging atherosclerotic lesions with magnetic resonance using antibodies that recognize oxidation-specific epitopes. Circulation. 2008; 117: 3206-3215.
[36] Uchida Y, Uchida Y, Kawai S, Kanamaru R, Sugiyama Y, Tomaru T, Maezawa Y, Kameda N. Detection of vulnerable coronary plaques by color fluorescent angioscopy. JACC Cardiovasc Imaging. 2010; 3: 398-408.
[37] Uchida Y, Uchida Y, Sugiyama Y, Kanai M, Sakurai T, Shirai S. Two-dimensional visualization of cholesterol and cholesteryl esters within human coronary plaques by near-infrared fluorescence angioscopy. Clinical Cardiology. 2010; 33: 322-325.
[38] Uchida Y, Uchida Y, Kawai S, Kanamaru R, Kameda N. Imaging of lysophosphatidylcholine in human coronary plaques by color fluorescence angioscopy. Int Heart J. 2010; 51: 129-133.
[39] Uchida Y, Uchida Y, Kameda N. Visualization of lipid components in human coronary plaques using color fluorescence angioscopy. Circ J. 2010; 74: 2181-2186.
[40] Uchida Y. Recent advances in coronary angioscopy. J Cardiol. 2011; 57: 18-30.
[41] Uchida Y. Angioscopy system. In Coronary angioscopy, Uchida Y (ed), Futura Publishing INC, Armonk, NY, 2001; 11-103.
[42] Uchida Y, Nakamura F, Tomaru T. Observation of atherosclerotic lesions by an intravascular microscope in patients with arteriosclerosis obliterance. Am Heart J. 1995; 130: 1114-1117.
[43] Uchida Y, Uchida Y, Sakurai T, Kanai M, Shirai S, Morita T.Characterization of coronary fibrin thrombus in patients with acute coronary syndrome using dye-staining angioscopy. ArteriosclerThromb Vasc Biol. 2011; 31: 1452-1460.
[44] Uchida Y, Uchida H. Therapeutic tool for vascular disease. United States Patent. US7025981 B2, 2006.
[45] Ralph P, Nakoinz I. Environmental and chemical dissociation of antibody-dependent phagocytosis from lysis mediated by macrophages: stimulation of lysis by sulfhydryl-blocking and elastase-inhibitory agents and depression by trypan blue and trypsin. Cell Immunol 1980; 50: 94-105.
[46] Brooks BO, Reed ND. The effect of trypan blue on the early control of Trypanosoma musculi parasitemia in mice. J Reticuloendothel Soc. 1979; 25: 325-328.
[47] Chen ZW, Balamurungan A, Chen SM. Detection of DNA by using bio-conducting polymer-Nile blue composite electrode; Nile blue as an indicator. Bioelectrochemistry. 2009; 75: 13-18.

12

Molecular Imaging of Tumor Angiogenesis

Shaunagh McDermott and Alexander Guimaraes
Massachusetts General Hospital, USA

1. Introduction

Molecular imaging has recently been defined by the Society of Nuclear Medicine as 'the visualization, characterization, and measurement of biological processes at the molecular and cellular levels in humans and other living systems' (Mankoff 2007). It usually exploits specific labeled molecular probes, as well as intrinsic tissue characteristics as the source of image contrast, and uses a number of molecular imaging modalities, including magnetic resonance imaging, optical imaging, targeted ultrasound, single photon emission tomography and positron emission tomography (Massoud and Gambhir 2003).

Angiogenesis is the development of new vasculature from pre-existing blood vessels and/or circulating endothelial calls (Bergers and Benjamin 2003). It is well established that angiogenesis is one of the key aspects in the growth and metastasis of solid tumors (Folkman 1995; Ferrara and Kerbel 2005). Typically tumor-associated angiogenesis goes through two phases, an avascular and a vascular phase that are separated by the 'angiogenic switch'. The avascular phase of tumors corresponds to small and occult lesions that stay dormant and subsist on diffusion of nutrients from the host microvasculature. After reaching a certain size (usually around 1-2mm), a small subset of dormant tumors enter the vascular phase in which exponential tumor growth ensues. Angiogenesis is a complex multistep process regulated by many factors. At the onset of angiogenesis, a number of pro-angiogenic growth factors (e.g. vascular endothelial growth factors, platelet derived growth factor, fibroblast growth factors) and proteolytic enzymes (e.g. metalloproteinases, cathepsin cysteine proteases, plasmin) are secreted into the interstitium. This leads to degradation of basal membrane surrounding the pre-existing vasculature, along with proliferation and migration of smooth muscle and endothelial cells. All these events lead to the alignment and organization of endothelial cells to form new vessels and a vascular network within the tumor (Ferrara and Kerbel 2005).

Tumor angiogenesis is not simply the production of an increased number of blood vessels to serve a growing mass. Although the main purpose of tumor angiogenesis can be considered to maintain a cancer's blood supply, the process occurs in an unmitigated fashion, and the resultant vascular network is highly abnormal. This profoundly aberrant vasculature dramatically alters the tumor microenvironment and influences heavily the ways in which cancers grow and progress, escape the host's immune system, metastasize, and respond to anticancer therapies.

The heterogeneity in vessel distribution and haphazard anatomical arrangement of the vasculature cause spatial and temporal heterogeneity in blood flow, with areas of hypervasularity adjacent to hypovascular ones (Tong, Boucher et al. 2004). Also, the structural abnormalities of the tumor vasculature lead to a marked increase in vessel leakiness. As a consequence, there is a protein and fluid build-up in the tumor interstitium. This excess extravasation of protein increases the extravascular oncotic pressure, dragging further fluid into the interstitial space (Stohrer, Boucher et al. 2000; Tong, Boucher et al. 2004). Furthermore, there is an absence of functional intratumoral lymphatic vessels, resulting in the impaired clearance of extracellular fluid and hence interstitial hypertension within tumors. The raised intratumoral interstitial fluid pressure (IFP) reduces the hydrostatic pressure gradient between the intravascular and extravascular compartments such that the two essentially equilibrate, which reduces transvascular flow. Also, the mechanical stress from the solid mass of proliferating cancer cells and the matrix is able to collapse tumor vessels, closing the lumen through compressive forces (Padera, Stoll et al. 2004). This combination of regional poor perfusion, raised IFP, and areas of vascular collapse produces regional hypoxia and acidosis within tumors (Helmlinger, Yuan et al. 1997). Aberrations in the tumor vasculature have great implications for tumor sensitivity to therapy. Hypoxia is a well-known mediator of cancer cell resistance to conventional radiotherapy and cytotoxics (Teicher 1996; Wouters and Brown 1997). Moreover, the poor blood supply and raised intratumoral IFP (leading to a reduction in transvacular flow) impair the delivery of systemically administered therapies to tumors such as conventional cytotoxics and monoclonal antibodies (Jain 1989; Tong, Boucher et al. 2004).

With the discovery of vascular endothelial growth factor (VEGF) as a major driver of tumor angiogenesis, efforts were focused on novel therapeutics aimed at inhibiting VEGF activity, with the goal of regressing tumors by starvation. Unfortunately, clinical trials of anti-VEGF monotherapy in patients with solid tumors have been largely negative (Jain, Duda et al. 2006). Intriguingly, the combination of anti-VEGF therapy with conventional chemotherapy has improved survival in cancer patients compared with chemotherapy alone (Sandler, Gray et al. 2006; Saltz, Clarke et al. 2008). In 2001, a 'vascular normalization' hypothesis was proposed to explain this paradox (Jain 2001). The normalization hypothesis suggests that by correcting the abnormalities in structure and function of tumor vessels (rather than destroying vessels completely) we can normalize the tumor microenvironment and ultimately control tumor progression and improve response to other therapies (Jain 2005).

Non-invasive imaging of tumor angiogenesis will allow for much earlier detection of tumors and also the development of surrogate markers for assessing response to treatment.

2. Imaging of angiogenesis

Imaging angiogenesis has been focused into three different arenas: 1) kinetic imaging using dynamic tracking of contrast administration; 2) steady state blood volume determinations of neovascular density; and 3) specific molecular markers of angiogenesis.

2.1 Kinetic imaging using dynamic tracking of contrast material

Dynamic contrast-enhanced imaging is a noninvasive technique that can provide parameters related to tissue perfusion and permeability for examination of the tumor vasculature.

2.1.1 Dynamic contrast-enhanced ultrasound

Contrast-enhanced ultrasound (CEU) imaging is based on the reception, analysis and display of acoustic signals produced by reflection or backscatter of sound (echo) with use of contrast agents. The most commonly used contrast agent are microbubbles that are gas-liquid emulsions consisting of a gaseous core (e.g. perfluorocarbon, sulfur hexfluoride, or nitrogen) that is enclosed by a shell composed of biocompatible materials (albumin, galactose, lipids, polymers). The gaseous core of the microbubbles causes a very high echogenic response following insonification with ultrasound, resulting in high contrast-to-tissue background ratio. Owing to their micron size (usually ranging in size between 1 and 4 μm in diameter), these microbubbles stay within the vascular compartment, and do not leak out into the extra-vascular space (Deshpande, Pysz et al. 2010). Thus, microbubbles are highly suitable for imaging angiogenic markers that are over expressed on tumor vascular endothelial cells (Deshpande, Needles et al. 2010).

Following intravenous administration, microbubbles do not coalesce to form emboli, but dissolve leaving remnants that are easily metabolized or excreted. Further, biodistribution studies revealed that microbubbles have low circulation residence times as they are rapidly removed by the reticuloendothelial system (Perkins, Frier et al. 1997; Weskott 2008; Willmann, Cheng et al. 2008). To increase the circulation time of the microbubbles in serum, additional coatings, such as polyethylene glycol polymer arms are added onto the microbubble shell. Additionally these coatings help stabilize the microbubble by providing additional steric protection, preventing aggregation and help escape immune surveillance by the body (Klibanov 2009).

To make ultrasound a molecular imaging tool, contrast microbubbles can be functionalized with ligands such as antibodies or peptides that bind molecular marker of interest with high affinity (Klibanov, Hughes et al. 1999). These binding ligands can either be coupled to the microbubbles using non-covalent attachment, or chemical conjugation (Klibanov 2005), or they can be integrated into the microbubble shell directly during the production process or after manufacturing (Pochon, Tardy et al. 2010; Pysz, Foygel et al. 2010).

The huge benefit of using microbubbles is that the microcirculation can be detected. Since the nonlinear signals from microbubbles occur regardless of their motion and equally when they are stationary, CE US detects the capillary bed, which is by far the largest part of the microcirculation. Of course, its spatial resolution is limited, so that individual capillaries cannot be discerned, but the microbubble content gives rise to a signal 'wash' whose intensity is proportional to the microbubble concentration and thus to the blood volume in that portion of tissue (Figure 1).

To estimate or measure perfusion, the essential tool is the transit or wash-in, wash-out curve, often referred to as the time-intensity curve (TIC) in which the time course of the transit of the microbubbles across a region of interest (ROI) is measured (Cosgrove and Lassau 2010). Two families of information are available from these TICs, those that depend on timing events, such as the arrival time and the time to peak enhancement, and those that depend on the amount of enhancement detected, such as the peak enhancement and the area under the TIC. These indices are rather more complex as they rely on a number of key assumptions. One is that the signal strength is proportional to the microbubble concentration (Blomley, Albrecht et al. 1997; Claassen, Seidel et al. 2001). Another assumption is that all the non-linear signals in the ROI do emanate from the microbubbles, rather than from tissue.

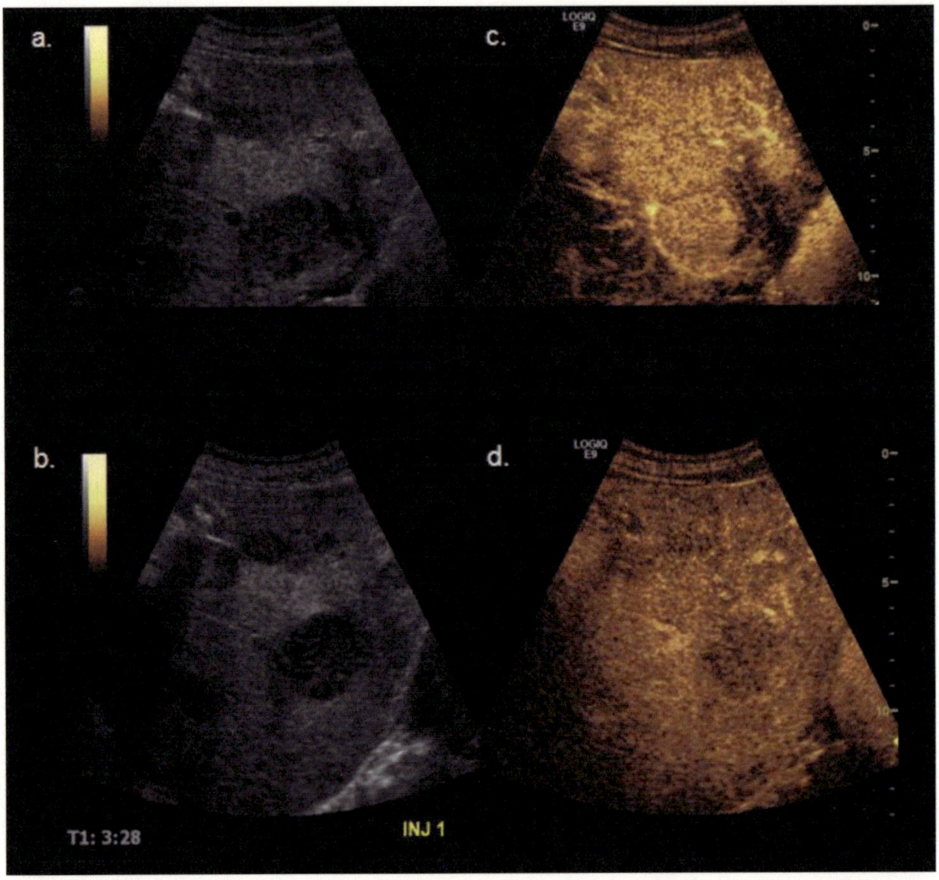

Fig. 1. Four images from a patient with pathologic proven rectal neuroendocrine tumor that is metastatic to the right lobe of the liver. (a) & (b) are conventional ultrasound images of the right lobe of the liver which demonstrates a well circumscribed, hypoechoic mass. (c) & (d) are contrast mode rapid ultrasound following injection of ~3 x 10^{-8} microbubbles that are approximately 2.5 microns in size in a volume of 2.4mL. Panels (c) and (d) demonstrate different timepoints which demonstrate enhancement of the tumor fairly homogenously in (c), and in (d) washout of the tumor with enhancement of the hepatic venous system. (Figure from Dhyani & Samir et. al. unpublished data)

The other way to generate boluses of contrast depends on the unique interaction between the imaging beam and the contrast agent: microbubbles are destroyed by higher intensity ultrasound which causes them to oscillate wildly and in complex patterns such that the gas escapes and the contrast effect is lost. The readiness with which this happens depends on the robustness of the shell, but for the commonly used clinical agent it is well within those licensed by regulatory agencies (usually a mechanical index (MI) of 1.9 is allowable). In a typical set-up, an infusion of microbubbles is used to achieve a steady blood concentration, and then a series of pulses at high MI is sent into the ROI before the system is switched back to a low MI microbubble-specific mode for imaging (Wei, Jayaweera et al. 1998). The progressive inflow of the microbubbles in the cleared region can then be observed and the accumulation plotted. It takes the form of a rising exponential whose initial slope, β, is related to the flow rate and whose maximum value, A, is related to the equilibrium concentration of the microbubbles, also known as the fractional vascular volume. The formula that is usually deployed is:

$$R = A\,(1\text{-}e^{(-\beta t)}) \tag{1}$$

though other approximations can be used (Lucidarme, Kono et al. 2003). An important difference between ultrasound and most other contrast agents should be stressed here: because of their relatively large size, microbubbles do not diffuse across the endothelium and into the interstitial space, unlike the ionic agents used for CT and MR. Advantages of this 'destruction reperfusion' method are its ready repeatability and the clean inflow function - there is no blurring effect from the upstream circulation as occurs following an iv bolus.

The breast was one of the first tumors studies when contrast agents became available and striking differences between benign and malignant masses were reported (Kedar, Cosgrove et al. 1995). Not only was there more enhancement in malignancies but also the pattern was more chaotic. A rather crude attempt to evaluate transit times in the masses suggested that the cancers had earlier enhancement and retained the contrast for longer. Subsequent studies of breast masses have been less positive, with only poor enhancement and little differences between benign and malignant lesions as well as false positives where highly vascular fibroadenomas caused confusion (Rizzatto, Martegani et al. 2001; Jung, Jungius et al. 2005). In a more recent study of 50 consecutive patients with histological proof, QLab software was used to calculate features from TICs after bolus injections of SonoVue (Barnard, Leen et al. 2008). The area under the curve (AUC) and the peak enhancement were larger in malignant than benign lesions.

The prostate has also been studied from early after the introduction of microbubbles, both to improve detection of cancers and to assess response to antiandrogen therapy (Eckersley, Sedelaar et al. 2002). Again, the techniques were crude, exploiting what was available. More recently, microbubble-specific modes and more durable microbubbles have become available, and reports of their usefulness in targeting biopsies promise to reduce the high proportion of negative biopsies (Frauscher, Klauser et al. 2003; Wink, Frauscher et al. 2008).

A study found that DCE US was a useful method for evaluating the neovascularization of gastric carcinomas, and enhanced intensity (enhanced intensity is equal to peak intensity minus baseline intensity) had a strongly positive linear correlation with microvessel density (MVD) (Shiyan, Pintong et al. 2009). Another study found that DCE US was a valuable method for evaluating angiogenesis in colorectal tumors in vivo (Zhuang, Yang et al. 2011). This study also found that the area under the curve (AUC) had a positive linear correlation with MVD and could form a new index for assessing angiogenesis and the biological behavior of colorectal tumors. A recent study also found that the peak intensity and AUC reflected the MVD in ovarian tumors (Wang, Lv et al. 2011).

In summary, DCE US is a powerful tool for studying neovascularization and the effect of anti-angiogenic therapy, with minimal morbidity.

2.1.2 CT perfusion

CT perfusion (CTP) is a theoretical tool able to objectively quantify (with the use of mathematical models and dedicated software) the 'real' perfusion of tissues in that it only measures the density difference produced by the contribution of contrast material (and therefore of blood) to tissues. CTP is based on two indispensable technical requirements.

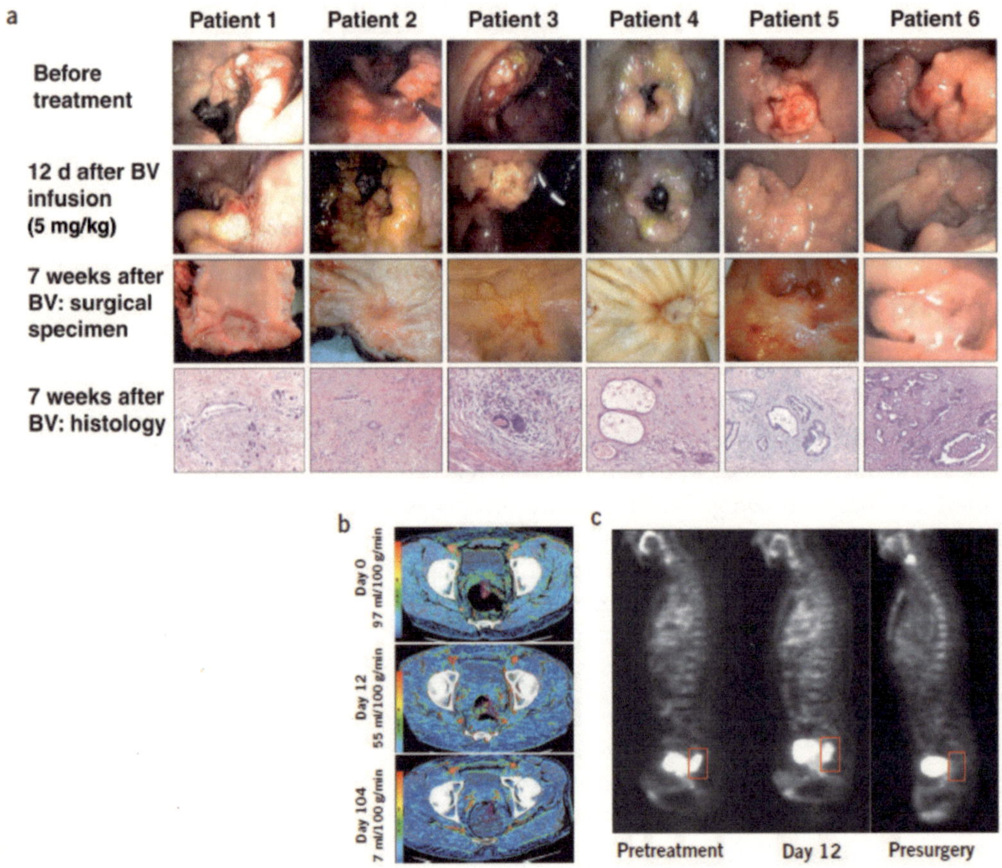

Fig. 2. Effect of treatment on tumors in patients who completed entire combined treatment regimen, and surgery. (a) Endoscopic and pathological evaluation of rectal tumors. Surgical specimens showed grade II tumor regression in patients 1-5 and grade III in patients 6, by Mandard criteria. Endoscopic image (instead of surgical specimen) was taken for patients 6, 3.5 weeks before surgery. BV, bevacizumab. (b) Representative functional CT images of blood perfusion before treatment (day 0), after bevacizumab (day 12) and after completion of treatment (day 104) in patient 5. (c) Tumor FDG uptake before treatment (pretreatment), 12d after bevacizumab treatment and 6-7 weeks after completion of all neoadjuvant therapy (presurgery). Saggital projections of FDG-PET scans for patient 1 are shown. Tumor is outlined in box, posterior to the bladder. (Reprinted with permission from Nature Medicine, 10(2), Willet et al. Direct evidence that the VEGF-specific antibody bevacizumab has antivascular effects in human rectal cancer., 145-7, Copyright 2004)

The first is the performance of repeated CT scans of the volume being analyzed (also known as dynamic, cine or perfusion scans). These need to be acquired before, during and after intravenous administration of iodinated contrast material to enable the study of density variations over time. The density measured by CT in the unit volume (voxel) is directly proportional to the quantity of contrast material present within it (Lee, Purdie et al. 2003). The contrast material contained within the tissue volume being studied is due to contrast material in vessels and contained in the extravascular/cellular space (or more simply, interstitial space) due to passive diffusion (Cenic, Nabavi et al. 2000). The second requirement is the selection of the arterial input. Placement of an ROI on an artery (arterial input) makes it possible to obtain a density/time curve, expressed in Hounsfield units (HU) per second (s), which is compared with the density/time curve of the tissues being studied, which is also obtained with placement of an ROI. Thanks to the comparison, the quantity of contrast material within vessels (vascular component) can be distinguished from contrast material within the interstitium (extravascular/cellular component). Lastly, with the use of a number of kinetic models, perfusion parameters can be calculated that quantify perfusion of the tissues being studied (Figure 2).

Two-compartment (or Patlak) analysis sees the vascular compartment and the extravascular/cellular compartment as distinct, and quantifies exchange between them (Patlak, Blasberg et al. 1983). It provides an estimate of blood volume (BV) within the microvasculature and the extraction fraction (EF), also known as the transit constant (K^{trans}), which is the sum of the flow within the microvasculature and capillary permeability. One-compartment analysis (or slope method) enables the calculation of perfusion with short-duration perfusion scans. Perfusion can be calculated as the ratio between the maximum slope of the density/time curve of tissue and the peak density reached by the artery selected as arterial input. The main advantage of this method is that it allows the calculation of perfusion with short-duration scans, in that the density/time curve of tissues reaches its maximum slope well before peak density. Short-duration scans are defined to include only the first pass of contrast material to avoid blood recirculation from interfering with perfusion quantification. In addition, they offer the advantage of being able to be performed in conditions of breath-hold in critical regions, thus limiting the possibility of motion artifacts. Nonetheless, this kinetic model is by its nature highly sensitive to noise present in the acquired images in that images are analyzed in a 'discontinuous' manner. Perfusion is, in fact, calculated by using only four images: the baseline image, the image obtained at peak density of the artery and the two subsequent images that show the greatest differences in tissue density. The presence of noise in one of these images can invalidate perfusion quantification (Miles and Griffiths 2003).

Deconvolution-based perfusion analysis applies a mathematical operation of deconvolution to compare the density/time curve obtained from the arterial input and from the tissue being studied to obtain a theoretical concentration curve (of contrast material in the tissue being studied/time), known as the residual impulse response function (IRF) (Bronikowski, Dawson et al. 1983). Using the first part of the concentration curve, it can reasonably be assumed that the contrast material lies solely within the vascular compartment. In this fashion, blood flow (BF), BV and mean transit time (MTT) of blood within the microvasculature can be calculated according to the central volume principle, whereby BF = BV/MTT. In reality, the contrast material is distributed in the vascular compartment only exclusively in the brain parenchyma (where the blood-brain barrier hinders it passage into the extravascular/cellular component), in the testicle and in the retina. In all other organs, the contrast material spreads via capillaries into the interstitium. Nonetheless, most contrast material diffuses in the interstitium late, and the amount that diffuses during the first pass is small. It can therefore be theoretically assumed that the contrast material is only in the vascular compartment in all other parenchyma if only the early scans are used for perfusion analysis (within the first 45-60s from contrast administration), with a maximum error of 15%(Purdie, Henderson et al. 2001). Using the last part of the curve and the St. Lawrence and Lee adiabatic approximation, passage of contrast material into the interstitium can be quantified, with inclusion in the perfusion analysis of the CT scan performed after the first phase (therefore known as the interstitial phase). Calculating the permeability surface area-product (PS) is done according to the following equation:

$$PS = -BF\ [in(1-E)], \qquad (2)$$

where E is the fraction of contrast that leaks into the interstitium from the vascular space (EF) (Petralia, Preda et al. 2010).

A study of 23 patients with colorectal adenocarcinoma found that tumor permeability surface-area product and blood volume correlate positively with MVD and may reflect the microvascularity of colorectal tumors (Goh, Halligan et al. 2008). A study in 6 patients with primary or locally advanced adenocarcinoma of the rectum found that after a single infusion of bevacizumab (a VEGF-specific antibody) there was a significant decrease in tumor blood flow (40-44%) and blood volume (16-39%), which was accompanied by a significant decreased in tumor MVD (Willett, Boucher et al. 2004). A study of 20 patients with resectable soft tissue sarcoma treated with neoadjuvant bevacizumab and radiotherapy found that the BV, BF and PS decreased by 62-72% (Yoon, Duda et al. 2010). A study in patients treated with antiangiogenic therapy for metastatic renal cell carcinoma found that the baseline perfusion parameters were higher in responders than in stable patients, and that after the first cycle of treatment there was a significant decrease in BF and BV in patients receiving antiangiogenic treatment. They concluded that perfusion parameters determined with DCE CT could help predict biological response to antiangiogenic drugs before beginning therapy and help detect an effect after a single cycle of treatment (Fournier, Oudard et al. 2010). A further study in patients with advanced lung adenocarcinoma found that BF, BV and permeability values were higher in responding patients than in the other patients, with a significant difference at second follow-up for BF, BV and permeability (Fraioli, Anzidei et al. 2011). A study in patients with advanced HCC treated with bevacizumab initially and then in combination with gemcitabine and oxaliplatin, found that there was a significant decrease in BF, BV, and PS and an increase in MTT from baseline. They also found that tumors with higher baseline MTT values correlated with favorable clinical outcome and had better 6 months progression-free survival. The baseline K^{trans} of responders was significantly higher than that of nonresponders. They concluded that CTP was a more sensitive image biomarker for monitoring early antiangiogenic treatment effects as well as in predicting outcome at the end of treatment and progression-free survival as compared with RECIST and tumor density (Jiang, Kambadakone et al. 2011). Another study found that perfusion MDCT can detect focal blood changes even when the tumor is shrinking, possibly indicating early reversal of tumor responsiveness to antiangiogenic therapy (Sabir, Schor-Bardach et al. 2008).

2.1.3 Dynamic contrast enhanced MRI

Functional dynamic contrast enhanced MRI (DCE-MRI) relies on the "leaky" nature of angiogenic blood vessels associated with malignancy. DCE-MRI is the acquisition of serial images before, during, and after the administration of an intravenous contrast agent, which produces time series images that enable pixel-by-pixel analysis of contrast kinetics within the tumor. PK models provide a means of summarizing contrast enhancement data in terms of parameters that relate to underlying vascular anatomy and physiology. Commonly used PK models assume that the contrast agent resides in and exchanges between two compartments in the tumor: the vascular space and the extravascular-extracellular space (EES) (Tofts 1997; Tofts, Brix et al. 1999). The contrast agent enters the tumor through the vascular space by perfusion, and diffuses between the vascular space and the EES. The rates of diffusion from the vascular space to the EES are determined by the concentrations of contrast agent in plasma and EES and the size and permeability of the capillary-EES interface (Brix, Semmler et al. 1991; Furman-Haran, Margalit et al. 1996; Knopp, Weiss et al. 1999; Tofts, Brix et al. 1999; Knopp, Giesel et al. 2001).

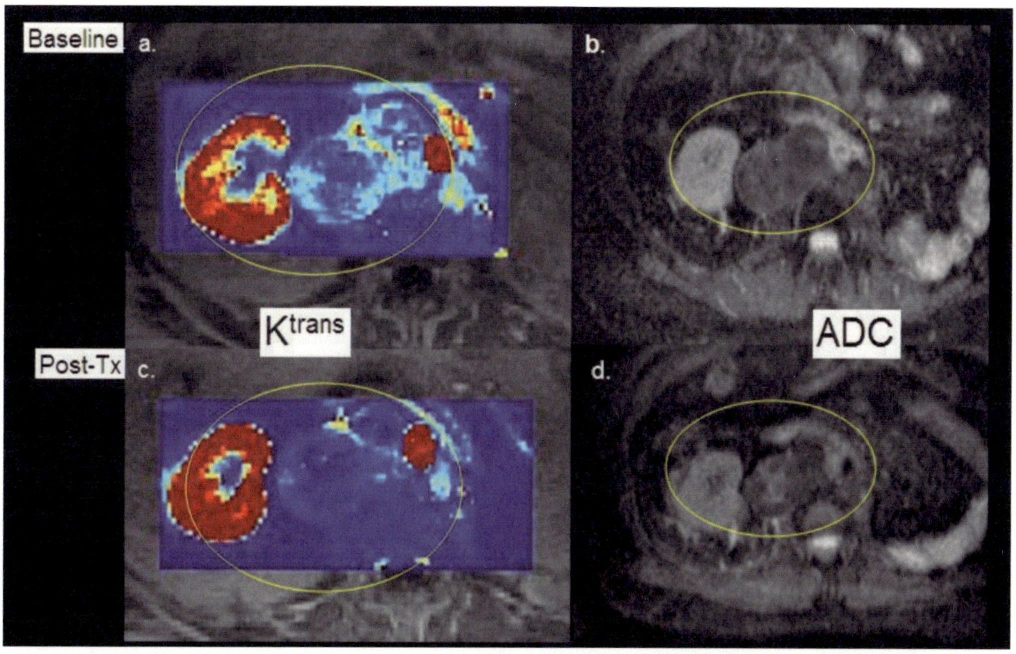

Fig. 3. Axial MR images from a patient with known metastatic renal cell carcinoma metastatic to retroperitoneal lymph nodes. (a) Overlying T1 weighted post contrast images are parametric permeability (K^{trans}) images derived from bolus injection of gadolinium DTPA mathematically derived from analysis schemes as described in section 2.1.3. Please note the increased permeability throughout the metastatic lymph node. (b) Parametric images representing the apparent diffusion coefficient (ADC) at approximately the same level. Please note the homogeneous decreased signal intensity on ADC maps throughout the metastatic lymph node. One week following sunitinib therapy, there is dramatically decreased permeability within the metastatic lymph node on the superimposed K^{trans} map (c), and there is heterogeneously increased ADC within the metastatic lymph node (d), both of which correspond to physiologic response to therapy. Figure from Rosen et al (unpublished data).

The majority of DCE-MRI studies are performed with small molecule, FDA approved Gadolinium based contrast agents. By mapping the T1 relaxation constant parametrically, and dynamically "following" the distribution of the contrast agent through the tumor microvasculature utilizing volumetric T1 weighted imaging, one can model the permeability and other parameters that may serve as surrogate biomarkers of angiogenesis (Figure 3 and 4). To do this, the change in tumor concentration with time is governed by the differential equation:

$$dC_{tumor}/dt=K^{trans}C_p-k_{ep}C_{tumor} \quad (3)$$

where C_{tumor} and C_p are the concentration of the agent in the EES and plasma space, respectively, K^{trans} is the transfer constant between the plasma and the EES, and K_{ep} + K^{trans}/v_e, where v_e is the fraction of tumor volume occupied by the EES. Thus the concentration of contrast agent within the tumor is determined by the blood plasma concentration curve and the two parameters, K^{trans}, the transfer constant, and the EES fractional volume index, v_e (Tofts, Brix et al. 1999).

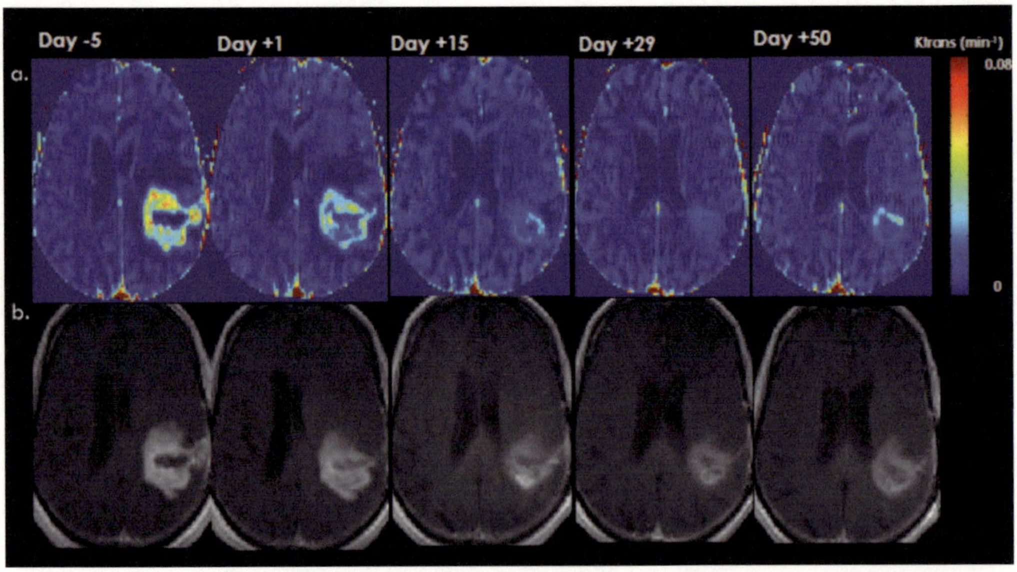

Fig. 4. (a) Maps of K^{trans}, a measure of blood-brain barrier permeability. (b) T1-weighted anatomic images after intravenous administration of a contrast agent (gadolinium-DTPA), demonstrating a region of bright signal corresponding to the recurrent brain tumor in the left frontal lobe. Note the reduction in K^{trans} following Gd-DTPA injection and kinetic analysis, and the accompanying shrinkage of the mass after injection of Cediranib (VEGF inhibitor). Figure from Jennings et. al. (unpublished data).

In relating the shape of the enhancement curve obtained from dynamic MRI studies, K^{trans} controls the height of the C_{tumor} curve and $k_{ep} = K^{trans}/v_e$ controls the shape of the curve; the smaller k_{ep}, the more delayed the enhancement. K^{trans} is a function of flow (perfusion) and permeability; the greater the flow and permeability, the greater the K^{trans} (Choyke, Dwyer et al. 2003) (Figure 5).

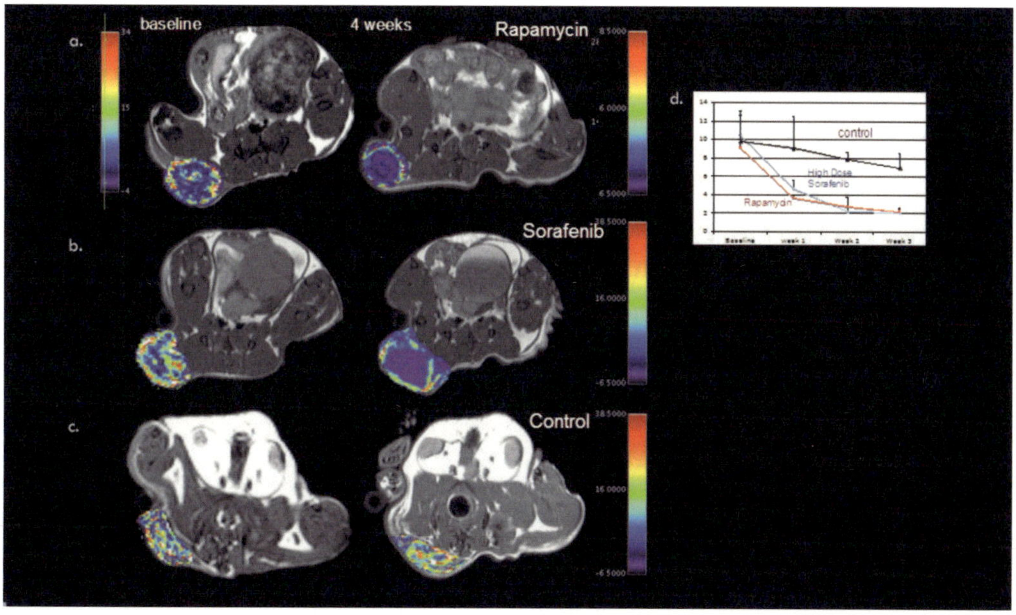

Fig. 5. T1-weighted MRI of mice with pseudocolorized VVF maps superimposed through the center of the tumor within the right flank for each treatment arm (rapamycin (a), sorafenib (b), and control (c)) at baseline and at the end of therapy. Note the heterogeneity of signal intensity and color spread throughout the cohorts at baseline, with marked decrease in vascularity in the rapamycin (a) and sorafenib (b) treated animals as compared to control (c). Of note, only 3 mice survived all 3 weeks of treatment within the rapamycin treated arm. VVF was quantified each week in each cohort and graphed (mean +/- SEM) (d). Note the parallel, rapid decrease in VVF in both the sorafenib and rapamycin treated cohorts as compared to control with a statistically significant decrease in VVF ($p<0.001$) at week 3 in both cohorts relative to control. Although there was a decrease in mean VVF in control mice, there was no statistically significant difference in VVF comparing week 3 to baseline measurements in control mice. Figure from Guimaraes et. al. (unpublished data).

Utilizing this approach in humans suffering from breast cancer, Hulka et al demonstrated a sensitivity of 86% and specificity of 93% for the diagnosis of malignancy (Hulka, Smith et al. 1995; Hulka, Edmister et al. 1997; Tofts, Brix et al. 1999). Knopp et al expanded on these results and were able to demonstrate, by correlative analysis with VEGF and CD31 analysis, significantly faster enhancement characteristics between histologic subtypes (invasive ductal carcinoma, invasive lobular carcinoma and ductal carcinoma in situ)(Knopp, Weiss et al. 1999). Subsequently, various groups have demonstrated, in vivo, in animal models and clinical trials, statistically significant differences in permeability transfer constants following the administration of angiogenesis inhibitors (Pham, Roberts et al. 1998; Morgan, Thomas et al. 2003). Morgan et al demonstrated a rapid reduction in enhancement within 26 to 33 hours after the first dose of the VEGF inhibitor PTK 787/ZK 222584 in a liver metastasis from colorectal carcinoma. This substantial reduction in enhancement is evident across all dose groups on day 2, with a mean reduction in permeability transfer constant of 43% (Morgan, Thomas et al. 2003).

Despite these sophisticated models and encouraging results, pharmacokinetics modeling has been utilized with varying success to calculate blood volume of fractional plasma volume, with reported values demonstrating a correlation coefficient of R^2 0.61, and most studies indicate high sensitivity (>90%), but wide variability in specificity, with published values as low as 30% (Piccoli 1997). This variability is demonstrated well in a study by Su et al who performed DCE MRI on 105 patients with breast cancer and correlated it to VEGF serum marker levels as well as microvascular density as assessed post CD31 staining. Although patients with increased VEGF demonstrated higher CD31 microvascular densities, no significant association between MRI parameters and these other surrogate markers was demonstrated (Su, Cheung et al. 2003). In a study of 38 patients with advanced hepatocellular carcinoma treated with sunitinib, the investigators found significant decreases in K^{trans} and K_{ep} to approximately half. Moreover, the extent of decrease in K^{trans} in patients who experienced partial response/stable disease was significantly greater (two-fold on average) compared with patients with progressive disease or who died during the first two cycles of therapy (Zhu, Sahani et al. 2009).

DCE-MRI, in summary, has exciting potential to study the early effects of anti-angiogenic therapy in various organ systems.

2.1.4 Positron emission tomography

PET has been used in some studies to assess tumor blood flow with $H_2\,^{15}O$ as a biological endpoint of response to antiangiogenic agents (Herbst, Mullani et al. 2002). The principal advantage of $H_2\,^{15}O$ is that it is a 'freely diffusible' tracer, meaning that its uptake by the tumor is not limited by vascular permeability. $H_2\,^{15}O$ PET has been used to measure blood flow in several tumor types, including breast (Beaney, Lammertsma et al. 1984) and brain tumors (Ito, Lammertsma et al. 1982). The first report of the use of PET to measure vascular pharmacodynamics in humans was part of a phase 1 dose-escalation study of the tumor vascular targeting agent combretastatin A4 phosphate (CA4P) (Anderson, Yap et al. 2003). $H_2\,^{15}O$ PET was used to measure tumor and normal tissue perfusion and blood volume, before and after the administration of CA4P. Significant reductions in tumor perfusion were measured 30 minutes after administration of CA4P. However, there are potential limitations. $H_2\,^{15}O$ has a short half-life (2 minutes) and therefore studies require an on-site cyclotron and a separate tracer synthesis for each injection. In small tumors, partial volume effects may be significant if the tumor size is less than twice the resolution of the scanner. Second, there is a phenomenon known as 'spill over' or 'spill in' of counts from surrounding structures with high blood flow, such as the heart and the aorta, or within areas of relatively high blood flow, such as the liver, therefore limiting the use of this technique in the lung, liver and mediastinum.

2.2 Steady state blood volume determinations of neovascular density

2.2.1 Magnetic resonance imaging

Ultrasmall super paramagnetic iron oxide (a.k.a. magnetic nanoparticle (MNP)) is a steady state blood pool agent that creates contrast through magnetic susceptibility variations proximal to the vascular network (Enochs, Harsh et al. 1999; Tropres, Grimault et al. 2001; Corot, Robert et al. 2006; Persigehl, Bieker et al. 2007), which results in changes in inherent and induced transverse relaxation times defined as T_2 and T_2^*, respectively. Accurate evaluation of R_2^* ($1/T_2^*$) or R_2 ($1/T_2$) necessitate defining two or more points on the natural or induced transverse relaxation decay curve. Addition of contrast agent increases R_2^* ($1/T_2^*$) thus causing limits on sampling as the T_2^* is shortened. It can be shown that:

$$\Delta R_2^* \text{ or } \Delta R_2 \propto \log\left[S^{post}/S^{pre}\right] \quad (4)$$

where, S^{pre} and S^{post} are pre- and post-contrast MRI signal intensity (Brown and Giaccia 1998). The change in transverse relaxation rate ΔR_2 ($1/\Delta T_2$) and changes in effective transverse relaxation rate ΔR_2^* ($1/\Delta T_2^*$) caused by the contrast agent are proportional to tumor blood volume (BV) fraction (Belliveau, Rosen et al. 1990; Dennie, Mandeville et al. 1998; Ostergaard, Smith et al. 1998). Therefore, the capability of MNP to modulate the effective transverse relaxation rate, R_2^*, is exploited where the difference of R_2^* before and after administration of MNP will be useful in determining microvessel density (Hyodo, Chandramouli et al. 2009).

Bremer et al first utilized intravital microscopy to determine whether a prototype magnetic nanoparticle (MION) agent truly had intravascular distribution in tumor microenvironment (Bremer, Mustafa et al. 2003). For these experiments a green fluorescent protein expressing 9L tumor model was utilized, in which tumor microvasculature is clearly outlined against fluorescent tumor cells, even at very high spatial resolution, which demonstrated that MION selectively enhanced the vascularity without any significant leakage into tumor interstitium during time of observation (30 minutes). They also found that steady state measures of vascular volume fraction (VVF) with MRI allow a volumetric, in vivo, non-invasive assay of microvascular density in experimental tumor models.

Pancreatic adenocarcinoma xenograft lines were subcutaneously implanted into nude mice, which were then therapies targeted to 3 loci of the sonic hedgehog signaling pathway. MRI imaging was performed 1 week after therapy, pre and post injection of MION-47. Following treatment, tumors showed a significant decrease in VVF compared to controls (Guimaraes, Rakhlin et al. 2008). A study on fibrosarcoma-bearing nude mice which were injection with a thrombogenic vascular targeting agent (VTA) found that the $\Delta R2^*$ values were significantly reduced shortly after treatment initiation and concluded that USPIO-enhanced MR imaging enable early monitoring of antiangiogenic treatment of tumors (Persigehl, Bieker et al. 2007).

A recently published study on rhabdomyosarcoma-bearing mice treated with bevacizumab or saline as control, found that multiecho $\Delta R2^*$ MR relaxometry allowed an early and quantitative assessment of tumor vascularization changes in response to an antiangiogenic treatment (Ring, Persigehl et al. 2011). Another study on renal cell carcinoma-bearing mice treated with rapamycin (mTOR inhibitor), sorafenib (VEGF inhibitor) or saline control, VVF correlated with MVD and that the VVF in all treatment arms differed from control and declined weekly with treatment. They also reported that VVF changes with rapamycin were similar to high-dose sorafenib (Guimaraes, Ross et al. 2011).

Although not FDA approved, MNP enhanced MRI measures allow for interrogation of altered tumor microvascular morphology, and may serve as a robust means of evaluating the microstructural microvascular changes associated with anti-angiogenic therapy in humans.

2.3 Specific molecular markers of angiogenesis

Advances in knowledge of tumor angiogenesis have resulted in the identification of several molecules in tumor angiogenic signaling. These molecules have been exploited for their use as targets for molecular imaging and quantification of tumor angiogenesis. Furthermore, discovery of these molecules has led to realization of the concept that tumor vessels can be selectively targeted for therapy. Non-invasive molecular imaging of tumor angiogenesis can allow for much easier diagnosis and better prognosis of cancer, as well as more accurate treatment monitoring, which will eventually lead to personalized molecular medicine.

2.3.1 Vascular endothelial growth factor

Vascular endothelial growth factor (VEGF) is one of the key factors regulating angiogenesis. Most of the vasculogenic and angiogenic effects of VEGF are mediated through two endothelium-specific receptor tyrosine kinases, VEGF receptor 1 (VEGFR-1) and VEGF receptor 2 (VEGFR-2)(Millauer, Wizigmann-Voos et al. 1993). VEGFR-1 is critical for physiologic and developmental angiogenesis, and VEGFR-2 is the major mediator of the mitogenic, angiogenic, and permeability-enhancing effects of VEGF (Ferrara 2004). In the imaging studies reported to date, however, specificity for ether VEGFR-1 or VEGFR-2 has rarely been achieved, because most of the tracers are based on $VEGF_A$ isoforms, which bind to both VEGFRs. Because of a high level of VEGFR-1 expression, rodent kidneys can take up a significant amount of a $VEGF_A$-based tracer, a fact that often makes the kidneys the dose-limiting organ. Because VEGFR-2 is generally accepted to be more functionally important than VEGFR-1 in cancer progression, this limits the use of current techniques.

Recently, in vivo CE US imaging of VEGF/VEGFR expression has been reported. In 2 murine tumor models, microbubbles conjugated to anti-VEGFR-2 monoclonal antibodies were used to image VEGFR-2 expression (Willmann, Paulmurugan et al. 2008). The targeted microbubbles produced a significantly higher average signal intensity than control microbubbles, and the signal intensity was significantly lower when anti-VEGFR-2 antibodies (blocking antibodies) were used, demonstrating target specificity.

^{99m}Tc-labelled human $VEGF_{121}$ (one of the homodimeric isoforms of $VEGFR_A$) has been used as a molecular imaging marker of VEGFR expression in an orthotopic mouse model of mammary adenocarcinoma, and for the imaging of tumor vasculature before and after tumoricidal cyclophosphamide treatment (Blankenberg, Backer et al. 2006). [^{123}I]$VEGF_{165}$ has also been reported as a potential tumor marker (Cornelissen, Oltenfreiter et al. 2005), but despite the high receptor affinity of this tracer, biodistribution in melanoma tumor-bearing mice indicated poor tumor-to-background ratios, most likely due to the low metabolic stability (deiodination) of the compound. Nonetheless, biodistribution, safety, and absorbed dose of $[^{123}I]VEGF_{165}$ was studied in patients with pancreatic carcinoma (Li, Peck-Radosavljevic et al. 2004). Following IV administration, sequential images were recorded during the initial 30 minutes after injection. Although a majority of primary pancreatic tumors and their metastases were visualized by the $[^{123}I]VEGF_{165}$ scan, the organ with the highest absorbed dose was the thyroid, indicating severe deiodination of the probe.

To target the VEGFR-2, Backer et al (Backer, Patel et al. 2006) used single chain VEGF (scVEGF) with an N-terminal cysteine-containing tag (Cys-tag), which can be used for site specific attachment of various agents (Backer, Levashova et al. 2008). The scVEGF-based family of probes has been validated to target the VEGF receptor in vitro and in vivo tumor angiogenesis (Blankenberg, Backer et al. 2006; Levashova, Backer et al. 2008)

^{64}Cu-labelled $VEGF_{121}$ has been used for PET imaging of tumor angiogenesis and VEGFR expression (Cai, Chen et al. 2006). DOTA-$VEGF_{121}$ (where DOTA denotes 1,4,7,10-tetraazacyclododecane-1,4,7,10-tetraacetic acid) exhibits nanomolar receptor affinity in vitro. In an animal model, microPET imaging revealed rapid, specific, and prominent uptake of $[^{64}Cu]$DOTA-$VEGF_{121}$ in highly vascularized small xenografts (high VEGFR-2 expression) but significantly lower and sporadic uptake in large tumors (low VEGFR-2 expression). Substantial tracer uptake in the kidneys was also observed, most likely due to the high VEGFR-1 expression in this organ.

A VEGFR-2-specific PET tracer based on mutant $VEGF_{121}$ has been recently developed (Wang, Cai et al. 2007). The D63AE64AE67A mutant of $VEGF_{121}$ ($VEGF_{DEE}$), compared with $VEGF_{121}$ had an affinity for binding to VEGFR-1 that was 20-fold lower, without a significant reduction in VEGFR-2-binding affinity.

HuMV833, a humanized mouse monoclonal anti-VEGF antibody was labeled with ^{124}I for PET imaging of solid tumors in phase 1 trial cancer patients (Jayson, Zweit et al. 2002). Antibody distribution and clearance were markedly heterogeneous between and within patients and between and within individual tumors, suggesting that dose escalation design of phase 1 studies with antiangiogenic antibodies such as HuMV833 would be problematic.

2.3.2 Integrins

Integrins are a family of cell adhesion molecules consisting of two noncovalently bound transmembrane subunits (α and β) that pair to create heterodimers with distinct adhesive capabilities. Integrin $\alpha_v\beta_3$ mediates the migration of endothelial cells through the basement membrane during blood-vessel formation (Josephs, Spicer et al. 2009). Imaging of integrin $\alpha_v\beta_3$ expression is promising for the assessment of angiogenesis, as integrin $\alpha_v\beta_3$ is significantly up-regulated on endothelium during angiogenesis, but not an quiescent endothelium (Brooks, Clark et al. 1994). In addition, in healthy tissue, expression of integrin $\alpha_v\beta_3$ is highly restricted with significant amounts only observed in osteoclasts (van der Flier and Sonnenberg 2001). Integrin $\alpha_v\beta_3$, which mediates the migration of endothelial cells through the basement membrane during blood-vessel formation, binds to peptides containing the amino-acid sequence arginine-glycine-aspartic acid (RGD) within the interstitial matrix (Haubner 2006). By labeling these peptides with ^{125}I, ^{111}In, ^{64}Cu, ^{99m}Tc, ^{18}F or fluorescence dyes, specific binding of imaging agents to integrin $\alpha_v\beta_3$ in tumors has been demonstrated (Haubner, Wester et al. 1999; van Hagen, Breeman et al. 2000; Haubner,

Wester et al. 2001; Janssen, Oyen et al. 2002; Chen, Conti et al. 2004; Beer, Lorenzen et al. 2008).

Targeted ultrasound imaging of integrin $\alpha_v\beta_3$ during tumor angiogenesis has been reported (Ellegala, Leong-Poi et al. 2003). In a rat model of human glioblastoma, CEU was performed with microbubbles coated with echistatin, an RGD-containing disintegrin, which binds specifically to integrin $\alpha_v\beta_3$. The CEU signal was found to be highest at the periphery of tumors, where integrin expression was most prominent as indicated by immunohistochemistry, and correlated well with tumor microvascular blood volume.

Gd3+-containing paramagnetic liposomes (300-350nm in diameter) have been used for MRI of integrin $\alpha_v\beta_3$ expression (Sipkins, Cheresh et al. 1998). In that study, mMRI of squamous cell carcinomas in a rabbit model was achieved with LM609, a mouse antihuman integrin $\alpha_v\beta_3$ monoclonal antibody, as the targeting ligand. Peptidomimetic integrin $\alpha_v\beta_3$ antagonist-conjugated magnetic magnetic nanoparticles were tested in a Vx-2 squamous cell carcinoma model with the common clinical field strength of 1.5 T(Winter, Caruthers et al. 2003). The targeted nanoparticles increased the MR signal dramatically in the periphery of the tumor at 2 hours after injection. Despite their relatively large size (~270nm in diameter), these nanoparticles penetrated into the leaky tumor neovasculature but did not migrate into the interstitum in appreciable amounts. In a later report, athymic nude mice bearing human melanoma tumors were successfully imaged with systemically injected integrin $\alpha_v\beta_3$-targeted paramagnetic nanoparticles (Schmieder, Winter et al. 2005). Very small regions (about 30mm^3) of angiogenesis associated with nascent melanoma tumors were visualized by this technique, which may enable phenotyping and staging of early melanomas in clinical settings.

Integrin $\alpha_v\beta_3$-targeted ultrasmall SPIO nanoparticles were used with a 1.5T RI scanner for the noninvasive differenciation of tumors with large and small fractions of integrin $\alpha_v\beta_3$-positive tumor vessels (Zhang, Jugold et al. 2007). After injection of RGD peptide-conjugated small SPIO nanoparticles, T2*-weighted MR images revealed the heterogeneous distribution of integrin -positive tumor vessels, as evidenced by an irregular signal intensity decrease. In contrast, the signal intensity decreased homogeneously in the control tumor, with predominantly small and uniformly distributed vessels.

In recent years, many fluorescently labeled cyclic RGD peptides have been developed for near infrared fluorescence imaging like RGD-Cy7, RGD-Cy5.5, RGD-QD705 (Chen, Conti et al. 2004; Cai, Shin et al. 2006; Wu, Cai et al. 2006) and cyclic RGD coupled to IRDye 800CW-labeled peptide which is even more shifted towards the infrared parts of the spectrum resulting in ideal fluorescent characteristics for in vivo use (Adams, Ke et al. 2007). Mulder et al (Mulder, Koole et al. 2006; Mulder, Castermans et al. 2009) recently described paramagnetic lipid-encapsulated quantum dots with RGD presented at the outside and a green fluorescent quantum dot at the inside of the micellar shell. These targeted particles are both suitable for fluorescence imaging as well as MRI, thus providing unique opportunities for the use of multimodality molecular imaging.

Several groups have improved $\alpha_v\beta_3$ integrin specificity, binding affinity, and possible targeted delivery of therapeutics, by coupling multiple RGD motifs on a backbone molecule (Kok, Schraa et al. 2002; Cheng, Wu et al. 2005; Mulder, Koole et al. 2006; Jin, Josserand et al.

2007; Mulder, Castermans et al. 2009). Although, many types of tumor cells are positive for $\alpha_v\beta_3$ integrin, RGD-modified proteins mainly localize at the tumor endothelium and not in the tumor itself (Schraa, Kok et al. 2002).

The commercially available near infrared fluorescent (NIRF) probe IntegriSense (Visen Medical) consists of a small molecule nonpeptide $\alpha_v\beta_3$ antangonist fused to the VivoTg-S680 near infrared fluorophore. IntegriSense has a much higher specificity for $\alpha_v\beta_3$ integrin compared to RGD-based probes. Unlike RGD-based probes, extravasation of IntegriSense does occur and the probe localizes at both the surface of $\alpha_v\beta_3$ integrin positive endothelial cells and the surface $\alpha_v\beta_3$ integrin positive tumor cells. Furthermore, IntegriSense is internalized by the $\alpha_v\beta_3$ integrin positive tumor cells leading to a slower clearance of the probe from tumors compared to the surrounding tissues. A drawback of the slower clearance from the tumor is the practical upper limit on the possible frequency of repeated measurements (Kossodo, Pickarski et al. 2010).

A dimeric RGD peptide E[c(RGDyK)]$_2$ (abbreviated as FRGD2) has been labeled with ^{18}F. A high accumulation of ^{18}F-FRGD2 in integrin $\alpha_v\beta_3$ –rich tumors was demonstrated with a high tumor/background ratio at late time points of imaging (Zhang, Xiong et al. 2006). A glycopeptides based on c(RGDyK) was later labeled with 18F and the resulting 18F-galacto-RGD was found to be safely administered to patients and allowed detection of integrin-positive tumors (Haubner, Weber et al. 2005). Despite the successful translation of 18F-galacto-RGD into clinical trials however, several key issues remain to be resolved, such as tumor-targeting efficacy, pharmacokinetics, and the ability to quantify integrin $\alpha_v\beta_3$ density in vivo. Indeed, other promising multimetric RDG peptides are being investigated and may give better localization than galacto-RGD (Cai, Niu et al. 2008)

Etaracizumab, a humanized murine monoclonal antibody against human integrin $\alpha_v\beta_3$ has been conjugated with a chelating agent DOTA and labeled with ^{64}Cu. The resulting [^{64}Cu]DOTA-etaracizumab correlated well with integrin $\alpha_v\beta_3$ in tumor xenografts via PET imaging (Cai, Wu et al. 2006). MicroPET studies revealed avid [^{64}Cu]DOTA-etaracizumab uptake in integrin $\alpha_v\beta_3$ -positive tumors. The receptor specificity of [^{64}Cu]DOTA-etaracizumab was confirmed by effective blocking of tumor uptake with co-administration of non-radioactive etaracizumab.

A nanoparticle-based probe has been used for both MRI and optical imaging of integrin $\alpha_v\beta_3$. MRI-detectable and fluorescent liposomes carrying RGD peptides were evaluated for in vivo tumor imaging (Mulder, Strijkers et al. 2005). Both RGD-conjugated liposomes and RAD (a control peptide that does not bind to integrin $\alpha_v\beta_3$)-conjugated liposomes provided enhanced T1-weighted MR contrast. Ex vivo fluorescence microscopy revealed that RGD-conjugated liposomes were specifically associated with the activated tumor endothelium, whereas RAD-conjugated liposomes were located in the extravascular compartment.

A quantum dot (QD)-based probe for NIRF imaging and PET of integrin $\alpha_v\beta_3$ has been developed (Cai, Chen et al. 2007). QD surface modification with RGD peptides allowed for integrin $\alpha_v\beta_3$ targeting, and DTA conjugation enabled PET after ^{64}Cu labeling. It was found that the majority of the probe in the tumor was within the vasculature, as evidenced by excellent overlay of the QD fluorescence signal and vasculature integrin $\alpha_v\beta_3$ staining. This dual-modality (PET/NIRF imaging) probe can confer sufficient tumor contrast at a concentration much lower than that required for in vivo NIRF imaging, significantly reduces the potential toxicity of cadmium-based QDs, and may hasten the future translation of QD-based imaging agents to clinical and biomedical applications.

2.3.3 Transforming growth factor β

Transforming growth factor β (TGF-β) signaling plays a role in several biological processes, including embryonic development, carcinogenesis, wound healing, and angiogenesis (Bernabeu, Lopez-Novoa et al. 2009). In normal cells, the TGF-β pathway restricts cell growth, differentiation and cell death. In contrast, in malignant cells, various components of the TGF-β signaling pathway become mutated thereby exploiting the ability of TGF-β to modulate growth promoting processes, including cell invasion and angiogenesis. TGF-β signaling is mediated by TGF-β binding to TGF-β receptors, of which, there are three classes: Type I and II are heterodimeric receptor whereas type III are homodimeric receptors . CD105, also known as endoglin, is a TGF-β type III receptor that has been shown to participate in signaling angiogenesis. Endoglin is predominantly expressed on proliferating endothelial cells (Fonsatti, Altomonte et al. 2003), and inhibition of its expression has been shown to restore the growth suppressing signals of the TGF-β signaling pathway (Ma, Labinaz et al. 2000). Thus, endoglin is an attractive molecular target of angiogenesis since it is over-expressed on tumor-associated endothelium (Bernabeu, Lopez-Novoa et al. 2009).

Avidin (Av) was incorporated into the shell of perfluorocarbon-exposed sonicated dextrose albumin micobubbles (Av-MBs) to anchor biotinylated monoclonal antibodies (mAbs) (Korpanty, Grayburn et al. 2005). A rat anti-mouse CD105 mAb (MJ7/18) and an isotype-matched control mAb were investigated for biotinylation, microbubbles incorporation, and cellular studies. It was found that MJ7/18-conjugated microbubbles bound specifically to endothelial cells but not fibroblasts, while the control mAb-conjugated Av-MBs did not exhibit CD105-specific targeting. After demonstrating the proof-of-principle, a follow-up study was carried out to follow the vascular response of therapy in mouse models of subcutaneous and orthotopic pancreatic adenocarcinoma (Korpanty, Carbon et al. 2007). For comprehensive investigation of angiogenesis in tumor-bearing mice treated with anti-VEGF mAbs and/or gemcitabine (a nucleoside analog with known activity against pancreatic adenocarcinoma), the localization of microbubbles targeting CD105, VEGFR-2, or VEGF-activated blood vessels 9the VEGF-VEGFR complex) was monitored by ultrasound (Di Marco, Di Cicilia et al. 2010). In the subcutaneous model, receptor-targeted microbubbles gave significantly better enhancement of tumor vasculature than the non-targeted or control mAbs-conjugated microbubbles. In addition, video intensity from targeted microbubbles correlated with the level of target expression (CD105, VEGFR-2, or the VEGF-VEGFR complex), as well as with MVD in tumors under either anti-angiogenesis or cytotoxic therapy.

One study investigated the applicability of a human umbilical vein endothelial cell (HUVEC)-based in vitro model to mimic physiological and angiogenic vasculature (Vag, Schramm et al. 2009). High fluorescence signal was observed in proliferating HUVECs due to CD105 expression.

Molecular MRI of CD105 expression in tumor-bearing rats was achieved with Gd-DTPA-containing stabilized liposomes (Gd-SLs) (Zhang, Feng et al. 2009). A series of targeted and non-targeted MRI contrast agents were compared in glioma-bearing rats: Gd-DTPA, Gd-SLs, Gd-SLs conjugated to anti-CD105 mAbs (CD105-Gd-SLs), and Gd-SLs conjugated to control mAbs (IgG-Gd-SLs). Serial T1-weighted MRI before and after contrast agent administration revealed that the area with enhanced MRI contrast was restricted for CD105-Gd-SLs but not for the other three groups. In addition, the degree of contrast enhancement over time also varied between different groups. For example, Gd-DTPA gave an early contrast enhancement which peaked at 30 minutes and declined to baseline values at 60 minutes, while the signal intensity for CD105-Gd-SLs continued to increase over a period of 120 minutes. The signal intensity of IgG-Gd-SLs and Gd-SLs both peaked at 60 minutes followed by a decline, yet the rate of decrease was quite different. Ex vivo histology further revealed that the enhancement in the CD105-Gd-SLs group resulted mainly from new microvessels. However, both mature microvessels and new microvasculature were responsible for contrast enhancement in the other three groups.

A study investigated an ^{111}In-labeled anti-CD105 mAb (MJ7/18) and compared its neovascular binding, tumor accumulation, and in vivo behavior in an isotype-matched control mAb (Bredlow, Lewin et al 2000) In a B16 melanoma model, the tumors in animals receiving 111In-labelled MJ7/18 were more easily identified than animals receiving the radiolabeled control mAb. However, the tumor contrast was only modest. Ex vivo autoradiography and histology experiments of the tumor sections corroborated the different patterns of in vivo tumoral accumulation for the two antibodies. MJ7/18 exhibited intense activity in the peripheral region of the tumor, where the highest concentration of vessels was found, and much lower activity in the tumor center. On the other hand, little accumulation of activity could be found in tumors of mice that had been injected with ^{111}In-labeled control mAb.

Another study tested a ^{125}I-labeled anti-CD105 mAb (MAEND3) in a canine mammary carcinoma model (Fonsatti, Jekunen et al. 2000). After demonstrating differential expression of CD105 on human breast cancer and endothelial cells, two dogs with spontaneous mammary tumors were intravenously injected with ^{125}I-laveled MAEND3 and imaged eight hours later. Rapid and intense uptake of the radiolabeled mAb with excellent tumor-to-background ratio was observed in the tumor areas of both dogs, which were confirmed as ductal mammary adenocarcinoma after surgical excision ten days later. Another study also explored the use of ^{125}I-labeled anti-CD105 mAb for radioimmunotherapy applications in mouse tumor models (Tabata, Kondo et al. 1999). Significant growth suppression of the tumors was observed while a ^{125}I-labeled control mAb did not show any significant anti-tumor efficacy.

A ^{99m}Tc-labelled anti-CD105 mAb (E9) was investigated in freshly excised kidneys from renal carcinoma patients (Costello, Li et al. 2004). After perfusion of ^{99m}Tc-E9 through the renal artery, immunoscintigraphy revealed the presence of well-defined radioactive hot spots, which matched the positions of the tumors as identified by pre-surgery MRI and subsequent histology. Gamma-counting revealed that the median values of radioactivity uptake per gram of wet weight were > 10 fold higher in the tumors than in normal kidney tissues. Not only was CD105 specificity of the tracer confirmed by blocking studies, immunoscintigraphy with ^{99m}Tc-E9 was also able to identify tumors that were not detected during pre-surgery MRI.

2.3.4 Matrix metalloprotienases

Expression of matrix metalloproteinases (MMPs) is associated with the removal of the extracellular matrix (ECM) barrier to allow cancer cells ad endothelial cells to invade the basement membrane. A number of MMPs are also specifically involved in angiogenesis, including MMPs 1, 2, 3, 9, and 14 (Stollman, Ruers et al. 2009).

One approach for monitoring MMP activity in tumor-bearing animal models is the use of 'smart' fluorescence probes that are bound to a synthetic graft copolymer consisting of a cleavable backbone that can act as an MMP substrate. When placed in close proximity, these polymeric fluorochromes quench each other and are not detectable. On enzymatic cleavage of the backbone by MMPs, the fluorochromes are spatially dissociated and begin to fluoresce (Bremer, Bredow et al. 2001)

3. Clinical relevance of the finding

The development of anti-angiogenic agents has been rapid to date. Although demonstrating provocative physiologic effects, the results to date have not demonstrated any significant improvements in patient outcome. This may be a result of various factors including a better understanding of the timing associated with the greatest changes occurring physiologically or morphologically within the microvasculature, a better understanding of whether the hypothesis of vascular normalization (Jain 2001; Jain 2005) (Goel, Duda et al. 2011) has bearing and may be a window into the introduction of other targeted cytotoxic agents, and improved, translatable targeted molecular imaging approaches to interrogating the tumor microenvironment. As these methods evolve in parallel, one may see come to fruition a true clinical benefit to the outstanding insight proposed from Dr. Folkman's (Folkman 1971) seminal article many years ago.

4. View to the future

In order to bridge this gap in understanding the effects of angiogenesis, significant improvements and developments will have to occur within the following areas: 1) improvements in quality assurance and quality control associated with the physiologic measurements on interrogate the permeability, blood flow, and blood volume values that MRI, CT and PET; 2) improvements in targeted, molecular imaging approaches that may reflect the molecular changes that are occurring following administration of extant and novel anti-angiogenic or vascular disrupting agents, and lastly; 3) utilizing both of these approaches to better investigate and have a more comprehensive understanding of the validity and regulation of vascular normalization as a hypothesis for improved chemotherapeutic delivery is crucial.

Perfusion imaging with MRI, CT or PET provides a unique window into the vascular morphology and physiologic changes associated with agents that disrupt the tumor microenvironment or microvasculature. As we have noted in this chapter thus far, these have had a profound impact on the initial evaluation of agents that target the tumor microvasculature. If performed with proper quality assurance/quality control, and critical understanding of baseline variance, measures will allow for a more robust understanding of the true effects of agents targeted to the tumor microvasculature. Although many studies have demonstrated that there is in general good concordance with preclinical data and with other angiogenesis biomarkers, and if studies are performed well, the observations gleaned from these studies might improve the biologic understanding of the mechanism of drug action, potential drug interactions, and the duration of effects, however, the high variance demonstrated in many of these studies (>20% in some instances), makes proper determination of biologic effect sometimes suspect. This fact becomes more important as we go forward trying to study the correlation of these physiologic changes with clinical outcomes and relevant serum biomarkers.

MRI molecular imaging may play a role in improving some of these problems illustrated above. As noninvasive molecular imaging methods evolve, there will be an increasing possibility to personalization of therapy. For instance, imaging of MRI reporter-labeled stem cells or endothelial progenitor cells will provide new insights into their role in tumor angiogenesis, as these cell types have been implicated in tumor vascularization and potential poor response to antiangiogenic therapies (Monzani and La Porta 2008) (van der Schaft, Seftor et al. 2004). Exciting developments have been made in identification of tumor vascular specific receptors, which opens up possibilities for imaging but also monitoring using nanodevices the delivery of therapeutic agents, or gene delivery. Likewise, similar advances have been made in siRNA technology, where image-guided delivery to tumor microvasculature, visualization of this delivery via liposome technology or other nanocarriers, and detection of a therapeutic response are well within the realm of current imaging capabilities (Pathak, Penet et al. 2010). Yet, these technologies to this point remain preclinical and successful translation to the clinic remains a hurdle.

With all of the advances in imaging technology demonstrating effects and possible benefits of antiangiogenic therapy, the future of this kind of work remains unclear. One concept that has come to the fore and deserves mention is that of vascular normalization. A concept introduced by Rakesh Jain (Izumi, Xu et al. 2002), which describes the morphologic and physiologic changes that occur to tumor microvasculature accompanying anti-angiogenic therapy. This factor may be key in modulating the proangiogenic and anti-angiogenic forces ongoing in maintenance of the tumor microenvironment in addition to providing key insights into potential temporal windows for the introduction of cytotoxic agents. These questions remain the key to further improvements in the delivery of chemotherapeutic agents. "As a result, the presence and timing of therapy-induced normalization must be carefully studied in a range of human tumors, and novel therapeutics are needed. This will in part be informed by preclinical work, and also by development and validation of noninvasive biomarkers that survey the normalization phenotype. Only then will treatment be applied in a rational and judicious fashion with the intent of maximizing therapeutic outcomes" (Goel, Duda et al. 2011).

5. Take home message

The studies and techniques described attest to the validity of these extant and novel imaging techniques to probe the microstructural and morphologic microvascular changes that occur both as a result of tumor angiogenesis, and more importantly, soon after the delivery of anti-angiogenic therapy. These can be performed indirectly, by measuring hemodynamic parameters associated and related to blood volume, permeability and blood flow through imaging. These measures have been indispensible in the rapid and noninvasive interrogation of the microvascular changes accompanying antiangiogenic therapy. As existing techniques (e.g. DCE-MRI, CT perfusion, DCE-US) become more refined and validated by multi-institutional trials, the associated biomarkers may play a more pro-active role in the personalized approach that oncology is likely to engender. Furthermore, with the recent development of novel hybrid MRI PET devices, the realization and translation of more novel, targeted imaging approaches that probe the altered signaling pathways associated with angiogenesis, may become a reality in humans.

6. References

Adams, K. E., Ke, S., Kwon, S., Liang, F., Fan, Z., Lu, Y., Hirschi, K., Mawad, M. E., Barry, M. A., & Sevick-Muraca, E. M. (2007). "Comparison of visible and near-infrared wavelength-excitable fluorescent dyes for molecular imaging of cancer." *Journal of biomedical optics* 12(2): 024017, 1083-3668

Anderson, H. L., Yap, J. T., Miller, M.P., Robbins, A., Jones, T., & Price, P.M. (2003). Assessment of pharmacodynamic vascular response in a phase I trial of combretastatin A4 phosphate. *Journal of clinical oncology : official journal of the American Society of Clinical Oncology* 21(15): 2823-2830, 0732-183X

Backer, M. V., Levashova, Z., Levenson, R., Blankenberg, F.G., & Backer, J. M. (2008). Cysteine-containing fusion tag for site-specific conjugation of therapeutic and imaging agents to targeting proteins. *Methods in molecular biology* 494: 275-294, 1064-3745

Backer, M. V., Patel, V., Jehning, B. T., Claffey, K. P., & Backer, J. M. (2006). Surface immobilization of active vascular endothelial growth factor via a cysteine-containing tag. *Biomaterials* 27(31): 5452-5458, 0142-9612

Barnard, S., Leen, E., Cooke, T., & Angerson, W. (2008). A contrast-enhanced ultrasound study of benign and malignant breast tissue. *South African medical journal* 98(5): 386-391, 0256-9574

Beaney, R. P., Lammertsma, A. A., Jones, T., McKenzie, C. G., & Halnan, K. E. (1984). Positron emission tomography for in-vivo measurement of regional blood flow, oxygen utilisation, and blood volume in patients with breast carcinoma. *Lancet* 1(8369): 131-134, 0140-6736

Beer, A. J., Lorenzen, S., Metz, S., Herrmann, K., Watzlowik, P., Wester, H. J., Peschel, C., Lordick, F., & Schwalger, M. (2008). Comparison of integrin alphaVbeta3 expression and glucose metabolism in primary and metastatic lesions in cancer patients: a PET study using 18F-galacto-RGD and 18F-FDG. *Journal of nuclear medicine : official publication, Society of Nuclear Medicine* 49(1): 22-29, 0161-5505

Belliveau, J. W., Rosen, B. R., Kantor, H. L., Rzedzian, R. R., Kennedy, D. N., McKinstry, R. C., Vevea, J. M., Cohen, M. S., Pykett, I. L., & Brady, T. J. (1990). Functional cerebral imaging by susceptibility-contrast NMR. *Magnetic resonance in medicine : official journal of the Society of Magnetic Resonance in Medicine / Society of Magnetic Resonance in Medicine* 14(3): 538-546, 0740-3194

Bergers, G., & Benjamin, L. E. (2003). Tumorigenesis and the angiogenic switch. *Nature reviews. Cancer* 3(6): 401-410, 1474-175X

Bernabeu, C., Lopez-Novoa, J. M., & Quintanilla, M. (2009). The emerging role of TGF-beta superfamily coreceptors in cancer. *Biochimica et biophysica acta* 1792(10): 954-973, 0006-3002

Blankenberg, F. G., Backer, M. V., Levashova, Z., Patel, V., & Backer, J. M. (2006). In vivo tumor angiogenesis imaging with site-specific labeled (99m)Tc-HYNIC-VEGF. *European journal of nuclear medicine and molecular imaging* 33(7): 841-848, 1619-7070

Blomley, M. J., Albrecht, T., Cosgrove, D. O., & Bamber, J. C. (1997). Can relative contrast agent concentration be measured in vivo with color Doppler US? *Radiology* 204(1): 279-281, 0033-8419

Bredow, S., Lewin, M., Hofmann, B., Marecos, E., & Weissleder, R. (2000). Imaging of tumour neovasculature by targeting the TGF-beta binding receptor endoglin. *European journal of cancer* 36(5): 675-681, 0959-8049

Bremer, C., Bredow, S., Mahmood, U., Weissleder, R. & Tung, C. H. (2001). Optical imaging of matrix metalloproteinase-2 activity in tumors: feasibility study in a mouse model. *Radiology* 221(2): 523-529, 0033-8419

Bremer, C., Mustafa, M., Bogdanov, A., Jr., Ntziachristos, V., Petrovsky, A., & Weissleder, R. (2003). Steady-state blood volume measurements in experimental tumors with different angiogenic burdens a study in mice. *Radiology* 226(1): 214-220, 0033-8419

Brix, G., Semmler, W., Port, R., Schad, L. R., Layer, G. & Lorenz, W. J. (1991). Pharmacokinetic parameters in CNS Gd-DTPA enhanced MR imaging. *Journal of computer assisted tomography* 15(4): 621-628, 0363-8715

Bronikowski, T. A., Dawson, C. A., & Linehan, J. H. (1983). Model-free deconvolution techniques for estimating vascular transport functions. *International journal of bio-medical computing* 14(5): 411-429, 0020-7101

Brooks, P. C., Clark, R. A., & Cheresh, D. A. (1994). Requirement of vascular integrin alpha v beta 3 for angiogenesis. *Science* 264(5158): 569-571, 0036-8075

Brown, J. M. ,& Giaccia, A. J. (1998). The unique physiology of solid tumors: opportunities (and problems) for cancer therapy. *Cancer research* 58(7): 1408-1416, 0008-5472

Cai, W., Chen, K., Li, Z. B., Gambhir, S. S., & Chen, X. (2007). Dual-function probe for PET and near-infrared fluorescence imaging of tumor vasculature. *Journal of nuclear medicine : official publication, Society of Nuclear Medicine* 48(11): 1862-1870, 0161-5505

Cai, W., Chen, K., Mohamedall, K. A., Cao, Q., Gambhir, S. S., Rosenblum, M. G., & Chen X. (2006). PET of vascular endothelial growth factor receptor expression. *Journal of nuclear medicine : official publication, Society of Nuclear Medicine* 47(12): 2048-2056, 0161-5505

Cai, W., Niu, G., & Chen, X. (2008). Imaging of integrins as biomarkers for tumor angiogenesis. *Current pharmaceutical design* 14(28): 2943-2973, 1873-4286

Cai, W., D. Shin, D. W., Chen, K., Gheysens, O., Cao, Q., Wang, S. X., Gambhir, S. S., & Chen, X. (2006). Peptide-labeled near-infrared quantum dots for imaging tumor vasculature in living subjects. *Nano letters* 6(4): 669-676, 1530-6984

Cai, W., Wu, Y., Chen, K., Cao, Q., Tice, D. A., & Chen, X. (2006). In vitro and in vivo characterization of 64Cu-labeled Abegrin, a humanized monoclonal antibody against integrin alpha v beta 3. *Cancer research* 66(19): 9673-9681, 1538-7445

Cenic, A., Nabavi, D. G., Craen, R. A., Gelb, A. W., & Lee, T. Y. (2000). A CT method to measure hemodynamics in brain tumors: validation and application of cerebral blood flow maps. *AJNR. American journal of neuroradiology* 21(3): 462-470, 0195-6108

Chen, X., Conti, P. S., & Moats, R. A. (2004). In vivo near-infrared fluorescence imaging of integrin alphavbeta3 in brain tumor xenografts. *Cancer research* 64(21): 8009-8014, 0008-5472

Cheng, Z., Wu, Y., Xiong, Z., Gambhir, S. S., & Chen, X. (2005). Near-infrared fluorescent RGD peptides for optical imaging of integrin alphavbeta3 expression in living mice. *Bioconjugate chemistry* 16(6): 1433-1441, 1043-1802

Choyke, P. L., Dwyer, A. J., & Knopp, M. V. (2003). Functional tumor imaging with dynamic contrast-enhanced magnetic resonance imaging. *Journal of magnetic resonance imaging : JMRI* 17(5): 509-520, 1053-1807

Claassen, L., Seidel, G., & Algermissen, C. (2001). Quantification of flow rates using harmonic grey-scale imaging and an ultrasound contrast agent: an in vitro and in vivo study. *Ultrasound in medicine & biology* 27(1): 83-88, 0301-5629

Cornelissen, B., Oltenfreiter, R., Kersemans, V., Staelens, L., Frankenne, F., Foidart, J. M., & Slegers, G. (2005). In vitro and in vivo evaluation of [123I]-VEGF165 as a potential tumor marker. *Nuclear medicine and biology* 32(5): 431-436, 0969-8051

Corot, C., Robert, P., Idee, J. M., & Port, M. (2006). Recent advances in iron oxide nanocrystal technology for medical imaging. *Advanced drug delivery reviews* 58(14): 1471-1504, 0169-409X

Cosgrove, D., & Lassau, N. (2010). Imaging of perfusion using ultrasound. *European journal of nuclear medicine and molecular imaging* 37 Suppl 1: S65-85, 1619-7089

Costello, B., Li, C., Duff, S., Butterworth, D., Khan, A., Perkins, M., Owens, S., Al-Mowallad, A. F., O'Dwyer, S., & Kumar, S. (2004). Perfusion of 99Tcm-labeled CD105 Mab into kidneys from patients with renal carcinoma suggests that CD105 is a promising vascular target. *International journal of cancer. Journal international du cancer* 109(3): 436-441, 0020-7136

Dennie, J., Mandeville, J. B., Boxerman, J. L., Packard, S. D., Rosen, B. R., & Weisskoff, R. M. (1998). NMR imaging of changes in vascular morphology due to tumor angiogenesis. *Magnetic resonance in medicine : official journal of the Society of Magnetic Resonance in Medicine / Society of Magnetic Resonance in Medicine* 40(6): 793-799, 0740-3194

Deshpande, N., Needles, A., & Willmann, J. K. (2010). Molecular ultrasound imaging: current status and future directions. *Clinical radiology* 65(7): 567-581, 1365-229X

Deshpande, N., Pysz, M. A., & Willmann, J. K. (2010). Molecular ultrasound assessment of tumor angiogenesis. *Angiogenesis* 13(2): 175-188, 1573-7209

Di Marco, M., Di Cicilia, R., Macchini, M., Nobili, E., Vecchiarelli, S., Brandi, G., & Biasco, G. (2010). Metastatic pancreatic cancer: is gemcitabine still the best standard treatment? (Review). *Oncology reports* 23(5): 1183-1192, 1791-2431

Eckersley, R. J., Sedelaar, J. P., Blomley, M. J., Wijkstra, H., deSouza, N. M., Cosgrove, D. O., & de la Rosette, J. J. (2002). Quantitative microbubble enhanced transrectal ultrasound as a tool for monitoring hormonal treatment of prostate carcinoma. *The Prostate* 51(4): 256-267, 0270-4137

Ellegala, D. B., Leong-Poi, H., Carpenter, J. E., Klibanov, A. L., Kaul, S., Shaffrey, M. E., Sklenar, J., & Lindner, J. R. (2003). Imaging tumor angiogenesis with contrast ultrasound and microbubbles targeted to alpha(v)beta3. *Circulation* 108(3): 336-341, 1524-4539

Enochs, W. S., Harsh, G., Hochberg, F, & Weissleder, R. (1999). Improved delineation of human brain tumors on MR images using a long-circulating, superparamagnetic iron oxide agent. *Journal of magnetic resonance imaging : JMRI* 9(2): 228-232, 1053-1807

Ferrara, N. 2004). Vascular endothelial growth factor: basic science and clinical progress. *Endocrine reviews* 25(4): 581-611, 0163-769X

Ferrara, N., & Kerbel R. S. (2005). Angiogenesis as a therapeutic target. *Nature* 438(7070): 967-974, 1476-4687

Folkman, J. (1971). Tumor angiogenesis: therapeutic implications. *The New England journal of medicine* 285(21): 1182-1186.

Folkman, J. (1995). Angiogenesis in cancer, vascular, rheumatoid and other disease. *Nature medicine* 1(1): 27-31, 1078-8956

Fonsatti, E., Altomonte, M., Arsian, P. & Maio, M. (2003). Endoglin (CD105): a target for anti-angiogenetic cancer therapy. *Current drug targets* 4(4): 291-296, 1389-4501

Fonsatti, E., Jekunen, A. P., Kairemo, K. J., Coral, S., Snellman, M., Nicotra, M. R., Natali, P. G., Altomonte, M., & Maio, M. (2000). Endoglin is a suitable target for efficient imaging of solid tumors: in vivo evidence in a canine mammary carcinoma model. *Clinical cancer research : an official journal of the American Association for Cancer Research* 6(5): 2037-2043, 1078-0432

Fournier, L. S., Oudard, S., Thiam, R., Trinquart, L., Banu, E., Medioni, J., Balvay, D., Chatellier, G., Frija, G., & Cuenod, C. A. (2010). Metastatic renal carcinoma: evaluation of antiangiogenic therapy with dynamic contrast-enhanced CT. *Radiology* 256(2): 511-518, 1527-1315

Fraioli, F., Anzidei, M., Zaccagna, F., Mennini, M. L., Serra, G., Gori, B., Longo, F., Catalano, C., & Passariello, R. (2011). Whole-tumor perfusion CT in patients with advanced lung adenocarcinoma treated with conventional and antiangiogenetic chemotherapy: initial experience. *Radiology* 259(2): 574-582, 1527-1315

Frauscher, F., Klauser, A., Berger, A. P., Halern, E. J., Feuchtner, G., Koppelstaetter, F., Pallwein, L., Pinggera, G. M., Weirich, H., Horninger, W., Bartsch, G., & zur Nedden, D. (2003). The value of ultrasound (US) in the diagnosis of prostate cancer. *Der Radiologe* 43(6): 455-463, 0033-832X

Furman-Haran, E., Margalit, R., Grobgeld, D., & Degani, H. (1996). Dynamic contrast-enhanced magnetic resonance imaging reveals stress-induced angiogenesis in MCF7 human breast tumors. *Proceedings of the National Academy of Sciences of the United States of America* 93(13): 6247-6251, 0027-8424

Goel, S., Duda, D. G., Xu, L., Munn, L. L., Boucher, Y., Fukumura, D., & Jain, R. K. (2011). Normalization of the vasculature for treatment of cancer and other diseases. *Physiological reviews* 91(3): 1071-1121.

Goh, V., Halligan, S., Daley, F., Wellsted, D. M., Guenther, T., & Bartram, C. I. (2008). Colorectal tumor vascularity: quantitative assessment with multidetector CT--do tumor perfusion measurements reflect angiogenesis? *Radiology* 249(2): 510-517, 1527-1315

Guimaraes, A. R., Rakhlin, E., Weissleder, R., & Thayer, S. P. (2008). Magnetic resonance imaging monitors physiological changes with antihedgehog therapy in pancreatic adenocarcinoma xenograft model. *Pancreas* 37(4): 440-444, 1536-4828

Guimaraes, A. R., Ross, R., Figuereido, J. L., Watermen, P., & Weissleder, R. (2011). MRI with magnetic nanoparticles monitors downstream anti-angiogenic effects of mTOR inhibition. *Molecular imaging and biology : MIB : the official publication of the Academy of Molecular Imaging* 13(2): 314-320, 1860-2002

Haubner, R. (2006). Alphavbeta3-integrin imaging: a new approach to characterise angiogenesis? *European journal of nuclear medicine and molecular imaging* 33 Suppl 1: 54-63, 1619-7070

Haubner, R., Weber, W. A., Beer, A. J., Vabuliene, E., Reim, D., Sarbia, M., Becker, K. F., Goebel, M., Hein, R., Wester, H. J., Kessler, H., & Schwaiger, M. (2005). Noninvasive visualization of the activated alphavbeta3 integrin in cancer patients by positron emission tomography and [18F]Galacto-RGD. *PLoS medicine* 2(3): e70, 1549-1676

Haubner, R., Wester, H. J., Reuning, U., Senekowitsch-Schmidtke, R., Diefenbach, B., Kessler, H., Stocklin, G., & Schwaiger, M. (1999). Radiolabeled alpha(v)beta3 integrin antagonists: a new class of tracers for tumor targeting. *Journal of nuclear medicine : official publication, Society of Nuclear Medicine* 40(6): 1061-1071, 0161-5505

Haubner, R., Wester, H. J., Weber, W. A., Mang, C., Ziegler, S. I., Goodman, S. L., Senekowitsch-Schmidtke, R., Kessler, H., & Schwaiger, M. (2001). Noninvasive imaging of alpha(v)beta3 integrin expression using 18F-labeled RGD-containing glycopeptide and positron emission tomography. *Cancer research* 61(5): 1781-1785, 0008-5472

Helmlinger, G., Yuan, F., Dellian, M., & Jain, R. K. (1997). Interstitial pH and pO2 gradients in solid tumors in vivo: high-resolution measurements reveal a lack of correlation. *Nature medicine* 3(2): 177-182, 1078-8956

Herbst, R. S., Mullani, N. A., Davis, D. W., Hess, K. R., McConkey, D. J., Charnsangavej, C., O'Reilly, M. S., Kim, H. W., Baker, C., Roach, J., Ellis, L. M., Rashid, A., Pluda, J., Bucana, C., Madden, T. L., Tran, H. T., & Abbruzzese, J. L. (2002). Development of biologic markers of response and assessment of antiangiogenic activity in a clinical trial of human recombinant endostatin. *Journal of clinical oncology : official journal of the American Society of Clinical Oncology* 20(18): 3804-3814, 0732-183X

Hulka, C. A., Edmister, W. B., Smith, B. L., Tan, L., Sgroi, D. C., Campbell, T., Kopans, D. B., & Weisskoff, R. M. (1997). Dynamic echo-planar imaging of the breast: experience in diagnosing breast carcinoma and correlation with tumor angiogenesis. *Radiology* 205(3): 837-842, 0033-8419

Hulka, C. A., Smith, B. L., Sgroi, D. C., Tan, L., Edmister, W. B., Semple, J. P., Campbell, T., Kopans, D. B., Brady, T. J., & Weisskoff, R. M. (1995). Benign and malignant breast lesions: differentiation with echo-planar MR imaging. *Radiology* 197(1): 33-38, 0033-8419

Hyodo, F., Chandramouli, G. V., Matsumoto, S., Matsumoto, K., Mitchell, J. B., Krishna, M. C., & Munasinghe, J. P. (2009). Estimation of tumor microvessel density by MRI using a blood pool contrast agent. *International journal of oncology* 35(4): 797-804, 1791-2423.

Ito, M., Lammertsma, A. A., Wise, R. J., Bernardi, S., Frackowiak, R. S., Heather, J. D., McKenzie, C. G., Thomas, D. G., & Jones, T. (1982). Measurement of regional cerebral blood flow and oxygen utilisation in patients with cerebral tumours using

150 and positron emission tomography: analytical techniques and preliminary results. *Neuroradiology* 23(2): 63-74, 0028-3940.

Izumi, Y., Xu, L., di Tomaso, E., Fukumura, D., & Jain, R. K. (2002). Tumour biology: herceptin acts as an anti-angiogenic cocktail. *Nature* 416(6878): 279-280.

Jain, R. K. (1989). Delivery of novel therapeutic agents in tumors: physiological barriers and strategies. *Journal of the National Cancer Institute* 81(8): 570-576, 0027-8874

Jain, R. K. (2001). Normalizing tumor vasculature with anti-angiogenic therapy: a new paradigm for combination therapy. *Nature medicine* 7(9): 987-989, 1078-8956

Jain, R. K. (2005). Normalization of tumor vasculature: an emerging concept in antiangiogenic therapy. *Science* 307(5706): 58-62.

Jain, R. K., Duda, D. G., Clark, J. W., & Loeffler, J. S. (2006). Lessons from phase III clinical trials on anti-VEGF therapy for cancer. *Nature clinical practice. Oncology* 3(1): 24-40, 1743-4254

Janssen, M. L., Oyen, W. J., Dijkgraaf, I., Massuger, L. F., Frielink, C., Edwards, D. S., Rajopadhye, M., Boonstra, H., Corstens, F. H., & Boerman, O. C. (2002). Tumor targeting with radiolabeled alpha(v)beta(3) integrin binding peptides in a nude mouse model. *Cancer research* 62(21): 6146-6151, 0008-5472

Jayson, G. C., Zweit, J, Jackson, A., Mulatero, C., Julyan, P., Ranson, M., Broughton, L., Wagstaff, J., Hakannson, L., Groenewegen, G., Bailey, J., Smith, N., Hastings, D., Lawrance, J., Haroon, H., Ward, T., McGown, A. T., Tang, M., Levitt, D., Marreaud, S., Lehmann, F. F., Herold, M. & Zwierzine, H. (2002). Molecular imaging and biological evaluation of HuMV833 anti-VEGF antibody: implications for trial design of antiangiogenic antibodies. *Journal of the National Cancer Institute* 94(19): 1484-1493, 0027-8874

Jiang, T., Kambadakone, A., Kulkarni, N. M., Zhu, A. X., & Sahani, D. V. (2011). Monitoring Response to Antiangiogenic Treatment and Predicting Outcomes in Advanced Hepatocellular Carcinoma Using Image Biomarkers, CT Perfusion, Tumor Density, and Tumor Size (RECIST). *Investigative radiology*, 1536-0210

Jin, Z. H., Josserand, V., Foillard, S., Boturyn, D., Dumy, P., Favrot, M. C., & Coll, J. L. (2007). In vivo optical imaging of integrin alphaV-beta3 in mice using multivalent or monovalent cRGD targeting vectors. *Molecular cancer* 6: 41, 1476-4598

Josephs, D., Spicer, J., & O'Doherty, M. (2009). Molecular imaging in clinical trials. *Targeted oncology* 4(3): 151-168, 1778-260X.

Jung, E. M., Jungius, K. P., Rupp, N., Gallegos, M., Ritter, G., Lenhart, M., Clevert, D. A., & Kubale, R. (2005). Contrast enhanced harmonic ultrasound for differentiating breast tumors - first results. *Clinical hemorheology and microcirculation* 33(2): 109-120, 1386-0291

Kedar, R. P., Cosgrove, D. o., Bamber, J. C., & Bell, D. S. (1995). Automated quantification of color Doppler signals: a preliminary study in breast tumors. *Radiology* 197(1): 39-43, 0033-8419

Klibanov, A. L. (2005). Ligand-carrying gas-filled microbubbles: ultrasound contrast agents for targeted molecular imaging. *Bioconjugate chemistry* 16(1): 9-17, 1043-1802

Klibanov, A. L. (2009). Preparation of targeted microbubbles: ultrasound contrast agents for molecular imaging. *Medical & biological engineering & computing* 47(8): 875-882, 1741-0444

Klibanov, A. L., Hughes, M. S., Villanueva, F. S., Jankowski, R. J., Wagner, W. R., Wojdyla, J. K., Wible, J. H., & Brandenburger, G. H. (1999). Targeting and ultrasound imaging of microbubble-based contrast agents. *Magma* 8(3): 177-184, 0968-5243

Knopp, M. V., Giesel, F.L., Marcos, H., von Tengg-Kobligk, H., & Choyke, P. (2001). Dynamic contrast-enhanced magnetic resonance imaging in oncology. *Topics in magnetic resonance imaging : TMRI* 12(4): 301-308, 0899-3459

Knopp, M. V., Weiss, E., Sinn, H. P., Mattern, J,. Junkermann, H., Radeleff, A., Magener, A., Brix, G., Delorme, S., Zuna, I., & van Kaick, G. (1999). Pathophysiologic basis of contrast enhancement in breast tumors. *Journal of magnetic resonance imaging : JMRI* 10(3): 260-266, 1053-1807

Kok, R. J., Schraa, A. J., Bos, E. J., Moorlag, H. E., Asgeirsdottir, S. A., Everts, M., Meijer, D. K., & Molema, G. (2002). Preparation and functional evaluation of RGD-modified proteins as alpha(v)beta(3) integrin directed therapeutics. *Bioconjugate chemistry* 13(1): 128-135, 1043-1802

Korpanty, G., Carbon, J. G., Grayburn, P. A., Fleming, J. B., & Brekken, R. A. (2007). Monitoring response to anticancer therapy by targeting microbubbles to tumor vasculature. *Clinical cancer research : an official journal of the American Association for Cancer Research* 13(1): 323-330, 1078-0432

Korpanty, G., Grayburn, P. A., Shohet, R. V., & Brekken, R. A. (2005). Targeting vascular endothelium with avidin microbubbles. *Ultrasound in medicine & biology* 31(9): 1279-1283, 0301-5629

Kossodo, S., Pickarski, M., Lin, S. A., Gleason, A., Gaspar, R., Buono, C., Ho, G., Blusztajn, A., Cuneo, G., Zhang, J., Jensen, J., Hargreaves, R., Coleman, P., Hartman, G., Rajopadhye, M., Duong le, T., Sur, C., Yared, W., Peterson, J., & Bednar, B. (2010). Dual in vivo quantification of integrin-targeted and protease-activated agents in cancer using fluorescence molecular tomography (FMT). *Molecular imaging and biology : MIB : the official publication of the Academy of Molecular Imaging* 12(5): 488-499, 1860-2002

Lee, T. Y., Purdie, T. G., & Stewart, E. (2003). CT imaging of angiogenesis. *The quarterly journal of nuclear medicine : official publication of the Italian Association of Nuclear Medicine* 47(3): 171-187, 1125-0135

Levashova, Z., Backer, M., Backer, J. M., & Blankenberg, F. G. (2008). Direct site-specific labeling of the Cys-tag moiety in scVEGF with technetium 99m. *Bioconjugate chemistry* 19(5): 1049-1054, 1520-4812

Li, S., Peck-Radosavljevic, M., Kienast, O., Preitfellner, J., Havlik, E., Schima, W., Traub-Weidinger, T., Graf, S., Beheshti, M., Schmid, M., Angelberger, P., & Dudczak, R. (2004). Iodine-123-vascular endothelial growth factor-165 (123I-VEGF165). Biodistribution, safety and radiation dosimetry in patients with pancreatic carcinoma. *The quarterly journal of nuclear medicine and molecular imaging : official publication of the Italian Association of Nuclear Medicine* 48(3): 198-206, 1824-4785

Lucidarme, O., Kono, Y., Corbell, J., Choi, S. H., & Mattrey, R. F. (2003). Validation of ultrasound contrast destruction imaging for flow quantification. *Ultrasound in medicine & biology* 29(12): 1697-1704, 0301-5629

Ma, X., Labinaz, M., Goldstein, J., Miller, H., Keon, W. J., Letarte, M., & O'Brien, E. (2000). Endoglin is overexpressed after arterial injury and is required for transforming growth factor-beta-induced inhibition of smooth muscle cell migration. *Arteriosclerosis, thrombosis, and vascular biology* 20(12): 2546-2552, 1524-4636

Mankoff, D. A. (2007). A definition of molecular imaging. *Journal of nuclear medicine : official publication, Society of Nuclear Medicine* 48(6): 18N, 21N, 0161-5505

Massoud, T. F., & Gambhir S. S. (2003). Molecular imaging in living subjects: seeing fundamental biological processes in a new light. *Genes & development* 17(5): 545-580, 0890-9369

Miles, K. A., & Griffiths, M. R. (2003). Perfusion CT: a worthwhile enhancement? *The British journal of radiology* 76(904): 220-231, 0007-1285

Millauer, B., Wizigmann-Voos, S., Schnurch, H., Martinez, R., Moller, N. P., Risau, W., & Ullrich, A. (1993). High affinity VEGF binding and developmental expression suggest Flk-1 as a major regulator of vasculogenesis and angiogenesis. *Cell* 72(6): 835-846, 0092-8674

Monzani, E., & and La Porta, C. A. (2008). Targeting cancer stem cells to modulate alternative vascularization mechanisms. *Stem cell reviews* 4(1): 51-56.

Morgan, B., Thomas, A. L., Drevs, J., Hennig, J., Buchert, M., Jivan, A., Horsfield, M. A., Mross, K., Ball, H. A., Lee, L., Mietlowski, W., Fuxuis, S., Unger, C., O'Byrne, K., Henry, A., Cherryman, G. R., Laurent, D., Dugan, M., Marme, D., & Steward, W. P. (2003). Dynamic contrast-enhanced magnetic resonance imaging as a biomarker for the pharmacological response of PTK787/ZK 222584, an inhibitor of the vascular endothelial growth factor receptor tyrosine kinases, in patients with advanced colorectal cancer and liver metastases: results from two phase I studies. *Journal of clinical oncology : official journal of the American Society of Clinical Oncology* 21(21): 3955-3964, 0732-183X

Mulder, W. J., Castermans, K., van Beijnum, J. R., Oude Egbrink, M. G., Chin, P. T., Fayad, Z. A., Lowik, C. W., Kaijzel, E. L., Que, I., Storm, G., Strijkers, G. J., Griffioen, A. W., & Nicolay, K. (2009). Molecular imaging of tumor angiogenesis using alphavbeta3-integrin targeted multimodal quantum dots. *Angiogenesis* 12(1): 17-24, 1573-7209

Mulder, W. J., Koole, R., Brandwijk, R. J., Storm, G., Chin, P. T., Strijkers, G. J., de Mello Donega, C., Nicolay, K., & Griffioen, A. W. (2006). Quantum dots with a paramagnetic coating as a bimodal molecular imaging probe. *Nano letters* 6(1): 1-6, 1530-6984

Mulder, W. J., Strijkers, G. J., Habets, J. W., Bleeker, E. J., van der Schaft, D. W., Storm, G., Koning, G. A., Griffioen, A. W., & Nicolay, K. (2005). MR molecular imaging and fluorescence microscopy for identification of activated tumor endothelium using a bimodal lipidic nanoparticle. *The FASEB journal : official publication of the Federation of American Societies for Experimental Biology* 19(14): 2008-2010, 1530-6860

Ostergaard, L., Smith, D. F., Vestergaard- Poulsen, P., Hansen, S. B., Gee, A. D., Gjedde, A., & Gyldensted, C. (1998). Absolute cerebral blood flow and blood volume measured by magnetic resonance imaging bolus tracking: comparison with positron emission tomography values. *Journal of cerebral blood flow and metabolism : official journal of the International Society of Cerebral Blood Flow and Metabolism* 18(4): 425-432, 0271-678X

Padera, T. P., Stoll, B. R., Tooredman, J. B., Capen, D., di Tomaso, E., & Jain, R. K. (2004). Pathology: cancer cells compress intratumour vessels. *Nature* 427(6976): 695, 1476-4687

Pathak, A. P., M. Penet, et al. (2010). MR Molecular Imaging of Tumor Vasculature and Vascular Targets. *Advances in Genetics*, Elsevier Inc. 69.

Patlak, C. S., Blasberg, R. G., & Fenstermacher, J. D. (1983). Graphical evaluation of blood-to-brain transfer constants from multiple-time uptake data. *Journal of cerebral blood flow and metabolism : official journal of the International Society of Cerebral Blood Flow and Metabolism* 3(1): 1-7, 0271-678X

Perkins, A. C., Frier, M., Hindle, A. J., Blackshaw, P. E., Bailey, S. E., Hebden, J. M., Middleton, S. M., & Wastie, M. L. (1997). Human biodistribution of an ultrasound contrast agent (Quantison) by radiolabelling and gamma scintigraphy. The *British journal of radiology* 70(834): 603-611, 0007-1285

Persigehl, T., Bieker, R., Matuszewski, L., Wall, A., Kessler, T., Kooijman, H., Meier, N., Ebert, W., Berdel, W. E., Heindel, W., Mesters, R. M., & Bremer, C. (2007). Antiangiogenic tumor treatment: early noninvasive monitoring with USPIO-enhanced MR imaging in mice. *Radiology* 244(2): 449-456, 0033-8419

Petralia, G., Preda, L., D'Andrea, G., Viotti, S., Bonello, L., De Filippi, R., & Bellomi, M. (2010). CT perfusion in solid-body tumours. Part I: Technical issues. *La Radiologia medica* 115(6): 843-857, 1826-6983

Pham, C. D., Roberts, T. P., van Bruggen, N., Melnyk, O., Mann, J., Ferrara, N., Cohen, R. L., & Brasch, R. C. (1998). Magnetic resonance imaging detects suppression of tumor vascular permeability after administration of antibody to vascular endothelial growth factor. *Cancer investigation* 16(4): 225-230, 0735-7907

Piccoli, C. W. (1997). Contrast-enhanced breast MRI: factors affecting sensitivity and specificity. *European radiology* 7 Suppl 5: 281-288, 0938-7994

Pochon, S., Tardy, I., Bussat, P., Bettinger, T., Brochot, J., von Wronski, M., Passantino, L., & Schneider, M. (2010). BR55: a lipopeptide-based VEGFR2-targeted ultrasound contrast agent for molecular imaging of angiogenesis. *Investigative radiology* 45(2): 89-95, 1536-0210

Purdie, T. G., Henderson, E., & Lee, T. Y. (2001). Functional CT imaging of angiogenesis in rabbit VX2 soft-tissue tumour. *Physics in medicine and biology* 46(12): 3161-3175, 0031-9155

Pysz, M. A., Foygel, K., Rosenberg, J., Gambhir, S. S., Schneider, M., & Willmann, J. K. (2010). Antiangiogenic cancer therapy: monitoring with molecular US and a clinically translatable contrast agent (BR55). *Radiology* 256(2): 519-527, 1527-1315

Ring, J., Persigehl, T., Remmele, S., Heindel, W., Dahnke, H., & Bremer, C. (2011). Monitoring of bevacizumab-induced antiangiogenic treatment effects by "steady state" ultrasmall superparamagnetic iron oxide particles magnetic resonance imaging using robust multiecho DeltaR2* relaxometry. *Investigative radiology* 46(5): 326-330, 1536-0210

Rizzatto, G., Martegani, A, Chersevani, R., Macorig, D., Vrtovec, M. Aiani, L., & Tufarulo, L. (2001). Importance of staging of breast cancer and role of contrast ultrasound. *European radiology* 11 Suppl 3: E47-51, 0938-7994

Sabir, A., Schor-Bardach, R., Wilcox, C. J., Rahmanuddin, S., Atkins, M. B., Kruskal, J. B., Signoretti, S., Raptopoulos, V. D., & Goldberg, S. N. (2008). Perfusion MDCT enables early detection of therapeutic response to antiangiogenic therapy. *AJR. American journal of roentgenology* 191(1): 133-139, 1546-3141

Saltz, L. B., Clarke, S., Diaz-Rubio, E., Scheithauer, W., Figer, A., Wong, R., Koski, S., Lichinitser, M., Yang, T. S., Rivera, F., Couture, F., Sirzen, F., & Cassidy, J. (2008). Bevacizumab in combination with oxaliplatin-based chemotherapy as first-line therapy in metastatic colorectal cancer: a randomized phase III study. *Journal of clinical oncology : official journal of the American Society of Clinical Oncology* 26(12): 2013-2019, 1527-7755

Sandler, A., Gray, R., Perry, M. C., Brahmer, J., Schiller, J. H., Dowlati, A., Lilenbaum, R., & Johnson, D. H. (2006). Paclitaxel-carboplatin alone or with bevacizumab for non-small-cell lung cancer. *The New England journal of medicine* 355(24): 2542-2550, 1533-4406

Schmieder, A. H., Winter, P. M., Caruthers, S. D., Harris, T. D., Williams, T. A., Allen, J. S., Lacy, E. K., Zhang, H., Scott, M. J., Hu, G., Robertson, J. D., Wickline, S. A., & Lanza, G. M. (2005). Molecular MR imaging of melanoma angiogenesis with alphanubeta3-targeted paramagnetic nanoparticles. *Magnetic resonance in medicine : official journal of the Society of Magnetic Resonance in Medicine / Society of Magnetic Resonance in Medicine* 53(3): 621-627, 0740-3194

Schraa, A. J., Kok, R. J., Moorlag, H. E., Bos, E. J., Proost, J. H., Meijer, D. K., de Leij, L. F., & Molema, G. (2002). Targeting of RGD-modified proteins to tumor vasculature: a pharmacokinetic and cellular distribution study. *International journal of cancer. Journal international du cancer* 102(5): 469-475, 0020-7136

Shiyan, L., Pintong, H., Zongmin, W., Fuguang, H., Zhiqiang, Z., Yan, Y., & Cosgrove, D. (2009). The relationship between enhanced intensity and microvessel density of gastric carcinoma using double contrast-enhanced ultrasonography. *Ultrasound in medicine & biology* 35(7): 1086-1091, 1879-291X

Sipkins, D. A., Cheresh, D. A., Kazemi, M. R., Nevin, L. M., Bednarski, M. D., & Li, K. C. (1998). Detection of tumor angiogenesis in vivo by alphaVbeta3-targeted magnetic resonance imaging. *Nature medicine* 4(5): 623-626, 1078-8956

Stohrer, M., Boucher, Y., Stangassinger, M., & Jain, R. K. (2000). Oncotic pressure in solid tumors is elevated. *Cancer research* 60(15): 4251-4255, 0008-5472

Stollman, T. H., Ruers, T. J., Oyen, W. J., & Boerman, O. C. (2009). New targeted probes for radioimaging of angiogenesis. *Methods* 48(2): 188-192, 1095-9130

Su, M. Y., Cheung, Y. C., Fruehauf, J. P., Yu, H., Nalcioglu, O., Mechetner, E., Kyshtoobayeva, A., Chen, S. C., Hsueh, S., McLaren, C. E., & Wan, Y. L. (2003). Correlation of dynamic contrast enhancement MRI parameters with microvessel density and VEGF for assessment of angiogenesis in breast cancer. *Journal of magnetic resonance imaging : JMRI* 18(4): 467-477, 1053-1807

Tabata, M., Kondo, M., Haruta, Y., & Seon, B. K. (1999). Antiangiogenic radioimmunotherapy of human solid tumors in SCID mice using (125)I-labeled anti-endoglin monoclonal antibodies. *International journal of cancer. Journal international du cancer* 82(5): 737-742, 0020-7136

Teicher, B. A. (1996). A systems approach to cancer therapy. (Antioncogenics + standard cytotoxics-->mechanism(s) of interaction). *Cancer metastasis reviews* 15(2): 247-272, 0167-7659

Tofts, P. S. (1997). Modeling tracer kinetics in dynamic Gd-DTPA MR imaging. *Journal of magnetic resonance imaging : JMRI* 7(1): 91-101, 1053-1807

Tofts, P. S., Brix, G, Buckley, D. L., Evelhoch, J. L., Henderson, E., Knopp, M. V., Larsson, H. B., Lee, T. Y., Mayr, N. A., Parker, G. J., Port, R. E., Taylor, J., & Weisskoff, R. M. (1999). Estimating kinetic parameters from dynamic contrast-enhanced T(1)-weighted MRI of a diffusable tracer: standardized quantities and symbols. *Journal of magnetic resonance imaging : JMRI* 10(3): 223-232, 1053-1807

Tong, R. T., Boucher, Y., Kozin, S. V., Winkler, F., Hicklin, D. J., & Jain, R. K. (2004). Vascular normalization by vascular endothelial growth factor receptor 2 blockade induces a pressure gradient across the vasculature and improves drug penetration in tumors. *Cancer research* 64(11): 3731-3736, 0008-5472

Tropres, I., Grimault, S., Vaeth, A., Grillon, E., Julien, C., Payen, J. F., Lamalle, L., & Decorps, M. (2001). Vessel size imaging. *Magnetic resonance in medicine : official journal of the Society of Magnetic Resonance in Medicine / Society of Magnetic Resonance in Medicine* 45(3): 397-408, 0740-3194

Vag, T., Schramm, T., Kaiser, W. A., & Hilger, I. (2009). Proliferating and quiescent human umbilical vein endothelial cells (HUVECs): a potential in vitro model to evaluate contrast agents for molecular imaging of angiogenesis. *Contrast media & molecular imaging* 4(4): 192-198, 1555-4317

van der Flier, A., & Sonnenberg, A. (2001). Function and interactions of integrins. *Cell and tissue research* 305(3): 285-298, 0302-766X

van der Schaft, D. W., Seftor, R. E., Seftor, E. A., Hess, A. R., Gruman, L. M., Kirschmann, D. A., Yokoyama, Y., Griffioen, A. W., & Hendrix, M. J. (2004). Effects of angiogenesis inhibitors on vascular network formation by human endothelial and melanoma cells. *Journal of the National Cancer Institute* 96(19): 1473-1477.

van Hagen, P. M., Breeman, W. A., Bernard, H. F., Schaar, M., Mooij, C. M., Srinivasan, A., Schmidt, M. A., Krenning, E. P., & de Jong, M. (2000). Evaluation of a radiolabelled cyclic DTPA-RGD analogue for tumour imaging and radionuclide therapy. *International journal of cancer. Journal international du cancer* 90(4): 186-198, 0020-7136

Wang, H., Cai, W., Chen, K., Li, Z. B., Kashefi, A., He, L., & Chen, X. (2007). A new PET tracer specific for vascular endothelial growth factor receptor 2. *European journal of nuclear medicine and molecular imaging* 34(12): 2001-2010, 1619-7070

Wang, J., Lv, F., Fei, X., Cui, Q., Wang, L., Gao, X., Yuan, Z., Lin, Q., Lv, Y., & Liu, A. (2011). Study on the characteristics of contrast-enhanced ultrasound and its utility in assessing the microvessel density in ovarian tumors or tumor-like lesions. *International journal of biological sciences* 7(5): 600-606, 1449-2288

Wei, K., Jayaweera, A. R., Firoozan, S., Linka, A., Skyba, D. M., & Kaul, S. (1998). Quantification of myocardial blood flow with ultrasound-induced destruction of microbubbles administered as a constant venous infusion. *Circulation* 97(5): 473-483, 0009-7322

Weskott, H. P. (2008). Emerging roles for contrast-enhanced ultrasound. *Clinical hemorheology and microcirculation* 40(1): 51-71, 1386-0291

Willett, C. G., Boucher, Y., di Tomaso, E., Duda, D. G., Munn, L. L., Tong, R. T., Chung, D. C., Sahani, D. V., Kalva, S. P., Kozin, S. V., Mino, M., Cohen, K. S., Scadden, D. T., Hartford, A. C., Fischman, A. J., Clark, J. W., Ryan, D. P., Zhu, A. X., Blaszkowsky, L. S., Chen, H. X., Shellito, P. C., Lauwers, G. Y., & Jain, R. K. (2004). Direct evidence that the VEGF-specific antibody bevacizumab has antivascular effects in human rectal cancer. *Nature medicine* 10(2): 145-147, 1078-8956

Willmann, J. K., Cheng, Z., Davis, C., Lutz, A. M., Schipper, M. L., Nielsen, C. H., & Gambhir, S. S. (2008). Targeted microbubbles for imaging tumor angiogenesis: assessment of whole-body biodistribution with dynamic micro-PET in mice. *Radiology* 249(1): 212-219, 1527-1315

Willmann, J. K., Paulmurugan, R., Chen, K., Gheysens, O., Rodriguez-Porcel, M., Lutz, A. M., Chen, I. Y., Chen, X., & Gambhir, S. S. (2008). US imaging of tumor angiogenesis with microbubbles targeted to vascular endothelial growth factor receptor type 2 in mice. *Radiology* 246(2): 508-518, 1527-1315

Wink, M., Frauscher, F., Cosgrove, D., Chapelon, J. Y., Palwein, L., Mitterberger, M., Harvey, C., Rouviere, O., de la Rosette, J., & Wijkstra, H. (2008). Contrast-enhanced ultrasound and prostate cancer; a multicentre European research coordination project. *European urology* 54(5): 982-992, 0302,2838

Winter, P. M., Caruthers, S. D., Kassner, A., Harris, T. D., Chinen, L. K., Allen, J. S., lacy, E. K., Zhang, H., Robertson, J. D., Wickline, S. A., & Lanza, G. M. (2003). Molecular imaging of angiogenesis in nascent Vx-2 rabbit tumors using a novel alpha(nu)beta3-targeted nanoparticle and 1.5 tesla magnetic resonance imaging. *Cancer research* 63(18): 5838-5843, 0008-5472

Wouters, B. G., & Brown, J. M. (1997). Cells at intermediate oxygen levels can be more important than the "hypoxic fraction" in determining tumor response to fractionated radiotherapy. *Radiation research* 147(5): 541-550, 0033-7587

Wu, Y., Cai, W., & Chen, X. (2006). Near-infrared fluorescence imaging of tumor integrin alpha v beta 3 expression with Cy7-labeled RGD multimers. *Molecular imaging and biology : MIB : the official publication of the Academy of Molecular Imaging* 8(4): 226-236, 1536-1632

Yoon, S. S., Duda, D. G., Karl, D. L., Kim, T. M., Kambadakone, A. R., Chen, Y. L., Rothrock, C., Rosenberg, A. E., Nielsen, G. P., Kirsch, D. G., Choy, E., Harmon, D. C., Hornicek, F. J., Dreyfuss, J., Ancukiewicz, M., Sahani, D. V., Park, P. J., Jain, R. K., & Delaney, T. F. (2010). Phase II Study of Neoadjuvant Bevacizumab and Radiotherapy for Resectable Soft Tissue Sarcomas. *International journal of radiation oncology, biology, physics,* 1879-355X

Zhang, C., Jugold, M., Woenne, E. C., Lammers, T., Morgenstern, B., Mueller, M. M., Zentgraf, H., Bock, M., Eisenhut, M., Semmler, W., & Kiessling, F. (2007). Specific targeting of tumor angiogenesis by RGD-conjugated ultrasmall superparamagnetic iron oxide particles using a clinical 1.5-T magnetic resonance scanner. *Cancer research* 67(4): 1555-1562, 0008-5472

Zhang, D., Feng, X. Y., Henning, T. D., Wen, L., Lu, W. Y., Pan, H., Wu, X., & Zou, L. G. (2009). MR imaging of tumor angiogenesis using sterically stabilized Gd-DTPA liposomes targeted to CD105. *European journal of radiology* 70(1): 180-189.

Zhang, X., Xiong, Z., Wu, Y., Cai, W., Tseng, J. R., Gambhir, S. S., & Chen, X. (2006). Quantitative PET imaging of tumor integrin alphavbeta3 expression with 18F-FRGD2. *Journal of nuclear medicine : official publication, Society of Nuclear Medicine* 47(1): 113-121, 0161-5505

Zhu, A. X., Sahani, D. V., Duda, D. G., di Tomaso, E., Ancukiewicz, M., Catalano, O. A., Sindhwani, V., Blaszkowsky, L. S., Yoon, S. S., Lahdenranta, J., Bhargava, P., Meyerhardt, J., Clark, J. W., Kwak, E. L., Hezel, A. F., Miksad, R., Abrams, T. A., Enzinger, P. C., Fuchs, C. S., Ryan, D. P., & Jain, R. K. (2009). Efficacy, safety, and potential biomarkers of sunitinib monotherapy in advanced hepatocellular carcinoma: a phase II study. *Journal of clinical oncology : official journal of the American Society of Clinical Oncology* 27(18): 3027-3035, 1527-7755

Zhuang, H., Yang, Z. G., Chen, H. J., Peng, Y. L., & Li, L. (2011). Time-intensity curve parameters in colorectal tumours measured using double contrast-enhanced ultrasound: correlations with tumour angiogenesis. *Colorectal disease : the official journal of the Association of Coloproctology of Great Britain and Ireland*, 1463-1318

13

PET and SPECT Imaging of Tumor Angiogenesis

Marcian E. Van Dort[1,3], Pedram Navid-Azarbaijani[2], Rajesh Ranga[2], Alnawaz Rehemtulla[2,3], Brian D Ross[1,3], Allan E David[4] and Mahaveer S Bhojani[1,3]

[1]Dept. of Radiology,
[2]Dept. of Radiation Oncology,
[3]Center for Molecular Imaging,
University of Michigan Medical School, Ann Arbor,
[4]College of Pharmacy,
USA

1. Introduction

1.1 PET and SPECT imaging

Positron Emission Tomography (PET) and Single Photon Emission Computed Tomography (SPECT) based functional imaging utilize radiolabeled tracers to provide information for real time visualization of physiological or biological processes in live animals or humans. Disease-related biomarkers involved in initiation and/or progression of a pathological condition are imaged by these nuclear imaging technologies which lead to early detection of abnormalities prior to the appearance of morphological changes visualized by other imaging modalities such as CT or MRI (1-3). Additional advantages of nuclear imaging approaches are high sensitivity of detection and high spatial resolution. Further they are either non- or minimally invasive and highly quantitative (4). Together, these characteristics of PET and SPECT make them an invaluable technique for monitoring some diseases and disorders.

There are significant differences between PET and SPECT, some of which are highlighted below. A major advantage of PET over SPECT is its 2-3 orders of magnitude greater sensitivity and quantitative capability (5). PET utilizes radioisotopes that decay via emission of positrons, whereas, SPECT radioisotopes decay by electron capture and/or gamma emission (5). Table **1** lists some of the most commonly used PET and SPECT radioisotopes and their physical properties. The synthetic chemistry behind development of these radioisotopes as tracers for imaging is dependent on the half-lives. For example, the short decay half-lives (2 - 20 min) of the PET radioisotopes: carbon-11, nitrogen-13 and oxygen-15 requires that radiotracer synthesis with these radioisotopes be conducted in close proximity to a cyclotron (3-5). On the other hand, radioisotopes such as fluorine-18, copper-64, indium-111, iodine-123 and iodine-124 are sufficiently long-lived to allow transportation from regional commercial sites (3-5). Additionally, the radioisotopes gallium-68, copper-62 and technetium-99m can be conveniently obtained from an in-house generator (3-5). At the present time, clinical SPECT imaging is more prevalent than PET imaging due to both its cost effectiveness and the greater availability of SPECT scanners at most nuclear medicine clinics.

Isotope	Imaging Mode	Production Method	Half-Life	Decay Mode(s)
^{11}C	PET	Cyclotron	20.4 min	β+ (99+%)
^{13}N	PET	Cyclotron	10 min	β+ (100%)
^{15}O	PET	Cyclotron	2.03 min	β+ (99.9%)
^{18}F	PET	Cyclotron	110 min	β+ (97%) EC (3%)
^{124}I	PET	Accelerator	4.2 days	EC (74.4%) β+ (25.6%)
^{68}Ga	PET	Generator	68.3 min	β+ (90%) EC (10%)
^{62}Cu	PET	Generator	9.73 min	β+ (98%) EC (2%)
^{64}Cu	PET	Reactor	12.7 hours	β+ (61%) β- (39%)
^{99m}Tc	SPECT	Generator	6.02 hours	IC (100%)
^{111}In	Gamma Scintigraphy	Accelerator	2.8 days	EC (100%)
^{123}I	SPECT	Accelerator	13.3 hours	β+ (100%)
^{192}Ir	SPECT	Reactor	73.8 days	EC (4.9%) β- (95.1%)
^{201}Tl	SPECT	Cyclotron	73 hours	EC (100%)
^{82}Rb	PET	Generator	1.27 min	β+ (100%)
^{89}Zr	PET	Cyclotron	3.3 days	β+ (100%)

β+ = positron emission; EC = electron capture; IC = isomeric conversion, β- = electron emission

Table 1. Common PET and SPECT Radioisotopes

In recent years, an effort has been made to combine anatomical imaging modalities (such as CT and MRI) with molecular imaging modalities in order to capitalize on the strengths of both techniques. These multi-modality approaches can provide both high structural detail and high detection sensitivity of pathophysiological changes giving greater insight into the dynamic processes of tumor growth and progression. Advances in this field have already been made and PET-CT technology is now available for use in many clinics (6-8). Further, the recent approval by the US Food and Drug Administration (FDA) of the first PET-MRI machine for clinical imaging (9) is a major step forward in multimodal imaging. Compared with PET-CT technology, PET-MRI scans demonstrate higher structural detail, especially of soft tissues, and additionally permit the use of MRI techniques such as perfusion imaging and MR spectroscopy (10). Furthermore, MRI scans (in PET-MRI) use magnetic fields instead of x-rays, thereby decreasing patient radiation doses in comparison to PET-CT scans

(10). Boss et al. showed the effectiveness and reliability of PET-MRI in scanning intracranial tumors using [^{11}C] methionine or [^{68}Ga] DOTATOC (11).

The past decade has seen the investigation and validation of several radiotracers with particular emphasis in oncology. These targets include molecular biomarkers such as growth factor receptors, protein kinases, specific receptor over-expression or biological events such as angiogenesis, apoptosis, hypoxia and tumor proliferation (1-3). This review will highlight recent PET and SPECT radiotracer development for angiogenesis imaging with a major focus on their application in oncology.

1.2 Biology of angiogenesis

Angiogenesis, the formation of new blood vessels, plays a central role in growth of tumors beyond 1-2 mm^3 as neovascularization is required to supply oxygen and nutrients and for removal of cellular wastes(12-14). Further, neo-angiogenesis is critical to the metastatic potential of tumors as it aids in the dispersion of cancer cells to distant organs. Recent advances in cellular and molecular biology have led to the identification of novel angiogenic biomarkers and molecular dissection of their signaling pathways(13, 15). One of the key signaling pathways involved in initiation of new tumor blood vessels is mediated by vascular endothelial growth factor (VEGF) and its receptor tyrosine kinase (VEGFR)(16-18). Pro-angiogenic signaling mediated by VEGF/VEGFR is critical when tumors outgrow their existing blood supply and frequently display oxygen deficiency (hypoxia). Hypoxia is known to trigger the secretion of VEGF (19-22). Binding of VEGF to its receptor initiates a signaling cascade that promotes the proliferation, migration and survival of endothelial cells, ultimately leading to angiogenesis (23-25). The angiogenic effects of the VEGF family are believed to be primarily mediated through VEGF-A. To date, VEGF-A (also referred to as VEGF) and its receptors are the most characterized signaling pathways in developmental and tumor angiogenesis(24, 26-35).

Alternative splicing of RNA has revealed the existence of at least nine different molecular isoforms for VEGF-A, comprising 121, 145, 148, 162, 165, 165b, 183, 189 or 206 amino acids(36-43). The angiogenic actions of VEGF-A are mediated primarily via two closely related endothelium-specific receptor tyrosine kinases (VEGFR-1 and VEGFR-2)(44-46). All of the VEGF-A isoforms bind to both VEGFR-1 and VEGFR-2, of which, VEGFR-2 is the major mediator of proliferation and angiogenesis (14). Thus, a variety of solid tumor cells overexpress VEGFR-2, which serves as poor prognostic marker for the survival of cancer patients (47, 48). Therefore, new therapies based on humanized monoclonal antibodies that inhibit VEGF-A are used to treat cancers of colorectal, lung, kidney and eye origin and there are many newer therapies under various stages of development (27, 49)

2. Molecular targets and ligands for PET/SPECT imaging of angiogenesis

2.1 VEGF receptor and ligands

PET imaging of VEGFR expression *in vivo* was first demonstrated using $VEGF_{121}$ radiolabeled with ^{64}Cu. Radiolabeling was achieved via ^{64}Cu chelation to a DOTA-$VEGF_{121}$ conjugate (DOTA is an abbreviation for 1,4,7,10-tetraazacyclododecane-*N,N′,N″,N‴*-tetraacetic acid). *In vivo* evaluation of ^{64}Cu-DOTA-$VEGF_{121}$ using microPET imaging of athymic nude mice bearing U87MG human glioblastoma xenografts showed rapid and high specific accumulation of the radioligand in small U87MG tumors (16% injected dose per gram [ID/g]) at 4 h post-injection. Larger tumors showed significantly lower uptake (1 - 3% ID/g). Differences in tumor localization between large and small tumors showed a good correlation with tumor VEGF receptor expression (VEGFR-2). *In vivo* VEGFR-2 specificity of the radioligand was also confirmed by pharmacological blocking experiments and *ex vivo* studies (immunofluorescence staining, western blot analysis). This study also demonstrated the dynamic nature of VEGFR signaling during tumor growth and proliferation. Subsequently, these authors also reported on the development of a ^{64}Cu-labeled vasculature-targeting fusion toxin ($VEGF_{121}$/rGel) composed of a $VEGF_{121}$ linked recombinant plant toxin gelonin construct (rGel) for multimodality imaging and therapy of glioblastoma. Sustained tumor accumulation and high signal-to-noise ratios were demonstrated by this radioligand in mice bearing glioblastoma xenografts up to 48 h post-injection. Based on the pharmacokinetic information obtained from the imaging studies, therapeutic administration of $VEGF_{121}$/rGel to mice bearing orthotopic U87MG glioblastomas revealed specific tumor neovasculature damage by histological analysis after a multiple dose treatment regimen.

Apart from their role in tumor angiogenesis, VEGF/VEGFR signaling plays a key role in other human pathologies. For example, myocardial infarction (MI) is known to activate VEGF/VEGFR signaling. PET imaging studies conducted in a rat model of MI with ^{64}Cu-DOTA-$VEGF_{121}$ revealed a 3 - 4 higher myocardial uptake of radioactivity for up to 2 weeks following infarction as compared to controls (50, 51). In addition, PET imaging of VEGFR expression with ^{64}Cu-DOTA-$VEGF_{121}$ in a rat stroke model showed peak tracer uptake in the stroke border zone at approximately 10 days post-surgery indicating neovascularization as confirmed by histopathology studies(52).

^{111}In-labeled recombinant VEGF isoform $VEGF_{165}$ (^{111}In-hn-Tf-VEGF) was reported by Chan and coworkers as a tumor angiogenic marker in experimental mice models. $VEGF_{165}$ was fused through a flexible polypeptide linker to the *n*-lobe of human transferrin(53). The latter construct permitted labeling of the radioligand with ^{111}In at a site remote from the VEGF receptor-binding domain. In radioligand stability studies, ^{111}In-hn-Tf-VEGF demonstrated a moderate loss of ^{111}In to transferrin in human plasma *in vitro* over a 72 h period (21.3% ± 3.4% per day). Radioligand biodistribution studies and whole-body gamma camera imaging were conducted in athymic mice bearing subcutaneous U87MG human glioblastoma xenografts. ^{111}In-hn-Tf-VEGF displayed tumor and blood radioactivity accumulations of 6.7 ± 1.1 %ID/g and 1.6 ± 0.4 %ID/g, respectively, at 72 h post-injection. Co-administration of a 100-fold excess of VEGF led to a 15-fold decrease in tumor uptake of radioactivity. High uptake of radioactivity was also observed in liver (45.5 ± 7.5 %ID/g), kidneys (39.4 ± 7.0 %ID/g) and spleen (35.6 ± 4.4 %ID/g) at this time interval. The authors present evidence to indicate that uptake of radioactivity in these organs is due to ^{111}In-hn-Tf-VEGF and not due to ^{111}In-transferrin via transchelation of ^{111}In from the radioligand to transferrin.

Along with labeling VEGF-A and its isoforms, efforts have also been made to create anti-VEGF-A antibodies for imaging and therapeutic purposes. Success in this field was achieved with the creation of bevacizumab, a humanized monoclonal antibody that blocks VEGF-induced endothelial cell proliferation. A radiolabeled form of bevacizumab, ^{89}Zr-bevacizumab, was demonstrated to have high tumor uptake in small animal PET imaging (54, 55). A phase 1 clinical trial with ^{124}I-labelled HuMV833 showed promising findings as well establishing the utility of radiolabeled antibodies in imaging VEGF(56, 57).

2.2 $\alpha_v\beta_3$ integrins and RGD peptide

An indirect approach to angiogenesis imaging has focused on radioligands targeting the $\alpha_v\beta_3$ class of cell adhesion molecule integrins. Integrin $\alpha_v\beta_3$ receptors are significantly up-regulated in endothelial cells during angiogenesis but not in mature vessels or non-neoplastic epithelium (Brooks PC, Science 1994; Pasqualini R, Nat Biotechnol, 1997). Integrin $\alpha_v\beta_3$ is also expressed in a variety of tumor cells, including melanoma, late-stage glioblastoma, ovarian, breast and prostate cancer. The ability to visualize and quantify integrin $\alpha_v\beta_3$ expression *in vivo* would allow for appropriate selection of patients for anti-integrin treatment and also monitor treatment efficacy in such patients.

Radioligand development for $\alpha_v\beta_3$ imaging has focused primarily on small RGD peptide antagonists. The tripeptide sequence motif, arginine-glycine-aspartate (RGD), is found in proteins of the extracellular matrix. Many integrins, including $\alpha_v\beta_3$, link the intracellular cytoskeleton of cells with the extracellular matrix via recognition and binding to this RGD motif. [^{18}F]GalactoRGD was the first radiotracer used for successful PET imaging of tumor $\alpha_v\beta_3$ expression in patients. Subsequently, a hydrophilic D-amino acid containing tetrapeptide analog was also developed which demonstrated improved pharmacokinetics and proteolytic stability. Wu and coworkers have reported on the enhanced $\alpha_v\beta_3$ receptor binding characteristics of dimeric and multimeric RGD peptides over monomeric peptides which has been attributed to an increased local concentration of RGD domains at the receptor vicinity (polyvalency effect). Accordingly, several [^{18}F]- and [^{64}Cu]-labeled dimeric and tetrameric RGD peptide analogs have been recently synthesized and evaluated by this group for integrin-targeted imaging in lung, brain and breast cancer. As an example, microPET imaging studies with a dimeric RGD peptide coupled to 4-[^{18}F]Fluorobenzoate {[^{18}F]-FB-E[c(RGDyK)]2} showed predominantly renal excretion and twice as much tumor uptake in the same animal model as the monomeric analog [^{18}F]-FB-c(RGDyK). Binding potentials derived from tracer kinetic modeling studies showed good correlation with tumor integrin expression levels as measured by SDS-PAGE/autoradiography in the six tumor models tested.

Recently, a disulfide-based cyclic RGD called iRGD (internalizing RGD) was reported that showed binding affinity to the $\alpha_v\beta_3$ integrin and neurophilin-1 (NRP-1) receptor and portrayed the ability to penetrate tumor tissue for both imaging and drug-delivery purposes(58). These characteristics of the peptide iRGD (CRGDKGPDC) are achieved through a sequence of steps. Initially, iRGD binds to the $\alpha_v\beta_3$ integrins expressed on the endothelium of tumor cells through its RGD motif(59). Subsequently, the peptide is proteolytically cleaved producing a C-terminal RGDK/R sequence that both increases the peptide's affinity to NRP-1 and decreases its binding activity to $\alpha_v\beta_3$ due to the CendR motif(59). This newfound affinity to NRP-1 provides iRGD its tumor penetrating capabilities(60). Not surprizingly, iRGD has become a major target for *in vivo* imaging as it can both home to tumor cells and also be internalized making the peptide a more effective imaging agent compared with other RGD peptides. iRGD imaging has been achieved using optical fluorescent and MRI agents, but a nuclear imaging agent has yet to be developed for this promising peptide(58, 59).

2.3 Matrix Metalloproteinases (MMP)

Matrix metalloproteinases (MMP's), a family of zinc- and calcium-dependent endopeptidases, facilitate endothelial cell migration during angiogenesis via the enzymatic degradation of connective tissue(61). Within the family of MMP's, MMP-2 and MMP-9 have been most associated with tumor aggressiveness and metastatic potential(62). Consequently, several MMP-specific peptides as well as small-molecule inhibitors (MMPI's) have been radiolabeled with ^{125}I, ^{123}I, ^{64}Cu, or ^{18}F for PET or SPECT imaging of angiogenesis(63). For example, Koivunen et al. discovered that the decapeptide *cyclo*(Cys-Thr-His-Trp-Gly-Phe-Thr-Leu-Cys)(CTT) selectively inhibited MMP-2 and MMP-9 thus suppressing the migration of endothelial and tumor cells(63, 64). Subsequent radiolabeling with ^{64}Cu and chelation to DOTA showed low tracer accumulation in tumors(63). Studies on other MMP imaging agents have shown similar results calling into question their utility for angiogenesis imaging due to their low tumor targeting capabilities, nonspecific activity in preclinical trials, and *in vivo* instability(62).

2.4 Nucleolin and F3 peptide

It is now commonly believed that different organs and tissues may have a distinct vasculature, and molecular profiling studies have revealed that this heterogeneity stems from expression of distinct functional biomarkers in endothelial cells and its milieu. Similarly, molecular dissections of tumor and tumor vasculature have revealed that the angiogenic network of blood vessels in tumor is unique both structurally and physiologically. Tumor vasculature expresses unique biomarkers that distinguish it from normal blood vessels and allow targeting of cargo of therapeutic or imaging agents (14).

Phage display peptide libraries contain peptide motifs that can home to the tumor vasculature and bind directly to the molecules expressed on tumor vessels (65, 66). Utilizing *in vivo* phage display technology, Ruoslahti's group identified F3 peptide (KDEPQRRSARLSAKPAPPKPEPKPKKAPAKK) as a sequence that specifically binds to tumor and its angiogenic endothelial cells (67). Later studies identified Nucleolin, as the receptor for F3 peptide. Nucleolin is localized both within the nucleus and the cytoplasm and is involved in RNA transport and processing. However, in proliferating tumor cells, it is cyclically transported from the nucleus to cell surface and back by a specific shuttle mechanism (68). Subcellular distribution of fluorescently-labeled F3 peptide shadowed nucleolin localization both in vitro and in vivo (Figure 1, (69, 70)). Further, we recently performed meta-analysis of microarray data from tumor samples and found that Nucleolin is upregulated in brain, head and neck and lung cancers when compared with respective normal tissue. Taken together, the overexpression of nucleolin and its unique localization at cell surface, suggest that nucleolin may be targeted for tumor imaging and delivery of therapeutic agents.

F3 peptide has been used to deliver fluorescent tags, siRNA, and therapeutic radionuclides to tumors (44, 71-75). We have recently demonstrated that this peptide sequence can carry a pay load of 80 nm multifunctional nanoparticles in a tumor specific manner (76) and that these reside at the tumor sites longer than the untargeted nanoparticles. Several groups have generated a variety of distinct F3-targeted nanoparticles and shown their efficacy in targeting mouse tumors or human xenografts in mouse (44, 71-75, 77). We recently reported the development of an new F3 peptide with cysteine at the c-terminus. Fluorescently or $[^{125}I]$-labeled conjugates of this peptide localized to tumors in a mouse model, when systemically administered (Figure 2).

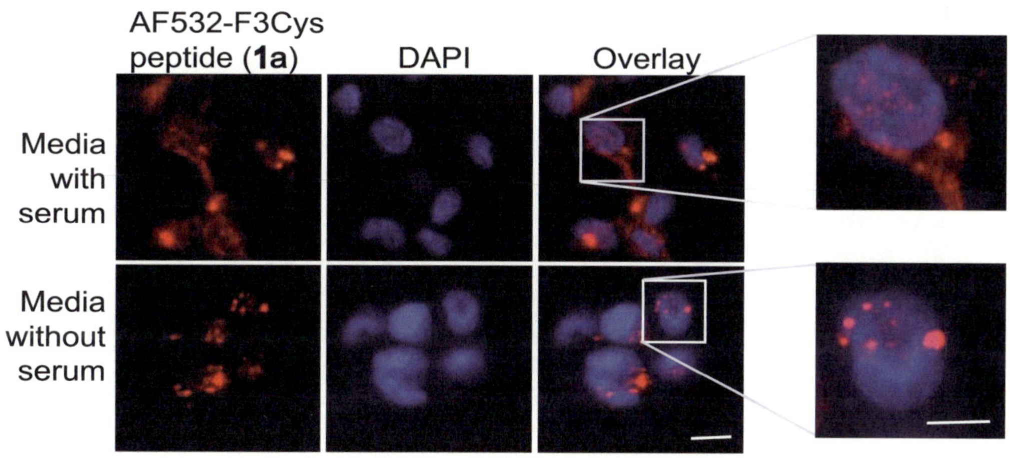

Fig. 1. **Subcellular localization of Fluorescent-labeled F3Cys peptides shadows that of nucleolin.** MDA-MB-435 cells, in optically clear bottom dishes, cultured in either serum free or serum containing media were stained with AF532-F3Cys, counterstained with DAPI and monitored under a fluorescent microscope. In cells grown in media containing 10% serum, cell surface and nuclear staining of F3Cys was observed while serum starved cells showed predominantly nuclear staining without significant membrane staining. This suggests that F3Cys localizes to cell surface in actively growing cells.

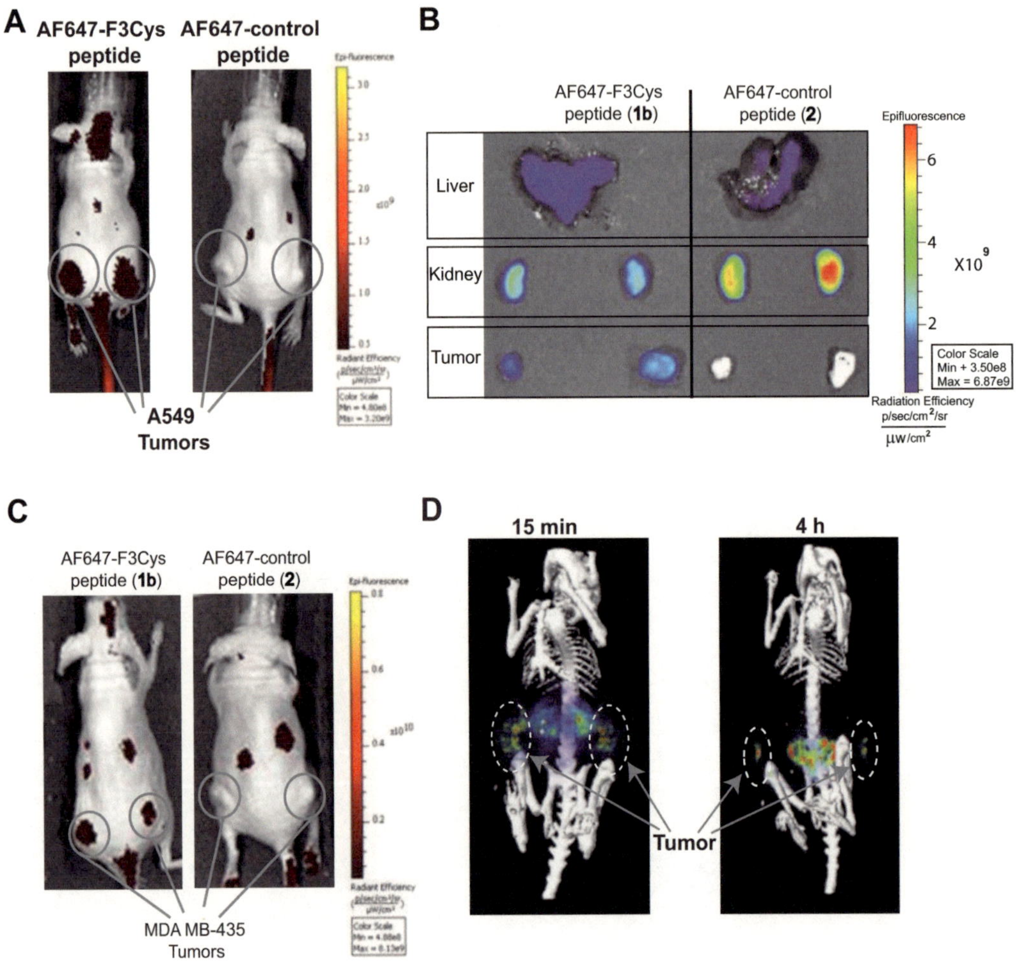

Fig. 2. **Fluorescent or SPECT imaging using tagged F3-cys peptide.** Mice bearing A549 (**A**) xenografts were injected i.v. via the tail vein with either AF647-F3Cys or AF647-Control peptide and fluorescence images were acquired over time. Tumor specific uptake at 2 h was observed only with AF647-F3Cys but not with AF647-Control peptide (A). *Ex vivo* fluorescence imaging of tumor, kidney and liver harvested 2 h after AF647-F3Cys peptide injection in animals bearing A549 Tumor xenografts show that F3 peptide is taken up by tumor, kidney and liver while AF647-Control peptide shows no tumor specific fluorescence (**B**). Tumor specific uptake was also seen with MDA-MB-435 (melanoma cancer cells) xenografts when AF647-F3Cys and not AF647-Control peptide was administered (**C**). SPECT imaging studies conducted following i.v. administration of [^{125}I]IBMF3 to nude mice bearing MDA-MB-435 tumor xenografts showed distinct uptake of radioactivity in tumor as early as 15 min post-injection and also at 4 h post-injection (**D**).

2.5 Miscellaneous alternate targets

Prostate-specific membrane antigen (PSMA) is expressed on the neovascular endothelium of a majority of solid type tumors and not on endothelial cells of normal tissue. Thus, radiolabelled PSMA may be utilized in the detection of tumor-specific angiogenesis(78-80). For the detection of nodal metastasis in prostate cancer, the FDA approved ProstaScint, a PSMA antibody labeled with ^{111}In (81, 82). Another ^{111}In-labeled PSMA antibody (J591) in a phase I clinical trial was reported to accumulate in malignant sites of tumors associated with kidney, liver, colon, breast and melanomas suggesting a potential of PSMA in imaging angiogenesis(81-84).. In a preclinical study, a ^{11}C-labeled small molecule ligand for prostate-specific antigen was shown to localize to prostate cancer in experimental animal models.

A number of extracellular matrix (ECM) proteins have also been targeted in the imaging of angiogenesis as some of the antigens in ECM have been discovered to be associated with neoangiogenic sites. Extra domain B of fibronectin and extra domain C of tenascin have been targeted in preclinical model systems to detect neoangiogenesis in malignant sites (63, 85, 86)

3. Clinical relevance of imaging angiogenesis

Radiotracer imaging techniques such as PET and SPECT offer unique advantages for investigation of angiogenesis in patients at the molecular level by virtue of its high sensitivity and adequate spatial and temporal resolution. At the clinical level, such approaches could be useful for lesion detection, to select patients likely to respond to therapies directed at such targets, to confirm successful targeting and dose optimization as well as treatment monitoring. Additionally, nuclear imaging techniques could also aid in the development of new angiogenesis-targeted drugs and their validation. For example, PET imaging can provide rapid characterization of a drugs pharmacokinetics and pharmacodynamic behavior in both pre-clinical studies and clinical trials thereby improving the speed, efficiency and cost of drug development. Taken together, these exciting developments will likely play an important clinical role in the management of human malignancies.

3.1 Future outlook on angiogenesis radiotracer design

The past decade has seen major advances in the field of PET and SPECT radiotracer development for visualizing the molecular events associated with angiogenesis. A vast majority of these approaches have either focused on radiolabeled analogs of vascular endothelial growth factor (VEGF) or RGD small peptide antagonists of the $\alpha_v\beta_3$ class of cell adhesion molecule integrins. Despite these achievements, there is still a need for improvements in synthetic strategies for existing radiotracers and the development of alternate radiotracers for angiogenesis imaging. For example, approaches using radiolabeled VEGF are complicated by several factors such as the presence of multiple VEGF isoforms, high renal expression of VEGF receptors and the mitogenic activity of VEGF. Additionally, clinical trials conducted with RGD-based radiotracers have shown wide heterogeneity in tumor binding both within the same patient and between patients (87). Furthermore, RGD peptides may have limitations for tumor imaging due to the limited number of $\alpha_v\beta_3$ integrin receptors available per tumor cell and their low binding affinity (87). Thus, new radiotracers with improved targeting efficacy and pharmacokinetics are indispensible for successful clinical translation.

Angiogenesis is involved in a multitude of biological processes including, embryogenesis, female reproductive cycle, tissue remodeling and wound healing (88). Furthermore, imbalances or upregulation of angiogenic processes are observed in numerous disorders including rheumatoid arthritis, psoriasis, cardiac restenosis and diabetic retinopathy. Accordingly, the future availability of clinically-validated angiogenesis imaging radiotracers could have broad applicability in disease management beyond that of oncology.

4. Summary

In this review, we have focused on recent developments in the design of new PET and SPECT radiotracers for imaging the tumor angiogenic process and their biological evaluation in pre-clinical animal models and initial clinical studies. Radiotracers based on VEGF and the cell adhesion molecule integrin $\alpha_v\beta_3$ currently form the major focus for imaging agent development. Additionally, alternate approaches that focus on radiolabeled matrix metalloproteinase and prostate specific membrane antigen (PSMA) inhibitors as well as the tumor-homing F3 peptide are described. Molecular imaging techniques such as PET and SPECT continue to play an increasingly important role in both disease diagnosis at the presymptomatic stage and the monitoring of its progression and response to therapeutic intervention. The future availability of improved imaging biomarkers for angiogenesis and appropriate animal models for their validation will be crucial for unraveling this complex process in health and disease and could lead to important advances in the treatment of cancer.

5. Acknowledgment

This work was supported by the following NIH research grants: P50CA093990 (BDR), PO1CA085878 (BDR), U24CA083099 (BDR), P50 CADE97248 (MSB), P50CA093990 (MSB) and CA136429 (MSB).

6. References

[1] Weber WA. Positron emission tomography as an imaging biomarker. J Clin Oncol 2006;24: 3282-92.

[2] Wu AM. Antibodies and antimatter: the resurgence of immuno-PET. J Nucl Med 2009;50: 2-5.

[3] O'Connor JP, Jackson A, Asselin MC, Buckley DL, Parker GJ, Jayson GC. Quantitative imaging biomarkers in the clinical development of targeted therapeutics: current and future perspectives. Lancet Oncol 2008;9: 766-76.

[4] Brandon D, Alazraki A, Halkar RK, Alazraki NP. The role of single-photon emission computed tomography and SPECT/computed tomography in oncologic imaging. Semin Oncol 2011;38: 87-108.

[5] Rahmim A, Zaidi H. PET versus SPECT: strengths, limitations and challenges. Nucl Med Commun 2008;29: 193-207.

[6] Kaufmann PA, Di Carli MF. Hybrid SPECT/CT and PET/CT imaging: the next step in noninvasive cardiac imaging. Semin Nucl Med 2009;39: 341-7.
[7] Di Carli MF. Hybrid imaging: integration of nuclear imaging and cardiac CT. Cardiol Clin 2009;27: 257-63, Table of Contents.
[8] Di Carli MF, Hachamovitch R. Hybrid PET/CT is greater than the sum of its parts. J Nucl Cardiol 2008;15: 118-22.
[9] PET-MRI F. http://www.fda.gov/NewsEvents/Newsroom/PressAnnouncements/ucm258700.htm.
[10] Fatemi-Ardekani A, Samavati N, Tang J, Kamath MV. Advances in multimodality imaging through a hybrid PET/MRI system. Critical reviews in biomedical engineering 2009;37: 495-515.
[11] Boss A, Bisdas S, Kolb A, *et al.* Hybrid PET/MRI of intracranial masses: initial experiences and comparison to PET/CT. J Nucl Med;51: 1198-205.
[12] Folkman J. Angiogenesis in cancer, vascular, rheumatoid and other disease. Nature medicine 1995;1: 27-31.
[13] Zhu AX, Duda DG, Sahani DV, Jain RK. HCC and angiogenesis: possible targets and future directions. Nat Rev Clin Oncol 2011;8: 292-301.
[14] Carmeliet P, Jain RK. Angiogenesis in cancer and other diseases. Nature 2000;407: 249-57.
[15] Chi AS, Sorensen AG, Jain RK, Batchelor TT. Angiogenesis as a therapeutic target in malignant gliomas. Oncologist 2009;14: 621-36.
[16] Kadambi A, Mouta Carreira C, Yun CO, *et al.* Vascular endothelial growth factor (VEGF)-C differentially affects tumor vascular function and leukocyte recruitment: role of VEGF-receptor 2 and host VEGF-A. Cancer research 2001;61: 2404-8.
[17] Tsuzuki Y, Fukumura D, Oosthuyse B, Koike C, Carmeliet P, Jain RK. Vascular endothelial growth factor (VEGF) modulation by targeting hypoxia-inducible factor-1alpha--> hypoxia response element--> VEGF cascade differentially regulates vascular response and growth rate in tumors. Cancer research 2000;60: 6248-52.
[18] Duda DG, Batchelor TT, Willett CG, Jain RK. VEGF-targeted cancer therapy strategies: current progress, hurdles and future prospects. Trends Mol Med 2007;13: 223-30.
[19] Detmar M, Brown LF, Berse B, *et al.* Hypoxia regulates the expression of vascular permeability factor/vascular endothelial growth factor (VPF/VEGF) and its receptors in human skin. J Invest Dermatol 1997;108: 263-8.
[20] Enholm B, Paavonen K, Ristimaki A, *et al.* Comparison of VEGF, VEGF-B, VEGF-C and Ang-1 mRNA regulation by serum, growth factors, oncoproteins and hypoxia. Oncogene 1997;14: 2475-83.
[21] Gu JW, Adair TH. Hypoxia-induced expression of VEGF is reversible in myocardial vascular smooth muscle cells. Am J Physiol 1997;273: H628-33.
[22] Baek JH, Jang JE, Kang CM, Chung HY, Kim ND, Kim KW. Hypoxia-induced VEGF enhances tumor survivability via suppression of serum deprivation-induced apoptosis. Oncogene 2000;19: 4621-31.
[23] Soltau J, Drevs J. Mode of action and clinical impact of VEGF signaling inhibitors. Expert Rev Anticancer Ther 2009;9: 649-62.
[24] Selleck SB. Signaling from across the way: transactivation of VEGF receptors by HSPGs. Mol Cell 2006;22: 431-2.
[25] McMahon G. VEGF receptor signaling in tumor angiogenesis. Oncologist 2000;5 Suppl 1: 3-10.
[26] Bagri A, Kouros-Mehr H, Leong KG, Plowman GD. Use of anti-VEGF adjuvant therapy in cancer: challenges and rationale. Trends Mol Med 2010;16: 122-32.

[27] Grothey A, Galanis E. Targeting angiogenesis: progress with anti-VEGF treatment with large molecules. Nat Rev Clin Oncol 2009;6: 507-18.
[28] Tortora G, Ciardiello F, Gasparini G. Combined targeting of EGFR-dependent and VEGF-dependent pathways: rationale, preclinical studies and clinical applications. Nat Clin Pract Oncol 2008;5: 521-30.
[29] Harper SJ, Bates DO. VEGF-A splicing: the key to anti-angiogenic therapeutics? Nature reviews 2008;8: 880-7.
[30] Ellis LM, Hicklin DJ. VEGF-targeted therapy: mechanisms of anti-tumour activity. Nature reviews 2008;8: 579-91.
[31] Schneider BP, Sledge GW, Jr. Drug insight: VEGF as a therapeutic target for breast cancer. Nat Clin Pract Oncol 2007;4: 181-9.
[32] Nagy JA, Dvorak AM, Dvorak HF. VEGF-A and the induction of pathological angiogenesis. Annu Rev Pathol 2007;2: 251-75.
[33] Olsson AK, Dimberg A, Kreuger J, Claesson-Welsh L. VEGF receptor signalling - in control of vascular function. Nat Rev Mol Cell Biol 2006;7: 359-71.
[34] Jain RK, Duda DG, Clark JW, Loeffler JS. Lessons from phase III clinical trials on anti-VEGF therapy for cancer. Nat Clin Pract Oncol 2006;3: 24-40.
[35] Rosen LS. VEGF-targeted therapy: therapeutic potential and recent advances. Oncologist 2005;10: 382-91.
[36] Patil AS, Sable RB, Kothari RM. Occurrence, biochemical profile of vascular endothelial growth factor (VEGF) isoforms and their functions in endochondral ossification. J Cell Physiol 2011.
[37] Giacca M. Non-redundant functions of the protein isoforms arising from alternative splicing of the VEGF-A pre-mRNA. Transcr 2010;1: 149-53.
[38] Carter JG, Cherry J, Williams K, Turner S, Bates DO, Churchill AJ. Splicing factor polymorphisms, the control of VEGF isoforms and association with angiogenic eye disease. Curr Eye Res 2011;36: 328-35.
[39] Rennel ES, Varey AH, Churchill AJ, *et al.* VEGF(121)b, a new member of the VEGF(xxx)b family of VEGF-A splice isoforms, inhibits neovascularisation and tumour growth in vivo. Br J Cancer 2009;101: 1183-93.
[40] Varey AH, Rennel ES, Qiu Y, *et al.* VEGF 165 b, an antiangiogenic VEGF-A isoform, binds and inhibits bevacizumab treatment in experimental colorectal carcinoma: balance of pro- and antiangiogenic VEGF-A isoforms has implications for therapy. Br J Cancer 2008;98: 1366-79.
[41] Yukata K, Matsui Y, Goto T, Kubo T, Yasui N. Differential expression of VEGF isoforms and VEGF receptors in cartilaginous tumors. Anticancer Res 2005;25: 955-7.
[42] Hofstaetter JG, Saad FA, Samuel RE, Wunderlich L, Choi YH, Glimcher MJ. Differential expression of VEGF isoforms and receptors in knee joint menisci under systemic hypoxia. Biochem Biophys Res Commun 2004;324: 667-72.
[43] Park JE, Keller GA, Ferrara N. The vascular endothelial growth factor (VEGF) isoforms: differential deposition into the subepithelial extracellular matrix and bioactivity of extracellular matrix-bound VEGF. Mol Biol Cell 1993;4: 1317-26.
[44] Zhang Z, Neiva KG, Lingen MW, Ellis LM, Nor JE. VEGF-dependent tumor angiogenesis requires inverse and reciprocal regulation of VEGFR1 and VEGFR2. Cell Death Differ 2010;17: 499-512.
[45] Tam J, Duda DG, Perentes JY, Quadri RS, Fukumura D, Jain RK. Blockade of VEGFR2 and not VEGFR1 can limit diet-induced fat tissue expansion: role of local versus bone marrow-derived endothelial cells. PLoS One 2009;4: e4974.

[46] Jinnin M, Medici D, Park L, *et al.* Suppressed NFAT-dependent VEGFR1 expression and constitutive VEGFR2 signaling in infantile hemangioma. Nature medicine 2008;14: 1236-46.
[47] Ferrara N. Vascular endothelial growth factor: basic science and clinical progress. Endocrine reviews 2004;25: 581-611.
[48] Rudlowski C, Pickart AK, Fuhljahn C, *et al.* Prognostic significance of vascular endothelial growth factor expression in ovarian cancer patients: a long-term follow-up. Int J Gynecol Cancer 2006;16 Suppl 1: 183-9.
[49] Fischer C, Mazzone M, Jonckx B, Carmeliet P. FLT1 and its ligands VEGFB and PlGF: drug targets for anti-angiogenic therapy? Nature reviews 2008;8: 942-56.
[50] Gambhir SS, Rodriguez-Porcel M, Cai WB, *et al.* Imaging of VEGF receptor in a rat myocardial infarction model using PET. Journal of Nuclear Medicine 2008;49: 667-73.
[51] Sinusas AJ, Dobrucki LW. PET and SPECT in cardiovascular molecular imaging. Nat Rev Cardiol 2010;7: 38-47.
[52] Chen XY, Cai WB, Guzman R, *et al.* Positron Emission Tomography Imaging of Poststroke Angiogenesis. Stroke 2009;40: 270-7.
[53] Chan C, Sandhu J, Guha A, *et al.* A human transferrin-vascular endothelial growth factor (hnTf-VEGF) fusion protein containing an integrated binding site for (111)In for imaging tumor angiogenesis. J Nucl Med 2005;46: 1745-52.
[54] Nagengast WB, de Korte MA, Oude Munnink TH, *et al.* 89Zr-bevacizumab PET of early antiangiogenic tumor response to treatment with HSP90 inhibitor NVP-AUY922. J Nucl Med;51: 761-7.
[55] Nagengast WB, de Vries EG, Hospers GA, *et al.* In vivo VEGF imaging with radiolabeled bevacizumab in a human ovarian tumor xenograft. J Nucl Med 2007;48: 1313-9.
[56] Jayson GC, Mulatero C, Ranson M, *et al.* Phase I investigation of recombinant anti-human vascular endothelial growth factor antibody in patients with advanced cancer. Eur J Cancer 2005;41: 555-63.
[57] Jayson GC, Zweit J, Jackson A, *et al.* Molecular imaging and biological evaluation of HuMV833 anti-VEGF antibody: implications for trial design of antiangiogenic antibodies. J Natl Cancer Inst 2002;94: 1484-93.
[58] Ye Y, Zhu L, Ma Y, Niu G, Chen X. Synthesis and evaluation of new iRGD peptide analogs for tumor optical imaging. Bioorg Med Chem Lett;21: 1146-50.
[59] Sugahara KN, Teesalu T, Karmali PP, *et al.* Tissue-penetrating delivery of compounds and nanoparticles into tumors. Cancer Cell 2009;16: 510-20.
[60] Sugahara KN, Teesalu T, Karmali PP, *et al.* Coadministration of a tumor-penetrating peptide enhances the efficacy of cancer drugs. Science;328: 1031-5.
[61] Josephs D, Spicer J, O'Doherty M. Molecular imaging in clinical trials. Targeted oncology 2009;4: 151-68.
[62] Haubner R, Beer AJ, Wang H, Chen X. Positron emission tomography tracers for imaging angiogenesis. Eur J Nucl Med Mol Imaging;37 Suppl 1: S86-103.
[63] Dijkgraaf I, Boerman OC. Radionuclide imaging of tumor angiogenesis. Cancer Biother Radiopharm 2009;24: 637-47.
[64] Koivunen E, Arap W, Valtanen H, *et al.* Tumor targeting with a selective gelatinase inhibitor. Nature biotechnology 1999;17: 768-74.
[65] Ruoslahti E. Vascular zip codes in angiogenesis and metastasis. Biochem Soc Trans 2004;32: 397-402.
[66] Ruoslahti E, Duza T, Zhang L. Vascular homing peptides with cell-penetrating properties. Current pharmaceutical design 2005;11: 3655-60.

[67] Porkka K, Laakkonen P, Hoffman JA, Bernasconi M, Ruoslahti E. A fragment of the HMGN2 protein homes to the nuclei of tumor cells and tumor endothelial cells in vivo. Proc Natl Acad Sci U S A 2002;99: 7444-9.
[68] Srivastava M, Pollard HB. Molecular dissection of nucleolin's role in growth and cell proliferation: new insights. Faseb J 1999;13: 1911-22.
[69] Bhojani MS, Ranga R, Luker GD, Rehemtulla A, Ross BD, Van Dort ME. Synthesis and Investigation of a Radioiodinated F3 Peptide Analog as a SPECT Tumor Imaging Radioligand. PLoS One;6: e22418.
[70] Christian S, Pilch J, Akerman ME, Porkka K, Laakkonen P, Ruoslahti E. Nucleolin expressed at the cell surface is a marker of endothelial cells in angiogenic blood vessels. J Cell Biol 2003;163: 871-8.
[71] Hah HJ, Kim G, Lee YE, *et al.* Methylene Blue-Conjugated Hydrogel Nanoparticles and Tumor-Cell Targeted Photodynamic Therapy. Macromol Biosci 2010.
[72] Bhojani MS, Van Dort M, Rehemtulla A, Ross BD. Targeted Imaging and Therapy of Brain Cancer Using Theranostic Nanoparticles. Molecular pharmaceutics 2010.
[73] Park JH, von Maltzahn G, Zhang L, *et al.* Systematic surface engineering of magnetic nanoworms for in vivo tumor targeting. Small 2009;5: 694-700.
[74] Derfus AM, Chen AA, Min DH, Ruoslahti E, Bhatia SN. Targeted quantum dot conjugates for siRNA delivery. Bioconjug Chem 2007;18: 1391-6.
[75] Akerman ME, Chan WC, Laakkonen P, Bhatia SN, Ruoslahti E. Nanocrystal targeting in vivo. Proc Natl Acad Sci U S A 2002;99: 12617-21.
[76] Reddy GR, Bhojani MS, McConville P, *et al.* Vascular targeted nanoparticles for imaging and treatment of brain tumors. Clin Cancer Res 2006;12: 6677-86.
[77] Orringer DA, Koo YE, Chen T, *et al.* In vitro characterization of a targeted, dye-loaded nanodevice for intraoperative tumor delineation. Neurosurgery 2009;64: 965-71; discussion 71-2.
[78] Bander NH. Technology insight: monoclonal antibody imaging of prostate cancer. Nature clinical practice 2006;3: 216-25.
[79] Zuckier LS, DeNardo GL. Trials and tribulations: oncological antibody imaging comes to the fore. Semin Nucl Med 1997;27: 10-29.
[80] Mease RC, Dusich CL, Foss CA, *et al.* N-[N-[(S)-1,3-Dicarboxypropyl]carbamoyl]-4-[18F]fluorobenzyl-L-cysteine, [18F]DCFBC: a new imaging probe for prostate cancer. Clin Cancer Res 2008;14: 3036-43.
[81] Yao D, Trabulsi EJ, Kostakoglu L, *et al.* The utility of monoclonal antibodies in the imaging of prostate cancer. Seminars in urologic oncology 2002;20: 211-8.
[82] Smith-Jones PM, Vallabahajosula S, Goldsmith SJ, *et al.* In vitro characterization of radiolabeled monoclonal antibodies specific for the extracellular domain of prostate-specific membrane antigen. Cancer research 2000;60: 5237-43.
[83] Chopra A. 123I-Labeled (S)-2-(3-((S)-1-carboxy-5-(4-iodobenzylamino)pentyl)ureido) pentanedoic acid. 2004.
[84] Chopra A. 123I-Labeled (S)-2-(3-((S)-1-carboxy-5-(3-(4-iodophenyl) ureido)pentyl) ureido)pentanedoic acid. 2004.
[85] Guttery DS, Shaw JA, Lloyd K, Pringle JH, Walker RA. Expression of tenascin-C and its isoforms in the breast. Cancer Metastasis Rev;29: 595-606.
[86] Stollman TH, Ruers TJ, Oyen WJ, Boerman OC. New targeted probes for radioimaging of angiogenesis. Methods (San Diego, Calif 2009;48: 188-92.
[87] Danen EH. Integrins: regulators of tissue function and cancer progression. Current pharmaceutical design 2005;11: 881-91.
[88] Carmeliet P. Angiogenesis in health and disease. Nature medicine 2003;9: 653-60.

14

Molecular Imaging Studies on CD133$^+$ Hematopoietic Stem Cells From Human Umbilical Cord Blood

L.F. Pavon[1], L.C. Marti[2], T.T. Sibov,[1]
M.I. Camargo-Mathias[3], Jr.E. Amaro[1,4] and L.F. Gamarra[1]
[1]*Instituto do Cérebro – Instituto Israelita de Ensino e Pesquisa Albert Einstein - IIEPAE, São Paulo,*
[2]*Centro de Pesquisa Experimental – Instituto Israelita de Ensino e Pesquisa Albert Einstein - IIEPAE, São Paulo,*
[3]*Departamento de Biologia, Instituto de Biociências – Universidade Estadual Paulista - UNESP, Rio Claro,*
[4]*Departamento de Radiologia, Universidade de São Paulo – USP, São Paulo, Brasil*

1. Introduction

During the last decade, there has been enormous progress in understanding both multipotent stem cells such as hematopoietic stem cells and pluripotent stem cells such as embryonic stem cells and induced pluripotent stem cells. However, it has been challenging to study developmental potentials of these stem cells because they reside in complex cellular environments and aspects of their distribution, migration, engraftment, survival, proliferation, and differentiation often could not be sufficiently elucidated based on limited snapshot images of location or environment or molecular markers (Jang et al., 2011). Therefore, reliable imaging methods to monitor or track the fate of the stem cells are highly desirable. Both short-term and more permanent monitoring of stem cells in cultures and in live organisms have benefited from recently developed imaging approaches that are designed to investigate cell behavior and function. Transmission electronic microscopy (TEM) and series of noninvasive imaging technologies enable us to investigate cell behavior in the context of a live organism. In turn, the knowledge gained has brought our understanding of stem cell biology to a new level.

Cell based therapeutics are emerging as powerful regimens. To better understand the migration and proliferation mechanisms of implanted cells, a means to track cells in living subjects is essential, and to achieve that, a number of cell labeling techniques have been developed. Nanoparticles, with their superior physical properties, have become the materials of choice in many investigations along this line. Owing to inherent magnetic, optical or acoustic attributes, these nanoparticles can be detected by corresponding imaging modalities in living subjects at a high spatial and temporal resolution. These features allow implanted cells to be separated from host cells; and have advantages over traditional histological methods, as they permit non-invasive, real-time tracking in vivo (Bhird et al., 2011).

Superparamagnetic iron oxide nanoparticles and magnetic resonance imaging provide a non-invasive method to detect and label hematopoietic stem cells. These nanoparticles exhibit unique properties of superparamagnetism and can be utilized as excellent molecular probes for magnetic resonance imaging. Neumaier et al., (2008) related that cell labeling by iron oxide nanoparticles has emerged as a potentially powerful tool to monitor trafficking of a large number of cells in the cell therapy field. Magnetic resonance imaging and iron magnetic nanoparticles are able to increase the accuracy and the specificity of imaging and represent new imaging opportunities in preclinical and translational research (Neumaier et al., 2008).

Superparamagnetic behaviour of the marker used (magnetic fluid), composed of iron oxide (Fe_3O_4), comes from particles where the magnetization is free to re-orient itself due to thermal fluctuations (Sastry et al. 1995), characterizing the presence of electron-dense granules detectable by TEM. As described above, the nanoparticles can also be detected by magnetic resonance techniques, both *in vitro* and *in vivo*. The fundamental state of the free ion (Fe^{3+}) has an electronic configuration of $3d^5$, having all its 5 spins bound (S=5/2 and total momentum orbital=null), giving a ^6S configuration for the fundamental state, 6 times degenerated, forming 3 pairs of Kramers levels separated by the local electrical field (Stark effect). Since Fe^{3+} is an ion with an odd number of unpaired electrons, the duplet's degeneration can only be possible by a magnetic field and then the electronic paramagnetic resonance (EPR) can be observed.

CD133 antigen is a surface molecule with unknown functions expressed by more primitive $CD34^+$ hematopoietic progenitor cells (HPCs) (Miraglia et al., 1997). The presence of antigen CD133 on a subset of very primitive HPCs such as CD34/CD133 cells points to this marker as an attracting tool to isolated human HPCs for biologic studies and clinical purposes (Peichev et al., 2000).

In humans, CD133 is expressed in stem cells (Yin et al., 1997) and in several cellular progenitors (Yin et al., 1997), including those derived from the hematopoietic and nervous systems (Yin et al., 1997; Miraglia et al, 1997). CD133 expression is also detected in other primitive cells (Gehling et al., 2000) and in some tumors, such as retinoblastoma, glioblastoma, and medulloblastoma (Yin et al., 1997; Pfenninger et al., 2007).

Human cord blood has been described as an excellent source of $CD133^+$ HPCs with a large application potential (Rubinstein et al., 1998; Kuci et al., 2003).

A large number of studies on stem cell biology and HPCs transplantation indicate that umbilical cord blood (UCB) is a suitable source of transplantable human HPCs (Gluckman et al. 1997; Rocha et al., 2001).

BONANNO et al. (2004) described the clinical isolation and functional characterization of cord blood $CD133^+$ HPCs with high hematopoietic activity and *in vitro* mesenchymal potential (differentiation mesoderm). Thus, the authors suggest that large-scale isolation of $CD133^+$ cells from human UCB could represent a primary step to again access to a stem pool useful for therapeutic hematopoietic transplants, stem cell expansion for clinical purposes and pre-clinical research on tissue regenerating therapies.

In 2007, the same group (BONANNO et al.) related another therapeutic use of $CD133^{+}$ cells from human UCB. They suggested the use of these cells as a treatment for myocardium ischemia due their potential to differentiate into endothelial and cardiomyocyte-like cells *in vitro*. *In vivo* studies showed vasculogenic potential of $CD133^{+}$ cells from UCB in response to ischemia in an animal injury model (Finney et al., 2005; Ma et al., 2005).

$CD133^{+}$ cells can be isolated *in vitro* with monoclonal antibody anti-CD133 bound to magnetic beads that are composed of superparamagnetic nanoparticles (Miltenyi Biotec) and purified by MACS (*magnetic activated cell sorting*).

The low levels of toxicity of the magnetic nanoparticles binding to magnetite (Fe_3O_4) used in the process of cellular selection (MACS - Miltenyi Biotec) can also be observed through studies that used hematopoetic stem cells obtained by the same selection procedure, in transplants of patients with cancer, obtaining satisfactory therapeutic results (Lang et al., 2003; Richel, et al., 2000).

This manuscript presents the study of molecular imaging on $CD133^{+}$ hematopoietic stem cells from human umbilical cord blood.

2. Materials and methods

2.1 Collection and selection of the $CD133^{+}$ hematopoetic stem cells from human umbilical cord blood (UCB)

The collection of the umbilical cord blood was obtained in the Obstetric Centre of the Albert Einstein Israelita Hospital, São Paulo, Brazil, from pregnancies at term (n=5) with written permission from the mother. The collection was performed with sterile equipment through a puncture of the umbilical cord vein, at the moment of birth and after the cord was cut.

Blood bags with a maximum volume of 250mL with 2mL of anticoagulant were used. The volume of the collected blood varied between 70 and 120mL. A sample of 80μL of blood was separated for cell count. The blood was then diluted in 1:2 proportion in a RPMI (Gibco) culture medium and the limpho-mononuclear cells were separated by the Ficoll-Paque™ Plus (Amersham - GE Healthcare) density gradient in a 1:3 proportion (Lehner & Holter, 2002). After 35 minutes in a 400g centrifuge, the fraction of the limpho-mononuclear cells were carefully isolated with the help of a 10mL pipette and washed in RPMI.

The $CD133^{+}$ cell population was purified following the separation protocol by MiniMACS microbeads affinity chromatography using anti-CD133 bound to magnetic beads (Miltenyi Biotec).

The cells were filtrated in 30μm nylon filters and the number of these cells were determined by the cell count in an automatic counter (Coulter), after which they were centrifuged (400g for 5 minutes) and resuspended in the proportion of 300μL of solution for each 10^8 cells in a PBS solution containing 2mM EDTA and 0.5% BSA (solution 1). For each 10^8 cells, 100μL of FcR blocker and 100μL of magnetic micro-spheres with $CD133^{+}$ antibodies (6°C) were added. The labelled cells were centrifuged and resuspended in solution 1 to be separated in the chromatography column to isolate only the $CD133^{+}$ cells.

2.2 Flow cytometry

After CD133+ cell separation, the cell population was characterized by flow cytometry using the following monoclonal antibodies (Becton Dickinson, San Jose, CA) and (Miltenyi Biotec): CD34 (clone: 581) FITC-conjugated, CD45 (clone: 2D1) PerCP Cy-5.5-conjugated and CD133/2 (clone: AC141) APC-conjugated and the respective isotype controls IgG1 FITC-conjugated, IgG1 PerCP Cy-5.5-conjugated and IgG1 APC-conjugated.

Cells were incubated with antibodies at 4°C, on dark for 30 minutes, and then washed with PBS and fixed with 1% paraformaldehyde. A total of 10^5 fluorescent cellular events were acquired on the FACSARIA flow cytometry (BD Bioscience) and analyzed by FACSDIVA software. Briefly, the analysis was performed by gating the cell population on forward scatter (FSC) versus side scatter (SSC) followed by gating only the CD45+ cells. Within the CD45+ cell population, cells were analyzed for expression of CD34 and CD133 markers.

2.3 Transmission Electron Microscopy (TEM)

CD133+ cell population (10^7 cells) was fixed in 0,5% glutaraldehyde in 0,2M cacodylate buffer for two hours at 4°C. Two 15 minute washes in cacodylate buffer followed this process. Post-fixation was performed in 1% osmium tetroxide for one hour at 4°C, followed by another two 15 minute washes in the same buffer. For contrast, the material was immersed in a solution of uranyl acetate in acetone for 30 minutes. After dehydration, the material was embedded in Epon resin diluted in acetone (1:1) and incubated at 4°C with agitation for 24 hours. The material was then transferred to pure Epon resin and incubated at 60° C for 72 hours, until completely polymerized. Semi and ultrathin sections were obtained with the aid of a Porter Blum ultramicrotome. The semithin sections were stained with azur II (1%) and methylene blue (1%). The ultrathin sections were placed on copper grids and stained with uranyl acetate and lead citrate. The grids were studied and photographed in a transmission electron microscope, PHILLIPS CM100.

2.4 Electron Paramagnetic Resonance (EPR)

In order to corroborate with the referred marking of the CD133+ cells bound to iron oxide superparamagnetic nanoparticles the EPR technique was used.

The EPR signal of the iron oxide nanoparticles (iron markers Fe_3O_4) describe a peculiar absorption curve of approximately g= 2,0 where the curve area (double integral of the EPR spectrum) is proportional to the concentration of the sample nanoparticles.

To perform a quantitative analysis of the Fe_3O_4 concentration, a calibration curve was first built based on different known concentrations between 2,6µm and 0,6mM.

The sample preparation was obtained from a suspension of 10^7 stem cells (CD133+), bound to iron oxide nanoparticles, in 0,5% glutaraldehyde fixative in a 2µL quartz tube. Following this, the EPR measurements were performed. The methodology of the quantification calibration was already described in previous studies Gamarra et al. (2007); Sadeghiani et al., (2005); Lacava et al., (2002).

The EPR measurements were taken using 20.166mW power, $1{,}6 \times 10^5$ receiver gain, 4 scanning and the measurements were taken at room temperature. The spectral composition of EPR absorption was obtained with a Bruker homodyne spectrophotometer, model EMX, operating with a frequency of 9,2 GHz in the band X and modulated to 100 kHz, utilizing one cavity of a rectangular microwave in the operating mode of the dominant cavity TE_{102}.

3. Results

3.1 Characterization by flow cytometry of CD133+ stem cells from UCB

After selection of CD133+ cells with monoclonal antibodies bound to superparamagnetic nanoparticles, flow cytometry analysis revealed that about 82% of the population is comprised by CD34+/CD133+ cells, most of them expressing CD133 (Figure 1). After this first analysis, the ultrastructural characterization of the CD133+ cells was performed.

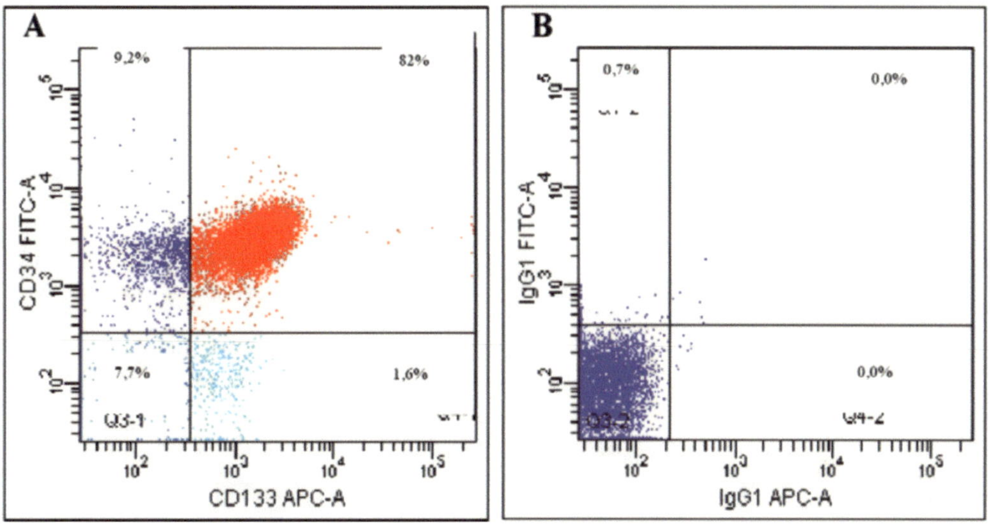

Fig. 1. (A) The Flow Cytometry graph shows that CD133+/CD34+ (82,0%), CD133/CD34+ (1,6%) and CD34+CD133- (9,2%). (B) Isotype control graph shows that wasn't unspecific staining.

3.2 Identification and ultrastructural characterization of CD133+ stem cells labelled with nanoparticles

Under the electron microscopy, ultrastructural analysis highlighted the presence of electrondense granules in the cell surface. This demonstrates the presence of anti-CD133 monoclonal antibodies bound to superparamagnetic nanoparticles recognizing the CD133 membrane protein (Figures 2A, B, C, D). This does not occur in the cells of the control group (CD133-) (Figures 3C, D) since similar electrondense signal surrounding cellular membrane of CD133- cells (control group) were not detected (Figures 3C, D).

Electrondense signals related to superparamagnetic nanoparticles were also observed in the cell cytoplasm, suggesting their internalization through the process of the endocytosis (pinocytosis) of nanoparticles bound to the antibodies (Figures 2C, D; 3A, B). CD133+ cells incorporated superparamagnetic nanoparticles through its small cytoplasmic projections forming the pinocytics vesicles, as shown in the figures 2C and 3B.

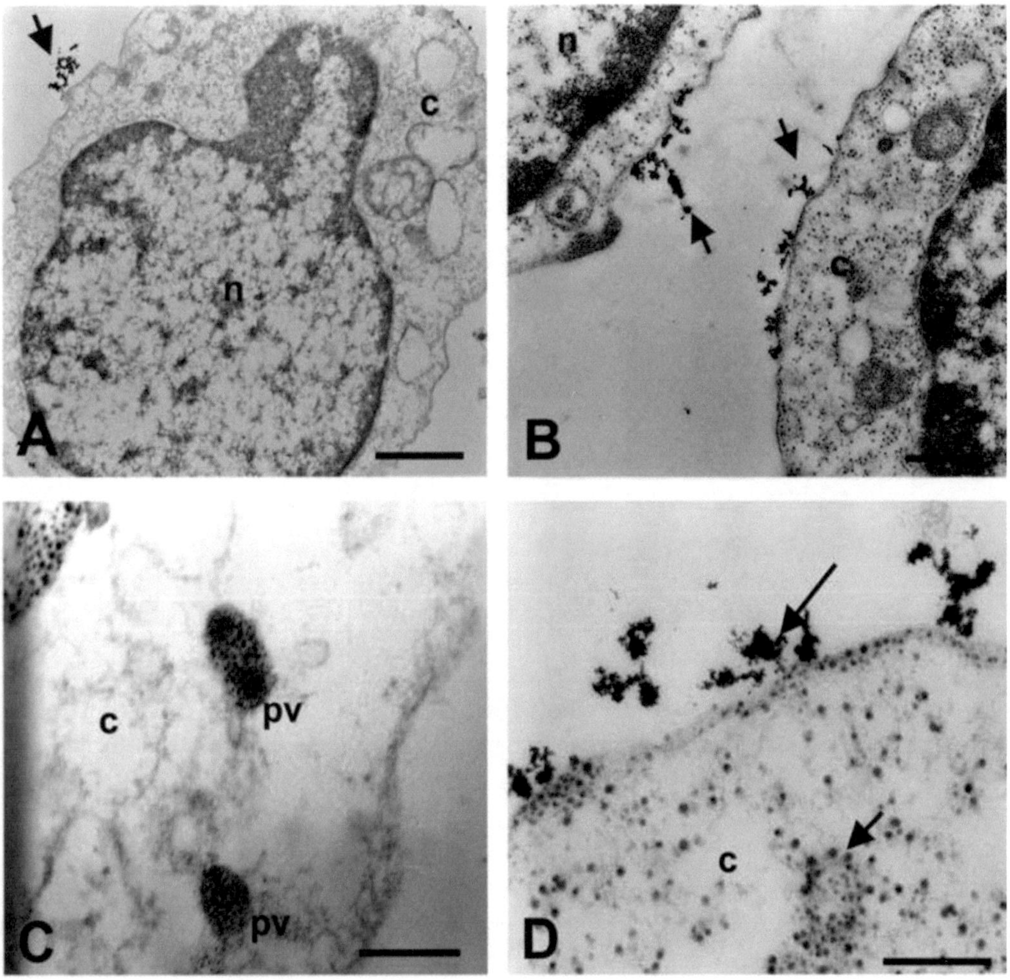

Fig. 2. Transmission electronic microscopy of CD133+ stem cells. n = nucleus, c = cytoplasm, arrow = electrondense granules or magnetic nanoparticles, pv = pinocytics vesicles. Scale: A) 1μm; B) 0,5μm; C) 0,25μm; D) 0,125 μm.

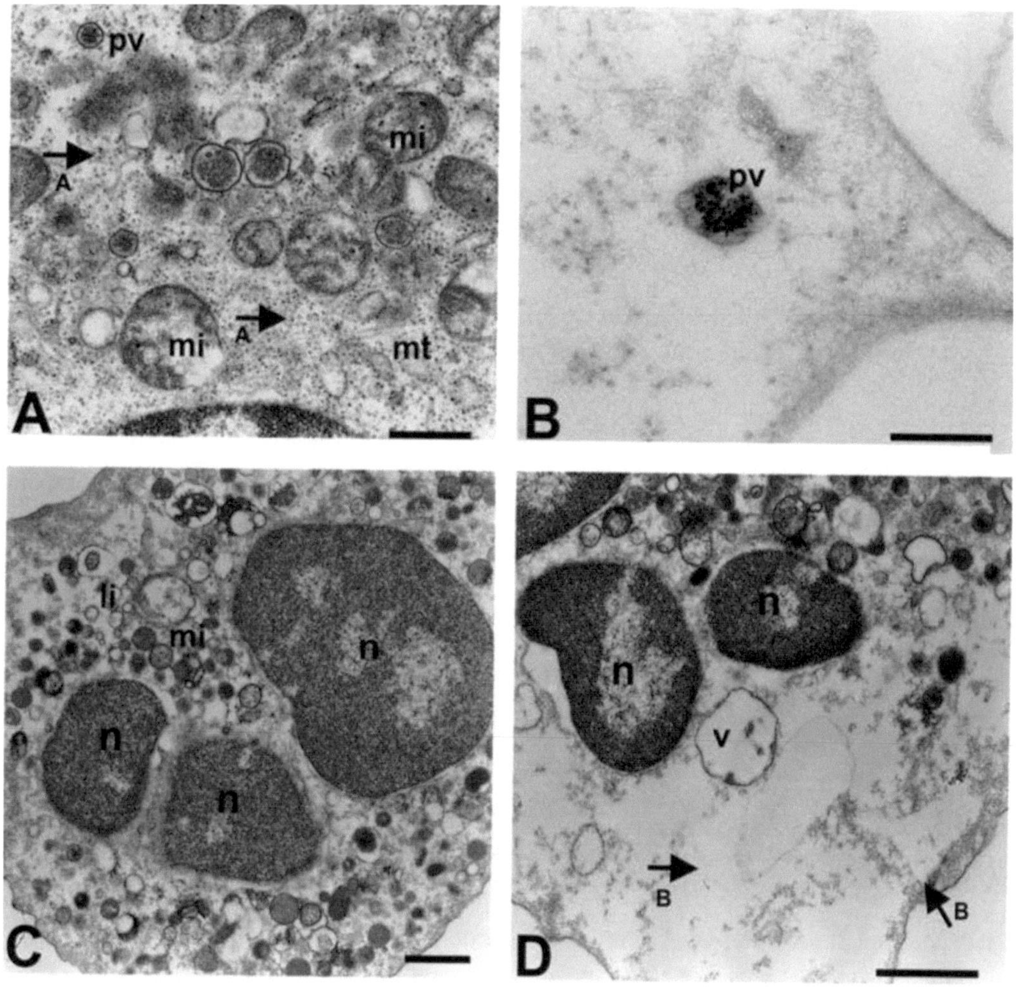

Fig. 3. (A, B) Transmission electronic microscopy of CD133^{+} stem cells. (C, D) Transmission electronic microscopy of CD133^{-} stem cells (control). n = nucleus, mi = mitochondria, mt = microtubules, arrow A = electrondense granules or magnetic nanoparticles, arrow B = absence of the electrondense granules or magnetic nanoparticles, pv = pinocytics vesicles, li = lipids, v = vacuoles. Scale: A) 1μm; B) 0,5μm; C) 0,25μm; D) 0,25μm.

3.3 Electron Paramagnetic Resonance (EPR) of the superparamagnetic nanoparticles labelled of CD133^{+} stem cells

To clearly show the expression of CD133 antigenic marker of the cell population under study, an EPR spectrum was first performed only with monoclonal antibodies anti-CD133 bound to magnetic nanoparticles composed of superparamagnetic nanoparticles. A resonance in g=2.0 (Figure 4) was observed, derived from Fe^{3+} spins that interact with themselves, but with a supermagnetic behavior that characterizes the presence of agglomerates (Gamarra et al., 2005; Hseih et al., 2002; Sharma & Waldner, 1977). This signal consists of a strong absorption, while the large width is attributed to the strong interaction between Fe^{3+} ions (Fe^{3+} ion cluster agglomerated by a strong exchange interaction).

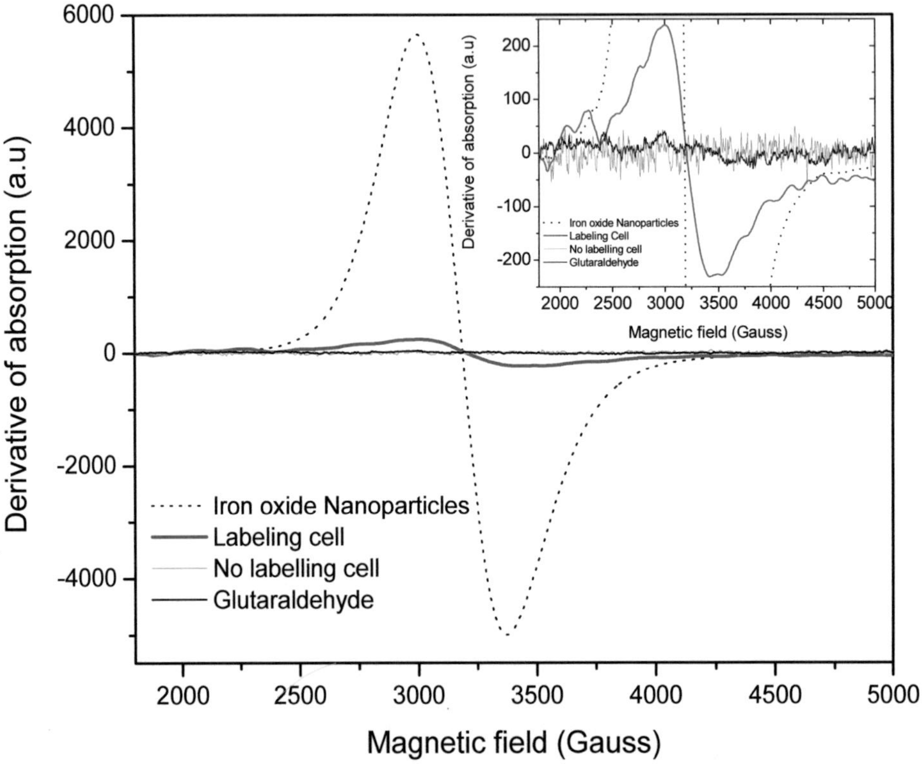

Fig. 4. EPR spectra, showing the resonance absorption curve of the superparamagnetic nanoparticles, labelled cells ($CD133^{+}$), unlabelled cells ($CD133^{-}$) and glutaraldehyde 0,5% fixative. The spectra are shown in the inset.

EPR spectrum of the labelled cells ($CD133^{+}$) was then performed, observing a resonance line in g=2.0 showing the presence of the magnetic nanoparticles bound to the cells, which were immersed in glutaraldehyde 0,5% fixative. This fixative was removed by centrifugation of the labelled cells and it was analyzed using the EPR spectrum. This spectrum showed the absence of resonance in glutaraldehyde fixative thus evidencing the absence of iron oxide superparamagnetic nanoparticles in the fixative.

As expected, the EPR spectrum of unlabelled cells ($CD133^{-}$), used as negative controls, did not present a resonance line.

4. Discussion

Modern imaging technologies that allow for in vivo monitoring of cells in intact research subjects have opened up broad new areas of investigation. In the field of hematopoiesis and stem cell research, studies of cell trafficking involved in injury repair and hematopoietic engraftment have made great progress using these new tools. Multiple imaging modalities are available, each with its own advantages and disadvantages, depending on the specific application. For mouse models, clinically validated technologies such as magnetic resonance imaging (MRI) and positron emission tomography (PET) have been joined by optical imaging techniques such as in vivo bioluminescence imaging (BLI) and fluorescence imaging, and all have been used to monitor bone marrow and stem cells after transplantation into mice. Each modality requires that the cells of interest be marked with a distinct label that makes them uniquely visible using that technology. For each modality, there are several labels to choose from. Finally, multiple methods for applying these different labels are available (Duda et al., 2007).

In this work was described the molecular imaging on CD133$^+$ hematopoietic stem cells from human umbilical cord blood through the nanobiotechnological applications. We were able to distinguish CD133$^+$ from CD133$^-$ cells by TEM, based on their attachment to nanoparticles, as well as by signal analysis of EPR generated by these nanoparticles. Our findings indicate potential nanobiotechnological applications for *in vivo* cell imaging and therapy.

In the hematopoietic system, CD133 is especially expressed in stem cells and progenitor cells found in the bone marrow, peripheral blood and human umbilical cord blood, which was used as the cellular source for this study (Yin et al., 1997; Miraglia et al. (1997). Recent data suggest that CD133$^+$ cells, besides having extensive hematopoietic plasticity (Wynter et al., 1998), can be used in different clinical applications, being an alternative in the utilization of CD34$^+$ cells, more commonly used in transplant protocols (Handgretinger et al., 2003). CD133$^+$ cellular fraction of bone marrow harbors precursors of granulocytes/macrophages and dendritic cells (Yin et al., 1997).

Studies performed by Gehling et al. (2000) demonstrated that CD133$^+$ cells have the capacity to differentiate in endothelial cells. After that, other researchers identified an endothelial progenitor (CD133$^+$) that co-expresses the receptor for vascular endothelial growth factor (VEGFR) (Gill et al., 2001). They also detected functional responses in these cells during vascular trauma, suggesting that these CD133$^+$ endothelial progenitors can be mobilized by VEFG, being useful in repairing vascular tissue injury (Gill et al., 2001).

Powell et al. (2005) related diseases of the coronary arteries with the reduction of fractions from three different sub-types of CD133$^+$ circulant cells: CD133$^+$CD34$^+$; CD133$^+$CXCR4$^+$ and CD133$^+$VEGFR2$^+$. These data indicated that the functional meaning of CD133 positive cellular fractions (CD133$^+$) transcends the hematopoietic tissue (Bhatia, 2001).

In the present study, after the previous analysis of flow cytometry confirming the significant expression (82%) of the CD133 cell surface antigen (CD133$^+$ phenotype) in the stem cells of the human umbilical cord blood (UCB), the analysis of these cells through Transmission Electronic Microscopy (TEM) was performed.

The electron micrographs highlighted the presence of electrondense granules in the cellular membrane, as well as dispersed in the cytoplasm of CD133$^+$ cells, which refers to the superparamagnetic nanoparticles bound to anti-CD133 monoclonal antibody. These electronic micrographs described an important ultrastructural finding related to the presence of vesicles that internalize of nanonoparticles conjugated to anti-CD133 by the process of pinocytosis for all antibodies tested. We suggest that in our study the pynocytisis occur by receptor-mediated endocytosis. The endocytosis process happens after the antibody biding to the receptor, and then a depression arises on the cell membrane which is followed by the formation of the pinocytic vesicles. These pinocytic vesicles that are surrounded by the cytoplasmic proteins called clatrines, are internalized (Pavon et al., 2010).

Electron Paramagnetic Resonance (EPR) analysis of the CD133+ stem cells from UCB detected that the signal (spectrum) generated by the labelled cells comes from the superparamagnetic nanoparticles composed of iron oxide bound to these cells.

For spectrum detection of the EPR of the superparamagnetic nanoparticles it was necessary to perform an earlier study of the qualitative visualization through TEM of these nanoparticles also bound to CD133+ stem cells. The micrographies showed that the anti-CD133 antibodies, bound to nanoparticles are bound to the cell surface antigens, thus demonstrating that the stem cell morphology, even after the selection process, was preserved. In this way the information of the analysis of the quantification by EPR of the iron content in the cells was validated (Billotey et al., 2003; Wilhelm et al., 2002), which is necessary for the intensity study of the image signal by magnetic resonance (MRI), to obtain the molecular image.

This findings may guide future research in the study of molecular imaging on CD133+ haematopoietic stem cells from human umbilical cord blood, highlighting the immunolocalization of monoclonal antibodies associated with superparamagnetic nanoparticles, as well as the signal detection generated by these nanoparticles (EPR) bound to the cells studied, suggest many biomedical applications using new resources in nanoscience as they become available. The EPR results, together with ultrastructural characterization of immunolocalized nanoparticles, strongly suggest that CD133+ cells labelled with nanoparticles can be considered for different nanobiotechnological applications, i.e., matter manipulation in a nanometric scale to help areas such as diagnosis, therapeutics or even bioengineering (Fargeas et al., 2006). This is because these CD133+ cells from human UCB could represent a primary step to again access to a stem pool useful for therapeutic hematopoietic transplants, stem cell expansion for clinical purposes and pre-clinical research on tissue regenerating therapies.

Recent developments are revolutionizing the understanding about hematopoietic stem-cell therapy. Over the past three decades, much knowledge has been accumulated to provide a sound basis for the optimal use of this approach in the treatment of hematopoietic cancers, especially acute myelogenous leukemia, Hodgkin's disease and other lymphomas and multiple myeloma (Verlinden et al., 1998; Thomas; Chift, 1999; Negrin et al., 2000; Childs et al., 2000; Sharp et al., 2000). This approach has also been used in the treatment of some solid tumors, most notably breast cancer, for which its value is still in dispute because of poor accrual in randomized trials and because it takes many years to obtain definitive answers, even from well-designed trials (Joshi et al., 2000). Hematopoietic stem-cell therapy is also being tried in sickle cell disease and thalassemia and recently in progressive multiple sclerosis, systemic scleroderma, severe systemic lupus erythematosus, and rheumatoid arthritis with a poor prognosis (Shichishima et al., 1983; Papanikolaou et al., 2011; Alderucciro et al., 2011).

The broadening therapeutic applications of hematopoietic stem cells also reflect an increased understanding of how to modulate the cells of the immune system to minimize both rejection and graft-versus-host disease and to improve the management of the infectious complications of immunosuppression (Verlinden et al., 1998; Sharp et al., 2000).

While much has been studied about hematopoietic stem-cell therapy several questions remain regarding the biology of stem cells in living subjects. For most therapeutic applications of regenerative medicine, critical issues such as stem cell type and delivery route of stem cells remain to be elucidated. In addition, after cells are transplanted to the living subject, it becomes critical to understand the biology of transplanted cells and how they interact with the microenvironment. Recent developments in molecular imaging modalities may likely permit investigators to answer some of these questions. Furthermore, some of these imaging strategies have the potential to be translated to patients, which makes them plausible to be used in the clinics.

5. Acknowledgements

We are grateful to the Laboratório de Microscopia Eletrônica, Departamento de Biologia, UNESP, Rio Claro, SP - Brasil, and Antonio T. Yabuki and Monika Iamonte for the technical support.

6. Funding provided by

Sociedade Beneficente Israelita Brasileira Hospital Albert Einstein - SBIBHAE (IEP 278-07), Instituto UNIEMP - Fórum Permanente das Relações Universidade Empresa.

7. Abbreviations

CD133: CD133 and the alternative tiles PROMININ, PROML1 and AC133 was originally identified as a protein that selectively localized at he apical surface of murine neuroepithelial cells, whereas PROML1 was identified as an antigenic marker (AC133 antigen) in hematopoietic stem cells.

Anti-CD133: monoclonal antibody against the CD133.

$CD133^+$: presence of CD133 antigen expression.

$CD133^-$: absence of CD133 antigen expression.

8. References

Alderuccio F, Nasa Z, Chung J, Ko HJ, Chan J, Toh BH. Hematopoietic Stem Cell Gene Therapy as a Treatment for Autoimmune Diseases. Rinsho Ketsueki.24(7):826-33, 1983.

Bhirde, A.; Xie, J.; Swierczewska, M. et al. Nanoparticles for cell labeling. Nanoscale, 2011, 3, 142-153

Bhatia M. (2001). CD133 expression in human stem cells. Leukemia. (11): 1685-1686.

Billotey C. et al. (2003). Cell internalization of anionic maghemite nanoparticles: quantitative effect on magnetic resonance imaging. Magn. Reson. Med. 49:646.

Bonanno, G. et al. (2004). Clinical isolation and functional characterization of cord blood CD133+ hematopoietic progenitor cells. Transplantation and Cellular Engineering. 44:1087-1097.

Bonanno, G. et al. (2007). Human cord blood CD133+ cells immunoselected by a clinical-grade apparatus differentiate in vitro into endothelial and cardiomyocyte-like cells. Transplantation and Cellular Engineering. 47:280-289.

Childs, R., Chernoff, A., Contentin, N., et al. (2000). Regression of metastatic renal-cell carcinoma after nonmyeloablative allogeneic peripheral-blood stem-cell transplantation. N. Engl. J. Med. *343,* 750–758.

Duda, J.; Karimi, M.; Negrin, R.S. et al. (2007). Methods for imaging cell fates in hematopoiesis. Methods Mol Med.134:17-34.

Fargeas, C.A. et al. (2006). Prominin-1 (CD133): from progenitor cells to human diseases. Future Lipidology. (1): 213–225.

Finney, M.R. et al. (2005). Characterization of umbilical cord blood CD133+ and in vivo functionality in response to ischemia in a murine hind-limb injury model. 106(11): 3693-3697.

Gamarra, L.F. et al. (2005). Biocompatible superparamagnetic iron oxide nanoparticles used for contrast agents: a structural and magnetic study. Journal of Magnetism and Magnetic Materials. 289: 439-441.

Gamarra, L.F. et al. (2007). Kinetics of elimination and distribution in blood and liver of biocompatible ferrofluids based on Fe_3O^4 nanoparticles: An EPR and XRF study. Materials Science & Engineering. C, Biomimetic Materials, Sensors and Systems doi:10.1016/j.msec.2007.06.005.

Gehling, U.M. et al. (2000). In vitro differentiation of endothelial cells from CD133 positive progenitor cells. Blood. 95(10): 3106-3112.

Gill M. et al. (2001). Vascular trauma induces rapid but transient mobilization of VEGFR2(+)CD133(+) endothelial precursor cells. Circ. Res. (88): 167-174.

Gluckman E. et al. (1997). Outcome of cord-blood transplantation from related and unrelated donors. N. Engl. J. Med. 337: 373-381.

Handgretinger, R. et al. (2003). Biology and plasticity of CD133+ hematopoietic stem cell. Annals New York Academy of Sciences. 996: 141-151.

Hseih, C.T. et al. (2002). The change from paramagnetic resonance to ferromagnetic resonance for iron nanoparticles made by the sol–gel method. Journal of Physics and Chemistry of Solids, v.63, p.733.

Jang, Y.Y; Ye, Z.; Cheng, L. (2011). Molecular imaging and stem cell research. Mol Imaging.10(2):111-22.

Joshi, S.S., Tarantolo, S.R., Kuszynski, C.A., and Kessinger, A. (2000). Antitumor therapeutic potential of activated human umbilical cord blood cells against leukemia and breast cancer. Clin. Cancer Res. 6, 4351–4358.

Kuci, S. et al. (2003). Identification of a novel class of human adherent $CD34^-$ stem cells that give rise to SCI repopulating cells. Blood. 101:869-876.

Lacava, L.M. et al. (2002). Use of magnetic resonance to study biodistribution of dextran-coated magnetic fluid intravenously administered in mice. J. Magn. Magn. Mater. 252:367.

Lehner, M. & Holter, W. (2002). Endotoxin-free purification of monocytes for dendritic cell generation via discontinuous density gradient centrifugation based on diluted Ficoll-Paque Plus. Int. Arch. Allergy Immunol. 128(1):73-76.

Ma, N. et al. (2005). Bone marrow vs. cord blood $CD133^+$ cells for myocardial regeneration. 53: 922-983.

Miraglia, S. et al. (1997). A novel five-transmembrana hematopoietic stem cell antigen: isolation, characterization and molecular cloning. Blood. (90): 5013-5021.

Neumaier, C.E.; Baio, G.;, Ferrini, S.; et al. (2008). MR and iron magnetic nanoparticles. Imaging opportunities in preclinical and translational research.Tumori. 94(2):226-33.

Negrin, R.S., Atkinson, K., Leemhuis, T., et al. (2000). Transplantation of highly purified CD34+ Thy-1+ hematopoietic stem cells in patients with metastatic breast cancer. Biol. Blood Marrow Transplant. 6, 262–271.

Papanikolaou E, Georgomanoli M, Stamateris E, et al. The new SIN-lentiviral vector for thalassemia gene therapy combining two HPFH activating elements corrects human thalassemic hematopoietic stem cells. Mol Pharm. 13:215:2554, 2011.

Pavon, L.F.; Gamarra, L.F.; Marti, L.C.; Sibov, T.T.; Oliveira, D.M.; Guilhen, D.D.; Amaro, E. Jr. (2010). Ultrastructural study of the tumorigenic cells used nanobiomarkers. Cancer Biotherapy & Radiopharmaceuticals. 25(3): 289-298.

Peichev, M. et al. (2000). Expression of VEGFR-2 and AC133 by circulating human CD43- cells identifies a population of functional endothelial precursors. Blood. 95: 952-958.

Pfenninger, C.V. et al. (2007). CD133 is not present on neurogenic astrocytes in the adult subventricular zone, but on embryonic neural stem cells, ependymal cells and glioblastoma cells. Cancer Research. 67(12): 5727-5736.

Powell, T.M. et al. (2005). Granulocyte colony-stimulating factor mobilizes functional endothelial progenitor cells in patients with coronary artery disease. Arterioscler. Thromb. Vasc. Biol. (25): 296-301.

Rocha, V. et al. (2001). Comparison of out-comes of unrelated bone marrow and umbilical cord blood transplants in children with acute leukemia. Blood. 97:2962-2971.

Rubinstein, P. et al. (1998). Outcomes among 562 recipients of placental blood transplant from unrelated donors. N. Engl. J. Med. 339:1565-177.

Sadeghiani, N. et al. (2005). Magnetic Resonance of Polyaspartic Acid-Coated Magnetite Nanoparticles Administered in Mice. IEEE Trans. Magn. 41(10):4108.

Sastry, M.D. et al. (1995). Electron magnetic resonance of ferrofluids: evidence for anisotropic resonance at 77 K in samples cooled in a magnetic field. Journal of Magnetism and Magnetic Materials, v.149, p.64.

Sharma, V.K. & Waldner, F. (1977). Superparamagnetic and ferromagnetic resonance of ultrafine Fe_3O_4 particles in ferrofluids. Journal of Applied Physics, v.48, p.4298.

Sharp, J.G., Kessinger, A., Lynch, J.C., Pavletic, Z.S., and Joshi, S.S. (2000). Blood stem cell transplantation: factors influencing cellular immunological reconstitution. J. Hematother. Stem Cell Res. 9, 971–981.

Shichishima T, Ishibashi T, Kanbayashi H, et al. (1983). [Hematopoietic stem cells in chronic rheumatoid arthritis].Rinsho Ketsueki. 24(7):826-33.

Simberg, D. et al. (2007). Biomimetic amplification of nanoparticle homing to tumors. PNAS, 104(3): 932-936.

Thomas, E.D. and Clift, R.A. (1999). Allogenic transplantation for chronic myeloid leukemia. Thomas, E.D., Blume, K.G., and Forman, S.J. eds. Blackwell Sci., 807–815.

Verlinden, S.F., Mulder, A.H., de Leeuw, J.P., and van Bekkum, D.W. (1998). T lymphocytes determine the development of xeno GVHD and of human hemopoiesis in NOD/SCID mice following human umbilical cord blood transplantation. Stem Cells. *16, Suppl. 1,* 205–217.

Watt, S.M. et al. (2000). Functionally defined CD164 epitopes are expressed on CD34+ cells throughout ontogeny but display distinct distribution patterns in adult hematopoietic and nonhematopoietic tissues. Blood. 65: 3113-3124.

Wilhelm, C. et al. (2002). Magnetophoresis and ferromagnetic resonance of magnetically labelled cells. Eur. Biophys (31):118.

de Wynter, E.A. et al. (1998). $CD34^{+}AC133^{+}$ cells isolated from cord blood are highly enriched in long-term culture-initiating cells, NOD/SCID-repopulating cells and dentritic cell progenitors. Stem Cells. (16): 387-396.

Yin, A.H. et al. (1997). CD133, a novel marker for human hematopoietic stem and progenitor cells. Blood. (90): 5002-5012.

15

Diagnostic and Treatment Response Imaging in Lymphomas

Xingchen Wu[1,2,3] and Pirkko-Liisa Kellokumpu-Lehtinen[1,3]
[1]*Department of Oncology, Tampere University Hospital, Tampere,*
[2]*Medical Imaging Centre, Department of Radiology,*
Tampere University Hospital, Tampere,
[3]*Medical School, University of Tampere, Tampere,*
Finland

1. Introduction

The lymphomas are a heterogeneous group of malignant diseases, which vary with respect to their molecular features, genetics, clinical presentations, treatment approaches and outcomes. They are divided into two broad groups on the basis of pathology: Hodgkin's disease (HD) and non-Hodgkin's lymphoma (NHL). They comprise approximately 5% - 6% of all malignancies and are the fifth most frequently occurring type of cancer in the Western world (Jemal A *et al.*, 2009). HD and many histological sub-types of NHL are potentially curable with appropriate chemotherapy and/or involved-field radiotherapy, and patients with disease relapse may be cured by second-line salvage treatments (Hampson FA and AS Shaw, 2008). Accurate staging and response assessment are essential to guide treatment decisions. Molecular imaging has become an essential tool in the early diagnosis (guiding biopsy), initial staging and risk stratification, monitoring response to therapy, and detection tumor recurrence of lymphomas. Research in molecular imaging is also contributing to our understanding of the disease pathogenesis of lymphomas and helping to direct more effective care of patients with the diseases.

Computed tomography (CT) once was the single imaging modality for staging and monitoring morphological changes after treatment. The relatively recent integration of positron emission tomography (PET) with the use of ^{18}F-fluorodeoxyglucose tracer (^{18}F-FDG) into oncologic imaging has further improved baseline staging and facilitated functional evaluation of disease behaviour (such as tumor malignancy grade), metabolic response to therapy, and earlier detection of disease recurrence (Ngeow JY *et al.*, 2009; Schoder H *et al.*, 2005; Spaepen K *et al.*, 2002). Particularly for conclusions of therapy response assessment, FDG-PET has been shown to be considerably more accurate than anatomical imaging by CT because of its ability to distinguish between viable tumor and necrosis or fibrosis in post-therapy residual masses.

The specificity of FDG-PET is improved with the addition of CT. Integrated PET/CT, with the advantage of combining functional and anatomical information and better attenuation correction, is regarded to be the current standard of practice for the management of lymphomas. However, PET/CT is expensive, time-consuming, involves exposure to ionizing radiation, and is not widely available because it requires support infrastructure, such as cyclotrons and radiochemistry laboratories (Huang B *et al.*, 2009). In contrast, magnetic resonance imaging (MRI) provides excellent tissue contrast and high spatial resolution, and lack of ionizing radiation. It may be a potential alternative for the surveillance of lymphoma patients with multiple follow-up examinations. Moreover, the rapidly evolving parallel imaging acquisition technique with multi-channel phased array surface coils has enabled a high spatial resolution whole-body MR examination within a reasonable time (Lauenstein TC and RC Semelka, 2006). The development of imaging modalities, which can encompass the entire body, is of great importance, especially for aggressive lymphomas, in which extensive disease involvement is common (Antoch G *et al.*, 2003; Ghanem N *et al.*, 2006).

Whole-body MRI has shown advantages for the detection of distant metastatic diseases, especially from tumors frequently spreading to the brain, liver, or bone marrow (Kwee TC *et al.*, 2009), and it has been introduced as a whole-body bone marrow screening application (Schmidt GP *et al.*, 2009). Within this context, whole-body MRI is highly accurate for staging of hematologic diseases, such as lymphomas. However, additional bone marrow biopsy is still considered mandatory.

Evaluation of nodal disease by CT and conventional MRI still relies on size criteria, lymph nodes with a short-axis diameter greater than 10 mm are generally considered positive. However, lymph nodes may be enlarged reactively and even small lymph nodes may be infiltrated by malignant cells. Thus, tumor in unenlarged lymph nodes may go undetected. Diffusion-weighted MRI (DWI) is a noninvasive technique that probes the random microscopic motion of water molecules *in vivo* (Le Bihan D, 1995). DWI with apparent diffusion coefficient (ADC) mapping provides quantitative physiological and functional information regarding characterization of lymphomas. Because of their high cellularity and high nuclear-to-cytoplasm ratio, aggressive lymphomas have relatively high signal intensity on DW images and low ADC values (Sumi M *et al.*, 2007). Recent studies have shown that DWI with ADC mapping could distinguish between benign and malignant lymphadenopathy (Holzapfel K *et al.*, 2009; Perrone A *et al.*, 2009), and it may have prognostic potential in patients with aggressive lymphomas (Wu X, PL Kellokumpu-Lehtinen *et al.*, 2011). An advantage of DWI over conventional MRI sequences in the evaluation of lymphoma is the high lesion-to-background contrast, which make it a valuable imaging modality for detecting metastasis and cancer relapse, and it has also been used to assess treatment response in various malignancies including lymphomas (Wu X, PL Kellokumpu-Lehtinen *et al.*, 2011). Our recent pilot study showed that DWI, in combination with whole-body MRI, yielded results comparable with those from integrated PET/CT in treatment evaluation of patients with diffuse large B-cell lymphoma (Wu X, PL Kellokumpu-Lehtinen *et al.*, 2011). DWI and PET/CT share similar applications in the field of clinical oncology. This is important when a patient is not suitable for PET/CT exams (e.g. diabetes) or PET/CT is not available.

This chapter will highlight the most important and potential applications of FDG-PET/CT and MRI including whole-body MRI and DWI emphasizing the strengths and pitfalls of each imaging approach in diagnosis, initial staging, and response assessment of lymphomas.

2. Classification of malignant lymphomas

The lymphoproliferative disorders encompass a collection of lymphoid neoplasms with different clinical and histological presentations. The classification of lymphoid malignant diseases has been beset by difficulties. In 1994, a census for universal lymphoma classification was published in the form of the Revised European-American Lymphoma (REAL) classification (Harris NL *et al.*, 1994). The current World Health Organization (WHO) classification was derived from the REAL criteria, in which NHL is categorized into more than 20 subtypes on the basis of cell origin (B- or T-cell precursor), morphological, and immunophenotypic data (Harris NL *et al.*, 2000). Diffuse large B-cell lymphoma and follicular lymphoma account for more than 50% of cases of NHL. The WHO classification helps to determine not only malignancy grade, but also prognosis. Systems in which NHL is grouped into indolent, aggressive, and very aggressive disorders are practically very useful (Cronin CG *et al.*, 2010).

3. Diagnosis, initial staging, and prognosis assessment of malignant lymphomas

Diagnosis is based on an integration of morphological (lymph nodes, blood and bone marrow), immunophenotypic, molecular, cytogenetic data, and clinical behavior. Many lymphomas have characteristic morphological features, but no specific biomarker is of diagnostic value. In patients suspected of malignant lymphoma, a surgical excision biopsy of an enlarged lymph node (or extra-nodal site) is mandatory to confirm the diagnosis and to define the histological subtypes.

Once the diagnosis of HD or NHL has been established by biopsy of a particular site, accurate determination of disease extent (staging) is crucial for appropriate treatment planning and prognosis prediction. In addition, knowing the sites of involvement at time of diagnosis makes it possible to accurately restage at the end of therapy and document a complete remission. Conventional staging techniques, considered the standard reference, include contrast-enhanced CT of the neck, chest, abdomen and pelvis, uni/bilateral bone marrow biopsy, and in some cases MRI. CT has been the most commonly used imaging modality for initial staging of lymphomas for decades. In patients with aggressive NHL and HD, FDG-PET and FDG-PET/CT are increasingly applied for the initial staging. Bone marrow biopsy is an invasive procedure and can be subject to sampling errors (Pelosi E *et al.*, 2008). Therefore, PET scan should be the first step in lymphoma staging workup so that it could be used to guide bone marrow biopsy in the presence of patchy bone marrow lesion (Figure 1). The role of FDG-PET in indolent lymphoma is still unclear, and not all indolent lymphomas are FDG-avid. In current clinical practice, the use of MRI for staging malignant lymphoma is still limited. It is mainly applied as an adjunct to CT in selected cases with soft tissue lesions, or suspected involvement of the central nervous system or bone marrow that need to be further evaluated (Vermoolen MA *et al.*, 2011).

Staging of both HD and NHL is based on the Ann Arbor classification, with the inclusion of a definition of bulky disease known as the Cotswold modification (Lister TA *et al.*, 1989). This staging system encompasses the number of sites of disease involved, the type of involvement (nodal or extra-nodal), and the distribution of disease. Whole-body imaging is

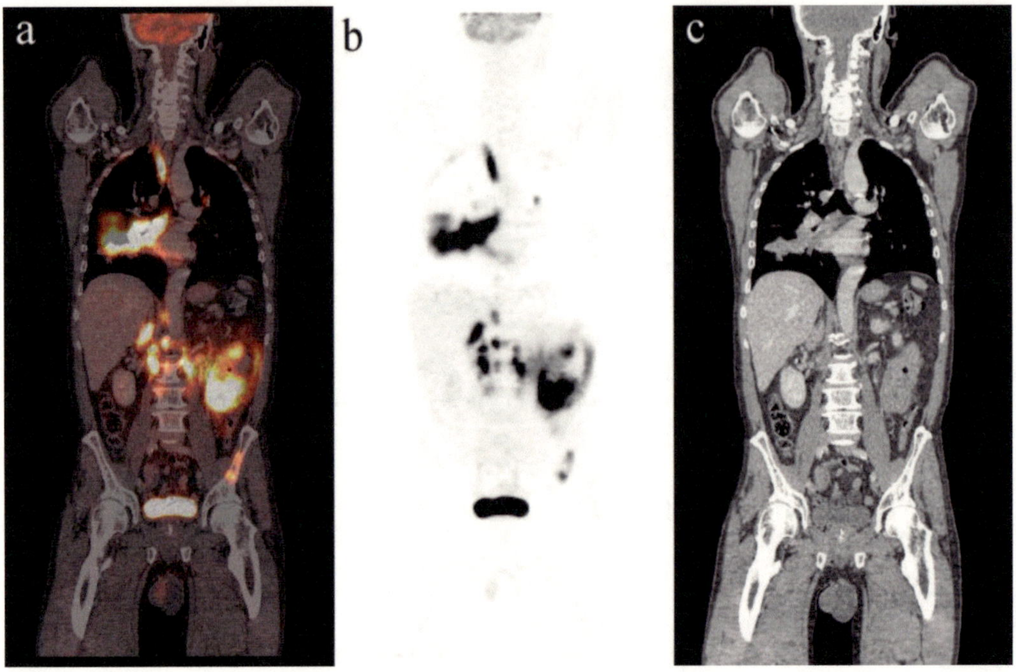

Fig. 1. A coronal slice of fused PET/CT image (a), the corresponding PET image (b) and CT image (c) in a 62-year-old male patient with diffuse large B-cell lymphoma
Multiple FDG avid lesions are showing in the cervical, mediastinum, abdominal region, and the left iliac on both the fused PET/CT image and the PET image. The iliac lesion was neither detected by the corresponding CT image, nor by bone marrow biopsy that was performed at the right side of the iliac.

therefore an indispensable tool. Ann Arbor stage I: Only one lymph node region or extra-nodal site is affected. Stage II: Multiple lymph node regions are affected, but limited to the same side of the diaphragm. Stage III: Involvement of lymph node regions on both sides of the diaphragm, which may be accompanied by local extra-nodal extension. Stage IV: Diffuse involvement of one or more extra-nodal organs or sites, including bone marrow, liver, and lung (Lister TA *et al.*, 1989). Accurate staging is critical for identifying patients with early stage (stage I or II) lymphoma, some of which might be treated with involved-field radiation therapy. Chemotherapy is performed in patients with more advanced stage disease (stage III or IV).

The International Prognostic Score (IPS) based on seven factors consisting of serum albumin, hemoglobin, gender, stage, age, leukocytosis, and lymphocytopenia is used for newly diagnosed HD patients. Whereas the International Prognostic Index (IPI) is the most widely used prognostic index for adult NHL, which is based on both clinical and imaging findings including age, serum lactate dehydrogenase (LDH) level, extent of disease, and performance status. The IPI is derived from an additive score of 0 to 5 points to stratify patients as having low (0 - 1 point), low-to-intermediate (2 points), high-to-intermediate (3 points), or high (4 - 5 points) prognostic risk (Shipp MA, 1994). However, considerable variations still remain in the outcome of individual patients within the same prognostic group because of the biological and clinical heterogeneity of the diseases. Currently, the paradigm of treatment in HD and NHL is moving towards a more risk-adapted therapy based on the individual patient's prognosis by advanced imaging techniques.

4. Response assessment of malignant lymphomas

The response to therapy of lymphomas shows a high variability, therefore, it is important to have knowledge of early chemotherapy efficacy for individual patient. Furthermore, assessment of early- or mid-treatment response to chemotherapy has been shown to be of prognostic value in patients with malignant lymphomas (MacManus MP *et al.*, 2007). Identification of nonresponders at an early stage allows for the adjustment of chemotherapy and radiotherapy regimens promptly and thereby may improve the outcomes and decrease the toxicity and costs that associated with ineffective treatment. However, the value of altering therapy based on early- or mid-treatment FDG-PET remains to be established (Cheson BD *et al.*, 2007). Response assessment at the end of treatment is performed to assess whether there is a partial or complete remission, which is important for determining the need for additional treatment and for determining prognosis. The International Working Group (IWG) criteria, published in 1999, have become the widely accepted standard for response assessment in NHL, and were subsequently adopted for HD (Cheson BD *et al.*, 1999). Although based primarily on CT findings, the IWG criteria take bone marrow biopsy, clinical, and biochemical information into account. The IWG criteria have proved extremely useful in the standardization of treatment response, but they do have a number of limitations. As a consequence of this, together with advances in functional imaging, revised criteria that incorporate both CT and FDG-PET were published in 2007 (Cheson BD *et al.*, 2007). Complete remission indicates disappearance of all evidence of disease, partial remission indicates regression of measurable disease and no new sites, stable disease indicates failure to attain complete remission or partial remission, and progressive disease indicates the appearance of new lesions or increase by ≥50% of previously involved sites (Cheson BD *et al.*, 2007). According to the revised criteria, a patient is considered to be complete remission even if a residual CT mass is present, provided the mass has changed from being FDG avid or PET-positive to PET-negative.

5. Different imaging modalities

5.1 Computed tomography

The introduction of CT in the mid 1970s was a tremendous breakthrough in noninvasive imaging, and its potential for staging malignant lymphoma was soon recognized and investigated. Since then, CT has gradually become the imaging modality of choice for staging malignant lymphomas. CT technology has continuously been developed and refined; major milestones include the introduction of spiral (helical) CT, and the advent of multi-detector row CT that increases the speed of data collection dramatically. In addition, current CT scanners have a faster gantry rotation. These properties enable acquisition of high resolution cross-sectional images of the whole-body within only a couple of seconds, which minimizes or eliminates breathing artifacts (Kwee TC, Kwee RM *et al.*, 2008; Rydberg J *et al.*, 2000). As a result, lymph nodes of 5 mm or less in diameter can be detected. In combination with powered injectors for rapid bolus administration of intravenous contrast medium, focal extra-nodal lesions on the order of a few millimeters can be identified (Lucey BC *et al.*, 2005; Vinnicombe SJ and RH Reznek, 2003). Intravenous contrast medium facilitates nodal recognition in the neck and in the retroperitoneum in patients with a paucity of adipose tissue. The importance of adequate bowel opacification with dilute oral contrast (so as to avoid confusion with intra-abdominal and pelvic masses) was well recognised (Kwee TC, Kwee RM *et al.*, 2008). However, contrast-enhanced CT is not very helpful in differentiating normal from malignant lymph nodes. CT has limitations in differentiating malignant from benign small lymph nodes or, after treatment, neoplastic tissue from fibrosis.

CT remains the basic imaging modality for initial staging malignant lymphomas because of its widespread availability and relatively low cost. However, the limited specificity of CT is still a fundamental problem in oncology, e.g. to detect pathological changes in normal-sized structures, to detect lesions that have poor contrast with surrounding tissue. At initial staging, determination of nodal involvement by CT is based on size criteria. Lymph nodes viewed on CT are considered as pathological if the maximum allowed long-axis diameter of 15 mm is exceeded, and/or if the short-axis diameter is more than 10 mm. In addition, nodal involvement is presumed if clustering of normal-sized lymph nodes is present in the anterior mediastinum or mesentery, or if lymph nodes of any size are visualized in areas where they normally are not observed (Vermoolen MA *et al.*, 2011). CT evaluation on the basis of nodal size has historically been regarded as the reference standard imaging technique for staging, with a reported sensitivity and specificity for nodal disease of 87.5% and 85.6%, respectively (la Fougere C *et al.*, 2006). General criteria for extra-nodal involvement are any focal density alterations or mass lesions involving soft tissues, bones, parenchymal organs and serosal cavities (Vermoolen MA *et al.*, 2011). Comparing current with previous CT scans may improve diagnostic reliability. Nevertheless, the use of CT alone in restaging malignant lymphoma can be limited, since it is not able to differentiate residual viable tumor tissue from therapy-induced fibrosis. Following treatment of lymphoma by chemotherapy and/or radiation, up to 40% of patients with nodal disease have a residual mass on CT. Previous studies have shown that only 10 - 20% of such patients will have disease in these residual masses (Hampson FA and AS Shaw, 2008). In early response assessment, CT is not an ideal diagnostic tool, as morphological changes may lag behind rapid functional changes in response to therapy. Another weakness of CT is the limited sensitivity for detecting bone marrow involvement, which, if present, by definition indicates stage IV disease (Vinnicombe SJ and RH Reznek, 2003) (Figure 1).

Major disadvantages of CT are exposure of the patient to ionizing radiation and the administration of iodinated contrast agents, which may induce secondary cancers and cause allergic reactions, respectively (Kwee TC *et al.*, 2009). Nevertheless, contrast-enhanced diagnostic CT remains the base for initial measurements of involved sites and detection of complications such as adjacent organ compression, although combined FDG-PET/CT is increasingly applied for initial staging of malignant lymphomas.

5.2 FDG-PET

Positron emission tomography was developed in the 1970s soon after CT (Phelps ME *et al.*, 1975). It is based on the use of positron-emitting radiopharmaceuticals and the detection in coincidence of the 2 nearly collinear 511 keV photons emitted following positron annihilation with an electron. Fluorodeoxyglucose (FDG), an analogue of glucose; is taken up by high-glucose-using cells. After transport into tumour cells, ^{18}F-FDG is phosphorylated to ^{18}F-FDG-6-phosphate that cannot be further metabolised. It will take approximately 60 minutes for the radiotracer to travel through the body and to be absorbed by the organ or tissue being studied. Thus, 60 minutes after intravenous injection, the concentrations of ^{18}F-FDG tracer give tissue glucose metabolic activity, in terms of regional glucose uptake. Cancer imaging by ^{18}F-FDG-PET is based on the observation that most cancers, including many lymphomas, metabolize glucose at an abnormally high rate (Warburg O, 1956). The most aggressive tumors require greater glucose consumption to maintain their accelerated growth. Imaging of malignant lymphoma with FDG was first described in the 1980s (Paul R, 1987), and the first reports on FDG-PET as a whole-body staging method in malignant lymphoma was published in the 1990s (Moog F *et al.*, 1997). PET technology has improved dramatically since its development. Initial patient imaging units had a system resolution greater than 15 mm, whereas current units have a 4 to 5 mm resolution. Raw data should be reconstructed by means of iterative expectation maximization algorithms, which provide superior signal-to-noise ratio compared with filtered back-projection images (Kwee TC, Kwee RM *et al.*, 2008). When one (or both) of the annihilation photos scatters in the body, it is prevented to be detected appropriately, which is called attenuation. Attenuation effects produce regional nonuniformities, distortions of intense structures, and edge effects. To improve anatomical delineation, additional transmission scanning for attenuation correction using an external radiation source is required. Attenuation correction also allows for semiquantitative evaluation, which offers a more objective way to assess FDG uptake. Nonattenuation corrected images should also be evaluated, because the attenuation correction itself may also introduce image artifacts (Rohren EM *et al.*, 2004).

FDG-PET imaging protocols vary from institution to institution, which highlights the need for standardization. In the most frequently used protocol, patients fast for 4 - 6 hours prior to the injection of FDG. Imaging commences approximately 60 minutes after the injection of a typical FDG dose of 370 MBq. Serum glucose levels of less than 150 mg/dl are desirable. Patients are also instructed to avoid any kind of strenuous activity prior to the examination and following injection of the radioisotope to avoid physiological muscle uptake of FDG.

Visual analysis of an FDG-PET scan can characterize the intensity of metabolic activity as low, moderate or high. In many cases visual image interpretation is sufficient to identify malignant lesions. Any focus of visually elevated FDG uptake relative to the background (surrounding normal tissue), not located in areas of physiologically increased uptake, is regarded as positive for malignant lymphomas (Vermoolen MA *et al.*, 2011). In organs with physiological FDG uptake (e.g., spleen and liver), focal or inhomogeneous uptake patterns are considered to be indicative of malignant lymphoma (Figure 1). Nevertheless, quantitative analysis of FDG uptake may complement visual image interpretation because it provides objective criteria, thus minimizing interobserver variability in image interpretation. The FDG uptake can also be assessed semiquantitatively using the standardized uptake value (SUV). The standardized uptake value, an index of glucose metabolism on FDG-PET image, is the ratio between the measured and expected uptake if FDG were distributed evenly throughout the body. The maximum standardized uptake value (SUVmax) has been used in daily clinical setting to evaluate the degree of malignancy, metabolic response to therapy, and early detection of disease recurrence (Ngeow JY *et al.*, 2009; Schoder H *et al.*, 2005; Spaepen K *et al.*, 2002; Wu X, P Dastidar *et al.*, 2011). Measurements of metabolic burden, which incorporate both FDG uptake and PET lesion volume may prove more useful for risk stratification and response assessment (Berkowitz A *et al.*, 2008).

Owing to its high diagnostic accuracy, FDG-PET has become an established imaging modality in addition to CT for the initial staging, response assessment, and detection recurrence of lymphomas [4]. Previous studies have demonstrated that FDG-PET is superior to CT in staging HD and high-grade NHL, with sensitivity, specificity, and accuracy reported at 85 - 98% (Hampson FA and AS Shaw, 2008; la Fougere C *et al.*, 2006). As a consequence a significant number of patients will have a change of stage, with many of these having their management revised (Hampson FA and AS Shaw, 2008). Most commonly this results in the disease being upstaged, since patients with true early stage disease are differentiated by FDG-PET from those with otherwise occult advanced disease.

FDG-PET is useful in lymphoma classification or grading, as well as guiding biopsy. Several studies have shown that standardized uptake value correlates with the degree of malignancy in lymphomas, and in patients with NHL and an standardized uptake value greater than 10 are quite likely to have aggressive disease (Okada M *et al.*, 2010). The degree of FDG uptake by lymphoma cells may be a biomarker for disease biology: e.g. different histopathological subtypes of HD who have exhibited significantly different levels of FDG uptake (Hutchings M *et al.*, 2006). Similarly, grade III follicular lymphomas appear to have significantly higher FDG uptake than grade I or II follicular lymphomas (Tang B *et al.*, 2009). FDG uptake is lower in indolent lymphoma compared to aggressive lymphoma. Histological transformation of indolent lymphoma occurs in 20 – 30% of the patients. Recent study has shown that FDG-PET can be used as an accurate guide for biopsies in suspected transformed tissues (Bodet-Milin C *et al.*, 2008). The standardized uptake value varies considerably in different tumors of the same lymphoma patients, and biopsies should be performed in the site with the maximum standardized uptake value of the whole body (the highest malignancy) that represents the malignancy of the disease (Bodet-Milin C *et al.*, 2008; Wu X, P Korkola *et al.*, 2011). However, histological analysis remains the gold standard to confirm the transformation, since there is considerable overlap in the range of maximum standardized uptake values for different subtypes of lymphomas.

The main advantage of FDG-PET over anatomical imaging techniques, such as CT, is its ability to detect metabolic changes in malignant lymphoma lesions before structural changes become visible. A pretreatment FDG-PET scan may identify additional focal bone marrow lesions that would be missed by bone marrow biopsy or CT examination (Figure 1). Furthermore, FDG-PET surpasses CT in differentiating residual viable tumor tissue from therapy-induced fibrosis, and this allows PET performed at the end of treatment to provide a more accurate response classification than assessment by CT. Therefore, when FDG-PET results are used to make treatment decisions at initial staging and response assessment, outcome may improve, particularly in patients with HD and aggressive NHL. In addition, early- and mid-treatment PET studies have been shown to be a good predictor of progression-free survival and overall survival. However, the value of FDG-PET for staging certain indolent NHLs that are not FDG-avid may be limited, and CT imaging remains the modality of choice in these subgroups (Vermoolen MA *et al.*, 2011). Routinely, FDG avid malignant lymphomas (HD, diffuse large B-cell lymphoma, follicular lymphoma, and mantle cell lymphoma) are well visualized both in initial staging and restaging. However, some subtypes of NHL, predominantly low-grade lymphomas, may have low or even no uptake of FDG. Nodal and extra-nodal marginal zone lymphomas, small lymphocytic lymphomas, primary duodenal follicular lymphoma, cutaneous T-cell lymphomas, and peripheral T-cell lymphomas all have been reported to be possibly FDG negative (Kwee TC, Kwee RM *et al.*, 2008). Caution is warranted in these histological subtypes of NHL because a negative FDG-PET scan could not rule out malignant lesions. It is also considered mandatory to perform a pretreatment FDG-PET scan in these variable FDG avid NHLs, since comparison of a post-treatment FDG-PET scan to a pretreatment FDG-PET scan will lead to more accurate restaging (Kwee TC, Kwee RM *et al.*, 2008).

A major drawback of FDG-PET is its lack of detailed anatomical information, which impedes precise localization of sites with FDG uptake. In addition, FDG-PET is not cancer specific; there is possibility of FDG uptake in benign conditions with increased glycolysis such as inflammation and granulomatous disease. Additionally, high physiological uptake within the brain, myocardium, gastrointestinal tract, urinary tract, muscle, brown fat, salivary glands, and thymus may obscure or mimic the presence of tumor deposits. Caution also is warranted in patients receiving chemotherapy in conjunction with cytokines, such as granulocyte colony stimulating factor, because these patients may have increased bone marrow FDG uptake up to 3 weeks after the last dose of cytokines (Kazama T *et al.*, 2005). Therefore, a careful evaluation of FDG-PET findings, along with a patient's accurate history and clinical examination, is necessary to minimize the number of false-positive interpretations. Another disadvantage of FDG-PET is exposure of the patient to ionizing radiation.

In conclusion, ^{18}F-FDG-PET is the imaging technique of choice for initial staging and end-of-treatment evaluation. However, ^{18}F-FDG is not specific for tumoral tissue. Several factors can make the interpretation of PET studies challenging. Chief among these factors are the variable physiological uptake of FDG by normal tissues, FDG uptake related to inflammation, occasional malignant lesions with low avidity for FDG, limited resolution of small lesions, altered biodistribution of FDG related to hyperglycemia or hyperinsulinemia, and, in particular, bone marrow activation commonly encountered in cancer patients after treatment. It should be kept in mind that also FDG-negative lymphomas exist, and a negative ^{18}F-FDG-PET cannot exclude minimal residual disease. The interpretation of PET information requires therefore a thorough understanding of the normal physiological distribution of FDG in the body, and one should always correlate PET findings with clinical and laboratory data, other imaging modalities, and/or a biopsy.

5.3 FDG-PET/CT fusion

Advances in the scanner and computer technology enabled the development of PET/CT hybrid systems with a hardware-oriented approach to image fusion. With this type of scanner, accurately registered anatomical and functional images can be acquired in a single examination, and CT data can be used for attenuation correction of PET images. Although performed in one imaging section, the two examinations are by no means performed simultaneously. Rather, it is typically for the CT scan to be performed first, and the PET scan performed immediately after the CT scan has finished (or vice versa). Obviously, any patient motion between the PET and CT scans would lead to inaccurate attenuation correction and unreliable fusion. Several manufacturers are now offering integrated FDG-PET/CT systems combining different models of high-resolution dedicated PET scanners and multidetector-row CT scanners in line with a common imaging bed (Blodgett TM *et al.*, 2007; von Schulthess GK *et al.*, 2006). A computer platform (workstation) is used to reconstruct CT and PET data and create fused PET/CT images in the transaxial, coronal, and sagittal planes for interpretation. CT attenuation value and the maximum standardized uptake value are calculated at this workstation. PET/CT has been shown to increase both the accuracy of interpretation and the confidence level of the readers, and it has already been proven as an important diagnostic tool in several cancer types, including lymphomas, for initial staging, assessing prognosis, therapy monitoring, as well as detection of recurrence.

FDG-PET and CT provide functional and anatomical information, respectively. Integration of both modalities may outperform both FDG-PET alone and CT alone in initial staging and restaging of malignant lymphoma. FDG-PET/CT fusion, using a combined PET/CT scanner, allows more accurate localization of foci with increased FDG uptake than stand-alone PET, and this may reduce the problems of physiological FDG uptake being misinterpreted as pathological and false localization of disease. An additional advantage of combined PET/CT is the use of the CT images for attenuation correction of the PET emission data, which reduces whole-body scanning time to 30 minutes. This approach also provides low-noise attenuation correction factors compared with those from standard PET transmission measurements using an external radiation source, and eliminates bias from emission contamination of post-injection transmission scans (Kwee TC, Kwee RM *et al.*, 2008). A pitfall of CT-based attenuation correction, however, is that the use of concentrated CT contrast agents, CT beam-hardening artifacts due to metallic implants, and physiological motion can result in the alterations of standardized uptake value in lesions or the appearance of artifactual lesions. Thus, images without attenuation correction also should be evaluated to avoid misinterpretations (Blodgett TM *et al.*, 2007; von Schulthess GK *et al.*, 2006). In general, integrated PET/CT without iodinated contrast material or contrast-enhanced CT without PET is used for initial staging of lymphomas. Previous study has shown that PET/CT is more sensitive and specific than contrast-enhanced CT and suggested that PET/CT performed without intravenous contrast media is sufficient for staging patients with HD and aggressive NHL (Schaefer NG *et al.*, 2004). PET/CT in particular is recommended for primary diagnosis and follow-up because it is a whole-body imaging modality and provides both anatomical and metabolic information. Furthermore, PET/CT allows earlier detection of relapse than does morphological imaging with CT or MRI alone, and it is frequently used to detect relapse at follow-up of patients with lymphomas. Radiation dose is a point of concern in FDG-PET/CT fusion, although the CT portion of a PET/CT scan is usually performed at different settings than a standard diagnostic CT to decrease the radiation burden.

5.4 Whole-body magnetic resonance imaging

The high spatial resolution and excellent soft-tissue contrast make MRI an ideal tool for the detection of parenchymal and osseous lesions. However, because of long imaging time, MRI was previously used only as a tool to image limited anatomical areas of the body. Recent improvements in MRI technology have resulted in the availability of sufficiently fast and with diagnostic image quality sequences for whole-body MRI. As a result, whole-body MRI has become feasible for staging malignancies, including malignant lymphomas (Lauenstein TC and RC Semelka, 2006). Similar to MRI of limited body regions, whole-body MRI is sensitive to susceptibility artifacts, predominantly in the thoracic region, and motion artifacts in the abdomen (breathing and peristalsis) and thorax (breathing and cardiac motion). Image acquisition under breath-holding or respiratory triggering should therefore be applied.

Several studies have shown that whole-body MRI is feasible in both adults and children, and it may play an important role in staging and follow-up of various cancers, including malignant lymphomas (Kwee TC *et al.*, 2009; Lauenstein TC and RC Semelka, 2006; Schmidt GP *et al.*, 2009). A major advantage of whole-body MRI in malignant lymphomas is the possibility of completely evaluating the spread of disease throughout the entire body, including nodal, extra-nodal, and bone marrow involvement, in one examination (Vermoolen MA *et al.*, 2011). A disadvantage of whole-body MRI is that the image quality may be inferior to that of MRI examinations of limited body regions because the former allows less time to acquire different MRI sequences and imaging planes, and generally employs a greater slice thickness and lower spatial resolution. The use of a phased-array surface coil is preferred because it provides an increased signal-to-noise ratio and spatial resolution compared with an integrated body coil. There is no standard whole-body MRI protocol for staging malignant lymphomas yet; data regarding preferred sequence and imaging plane are lacking. A commonly recommended approach for tumor staging in general is the application of fat-suppressed T1-weighted gradient echo sequences before and after the administration of intravenous gadolinium, and fat suppressed T2-weighted sequence (Figure 2). Previous studies has shown that the fluid-sensitive fat-suppressed T2-weighted short-tau-inversion-recovery (STIR) sequence is useful for the assessment of the skeletal system and the pelvis (Lauenstein TC and RC Semelka, 2006). STIR is a particularly sensitive for detecting parenchymal and bone marrow lesions, which are generally visualized as structures of high signal intensity on images acquired with this sequence (Kwee TC, Kwee RM *et al.*, 2008). However, malignant lymph nodes can not be differentiated from benign nodes on the basis of signal intensity, neither on T1- nor on T2-weighted images.

Although MRI inherently provides superior soft-tissue contrast to CT and has the potential to characterize lesions on the basis of signal characteristics, assessment of nodal involvement is still based on size criteria. General criteria for extra-nodal involvement are any signal abnormalities or mass lesions involving soft tissues, bones, parenchymal organs, and serosal cavities. MRI is superior to CT for imaging the liver, whereas CT is superior to MRI for the assessment of mediastinal and pulmonary lymphomatous lesions (Lauenstein TC and RC Semelka, 2006). In addition, CT may be more attractive than MRI in patients with reduced health status, as it is a faster study and requires less patient cooperation.

Whole-body MRI is a feasible technique for staging malignant lymphomas, and whole-body MR imaging after gadolinium contrast injection can improve contrast and may facilitate detection of nodal and extra-nodal lymphomatous lesions (Schmidt GP *et al.*, 2009). However, disadvantages of gadolinium application include increased examination time and costs, and the potential risk of developing nephrogenic systemic fibrosis in patients with renal failure (Vermoolen MA *et al.*, 2011). In contrast to CT, FDG-PET, and FDG-PET/CT fusion, MRI has the advantage of not exposing the patient to ionizing radiation, which is

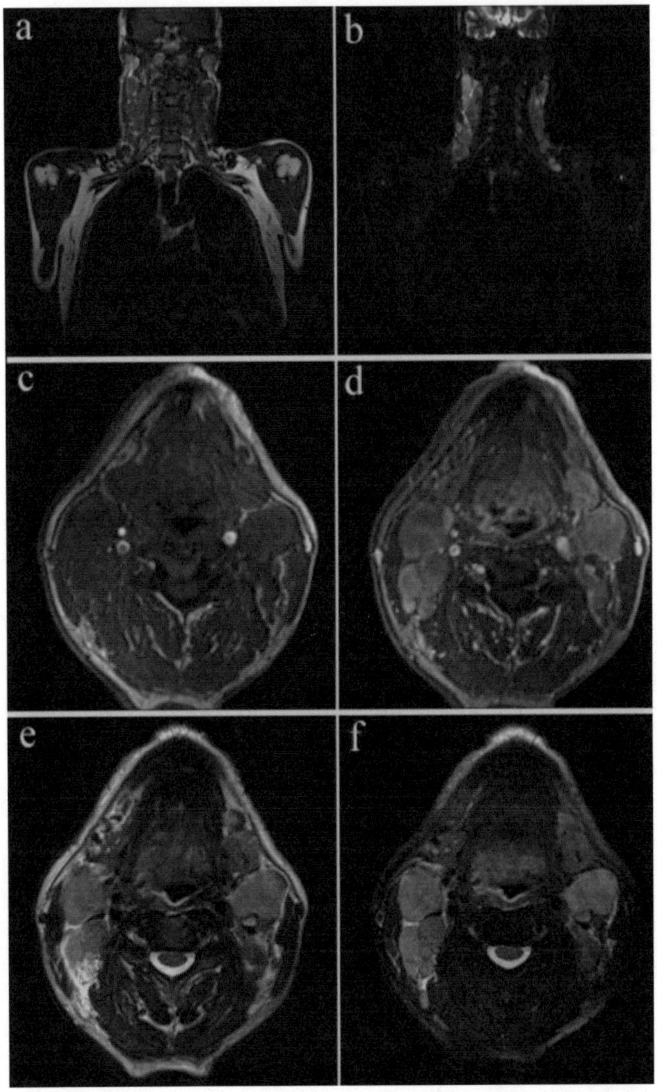

Fig. 2. MR images in a 57 year-old male patient with diffuse large B-cell lymphoma. Multiple lymph node lesions in the cervical region are shown: A coronal slice of T2-weighted image without fat-suppression (a) and the corresponding coronal slice of T2-weighted image with fat suppression (b). An axial slice of T1-weighted image before contrast agent injection and the corresponding axial slice of T1-weighted image with contrast enhancement (d). An axial slice of T2-weighted image without fat suppression (e) and the corresponding axial slice of T2-weighted image with fat suppression (f).

especially important in children. However, MRI cannot be performed in patients with pacemakers, defibrillators, or other implanted electronic devices, and in case of claustrophobia. Another limitation of conventional (anatomical) MRI is the lack of functional information, which may result in failure to detect pathological changes in normal-sized structures. However, it may be overcome with recently developed functional

MRI techniques, such as DWI. DWI highlights areas with restricted diffusion that occurs in many malignant tumors, including malignant lymphoma, without using contrast agent (Schmidt GP *et al.*, 2009; Wu X, PL Kellokumpu-Lehtinen *et al.*, 2011).

5.5 Diffusion-weighted imaging

Diffusion-weighted imaging enables the visualization of the random extra, intra, and transcellular motion of water molecules in biological tissues (Le Bihan D, 1995). DWI provides information on extracellular space tortuosity, tissue cellularity, and the integrity of cellular membranes. It can be used for the detection and characterization of pathological processes, including determination of lesion aggressiveness and monitoring response to therapy of malignant tumors, and it may therefore be of value in staging and follow-up evaluation of malignant lymphomas. The signal properties of DWI indicate both the T2 relaxation time and water diffusion, and reflect the microstructure and physiological state of tissue. Thus, subtle changes in tissue architecture can be seen by DWI. In order to create an ADC map, at least two datasets with different degrees of diffusion-weighting (i.e. *b*-values) have to be acquired. The ADC value derived from DWI is independent of the magnetic field strength and can overcome the effects of 'T2 shine-through` (an area with a very high T2 relaxation time may remain as a high signal in DWI and may be mistaken for restricted diffusion), thus allowing a more meaningful comparison of results from different studies. In general, malignant tissues tend to be hypercellular, with enlarged hyperchromatic nuclei and abundant macromolecular proteins (Wang J *et al.*, 2001). These factors reduce the diffusion space for water molecules in the extra and intracellular compartments, resulting in a decrease in ADC values (Herneth AM *et al.*, 2003; Sumi M *et al.*, 2007). In contrast, the breakdown of diffusion barriers in necrotic tissue allows the relatively unhindered diffusion of water molecules, resulting in high ADC values (Herneth AM *et al.*, 2003).

DWI using single-shot echo-planar imaging (EPI) is a well-established method to examine the brain. Extra-cranial DWI, however, did not become a clinical standard because the use of EPI was complicated by magnetic susceptibility artifacts and severe image distortion in the body (Ichikawa T *et al.*, 1998, 1999; Muller MF *et al.*, 1994). Recently introduced parallel imaging techniques, such as sensitivity encoding (Bammer R, 2003; Glockner JF *et al.*, 2005), and the development of stronger gradients and multichannel coils have largely overcome this problem; DWI of adequate quality can now be performed in the body at *b*-values of 500 - 1000 s/mm^2 (Koh DM and DJ Collins, 2007; Thoeny HC and F De Keyzer, 2007). Despite the above-mentioned breakthroughs in DWI, breathhold or respiratory triggered scanning was still considered necessary, since it was widely accepted that respiratory motion was an impediment for DWI of (moving) visceral organs (Low RN and J Gurney, 2007) .

DWI can be performed quickly and does not require a contrast agent. DW-MRI is not just sensitive to microscopic water movements but also to physiological motions of greater magnitude, such as blood, cerebrospinal fluid and ductal flows. At low *b*-values ($< 50 - 100$ s/mm^2) bulk water movement will be the predominant factor determining the ADC; at higher *b*-values, bulk water motion has less a role in the continued signal attenuation. Thus, it is possible to differentiate between the contributions made by water populations of high and low mobility by varying the experimental conditions for calculation of the ADC. It is generally accepted that with the high *b*-values used on clinical scanners (up to 500 - 1000 s/mm^2), ADC reflects water diffusion in the extracellular space (Patterson DM *et al.*, 2008).

The limitations of DWI include the sensitivity to artifacts (e.g. respiration and peristalsis movements), and therefore optimization is required to maximize the signal-to-noise ratio and to minimize artifacts. Above all, DWI is not specific to cancer. In order to interpret DWI correctly, both DW images and ADC maps should be evaluated with caution and compared with corresponding anatomical images when necessary.

Takahara *et al.* reported a unique concept of whole-body DWI, called "diffusion-weighted whole-body imaging with background body signal suppression" (DWIBS) (Takahara T *et al.*, 2004). This technique intentionally uses free breathing scanning rather than breathholding or respiratory triggering to visualize (moving) visceral organs and their lesions. In a study comparing pre- and post-chemotherapy FDG-PET with DWIBS, Kwee *et al.* found that DWIBS has higher spatial resolution for the imaging of patients with lymphomas, although it has only limited ability to help detect mediastinal lesions (Kwee TC, T Takahara *et al.*, 2008). In addition, whole-body DWI offers a high lesion-to-background contrast, making it a sensitive technique for the detection of lesions (Kwee TC *et al.*, 2009). When DWIBS is added to whole-body MRI, both anatomical and functional information can be provided within a single examination. A limitation of DWIBS is that the evaluation of structures close to the heart, such as mediastinal lymph nodes and the left liver lobe, may be compromised because of signal loss and artifacts due to cardiac motion (Vermoolen MA *et al.*, 2011).

6. View to future

6.1 Novel PET tracers

The development of new tracers and smart probes are the two key points in the development of multimodality image and diagnostic imaging in future. FDG is in routine diagnostics the most commonly used tracer for lymphoma detection and therapy follow-up, but it should be kept in mind that also FDG-negative lymphomas exist. A number of new radiotracers have been developed and are under clinical evaluation, e.g. [11C]choline, ^{18}F-fluorothymidine (^{18}F-FLT). One characteristic of malignant cells is an increased rate of cellular proliferation. There is good evidence that ^{18}F-FLT uptake is closely correlated with cellular proliferation (Buck AK *et al.*, 2006). However, high uptake in normal bone marrow and the liver may limit the sensitivity of FLT-PET for detection of extra-nodal involvement. ^{18}F-fluoride is a positron-emitting bone-seeking agent that reflects blood flow and remodelling of bone, it is also sensitive for detection of lytic and early marrow-based metastases. The instant fusion of increased ^{18}F-fluoride uptake with morphological data of CT improves the specificity in cancer patients by accurately differentiating between benign and malignant uptake sites (Even-Sapir E *et al.*, 2007).

6.2 Combination of PET with other modalities than CT: PET/MRI

Among the above-mentioned imaging techniques, no single modality is perfect and sufficient to gain all the necessary information. Therefore, the combination of multiple imaging techniques can offer synergistic advantages. Multi-modal imaging can be achieved either through the combination of imaging hardware such as PET/CT, through the combination of different contrast agents, or through co-registration of images acquired with different modalities. With regard to lymphatic imaging, this leads to improved accuracy and sensitivity of lymph nodes detection. PET/CT has been matured into an important clinical diagnostic tool. Clinical studies have shown that the combination of anatomical structures revealed from CT and the functional information from PET into one image, with high fusion accuracy, provides an advanced diagnostic tool and research platform. Although PET/CT is already an established clinical tool, it still bears some limitations. A major drawback is that CT provides only limited soft tissue contrast and exposes the studied patient to a significant radiation dose. Since PET and CT scanner are hard-wired back to back and share a common patient bed, PET/CT does not allow simultaneous data acquisition. This temporal mismatch causes image artifacts by patient movement or respiration motion between the two scans. To overcome these limitations, recent research concentrates on the combination of PET and MRI into one single machine. The goal of this development is to integrate the PET detectors into the MRI scanner which would allow simultaneous data acquisition, resulting in combined functional and morphological images with an excellent soft tissue contrast, good spatial resolution of the anatomy, and accurate temporal and spatial image fusion. Additionally, since MRI provides also functional information such as DWI, blood oxygenation level dependant (BOLD) imaging, or spectroscopy, PET/MRI could even provide multi-functional information of pathophysiological processes *in vivo*. Furthermore, the radiation dose for PET/MR will be lower than that for PET/CT, being of particular importance for repeated studies aimed to evaluate disease progression and therapy response. First experiments with PET/MRI prototypes showed promising results, indicating its great potential for clinical imaging (Shao Y *et al.*, 1997; Wagenaar DJ *et al.*, 2006). Multimodality imaging techniques will play a leading role in clinical applications and development of diagnostic imaging in oncology.

6.3 High field MRI and new MR contrast agent

As MRI systems operating at 1.5 T are now widely available and provide high-quality whole-body images in a reasonable acquisition time, implementation of whole-body MRI into diagnostic protocols for malignant lymphomas is expected in the near future. In particular, MRI may be expected to be suitable to replace CT for initial staging and response evaluation, as part of radiation-minimizing policies, especially in children and pregnant women. Whole-body MRI at higher field strength (3.0 T) may increase the image quality and lesion conspicuity with a reduced scan time, since it has higher signal-to-noise ratio. However, whole-body MRI at 3.0 T is more sensitive to artifacts and has not yet been proven to be diagnostically superior to whole-body MRI at 1.5 T (Schmidt GP *et al.*, 2007).

Superparamagnetic iron oxide nanoparticles, which are MRI-specific lymphographic agents, are currently under investigation and can potentially play a role in staging of malignant lymphoma by identifying involved lymph nodes independent of lymph node size (Will O *et al.*, 2006).

7. Conclusion

In conclusion, making the diagnosis of lymphoma often requires multiple imaging modalities, and CT is currently the most commonly used means for staging patients with malignant lymphomas. However, CT lacks functional information, which impedes identification of disease in normal-sized organs. ^{18}F-FDG-PET and hybrid FDG-PET/CT are good alternative diagnostic tools for the initial staging and treatment response assessment of malignant lymphomas. MRI techniques such as whole-body MRI and DW-MRI may be good radiation-free alternatives to FDG-PET/CT in lymphoma patients with multiple follow-up examinations, which may be particularly relevant for children and those who are not suitable for PET/CT exams. Furthermore, in assessment of patients with non-FDG-avid lymphomas MRI could become the imaging modality of choice. However, well-designed studies are needed to validate the accuracy of whole-body MRI and DWIBS for the staging and response assessment of malignant lymphomas.

8. Take home message

- Computed tomography remains the most commonly used modality for initial staging patients with malignant lymphomas because of its widespread availability and relatively low cost.
- FDG-PET and integrated FDG-PET/CT are the established imaging modalities for initial staging and response assessment of lymphomas. Integrated PET/CT has higher diagnostic accuracy than CT and FDG-PET alone.
- Whole-body MRI and DW-MRI are emerging radiation-free alternative imaging techniques for initial staging and treatment response evaluation of lymphomas. However, large studies are needed to determine the value of whole-body MRI and DWIBS.
- MRI at 3 T and combined PET/MRI may have potential for future clinical applications.

9. Acknowledgement

This work was supported by the Science Center of Pirkanmaa Hospital District, Tampere, Finland.

10. References

Antoch G, Vogt FM, Freudenberg LS, Nazaradeh F, Goehde SC, Barkhausen J, Dahmen G, Bockisch A, Debatin JF, Ruehm SG (2003) Whole-body dual-modality PET/CT and whole-body MRI for tumor staging in oncology. Jama 290: 3199-3206.

Bammer R (2003) Basic principles of diffusion-weighted imaging. European journal of radiology 45: 169-184.

Berkowitz A, Basu S, Srinivas S, Sankaran S, Schuster S, Alavi A (2008) Determination of whole-body metabolic burden as a quantitative measure of disease activity in lymphoma: a novel approach with fluorodeoxyglucose-PET. Nuclear medicine communications 29: 521-526.

Blodgett TM, Meltzer CC, Townsend DW (2007) PET/CT: form and function. Radiology 242: 360-385.

Bodet-Milin C, Kraeber-Bodere F, Moreau P, Campion L, Dupas B, Le Gouill S (2008) Investigation of FDG-PET/CT imaging to guide biopsies in the detection of histological transformation of indolent lymphoma. Haematologica 93: 471-472.

Buck AK, Bommer M, Stilgenbauer S, Juweid M, Glatting G, Schirrmeister H, Mattfeldt T, Tepsic D, Bunjes D, Mottaghy FM, Krause BJ, Neumaier B, Dohner H, Moller P, Reske SN (2006) Molecular imaging of proliferation in malignant lymphoma. Cancer research 66: 11055-11061.

Cheson BD, Horning SJ, Coiffier B, Shipp MA, Fisher RI, Connors JM, Lister TA, Vose J, Grillo-Lopez A, Hagenbeek A, Cabanillas F, Klippensten D, Hiddemann W, Castellino R, Harris NL, Armitage JO, Carter W, Hoppe R, Canellos GP (1999) Report of an international workshop to standardize response criteria for non-Hodgkin's lymphomas. NCI Sponsored International Working Group. J Clin Oncol 17: 1253.

Cheson BD, Pfistner B, Juweid ME, Gascoyne RD, Specht L, Horning SJ, Coiffier B, Fisher RI, Hagenbeek A, Zucca E, Rosen ST, Stroobants S, Lister TA, Hoppe RT, Dreyling M, Tobinai K, Vose JM, Connors JM, Federico M, Diehl V (2007) Revised response criteria for malignant lymphoma. J Clin Oncol 25: 579-586.

Cronin CG, Swords R, Truong MT, Viswanathan C, Rohren E, Giles FJ, O'Dwyer M, Bruzzi JF (2010) Clinical utility of PET/CT in lymphoma. Ajr 194: W91-W103.

Even-Sapir E, Mishani E, Flusser G, Metser U (2007) 18F-Fluoride positron emission tomography and positron emission tomography/computed tomography. Seminars in nuclear medicine 37: 462-469.

Ghanem N, Lohrmann C, Engelhardt M, Pache G, Uhl M, Saueressig U, Kotter E, Langer M (2006) Whole-body MRI in the detection of bone marrow infiltration in patients with plasma cell neoplasms in comparison to the radiological skeletal survey. European radiology 16: 1005-1014.

Glockner JF, Hu HH, Stanley DW, Angelos L, King K (2005) Parallel MR imaging: a user's guide. Radiographics 25: 1279-1297.

Hampson FA, Shaw AS (2008) Response assessment in lymphoma. Clinical radiology 63: 125-135.

Harris NL, Jaffe ES, Diebold J, Flandrin G, Muller-Hermelink HK, Vardiman J, Lister TA, Bloomfield CD (2000) The World Health Organization classification of neoplastic diseases of the haematopoietic and lymphoid tissues: Report of the Clinical Advisory Committee Meeting, Airlie House, Virginia, November 1997. Histopathology 36: 69-86.

Harris NL, Jaffe ES, Stein H, Banks PM, Chan JK, Cleary ML, Delsol G, De Wolf-Peeters C, Falini B, Gatter KC, *et al.* (1994) A revised European-American classification of lymphoid neoplasms: a proposal from the International Lymphoma Study Group. Blood 84: 1361-1392.

Herneth AM, Guccione S, Bednarski M (2003) Apparent diffusion coefficient: a quantitative parameter for in vivo tumor characterization. European journal of radiology 45: 208-213.

Holzapfel K, Duetsch S, Fauser C, Eiber M, Rummeny EJ, Gaa J (2009) Value of diffusion-weighted MR imaging in the differentiation between benign and malignant cervical lymph nodes. European journal of radiology 72: 381-387.

Huang B, Law MW, Khong PL (2009) Whole-body PET/CT scanning: estimation of radiation dose and cancer risk. Radiology 251: 166-174.

Hutchings M, Loft A, Hansen M, Ralfkiaer E, Specht L (2006) Different histopathological subtypes of Hodgkin lymphoma show significantly different levels of FDG uptake. Hematological oncology 24: 146-150.

Ichikawa T, Haradome H, Hachiya J, Nitatori T, Araki T (1998) Diffusion-weighted MR imaging with a single-shot echoplanar sequence: detection and characterization of focal hepatic lesions. Ajr 170: 397-402.

Ichikawa T, Haradome H, Hachiya J, Nitatori T, Araki T (1999) Diffusion-weighted MR imaging with single-shot echo-planar imaging in the upper abdomen: preliminary clinical experience in 61 patients. Abdominal imaging 24: 456-461.

Jemal A, Siegel R, Ward E, Hao Y, Xu J, Thun MJ (2009) Cancer statistics, 2009. CA: a cancer journal for clinicians 59: 225-249.

Kazama T, Swanston N, Podoloff DA, Macapinlac HA (2005) Effect of colony-stimulating factor and conventional- or high-dose chemotherapy on FDG uptake in bone marrow. European journal of nuclear medicine and molecular imaging 32: 1406-1411.

Koh DM, Collins DJ (2007) Diffusion-weighted MRI in the body: applications and challenges in oncology. Ajr 188: 1622-1635.

Kwee TC, Kwee RM, Nievelstein RA (2008) Imaging in staging of malignant lymphoma: a systematic review. Blood 111: 504-516.

Kwee TC, Takahara T, Ochiai R, Nievelstein RA, Luijten PR (2008) Diffusion-weighted whole-body imaging with background body signal suppression (DWIBS): features and potential applications in oncology. European radiology 18: 1937-1952.

Kwee TC, van Ufford HM, Beek FJ, Takahara T, Uiterwaal CS, Bierings MB, Ludwig I, Fijnheer R, Nievelstein RA (2009) Whole-body MRI, including diffusion-weighted imaging, for the initial staging of malignant lymphoma: comparison to computed tomography. Investigative radiology 44: 683-690.

la Fougere C, Hundt W, Brockel N, Pfluger T, Haug A, Scher B, Hacker M, Hahn K, Reiser M, Tiling R (2006) Value of PET/CT versus PET and CT performed as separate investigations in patients with Hodgkin's disease and non-Hodgkin's lymphoma. European journal of nuclear medicine and molecular imaging 33: 1417-1425.

Lauenstein TC, Semelka RC (2006) Emerging techniques: whole-body screening and staging with MRI. J Magn Reson Imaging 24: 489-498.

Le Bihan D (1995) Molecular diffusion, tissue microdynamics and microstructure. NMR in biomedicine 8: 375-386.

Lister TA, Crowther D, Sutcliffe SB, Glatstein E, Canellos GP, Young RC, Rosenberg SA, Coltman CA, Tubiana M (1989) Report of a committee convened to discuss the evaluation and staging of patients with Hodgkin's disease: Cotswolds meeting. J Clin Oncol 7: 1630-1636.

Low RN, Gurney J (2007) Diffusion-weighted MRI (DWI) in the oncology patient: value of breathhold DWI compared to unenhanced and gadolinium-enhanced MRI. J Magn Reson Imaging 25: 848-858.

Lucey BC, Stuhlfaut JW, Soto JA (2005) Mesenteric lymph nodes: detection and significance on MDCT. Ajr 184: 41-44.

MacManus MP, Seymour JF, Hicks RJ (2007) Overview of early response assessment in lymphoma with FDG-PET. Cancer Imaging 7: 10-18.

Moog F, Bangerter M, Diederichs CG, Guhlmann A, Kotzerke J, Merkle E, Kolokythas O, Herrmann F, Reske SN (1997) Lymphoma: role of whole-body 2-deoxy-2-[F-18]fluoro-D-glucose (FDG) PET in nodal staging. Radiology 203: 795-800.

Muller MF, Prasad P, Siewert B, Nissenbaum MA, Raptopoulos V, Edelman RR (1994) Abdominal diffusion mapping with use of a whole-body echo-planar system. Radiology 190: 475-478.

Ngeow JY, Quek RH, Ng DC, Hee SW, Tao M, Lim LC, Tan YH, Lim ST (2009) High SUV uptake on FDG-PET/CT predicts for an aggressive B-cell lymphoma in a prospective study of primary FDG-PET/CT staging in lymphoma. Ann Oncol 20: 1543-1547.

Okada M, Sato N, Ishii K, Matsumura K, Hosono M, Murakami T (2010) FDG PET/CT versus CT, MR imaging, and 67Ga scintigraphy in the posttherapy evaluation of malignant lymphoma. Radiographics 30: 939-957.

Patterson DM, Padhani AR, Collins DJ (2008) Technology insight: water diffusion MRI--a potential new biomarker of response to cancer therapy. Nature clinical practice 5: 220-233.

Paul R (1987) Comparison of fluorine-18-2-fluorodeoxyglucose and gallium-67 citrate imaging for detection of lymphoma. J Nucl Med 28: 288-292.

Pelosi E, Pregno P, Penna D, Deandreis D, Chiappella A, Limerutti G, Vitolo U, Mancini M, Bisi G, Gallo E (2008) Role of whole-body [18F] fluorodeoxyglucose positron emission tomography/computed tomography (FDG-PET/CT) and conventional techniques in the staging of patients with Hodgkin and aggressive non Hodgkin lymphoma. La Radiologia medica 113: 578-590.

Perrone A, Guerrisi P, Izzo L, D'Angeli I, Sassi S, Mele LL, Marini M, Mazza D, Marini M (2011) Diffusion-weighted MRI in cervical lymph nodes: Differentiation between benign and malignant lesions. European journal of radiology 77:281-6.

Phelps ME, Hoffman EJ, Mullani NA, Ter-Pogossian MM (1975) Application of annihilation coincidence detection to transaxial reconstruction tomography. J Nucl Med 16: 210-224.

Rohren EM, Turkington TG, Coleman RE (2004) Clinical applications of PET in oncology. Radiology 231: 305-332.

Rydberg J, Buckwalter KA, Caldemeyer KS, Phillips MD, Conces DJ, Jr., Aisen AM, Persohn SA, Kopecky KK (2000) Multisection CT: scanning techniques and clinical applications. Radiographics 20: 1787-1806.

Schaefer NG, Hany TF, Taverna C, Seifert B, Stumpe KD, von Schulthess GK, Goerres GW (2004) Non-Hodgkin lymphoma and Hodgkin disease: coregistered FDG PET and CT at staging and restaging--do we need contrast-enhanced CT? Radiology 232: 823-829.

Schmidt GP, Reiser MF, Baur-Melnyk A (2009) Whole-body MRI for the staging and follow-up of patients with metastasis. European journal of radiology 70: 393-400.

Schmidt GP, Wintersperger B, Graser A, Baur-Melnyk A, Reiser MF, Schoenberg SO (2007) High-resolution whole-body magnetic resonance imaging applications at 1.5 and 3 Tesla: a comparative study. Investigative radiology 42: 449-459.

Schoder H, Noy A, Gonen M, Weng L, Green D, Erdi YE, Larson SM, Yeung HW (2005) Intensity of 18fluorodeoxyglucose uptake in positron emission tomography distinguishes between indolent and aggressive non-Hodgkin's lymphoma. J Clin Oncol 23: 4643-4651.

Shao Y, Cherry SR, Farahani K, Meadors K, Siegel S, Silverman RW, Marsden PK (1997) Simultaneous PET and MR imaging. Physics in medicine and biology 42: 1965-1970.

Shipp MA (1994) Prognostic factors in aggressive non-Hodgkin's lymphoma: who has "high-risk" disease? Blood 83: 1165-1173.

Spaepen K, Stroobants S, Dupont P, Vandenberghe P, Thomas J, de Groot T, Balzarini J, De Wolf-Peeters C, Mortelmans L, Verhoef G (2002) Early restaging positron emission tomography with (18)F-fluorodeoxyglucose predicts outcome in patients with aggressive non-Hodgkin's lymphoma. Ann Oncol 13: 1356-1363.

Sumi M, Ichikawa Y, Nakamura T (2007) Diagnostic ability of apparent diffusion coefficients for lymphomas and carcinomas in the pharynx. European radiology 17: 2631-2637.

Takahara T, Imai Y, Yamashita T, Yasuda S, Nasu S, Van Cauteren M (2004) Diffusion weighted whole body imaging with background body signal suppression (DWIBS): technical improvement using free breathing, STIR and high resolution 3D display. Radiation medicine 22: 275-282.

Tang B, Malysz J, Douglas-Nikitin V, Zekman R, Wong RH, Jaiyesimi I, Wong CY (2009) Correlating metabolic activity with cellular proliferation in follicular lymphomas. Mol Imaging Biol 11: 296-302.

Thoeny HC, De Keyzer F (2007) Extracranial applications of diffusion-weighted magnetic resonance imaging. European radiology 17: 1385-1393.

Wagenaar DJ, Kapusta M, Li J, Patt BE (2006) Rationale for the combination of nuclear medicine with magnetic resonance for pre-clinical imaging. Technology in cancer research & treatment 5: 343-350.

Wang J, Takashima S, Takayama F, Kawakami S, Saito A, Matsushita T, Momose M, Ishiyama T (2001) Head and neck lesions: characterization with diffusion-weighted echo-planar MR imaging. Radiology 220: 621-630.

Warburg O (1956) On the origin of cancer cells. Science (New York, NY 123: 309-314.

Vermoolen MA, Kersten MJ, Fijnheer R, van Leeuwen MS, Kwee TC, Nievelstein RA (2011) Magnetic resonance imaging of malignant lymphoma. Expert review of hematology 4: 161-171.

Will O, Purkayastha S, Chan C, Athanasiou T, Darzi AW, Gedroyc W, Tekkis PP (2006) Diagnostic precision of nanoparticle-enhanced MRI for lymph-node metastases: a meta-analysis. The lancet oncology 7: 52-60.

Vinnicombe SJ, Reznek RH (2003) Computerised tomography in the staging of Hodgkin's disease and non-Hodgkin's lymphoma. European journal of nuclear medicine and molecular imaging 30 Suppl 1: S42-55.

von Schulthess GK, Steinert HC, Hany TF (2006) Integrated PET/CT: current applications and future directions. Radiology 238: 405-422.

Wu X, Dastidar P, Pertovaara H, Korkola P, Jarvenpaa R, Rossi M, Koobi T, Eskola H, Kellokumpu-Lehtinen PL (2011) Early Treatment Response Evaluation in Patients with Diffuse Large B-Cell Lymphoma-A Pilot Study Comparing Volumetric MRI and PET/CT. Mol Imaging Biol 13:785-92.

Wu X, Kellokumpu-Lehtinen PL, Pertovaara H, Korkola P, Soimakallio S, Eskola H, Dastidar P (2011) Diffusion-weighted MRI in early chemotherapy response evaluation of patients with diffuse large B-cell lymphoma - a pilot study: comparison with 2-deoxy-2-fluoro-D-glucose-positron emission tomography/computed tomography. NMR in biomedicine doi: 10.1002/nbm.1689.

Wu X, Korkola P, Pertovaara H, Eskola H, Jarvenpaa R, Kellokumpu-Lehtinen PL (2011) No correlation between glucose metabolism and apparent diffusion coefficient in diffuse large B-cell lymphoma: A PET/CT and DW-MRI study. European journal of radiology 79:e117-121.

16

Targeting EGFR and HER2 for Molecular Imaging of Cancer

Haibiao Gong, Lakshmi Sampath,
Joy L. Kovar and D. Mike Olive
LI-COR Biosciences, Lincoln,
USA

1. Introduction

The epidermal growth factor (EGF) receptor (EGFR, HER1, ErbB1) and human epidermal growth factor receptor type 2 (HER2, ErbB2) belong to the ErbB family of type I tyrosine kinases (TKs). This family of receptor TKs also includes another two closely related members HER3/ErbB3 and HER4/ErbB4. The general structure of these cell surface receptor proteins contains an extracellular ligand-binding domain, a hydrophobic transmembrane domain, an intracellular tyrosine kinase domain and a non-catalytic carboxyl terminal tail (Ferguson et al., 2000; Kari et al., 2003; Mitsudomi & Yatabe, 2010; Pines et al., 2010). Various ligands for EGFR, HER3 and HER4 have been identified, with EGF the most extensively characterized for its binding and activation of EGFR. These ErbB proteins are present in the plasma membrane as monomers. Upon ligand binding, the ErbB receptors can associate with each other to form different receptor dimers, which may be homodimers (e.g., EGFR-EGFR) or heterodimers (e.g., EGFR-HER2). The dimerization results in the activation of kinase activity and downstream signaling pathways, which often leads to cell proliferation and malignant tumor growth. HER2 is an exception, with no compatible ligand identified. However, it is the preferred heterodimerization partner for all other ErbB members (Mishani & Hagooly, 2009; Niu et al., 2008; Tzahar et al., 1996; Yarden & Sliwkowski, 2001).

As EGFR and HER2 play important roles in many physiological and pathological processes, it is not surprising that deregulation of EGFR and HER2 is associated with various types of malignancies (Kari et al., 2003; Niu et al., 2008; Yarden & Sliwkowski, 2001). Both overexpression and mutation of EGFR have been identified in various types of cancers, while overexpression is a more commonly employed mechanism in the case of HER2 (Yarden & Sliwkowski, 2001). In these cancer cells, the TK activity is either elevated or constitutively activated. EGFR- and HER2-targeted anti-cancer medicines have been developed by either targeting the extracellular ligand-binding domain through antibody blocking, or by inhibiting the tyrosine kinase activity using low-molecular-weight molecules (Baselga, 2006; Pines et al., 2010; Speake et al., 2005). Cetuximab (a humanized mouse antibody) and panitumumab (a fully human antibody) have been approved for selected EGFR-targeted cancer treatment. Although these antibodies are designed to down-regulate EGFR signaling by inhibiting ligand-binding, preventing receptor dimerization and accelerating receptor degradation, antibody-dependent cell-mediated cytotoxicity is also considered as an important mechanism for IgG1 isotype antibody cetuximab (Cai et al., 2008; Okamoto, 2010). Trastuzumab (a humanized mouse antibody) is a widely used treatment for breast cancer patients with HER2 overexpression (Niu et al., 2008). Because TKs depend on ATP to provide phosphate for the phosphorylation process, small molecules that bind to the ATP-binding pocket of the kinase domain can inhibit its enzymatic activity. These TK inhibitors (TKIs) may bind either reversibly or irreversibly. Reversible TKIs erlotinib and gefitinib are EGFR-specific, while lapatinib inhibits both EGFR and HER2 (Pines et al., 2010).

Molecular imaging agents with specific targets can provide information regarding biological processes at a cellular level before anatomical changes occur. Similar to the approaches used to develop EGFR and HER2 therapeutic agents, two strategies could be used for EGFR- and HER2-targeted tumor imaging. The first class of imaging agents targets extracellular domain of the receptor. Examples of these imaging agents include whole antibodies, antibody fragments, affibodies and nanobodies. The EGFR ligands, which bind to EGFR extracellular domain at high affinity, could also be used for this purpose. The second class of molecules includes TKIs and analogs that bind reversibly or irreversibly to the kinase domain of the receptor. Actually, some of the EGFR- and HER2-targeted therapeutic agents mentioned above have been used for tumor imaging after labeling with different functional groups, such as radionuclides for positron emission tomography (PET) and single-photon emission computed tomography (SPECT) imaging, and fluorescent dyes for optical imaging (Mishani et al., 2008; Mishani & Hagooly, 2009; Niu et al., 2008).

2. Imaging agents targeting EGFR

2.1 Anti-EGFR antibodies

PET imaging with ^{64}Cu ($t_{1/2}$ = 12.7 h)-labeled cetuximab (^{64}Cu-DOTA-cetuximab) was employed to measure the EGFR expression in seven xenograft tumor models *in vivo*. The data was compared with EGFR levels in the tumors determined by Western blot. A reasonable linear correlation ($R^2 = 0.80$) between the tumor uptake of ^{64}Cu-DOTA-cetuximab (measured by PET) and the EGFR protein expression level (measured by Western blot) was discovered. It was also found that ^{64}Cu-DOTA-cetuximab had increasing tumor accumulation over time in EGFR-positive tumors but relatively low uptake in EGFR-negative tumors (Cai et al., 2007). In a following study, ^{64}Cu-DOTA-cetuximab was used to monitor the early response of EGFR degradation induced by 17-allyamino-17-demethoxygeldanamycin (17-AAG) treatment (Niu et al., 2008). 17-AAG is an Hsp90 inhibitor, which induces the degradation of EGFR protein (Lang et al., 2007). In a PC-3 prostate tumor model, 17-AAG treatment induced significant reduction of ^{64}Cu-DOTA-cetuximab uptake in the tumor. The reduction of ^{64}Cu-DOTA-cetuximab uptake correlated well with the lower EGFR protein level in the treated tumor as determined by immunofluorescence staining and Western blot (Niu et al., 2008).

Cetuximab has also been labeled with fluorescent dyes for optical imaging. Cy5.5 (Ex/Em: 675/695 nm)-labeled cetuximab (cetuximab-Cy5.5) was taken up specifically by head and neck squamous cell carcinoma (HNSCC) xenografts. The fluorescence from mouse tumors treated with cetuximab-Cy5.5 was significantly higher compared to a control probe IgG1-

Cy5.5 (Rosenthal et al., 2007). To reduce the background fluorescence signal, a two-step activation strategy was designed. EGFR-overexpressing tumors (A431) were pre-targeted with biotinylated cetuximab, followed by administration of neutravidin conjugated with BODIPY-FL fluorescent dye (nAv-BDPfl). As the fluorescence of nAv-BDPfl increases dramatically (~ 10-fold) upon binding to biotin, the nAv-BDPfl signal will be specifically activated at the tumor site, where the biotinylated cetuximab was concentrated. Not surprisingly, this approach produced a higher tumor-to-background ratio (Hama et al., 2007). Another activatable probe employed the fluorescence quenching of ICG after conjugation with antibodies. The fluorescence could be restored by disrupting the molecular interaction between ICG and antibodies either *in vitro* (SDS plus 2-ME treatment) or *in vivo* (target binding and internalization). ICG-labled panitumumab (labeling ratio 1:5) exhibited a 58-fold signal increase upon SDS/2-ME treatment. EGFR-overexpressing tumors (A431 and MDA-MB-468) could be identified by this probe. Two other antibodies, trastuzumab (anti-HER2) and daclizumab (anti-CD25) were also labeled with ICG and used to image their respective targets in this study (Ogawa et al., 2009).

In an attempt to extend EGFR-targeted imaging with cetuximab to clinical scenario, cetuximab was labeled with ^{99m}Tc ($t_{1/2}$ = 6 h). The resulting imaging probe ^{99m}Tc-EC-C225 was evaluated by cell uptake assay, and in tumor-bearing mice and rats. SPECT imaging on a patient with squamous cell carcinoma visualized the tumor 2 h after ^{99m}Tc-EC-C225 administration (Schechter et al., 2003). Assessment of the radiation dosimetry of this probe indicated that it has reasonable dosimetric properties for a diagnostic nuclear medicine agent (Schechter et al., 2004).

EGFR variant III (EGFRvIII) is a common in-frame deletion mutant that lacks a large part of the extracellular portion (exons 2-7), including components of the ligand-binding domain (Ekstrand et al., 1992). EGFRvIII is constitutively activated, and associated with glioblastoma and some other tumors, such as prostate and breast cancer (Wikstrand et al., 1998). EGFRvIII could be recognized by ch806, a chimeric anti-EGFR antibody that selectively binds an EGFR epitope exposed only on mutant, overexpressed, or ligand-activated forms of the receptor (Panousis et al., 2005). ^{124}I ($t_{1/2}$ = 4.2d)-labeled ch806 (^{124}I -IMP-R4-ch806) was able to detect EGFRvIII expressing tumors (U87MG.EGFRvIII) at 24 h after probe injection, and prolonged retention was evident up to 168 h post-injection. There was a good correlation between *in vivo* tumor PET quantitation of ^{124}I -IMP-R4-ch806 and *ex vivo* measurement from dissected tissues. Remarkably, this probe was tumor-specific, and no significant binding to normal tissue was observed (Lee et al., 2010). This is in contrast to cetuximab, which accumulates in EGFR-expressing tissues such as liver (Niu et al., 2008).

2.2 EGFR-specific antibody fragments

Due to their large size (~150 kDa), the antibody-based imaging agents suffer from drawbacks such as long biodistribution time, poor penetrating capability, and slow clearance from the blood and normal tissues, which causes limited imaging contrast early post-injection, high background signal and non-uniform tumor penetration (Gong et al., 2010; Schier et al., 1996). Antibodies could be dissected into minimal monovalent binding fragments, such as Fab (~55 kDa) and scFv (~28 kDa), which retain the binding specificity (Holliger & Hudson, 2005). These antibody fragments have also been used for molecular imaging studies.

The Fab fragment of a fully human antibody that recognizes the native extracellular domain of EGFR was labeled with ^{125}I ($t_{1/2}$ =59.4 d). The binding of ^{125}I-Fab to EGFR was confirmed by immunoprecipitation (IP) and fluorescence-activated cell sorting (FACS). In an animal imaging study, ^{125}I-Fab was able to distinguish the tumors with different levels of EGFR expression (Xu et al., 2009). An EGFR-specific scFv was isolated from a phage display library, and labeled with either quantum dot (QD) for fluorescence imaging, or magnetic iron oxide (IO) for magnetic resonance imaging (MRI). The resulting EGFR-targeted nanoparticles were discovered to accumulate in pancreatic xenograft tumors by tissue section fluorescence imaging and whole animal MRI (Yang et al., 2009). To achieve site-specific labeling, an anti-EGFR scFv was fused to the SNAP-tag creating a fusion protein 425(scFv)SNAP (~48 kDa) (Kampmeier et al., 2010). SNAP-tag is a 20-kDa protein derived from the human DNA repair protein O^6-alkylguanine-DNA-alkyltransferase (hAGT), which reacts with the fluorescent dye conjugated benzylguanine (BG) substrate, leading to covalent labeling of the fluorescent dye on the fusion protein (Keppler et al., 2004). The fusion protein 425(scFv)SNAP labeled with the near-infrared (NIR) substrate BG-747 accumulated rapidly and specifically at the tumor site. Due to the efficient clearance, the tumor to background ratio (TBR) of this probe was significantly higher compared to the full-length antibody cetuximab (Kampmeier et al., 2010).

Camelids contain a unique type of antibodies lacking the light chain (Hamers-Casterman et al., 1993). The single variable domain of heavy chain (VHH) has been isolated, and termed nanobody (~15 kDa). Several EGFR-specific nanobodies were labeled with ^{99m}Tc for SPECT imaging. These ^{99m}Tc-lableded nanobody molecules showed high specificity towards EGFR-overexpressing A431 tumors. The clearance from the blood was fast. The probe accumulation in the kidney was much higher than that in the liver, indicating a kidney clearance route (Gainkam et al., 2008; Huang et al., 2008). We labeled an EGFR-specific nanobody molecule (a kind gift from Dr. Paul van Bergen en Henegouwen at Utrecht University) with a NIR fluorescent dye IRDye® 800CW (Ex/Em: 774/789 nm) and used it for *in vivo* optical imaging. A431 xenograft tumors could be clearly identified at 1d post-injection with different dosages (0.4, 0.8 and 1.6 nmol per mouse) (Fig. 1). Consistent with SPECT results, the kidney accumulation of this fluorescent probe was high (Gong *et al.*, unpublished data). To increase the binding affinity and optimize the pharmacokinetic properties, a bivalent form of nanobody molecule was created by fusing two monovalent

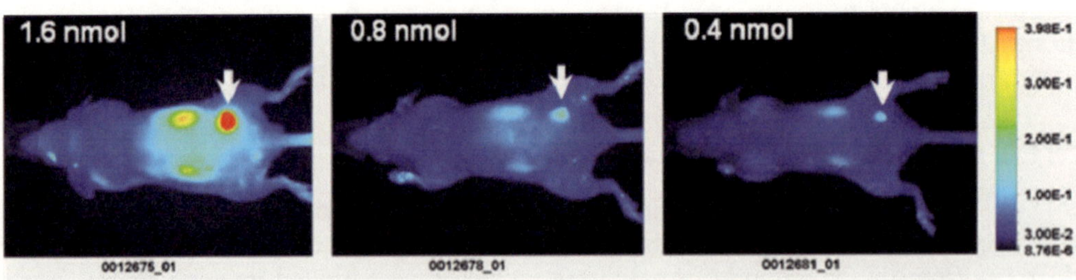

Fig. 1. *In vivo* fluorescence imaging of nude mice bearing A431 tumors using an EGFR-specific nanobody labeled with IRDye 800CW. Images (dorsal view) were acquired at 1 d after injection of 1.6 nmol, 0.8 nmol or 0.4 nmol imaging agents, respectively. Arrows indicate A431 tumors. The nanobody was a gift from Dr. Paul van Bergen en Henegouwen, Utrecht University.

nanobody (EG_2) molecules to the human Fc fragment. The resulting molecule, EG_2-hFc (80 kDa) was labeled with the fluorescent dye Cy5.5, and compared with Cy5.5-labeled monovalent EG_2, and Cy5.5-labeled pentavalent derivative V2C- EG_2 (128 kDa). *In vivo* pharmacokinetic and biodistribution studies in mice revealed that the plasma half life of EG_2-hFc-Cy5.5 was much prolonged compared to the other two probes. The retention of EG_2-hFc-Cy5.5 in EGFR/EGFRvIII-expressing orthotopic brain tumors was also significantly higher, resulting in an improved tumor fluorescence signal (Iqbal et al., 2010).

2.3 Natural ligand EGF

EGF (MW: 6045 Da) is a small polypeptide that binds with high affinity to EGFR on the cell surface (Stoscheck & King, 1986; Yarden & Sliwkowski, 2001). ^{111}In ($t_{1/2}$ = 2.8 d)-labeled hEGF (^{111}In-DTPA-hEGF) was compared with an ^{111}In-labeled monoclonal antibody (^{111}In-DTPA-MAb528) for *in vivo* tumor imaging. The blood clearance of ^{111}In-DTPA-hEGF was much faster (< 0.2%ID/g for ^{111}In-DTPA-hEGF *vs* 3%ID/g for ^{111}In-DTPA-MAb528 in the blood at 72 h post injection). The tumor accumulation of ^{111}In-DTPA-hEGF was lower. Although both probes could visualize EGFR-expressing tumors, the signal from ^{111}In-DTPA-MAb528 was more prominent at 72 h post-injection (Reilly et al., 2000). The fast clearance of EGF makes it advantageous over antibodies for radionuclides with shorter half-lives such as ^{68}Ga ($t_{1/2}$ = 68 min). ^{68}Ga-labeled hEGF (^{68}Ga-DOTA-hEGF) was used in a microPET imaging study. A quick localization of radioactivity in tumors (within 5 min) was demonstrated (Velikyan et al., 2005).

Both Cy5.5- and IRDye 800CW-labeled EGF (named as EGF-Cy5.5 and EGF800 respectively) have been successfully used for fluorescence optical imaging of EGFR-expressing tumors. The specificity of both probes was verified by competition with excess cetuximab (Ke et al., 2003; Kovar et al., 2006). However, a direct comparison between these two probes revealed that EGF800 produced a significantly lower background and a higher tumor-to-background ratio, implying that IRDye 800CW is superior to Cy5.5 for this application (Adams et al., 2007). Analysis of the excised tumors from EGF800-treated mice demonstrated a good correlation between tumor wet weight and *in vivo* tumor fluorescence signal. Repeated administration of EGF800 probe allowed for the non-invasive tracking of orthotopic prostate tumor growth (Fig. 2) (Kovar et al., 2006). Another study with EGF800 showed that probe accumulation in tumors reflected relative EGFR expression and EGFR occupancy by cetuximab (Manning et al., 2008).

QDs have also been used to label EGF for fluorescence optical imaging. An EGFR targeting nanoprobe was formed by coupling NIR QDs to EGF. The tumor-specific accumulation of this nanoprobe was demonstrated by both whole animal imaging and *ex vivo* tissue analysis (Diagaradjane et al., 2008).

2.4 EGFR-specific affibody

Affibody molecules are a class of affinity proteins composed of 58 amino acid residues that are derived from one of the IgG-binding domains of staphylococcal protein A. EGFR-specific affibody molecules (~7 kDa) have been selected by phage display technology (Friedman et al., 2007). A head-to-tail dimeric form $(Z_{EGFR:955})_2$ that has a higher binding affinity was labeled with ^{111}In and successfully used for *in vivo* imaging of A431 tumors

(Nordberg et al., 2008). To further improve the binding affinity and specificity, the affibody was optimized by affinity maturation process (Friedman et al., 2008). The second generation of EGFR-specific affibody has been conjugated with various labels, and characterized in detail.

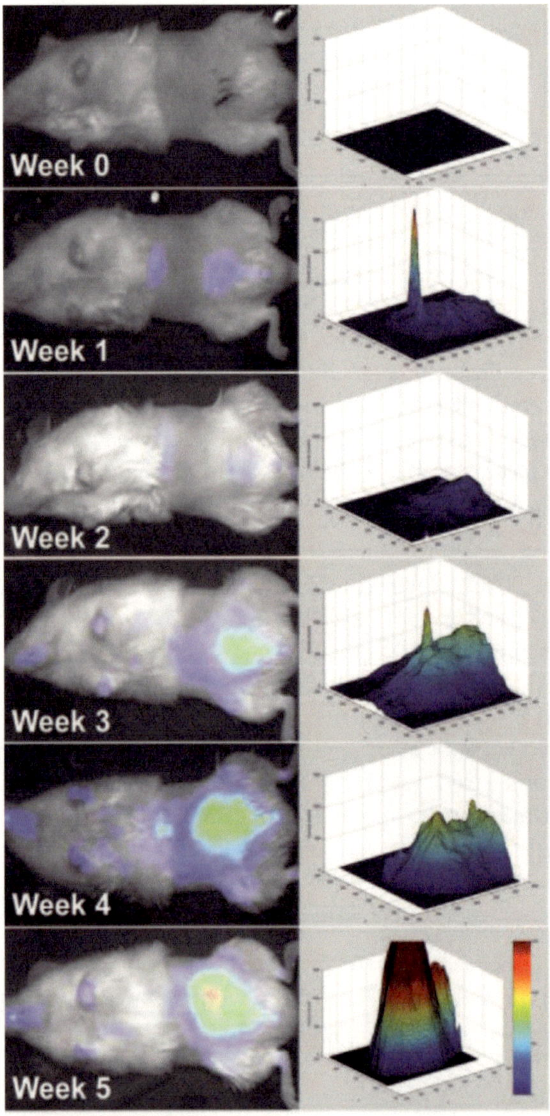

Fig. 2. Tracking of orthotopic prostate tumor growth with EGF800. Male NOD/SCID mice were injected orthotopically with 22Rv1 tumor cells. Animals were injected with EGF800 at different time points and imaged. The left column shows the tumor progression of a representative mouse in color-coded fluorescence images superimposed on the white light images. In the right column, total fluorescence in an ROI encompassing the tumor region was quantified. Fluorescence intensity is color-coded to assist visualization. Adapted from (Kovar et al., 2006) with permission.

In vivo imaging with ^{64}Cu- or Cy5.5-labeled $Z_{EGFR:1907}$ showed fast tumor (A431) targeting and good tumor-to-normal tissue contrast. Both agents accumulated at a high level in tumor, liver and kidney as revealed by biodistribution study (Miao et al., 2010, 2010). A dimeric form of EGFR-specific affibody (13.7 kDa) was labeled with IRDye 800CW (named as Eaff800), and used to image A431 xenograft tumors. The tumor could be visualized 1 h post-injection, and it became most prominent after 1 d (Fig. 3). The binding and uptake of Eaff800 was EGFR-specific because it only produced minimal signal when reacted with SK-OV-3 cells (HER2-overexpressing) in both cell-based assay and *in vivo* imaging study. It is notable that the liver uptake of Eaff800 was high, possibly due to the cross-reaction between Eaff800 and murine EGFR expressed in the liver (Gong et al., 2010).

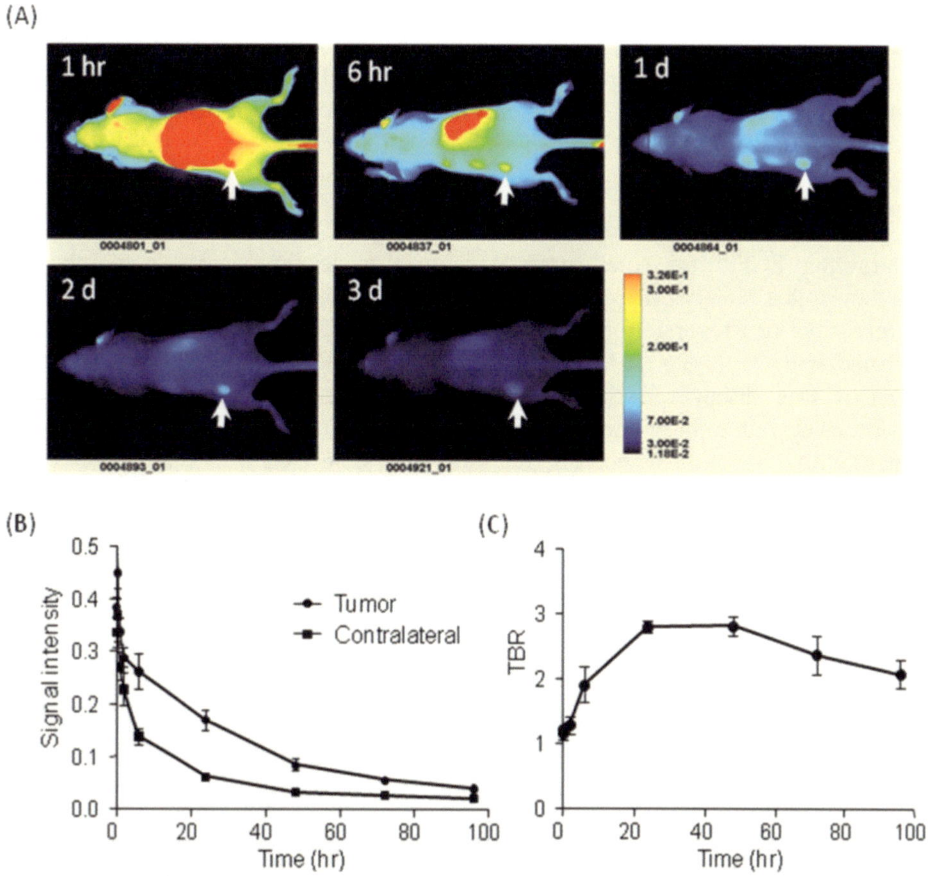

Fig. 3. *In vivo* optical imaging of nude mice bearing A431 tumors using Eaff800. (A) A representative series of whole body images (dorsal view) acquired at different time points following injection of 0.5 nmol Eaff800. The tumors were indicated with arrows. (B) Clearance of Eaff800 from the tumor and normal tissue. Average signal intensities were quantified using ROIs of equivalent sized areas from the tumor sites and contralateral sites at indicated time points. Data were presented as mean ± SD of three individual mice. (C) Tumor-to-background ratio (TBR) at different time points after probe injection. TBR was calculated by dividing mean tumor signal by mean background signal of the contralateral site. Adapted from (Gong et al., 2010) with permission.

The monomer $Z_{EGFR:1907}$ and dimer $(Z_{EGFR:1907})_2$ were labeled with ^{111}In and ^{125}I, respectively. The resulting four variants, ^{111}In-Bz-DTPA-$Z_{EGFR:1907}$, ^{111}In-Bz-DTPA-$(Z_{EGFR:1907})_2$, ^{125}I-PIB-$Z_{EGFR:1907}$ and ^{125}I-PIB-$(Z_{EGFR:1907})_2$ were compared in A431 tumor bearing nude mice. At 24 h after injection, the use of ^{111}In provided higher tumor radioactivity level than did ^{125}I for both the monomer and the dimer. It was also discovered that the tumor uptake of monomer was higher than that of dimer, despite a superior cellular retention of radioactivity for dimer in cell-based assays. The best probe, ^{111}In-Bz-DTPA-$Z_{EGFR:1907}$, produced a tumor-to-blood ratio of 100 at 24 h after injection (Tolmachev et al., 2009). To investigate the effect of injected protein dose, an aliquot of labeled affibody ^{111}In-DOTA-$Z_{EGFR:2377}$ was diluted in different amounts of unlabeled affibody before injection to A431 tumor bearing mice. A bell-shaped dose-responsive curve was observed. The initial increase in uptake was reasoned to be associated with saturation of EGFR in normal tissues, resulting in more ^{111}In-DOTA-$Z_{EGFR:2377}$ available for tumor targeting. Further increase in the unlabeled affibody caused the competition of EGFR in the tumor site and reduced ^{111}In-DOTA-$Z_{EGFR:2377}$ uptake (Tolmachev et al., 2010).

2.5 TKI derivatives

TKIs targeting EGFR are small organic molecules developed based mainly on the anilinoquinazoline moiety. These molecules bind to ATP-binding site of the kinase domain either reversibly or irreversibly (Mishani & Hagooly, 2009). Reversible TKI agent gefitinib was labeled with ^{18}F ($t_{1/2}$ = 110 min) to image the EGFR status of different cancer cells. However it was discovered that [^{18}F]-gefitinib uptake did not correlate with EGFR expression levels due to high non-specific cellular uptake (Su et al., 2008). This finding is in agreement with other studies showing that most reversible TKIs were inadequate for *in vivo* imaging despite impressive *in vitro* profile, including high affinity and specificity toward EGFR. These radio-labeled reversible agents often exhibit low uptake in targeted tumors and high uptake in non-targeted tissues (Mishani & Hagooly, 2009). Nevertheless, a recent study with ^{11}C ($t_{1/2}$ = 20 min)-labeled erlotinib, another reversible TKI, showed that [^{11}C]-erlotinib accumulated in HCC827 tumors that expresses high level of EGFR and is sensitive to erlotinib treatment. HCC827 xenograft tumors could be visualized by micro-PET scanning with [^{11}C]-erlotinib, whereas A549 and NCI358 xenografts (both express low level of EGFR) could not. However HCC827 cells also harbor an in-frame deletion mutation in exon 19 that contributes to the enhanced sensitivity to erlotinib. It is not clear whether this mutation causes the accumulation of [^{11}C]-erlotinib in the tumor (Memon et al., 2009).

To enhance binding efficacy, much effort has been invested in the development of irreversible TKIs as therapeutic drugs and imaging agents (Mishani et al., 2008; Mishani & Hagooly, 2009). An irreversible TKI-based radiotracer, morpholino-[^{124}I]-IPQA, has been developed and characterized. Morpholino-[^{124}I]-IPQA covalently binds to the ATP-binding site of the activated (phosphorylated) EGFR, but not the inactive EGFR. A431 tumors on immunocompromised rats and mice were successfully visualized by PET imaging with this probe (Pal et al., 2006). A newer version of this probe, [^{18}F]F-PEG6-IPQA, which has better water solubility, has also been developed. [^{18}F]F-PEG6-IPQA could detect NSCLC xenograft tumors harboring L858R activating EGFR mutations, and did not recognize NSCLC xenografts expressing either wild type or L858R/T790M dual mutant EGFR (Yeh et al., 2011). Another irreversible TKI analog ML04 exhibited excellent specificity to EGFR *in vitro.*

However, *in vivo* biodistribution analysis of [^{18}F]ML04 showed that the probe uptake in EGFR-positive tumors was mainly non-specific, suggesting that further optimization of this probe is needed (Abourbeh et al., 2007; Mishani et al., 2008).

3 Imaging HER2-overexpressing tumors

3.1 Anti-HER2 antibodies

HER2 amplification was initially observed in human breast cancer and was subsequently identified in ovarian cancer and other types of cancers (Niu et al., 2008; Slamon et al., 1989; Zhang et al., 1989). HER2 expression is highly conserved between primary breast lesions and metastases in lymph node, bone marrow as well as distant locations (Gancberg et al., 2002; Lopez-Guerrero et al., 2006; Regitnig et al., 2004; Simmons et al., 2009; Simon et al., 2001; Tapia et al., 2007; Vincent-Salomon et al., 2007); and remains so throughout therapy (Carlsson et al., 2004; Gong et al., 2005; Pectasides et al., 2006). Thus, accurate assessment of HER2 expression levels is of great interest for identifying breast cancer patients who will benefit from HER2-targeted therapy.

Trastuzumab (Herceptin; Genentech, CA), a recombinant humanized monoclonal antibody directed against the extracellular domain of the HER2 protein, was engineered by inserting the complementarity determining region of a murine antibody (clone 4D5) into the framework of a consensus human IgG1 (Carter et al., 1992). Tratuzumab has been shown to be effective in early-stage breast cancer that overexpresses HER2. Clinical trials indicate that combining tratuzumab treatment with standard chemotherapy for early-stage HER2 positive breast cancer reduces the risk of recurrence and death when compared to chemotherapy alone, thereby improving disease-free and overall survival rates in patients (Baselga et al., 2006; Romond et al., 2005).

Trastuzumab was radio-labeled with ^{111}In using DTPA as a chelator. ^{111}In-DTPA-trastuzumab selectively bound to the human HER2 receptor in *in vitro* analysis. Biodistribution and tumor targeting were studied in SK-OV-3 (HER2+) and GLC4 (HER2-) tumor-bearing athymic mice. The SK-OV-3 tumor showed substantial uptake of the labeled antibody after 5 h. The difference in uptake between SK-OV-3 and GLC4 tumors was even more pronounced 3 d after injection. At that time, the SK-OV-3 tumor was clearly visualized by radioimmunoscintigraphy (Lub-de Hooge et al., 2004). Research has also demonstrated that fluorescent dye-labeled trastuzumab enabled differentiation between breast cancer cells expressing high and low levels of HER2. Serial imaging before and during trastuzumab therapy revealed a significant reduction in probe uptake with treatment (Gee et al., 2008). Trastuzumab was also used to mediate the cellular internalization of pH-activatable fluorephores. These probes produced minimal fluorescence outside of the cell, and were activated by sensing the pH change in the lysosome after internalization (Urano et al., 2009). Other optical imaging based applications include imaging SK-BR-3 tumors with Cy5.5-labeled trastuzumab (Hilger et al., 2004), and distinguishing between HER2+ pulmonary metastases and HER2- pulmonary metastases using rhodamine green-conjugated trastuzumab (Koyama et al., 2007).

Another antibody against HER2 used for imaging applications is pertuzumab, a humanized antibody derived from the murine antibody 2C4. Unlike trastuzumab, pertuzumab sterically hinders HER2 hetero-dimerization with EGFR and HER3. Pertuzumab conjugated with ^{177}Lu showed significant tumor uptake in an *in vivo* study using gamma camera imaging (Persson et al., 2005).

3.2 HER2-specific antibody fragments

Trastuzumab-derived antibody fragments Fab and $F(ab')_2$ have also been employed for molecular imaging. ^{111}In- or ^{99m}Tc-labeled trastuzumab Fab conjugates were used to detect HER2-expressing tumors using whole-body scintigraphy. Tumors were visualized 6 h post-injection (Tang et al., 2005; Tang et al., 2005). Trastuzumab and trastuzumab-derived Fab fragment (Fab4D5) labeled with ^{111}In were compared in a MMTV/HER2 mouse allograft model. Although Fab4D5 showed accumulation in the tumor as early as 2 h, rapid wash-out through the kidneys was observed by 6 h. On the contrary, trastuzumab was slow for tumor deposition and slow for clearance from the normal tissues. To improve the pharmacokinetic properties of the Fab fragment, an albumin binding sequence was introduced to generate a bifunctional molecule (AB.Fab4D5). Similar to Fab4D5 alone, AB.Fab4D5 visualized the tumor at 2 h post-injection, but its presence was sustained beyond 24 h, which resembles trastuzumab. Intravital microscopy revealed that tumor cell staining by AB.Fab4D5 was more uniform than for Fab4D5 or trastuzumab. The association of AB.Fab4D5 with albumin altered the clearance route of the probe, and minimal probe accumulation in the kidney was observed (Dennis et al., 2007). In another report, trastuzumab $F(ab')_2$ fragment labeled with ^{68}Ga was successfully used to quantify the loss and recovery of HER2 induced by HSP90 inhibitor 17-AAG in mice bearing BT-474 tumors (Smith-Jones et al., 2004). Table 1 summarizes trastuzumab-based agents for nuclear, optical and dual-modality imaging. This table includes only representative agents in each class, thus is in no way a complete list. The dual-labeled probes listed here will be discussed in detail later.

Imaging modality	Imaging agents	Animal model and cell lines	Dosage	Reference
Nuclear medicine				
PET	^{64}Cu-DOTA-Herceptin, ^{68}Ga-DOTA-$F(ab')_2$	Mouse xenograft; BT-474, MCF-7, MDA-MB-468	4 MBq 309 MBq	(Smith-Jones et al., 2004)
	^{89}Zr-trastuzumab	Mouse xenograft; SKOV3, GLC4	100 µg of trastuzumab (1 MBq)	(Dijkers et al., 2009)
SPECT/CT	^{111}In-DOTA-Fab4D5, ^{111}In-DOTA-AB.Fab4D5	Mouse allograft; tumors derived from MMTV/HER2 transgenic mice	4 mg/kg (300-500 µCi)	(Dennis et al., 2007)

Scintigraphy (whole body)	[^{99m}Tc]-HYNIC-trastuzumab Fab, ^{111}In-trastuzumab Fab, ^{111}In-DTPA-trastuzumab	Mouse xenograft; BT-474, SK-OV-3 human	25 MBq (30μg) 3.7 MBq (30μg) Mice: 450 ± 25 kBq (25 μg); Human: 100-150 MBq (5mg)	(Lub-de Hooge et al., 2004; Tang et al., 2005; Tang et al., 2005)
Optical imaging				
Fluorescent dyes	Herceptin-RhodG	Mouse xenograft; SK-BR-3, PE/CA-PJ34	50 μg in 200 μl PBS	(Koyama et al., 2007)
	Tra-Cy5.5 (SQ), Tra-Alexa680(SQ)	Mouse xenograft; 3T3/HER2+, Balb/3T3/HER2-	50 μg/100 μL PBS	(Ogawa et al., 2009)
	Trastuzumab-Cy5.5, Trastuzumab-AF750	Mouse xenograft; 9L, MCF-7, BT-474, SK-BR-3	0.4 nmol	(Gee et al., 2008)
Quantum dots (QDs)	Trastuzumab-QD	Mouse xenograft; 3T3/HER2+, Balb/3T3/HER2-	2 μM (100 μl)	(Li-Shishido et al., 2006; Tada et al., 2007)
Dual-modality				
Nuclear and optical agents	(^{111}In-DTPA)$_n$-trastuzumab-(IRDye800)$_m$	Mouse xenograft; SKBr3-luc	80-200 μg (70-200 μCi)	(Sampath et al., 2007)
	(^{64}Cu-DOTA)$_n$-trastuzumab-(IRDye800)$_m$	Mouse allograft; 4T1.2/R, 4T1.2neu/R	150 μg (150 μCi)	(Sampath et al., 2010)
	^{111}In-trastuzumab-ICG	Mouse xenograft; 3T3/HER2, MDA-MB-468	60 μg (3.8 MBq)	(Ogawa et al., 2009)

Table 1. Summary of molecular imaging agents based on trastuzumab (Herceptin) or trastuzumab fragments

3.3 HER2-specific affibody

Phage display selection yielded affibody molecules that specifically bind to HER2 extracellular domain. One of these molecules, His_6-$Z_{HER2:4}$ (affibody $Z_{HER2:4}$ linked to a histidine tag) targets the extracellular domain of HER2 with an affinity (K_D) at about 50 nM. The affibody does not interfere with trastuzumab binding to HER2, since the binding sites are different (Wikman et al., 2004). The specificity of the affibody was illustrated by the uptake of ^{125}I- His_6-$Z_{HER2:4}$ in HER2-overexpressing SK-BR-3 breast cancer cells (Tran et al., 2007; Wikman et al., 2004). A bivalent version of the affibody $(Z_{HER2:4})_2$, which has an increased binding affinity (K_D = 3 nM) was later created (Steffen et al., 2005). When ^{125}I-labeled $(Z_{HER2:4})_2$ was investigated in an animal study, a tumor-to-blood ratio of about 10:1 was obtained 8 h after injection, and the tumor region could be visualized using gamma camera imaging (Steffen et al., 2006). However a comparison of ^{125}I-labeled (Tolmachev et al., 2009) or ^{18}F-labeled (Cheng et al., 2008) second generation affibody molecules (see below) demonstrated that the monomeric form provided better tumor targeting than the dimeric form, which is the same as EGFR-specific affibody molecules (Tolmachev et al., 2009).

The second generation of HER2-specific affibody was generated through a single-library affinity maturation step. One of them, $Z_{HER2:342}$, showed a >2200-fold increase in affinity (22 pM for $Z_{HER2:342}$ *vs* 50 nM for $Z_{HER2:4}$). SK-OV-3 tumor xenografts were imaged 6 h after injection of ^{125}I-labeled $Z_{HER2:342}$. The tumor uptake at 4 h post-injection was improved by a factor of 4 compared to the parental molecule $Z_{HER2:4}$ (Orlova et al., 2006). Comparison of ^{124}I-labeled $Z_{HER2:342}$ and trastuzumab demonstrated that better tumor-to-organ ratios were obtained with $Z_{HER2:342}$ due to the more rapid clearance (Orlova et al., 2009). By changing the radioisotope to ^{111}In, the labeled molecule ^{111}In-Benzyl-DTPA- $Z_{HER2:342}$ maintain a K_D of 21 pM. Detection of SK-OV-3 tumors was achieved at 4 h post-injection with a gamma-camera. Biodistribution analysis revealed a tumor-to-blood ratio of 100 (Tolmachev et al., 2006). HER2-specific affibody molecules were also labeled with fluorescent dyes. The binding affinities and specificities of the conjugated molecules were unchanged or minimally affected by the modifications. *In vivo* NIR optical imaging revealed that affibody fused with an albumin-binding domain (ABD-$(Z_{HER2:342})_2$) exhibited a better performance compared to either monomer or dimer alone (Lee et al., 2008).

Site-specific radio-labeling of $Z_{HER2:342}$ was achieved by synthetic chemistry. The resulting ^{111}In-DOTA-$Z_{HER2:342\text{-}pep2}$ has a binding affinity of 65 pM. High contrast gamma camera images were obtained in the tumor region as early as 1 h after injection. Although pre-treatment with trastuzumab did not compete with the binding of ^{111}In-DOTA-$Z_{HER2:342\text{-}pep2}$ in tumors, degradation of the HER2 receptor using the heat-shock 90 inhibitor 17-AAG before probe administration reduced tumor uptake (Orlova et al., 2007). These data taken together indicate that, similar to the first generation affibody $Z_{HER2:4}$, the binding site of $Z_{HER2:342}$ is different from that of trastuzumab, but specific to the HER2 receptor. Site-specific labeling of ^{99m}Tc was mediated by incorporation of either histidine tag (His_6), natural peptide sequences CCG, CGGG, or maGGG, maSSS, maSKS, maESE chelators into the $Z_{HER2:342}$ sequence. All ^{99m}Tc-labeled probes showed tumor-specific uptake at 6 h post-injection or earlier using gamma camera imaging (Engfeldt et al., 2007; Engfeldt et al., 2007; Orlova et al., 2006; Tran et al., 2007; Tran et al., 2008).

^{111}In and ^{68}Ga-labeled $Z_{HER2:342}$ were tested in patients with recurrent metastatic breast cancer. These agents detected 9 out of 11 ^{18}F-FDG-positive metastases at 2-3 h after injection, suggesting their potential to localize HER2-positive metastases not amenable to biopsy (Baum et al., 2010).

The HER2-specific affibody was further optimized by reengineering the nonbinding surface of $Z_{HER2:342}$ to improve its properties such as storage stability, surface hydrophilicity, melting point and amenability for peptide synthesis. The new generation of affibody was created and characterized (Ahlgren et al., 2010; Feldwisch et al., 2010).

The fact that HER2-specific affibodies and trastuzumab target separate epitopes might be advantageous when developing these affibodies as imaging agents. These imaging agents will not interfere with trastuzumab binding when being used to monitor the therapeutic effect of trastuzumab (Baum et al., 2010; Orlova et al., 2007). One cause of concern of these affibody-base imaging agents is the high non-specific kidney accumulation. This is due to the small molecular weight of the affibody molecules which renders their clearance mainly through the kidney.

3.4 Dual-labeled trastuzumab

Probes dual-labeled with a radionuclide and a NIR fluorophore enhance the advantages and compensate the disadvantages of each modality, and could offer unique opportunities for the combination of non-invasive whole body imaging and subsequent intraoperative guidance during surgery. To investigate this possibility, trastuzumab was conjugated with either ^{111}In (for SPECT imaging) or ^{64}Cu (for PET imaging), and IRDye 800CW to image HER2 overexpression in mouse xenograft tumors (Sampath et al., 2010; Sampath et al., 2007).

$(^{111}\text{In-DTPA})_n$-trastuzumab-$(\text{IRDye800})_m$ was synthesized using a three step process wherein, trastuzumab was first conjugated to DTPA and then with IRDye 800CW. Prior to animal imaging, radio-labeling with ^{111}In was performed. The agent was validated for binding specificity *in vitro* using the fluorescence microscopy. High probe uptake in HER2-overexpressing SKBr3-luc tumors was demonstrated using NIR fluorescence, SPECT and planar scintigraphy imaging. The tumor-to-muscle ratios were comparable between optical and nuclear imaging modalities, but NIR fluorescence imaging had a higher signal-to-noise ratio. Since NIR fluorescence imaging has improved sensitivity due to high photon count, it can be used to monitor the lymphatic uptake of the dual-labeled antibody after intradermal administration into the dorsal aspect of the foot pad. Accumulation into the lymph nodes was observed at picomole doses within 1 h after administration, while clearance was observed by 24 h (Sampath et al., 2007).

To test the ability of dual-labeled $(^{64}\text{Cu-DOTA})_n$-trastuzumab-$(\text{IRDye800})_m$ to detect metastasis, Balb/c mice bearing 4T1.2/R (murine breast cancer cell, HER-) and 4T1.2neu/R (murine breast cancer cell, HER+) tumors were used. The diagnostic capability of this dual-labeled probe was also compared with PET imaging agent ^{18}FDG. $(^{64}\text{Cu-DOTA})_n$-trastuzumab-$(\text{IRDye800})_m$ showed significantly higher uptake in 4T1.2neu/R primary tumors compared to 4T1.2/R tumors, indicating *in vivo* specificity of the dual-labeled imaging agent. In contrast ^{18}FDG did not show any preferential uptake between the two tumor types. Lung metastases of HER2-overexpressing 4T1.2neu/R cells were successfully detected with whole body PET imaging after administration of $(^{64}\text{Cu-DOTA})_n$-trastuzumab-

$(IRDye800)_m$. Unfortunately, due to its limited penetration capability, whole body NIR fluorescence imaging could not detect lung metastases although it detected superficial skin metastases successfully. But agent uptake was evident with *ex vivo* NIR fluorescence imaging. *Ex vivo* NIR fluorescence imaging also visualized the trafficking of imaging agent from the primary tumor to lymph nodes, which was not possible for nuclear imaging with ^{64}Cu. When ^{18}FDG was investigated, it could not detect metastases under these conditions (Sampath et al., 2010).

In another study, it was found that trastuzumab labeled with both ICG and ^{111}In mimicked the cocktail of ICG-trastuzumab and ^{111}In-trastuzumab when injected into 3T3/HER2 tumor-bearing mice. As the fluorescence of ICG in this probe was only activated after binding to the HER2 receptor on the cell surface and being internalized, the HER2-overexpressing tumor could be visualized with minimal background signal (Ogawa et al., 2009).

4 Imaging EGFR and HER2 simultaneously

4.1 Antibodies labeled with fluorescent dyes

Fluorescence optical imaging has the advantage of multiple channels, which can be employed to image two or more targets simultaneously. Cetuximab and trastuzumab were labeled with Cy5.5 and Cy7, respectively. The binding and internalization of cetuximab-Cy5.5 by A431, and trastuzumab-Cy7 by 3T3/HER2+ cells were confirmed by fluorescence microscopy. On the contrary, no binding of cetuximab-Cy5.5 to 3T3/HER2+, and trastuzumab-Cy7 to A431 was observed. When mice were injected with a cocktail of cetuximab-Cy5.5 and trastuzumab-Cy7, A431 and 3T3/HER2+ tumors could be detected distinctly based on the Cy5.5 and Cy7 spectral images (Barrett et al., 2007). In a subsequent study three antibodies (cetuximab, trastuzumab and daclizumab) were labeled with three different fluorophores (Cy5, Cy7 and AlexaFluor700), respectively. Spectrally resolved fluorescence imaging showed that these probes clearly distinguished their respective targeting tumors (A431, 3T3/HER2+ and SP2-Tac) based on their distinct optical spectra (Koyama et al., 2007).

4.2 Affibody molecules labeled with fluorescent dyes

The EGFR- or HER2-specific Affibody molecules were labeled with IRDye 800CW and DY-682, respectively. The labeled probes, Eaff800 and Haff682, were taken up at high levels by EGFR-overexpressing A431 and HER2-overexpressing SK-OV-3 cells, respectively. Whole animal imaging showed that Eaff800 mainly accumulated in A431 tumor, while more Haff682 signal was found in SK-OV-3 tumor (Fig. 4A). Scanning tissue sections of dissected tumors confirmed the *in vivo* data. The liver uptake of Eaff800 was much higher than that of Haff682, suggesting a role of murine liver EGFR in the uptake of Eaff800. When the labeled fluorophores on the affibody molecules were exchanged (i.e. EGFR-specific affibody labeled with DY-682 and HER-specific affibody labeled with IRDye 800CW), the specificities of the affibody molecules were not affected (Fig. 4B). These results demonstrated that the tumor uptake of these imaging agents is receptor-mediated, and is independent of the fluorophore labeled on the affibody molecules (Gong et al., 2010).

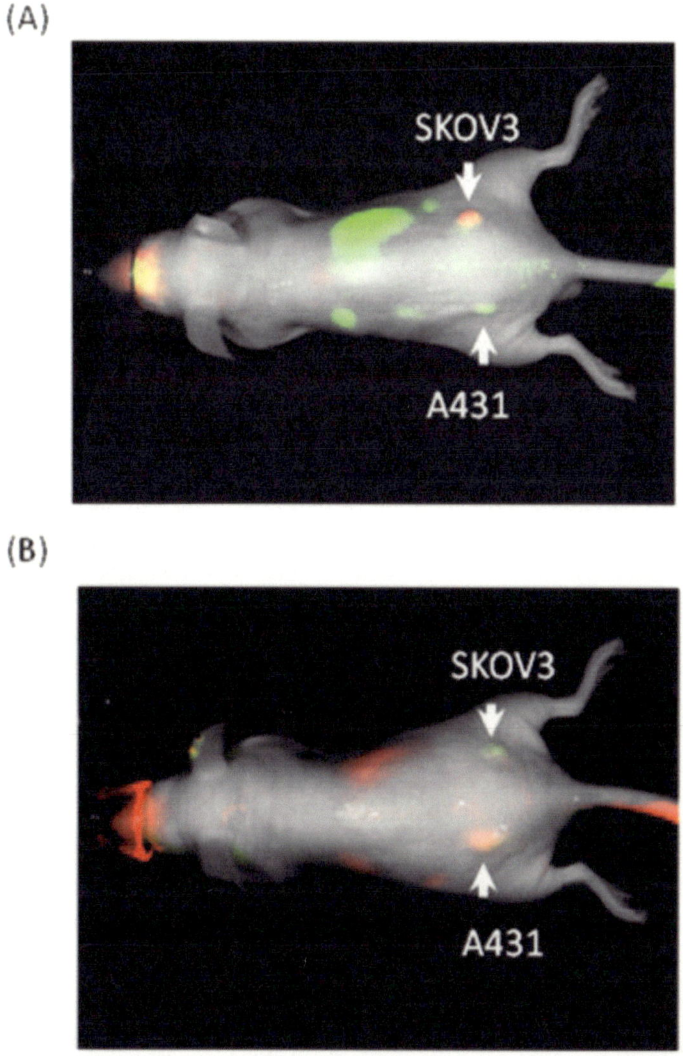

Fig. 4. Dual-color *in vivo* optical imaging with EGFR- and HER2-specific affibody molecules. Nude mice bearing A431 and SK-OV-3 tumors on the left side and right side, respectively, were injected with 100 µl PBS containing (A) 0.5 nmol Eaff800 and 0.5 nmol Haff682, or (B) 0.5 nmol Haff800 and 0.5 nmol Eaff682. Whole body images (dorsal view) were acquired at 1d following agent injection. The green color and red color represent IRDye800CW and DY-682 fluorescence signals, respectively. The tumors were indicated with arrows. Modified from (Gong et al., 2010) with permission.

5. Closing remarks

In vivo molecular imaging has become a valuable tool in biomedical research and drug development (Weissleder & Pittet, 2008; Willmann et al., 2008). The radionuclide-based imaging technology, such as PET and SPECT, has been used in clinical applications. In the research field, fluorescence optical imaging is becoming more and more popular due to its low cost, ease of use, longer time window for image capture and ability to track multiple probes simultaneously. Compared to fluorophores in the visible spectra, imaging with NIR fluorophores could reduce the autofluorescence, maximize tissue penetration, and are ideally suitable for non-invasive animal imaging applications (Kovar et al., 2007; Weissleder, 2001). However, even with NIR fluorophores, the direct clinical application of fluorescence imaging may be limited to superficial tissues such as breast and skin, or for visualization during endoscopy and image-guided-surgery procedures (Kampmeier et al., 2010).

EGFR- and HER2-targeted molecular imaging may aid in the selection of patients for individualized therapy by noninvasively assessing the expression level of EGFR and HER2 in tumors, and guide drug dosage and regime by measuring target-drug interaction and receptor occupancy. It can also be used to assess the responses to therapy in pre-clinical and clinical research, and provide valuable information for drug development and validation (Kampmeier et al., 2010).

EGFR and HER2 mediate a complex network of signaling pathways that interweaves with many other signaling networks. Interpretation of therapeutic output based solely on EGFR- and HER2-targeted imaging results might be oversimplified. Analysis of downstream molecules such as p-Erk1/2 may complement EGFR- and HER2-targeted imaging and provide new insights for cancer treatment (Cai et al., 2008). For EGFR-targeted therapy, it is not uncommon that drug effects are independent of EGFR expression levels in cancer cells. In these situations, targeting activated forms of the receptor instead of total receptor level may be a more reliable method to predict drug responsiveness (Pantaleo et al., 2009; Pantaleo et al., 2009).

6. References

Abourbeh G, Dissoki S, Jacobson O, Litchi A, Ben Daniel R, Laki D, Levitzki A & Mishani E (2007) Evaluation of radiolabeled ML04, a putative irreversible inhibitor of epidermal growth factor receptor, as a bioprobe for PET imaging of EGFR-overexpressing tumors. *Nucl Med Biol* 34: 55-70

Adams KE, Ke S, Kwon S, Liang F, Fan Z, Lu Y, Hirschi K, Mawad ME, Barry MA & Sevick-Muraca EM (2007) Comparison of visible and near-infrared wavelength-excitable fluorescent dyes for molecular imaging of cancer. *J Biomed Opt* 12: 024017

Ahlgren S, Orlova A, Wallberg H, Hansson M, Sandstrom M, Lewsley R, Wennborg A, Abrahmsen L, Tolmachev V & Feldwisch J (2010) Targeting of HER2-expressing tumors using 111In-ABY-025, a second-generation affibody molecule with a fundamentally reengineered scaffold. *J Nucl Med* 51: 1131-1138

Barrett T, Koyama Y, Hama Y, Ravizzini G, Shin IS, Jang BS, Paik CH, Urano Y, Choyke PL & Kobayashi H (2007) *In vivo* diagnosis of epidermal growth factor receptor expression using molecular imaging with a cocktail of optically labeled monoclonal antibodies. *Clin Cancer Res* 13: 6639-6648

Baselga J (2006) Targeting tyrosine kinases in cancer: the second wave. *Science* 312: 1175-1178

Baselga J, Perez EA, Pienkowski T & Bell R (2006) Adjuvant trastuzumab: a milestone in the treatment of HER-2-positive early breast cancer. *Oncologist* 11 Suppl 1: 4-12

Baum RP, Prasad V, Muller D, Schuchardt C, Orlova A, Wennborg A, Tolmachev V & Feldwisch J (2010) Molecular imaging of HER2-expressing malignant tumors in breast cancer patients using synthetic 111In- or 68Ga-labeled affibody molecules. *J Nucl Med* 51: 892-897

Cai W, Chen K, He L, Cao Q, Koong A & Chen X (2007) Quantitative PET of EGFR expression in xenograft-bearing mice using 64Cu-labeled cetuximab, a chimeric anti-EGFR monoclonal antibody. *Eur J Nucl Med Mol Imaging* 34: 850-858

Cai W, Niu G & Chen X (2008) Multimodality imaging of the HER-kinase axis in cancer. *Eur J Nucl Med Mol Imaging* 35: 186-208

Carlsson J, Nordgren H, Sjostrom J, Wester K, Villman K, Bengtsson NO, Ostenstad B, Lundqvist H & Blomqvist C (2004) HER2 expression in breast cancer primary tumours and corresponding metastases. Original data and literature review. *Br J Cancer* 90: 2344-2348

Carter P, Presta L, Gorman CM, Ridgway JB, Henner D, Wong WL, Rowland AM, Kotts C, Carver ME & Shepard HM (1992) Humanization of an anti-p185HER2 antibody for human cancer therapy. *Proc Natl Acad Sci U S A* 89: 4285-4289

Cheng Z, De Jesus OP, Namavari M, De A, Levi J, Webster JM, Zhang R, Lee B, Syud FA & Gambhir SS (2008) Small-animal PET imaging of human epidermal growth factor receptor type 2 expression with site-specific 18F-labeled protein scaffold molecules. *J Nucl Med* 49: 804-813

Dennis MS, Jin H, Dugger D, Yang R, McFarland L, Ogasawara A, Williams S, Cole MJ, Ross S & Schwall R (2007) Imaging tumors with an albumin-binding Fab, a novel tumor-targeting agent. *Cancer Res* 67: 254-261

Diagaradjane P, Orenstein-Cardona JM, Colon-Casasnovas NE, Deorukhkar A, Shentu S, Kuno N, Schwartz DL, Gelovani JG & Krishnan S (2008) Imaging epidermal growth factor receptor expression *in vivo*: pharmacokinetic and biodistribution characterization of a bioconjugated quantum dot nanoprobe. *Clin Cancer Res* 14: 731-741

Dijkers EC, Kosterink JG, Rademaker AP, Perk LR, van Dongen GA, Bart J, de Jong JR, de Vries EG & Lub-de Hooge MN (2009) Development and characterization of clinical-grade 89Zr-trastuzumab for HER2/neu immunoPET imaging. *J Nucl Med* 50: 974-981

Ekstrand AJ, Sugawa N, James CD & Collins VP (1992) Amplified and rearranged epidermal growth factor receptor genes in human glioblastomas reveal deletions of sequences encoding portions of the N- and/or C-terminal tails. *Proc Natl Acad Sci U S A* 89: 4309-4313

Engfeldt T, Orlova A, Tran T, Bruskin A, Widstrom C, Karlstrom AE & Tolmachev V (2007) Imaging of HER2-expressing tumours using a synthetic Affibody molecule containing the 99mTc-chelating mercaptoacetyl-glycyl-glycyl-glycyl (MAG3) sequence. *Eur J Nucl Med Mol Imaging* 34: 722-733

Engfeldt T, Tran T, Orlova A, Widstrom C, Feldwisch J, Abrahmsen L, Wennborg A, Karlstrom AE & Tolmachev V (2007) 99mTc-chelator engineering to improve tumour targeting properties of a HER2-specific Affibody molecule. *Eur J Nucl Med Mol Imaging* 34: 1843-1853

Feldwisch J, Tolmachev V, Lendel C, Herne N, Sjoberg A, Larsson B, Rosik D, Lindqvist E, Fant G, Hoiden-Guthenberg I, Galli J, Jonasson P & Abrahmsen L (2010) Design of an optimized scaffold for affibody molecules. *J Mol Biol* 398: 232-247

Ferguson KM, Darling PJ, Mohan MJ, Macatee TL & Lemmon MA (2000) Extracellular domains drive homo- but not hetero-dimerization of erbB receptors. *EMBO J* 19: 4632-4643

Friedman M, Nordberg E, Hoiden-Guthenberg I, Brismar H, Adams GP, Nilsson FY, Carlsson J & Stahl S (2007) Phage display selection of Affibody molecules with specific binding to the extracellular domain of the epidermal growth factor receptor. *Protein Eng Des Sel* 20: 189-199

Friedman M, Orlova A, Johansson E, Eriksson TL, Hoiden-Guthenberg I, Tolmachev V, Nilsson FY & Stahl S (2008) Directed evolution to low nanomolar affinity of a tumor-targeting epidermal growth factor receptor-binding affibody molecule. *J Mol Biol* 376: 1388-1402

Gainkam LO, Huang L, Caveliers V, Keyaerts M, Hernot S, Vaneycken I, Vanhove C, Revets H, De Baetselier P & Lahoutte T (2008) Comparison of the biodistribution and tumor targeting of two 99mTc-labeled anti-EGFR nanobodies in mice, using pinhole SPECT/micro-CT. *J Nucl Med* 49: 788-795

Gancberg D, Di Leo A, Cardoso F, Rouas G, Pedrocchi M, Paesmans M, Verhest A, Bernard-Marty C, Piccart MJ & Larsimont D (2002) Comparison of HER-2 status between primary breast cancer and corresponding distant metastatic sites. *Ann Oncol* 13: 1036-1043

Gee MS, Upadhyay R, Bergquist H, Alencar H, Reynolds F, Maricevich M, Weissleder R, Josephson L & Mahmood U (2008) Human breast cancer tumor models: molecular imaging of drug susceptibility and dosing during HER2/neu-targeted therapy. *Radiology* 248: 925-935

Gong H, Kovar J, Little G, Chen H & Olive DM (2010) *In vivo* imaging of xenograft tumors using an epidermal growth factor receptor-specific affibody molecule labeled with a near-infrared fluorophore. *Neoplasia* 12: 139-149

Gong Y, Booser DJ & Sneige N (2005) Comparison of HER-2 status determined by fluorescence in situ hybridization in primary and metastatic breast carcinoma. *Cancer* 103: 1763-1769

Hama Y, Urano Y, Koyama Y, Choyke PL & Kobayashi H (2007) Activatable fluorescent molecular imaging of peritoneal metastases following pretargeting with a biotinylated monoclonal antibody. *Cancer Res* 67: 3809-3817

Hamers-Casterman C, Atarhouch T, Muyldermans S, Robinson G, Hamers C, Songa EB, Bendahman N & Hamers R (1993) Naturally occurring antibodies devoid of light chains. *Nature* 363: 446-448

Hilger I, Leistner Y, Berndt A, Fritsche C, Haas KM, Kosmehl H & Kaiser WA (2004) Near-infrared fluorescence imaging of HER-2 protein over-expression in tumour cells. *Eur Radiol* 14: 1124-1129

Holliger P & Hudson PJ (2005) Engineered antibody fragments and the rise of single domains. *Nat Biotechnol* 23: 1126-1136

Huang L, Gainkam LO, Caveliers V, Vanhove C, Keyaerts M, De Baetselier P, Bossuyt A, Revets H & Lahoutte T (2008) SPECT imaging with 99mTc-labeled EGFR-specific nanobody for *in vivo* monitoring of EGFR expression. *Mol Imaging Biol* 10: 167-175

Iqbal U, Trojahn U, Albaghdadi H, Zhang J, O'Connor-McCourt M, Stanimirovic D, Tomanek B, Sutherland G & Abulrob A (2010) Kinetic analysis of novel mono- and multivalent VHH-fragments and their application for molecular imaging of brain tumours. *Br J Pharmacol* 160: 1016-1028

Kampmeier F, Niesen J, Koers A, Ribbert M, Brecht A, Fischer R, Kiessling F, Barth S & Thepen T (2010) Rapid optical imaging of EGF receptor expression with a single-chain antibody SNAP-tag fusion protein. *Eur J Nucl Med Mol Imaging* 37: 1926-1934

Kari C, Chan TO, Rocha de Quadros M & Rodeck U (2003) Targeting the epidermal growth factor receptor in cancer: apoptosis takes center stage. *Cancer Res* 63: 1-5

Ke S, Wen X, Gurfinkel M, Charnsangavej C, Wallace S, Sevick-Muraca EM & Li C (2003) Near-infrared optical imaging of epidermal growth factor receptor in breast cancer xenografts. *Cancer Res* 63: 7870-7875

Keppler A, Pick H, Arrivoli C, Vogel H & Johnsson K (2004) Labeling of fusion proteins with synthetic fluorophores in live cells. *Proc Natl Acad Sci U S A* 101: 9955-9959

Kovar JL, Johnson MA, Volcheck WM, Chen J & Simpson MA (2006) Hyaluronidase expression induces prostate tumor metastasis in an orthotopic mouse model. *Am J Pathol* 169: 1415-1426

Kovar JL, Simpson MA, Schutz-Geschwender A & Olive DM (2007) A systematic approach to the development of fluorescent contrast agents for optical imaging of mouse cancer models. *Anal Biochem* 367: 1-12

Koyama Y, Barrett T, Hama Y, Ravizzini G, Choyke PL & Kobayashi H (2007) *In vivo* molecular imaging to diagnose and subtype tumors through receptor-targeted optically labeled monoclonal antibodies. *Neoplasia* 9: 1021-1029

Koyama Y, Hama Y, Urano Y, Nguyen DM, Choyke PL & Kobayashi H (2007) Spectral fluorescence molecular imaging of lung metastases targeting HER2/neu. *Clin Cancer Res* 13: 2936-2945

Lang SA, Klein D, Moser C, Gaumann A, Glockzin G, Dahlke MH, Dietmaier W, Bolder U, Schlitt HJ, Geissler EK & Stoeltzing O (2007) Inhibition of heat shock protein 90 impairs epidermal growth factor-mediated signaling in gastric cancer cells and reduces tumor growth and vascularization *in vivo*. *Mol Cancer Ther* 6: 1123-1132

Lee FT, O'Keefe GJ, Gan HK, Mountain AJ, Jones GR, Saunder TH, Sagona J, Rigopoulos A, Smyth FE, Johns TG, Govindan SV, Goldenberg DM, Old LJ & Scott AM (2010) Immuno-PET quantitation of de2-7 epidermal growth factor receptor expression in glioma using 124I-IMP-R4-labeled antibody ch806. *J Nucl Med* 51: 967-972

Lee SB, Hassan M, Fisher R, Chertov O, Chernomordik V, Kramer-Marek G, Gandjbakhche A & Capala J (2008) Affibody molecules for *in vivo* characterization of HER2-positive tumors by near-infrared imaging. *Clin Cancer Res* 14: 3840-3849

Li-Shishido S, Watanabe TM, Tada H, Higuchi H & Ohuchi N (2006) Reduction in nonfluorescence state of quantum dots on an immunofluorescence staining. *Biochem Biophys Res Commun* 351: 7-13

Lopez-Guerrero JA, Llombart-Cussac A, Noguera R, Navarro S, Pellin A, Almenar S, Vazquez-Alvadalejo C & Llombart-Bosch A (2006) HER2 amplification in recurrent breast cancer following breast-conserving therapy correlates with distant metastasis and poor survival. *Int J Cancer* 118: 1743-1749

Lub-de Hooge MN, Kosterink JG, Perik PJ, Nijnuis H, Tran L, Bart J, Suurmeijer AJ, de Jong S, Jager PL & de Vries EG (2004) Preclinical characterisation of 111In-DTPA-trastuzumab. *Br J Pharmacol* 143: 99-106

Manning HC, Merchant NB, Foutch AC, Virostko JM, Wyatt SK, Shah C, McKinley ET, Xie J, Mutic NJ, Washington MK, LaFleur B, Tantawy MN, Peterson TE, Ansari MS, Baldwin RM, Rothenberg ML, Bornhop DJ, Gore JC & Coffey RJ (2008) Molecular imaging of therapeutic response to epidermal growth factor receptor blockade in colorectal cancer. *Clin Cancer Res* 14: 7413-7422

Memon AA, Jakobsen S, Dagnaes-Hansen F, Sorensen BS, Keiding S & Nexo E (2009) Positron emission tomography (PET) imaging with [11C]-labeled erlotinib: a micro-PET study on mice with lung tumor xenografts. *Cancer Res* 69: 873-878

Miao Z, Ren G, Liu H, Jiang L & Cheng Z (2010) Cy5.5-labeled Affibody molecule for near-infrared fluorescent optical imaging of epidermal growth factor receptor positive tumors. *J Biomed Opt* 15: 036007

Miao Z, Ren G, Liu H, Jiang L & Cheng Z (2010) Small-animal PET imaging of human epidermal growth factor receptor positive tumor with a 64Cu labeled affibody protein. *Bioconjug Chem* 21: 947-954

Mishani E, Abourbeh G, Eiblmaier M & Anderson CJ (2008) Imaging of EGFR and EGFR tyrosine kinase overexpression in tumors by nuclear medicine modalities. *Curr Pharm Des* 14: 2983-2998

Mishani E & Hagooly A (2009) Strategies for molecular imaging of epidermal growth factor receptor tyrosine kinase in cancer. *J Nucl Med* 50: 1199-1202

Mitsudomi T & Yatabe Y (2010) Epidermal growth factor receptor in relation to tumor development: EGFR gene and cancer. *FEBS J* 277: 301-308

Niu G, Cai W, Chen K & Chen X (2008) Non-invasive PET imaging of EGFR degradation induced by a heat shock protein 90 inhibitor. *Mol Imaging Biol* 10: 99-106

Niu G, Cai W & Chen X (2008) Molecular imaging of human epidermal growth factor receptor 2 (HER-2) expression. *Front Biosci* 13: 790-805

Nordberg E, Orlova A, Friedman M, Tolmachev V, Stahl S, Nilsson FY, Glimelius B & Carlsson J (2008) *In vivo* and *in vitro* uptake of 111In, delivered with the affibody molecule (ZEGFR:955)2, in EGFR expressing tumour cells. *Oncol Rep* 19: 853-857

Ogawa M, Kosaka N, Choyke PL & Kobayashi H (2009) *In vivo* molecular imaging of cancer with a quenching near-infrared fluorescent probe using conjugates of monoclonal antibodies and indocyanine green. *Cancer Res* 69: 1268-1272

Ogawa M, Regino CA, Choyke PL & Kobayashi H (2009) *In vivo* target-specific activatable near-infrared optical labeling of humanized monoclonal antibodies. *Mol Cancer Ther* 8: 232-239

Ogawa M, Regino CA, Seidel J, Green MV, Xi W, Williams M, Kosaka N, Choyke PL & Kobayashi H (2009) Dual-modality molecular imaging using antibodies labeled with activatable fluorescence and a radionuclide for specific and quantitative targeted cancer detection. *Bioconjug Chem* 20: 2177-2184

Okamoto I (2010) Epidermal growth factor receptor in relation to tumor development: EGFR-targeted anticancer therapy. *FEBS J* 277: 309-315

Orlova A, Magnusson M, Eriksson TL, Nilsson M, Larsson B, Hoiden-Guthenberg I, Widstrom C, Carlsson J, Tolmachev V, Stahl S & Nilsson FY (2006) Tumor imaging using a picomolar affinity HER2 binding affibody molecule. *Cancer Res* 66: 4339-4348

Orlova A, Nilsson FY, Wikman M, Widstrom C, Stahl S, Carlsson J & Tolmachev V (2006) Comparative *in vivo* evaluation of technetium and iodine labels on an anti-HER2 affibody for single-photon imaging of HER2 expression in tumors. *J Nucl Med* 47: 512-519

Orlova A, Tolmachev V, Pehrson R, Lindborg M, Tran T, Sandstrom M, Nilsson FY, Wennborg A, Abrahmsen L & Feldwisch J (2007) Synthetic affibody molecules: a novel class of affinity ligands for molecular imaging of HER2-expressing malignant tumors. *Cancer Res* 67: 2178-2186

Orlova A, Wallberg H, Stone-Elander S & Tolmachev V (2009) On the selection of a tracer for PET imaging of HER2-expressing tumors: direct comparison of a 124I-labeled affibody molecule and trastuzumab in a murine xenograft model. *J Nucl Med* 50: 417-425

Pal A, Glekas A, Doubrovin M, Balatoni J, Namavari M, Beresten T, Maxwell D, Soghomonyan S, Shavrin A, Ageyeva L, Finn R, Larson SM, Bornmann W & Gelovani JG (2006) Molecular imaging of EGFR kinase activity in tumors with 124I-labeled small molecular tracer and positron emission tomography. *Mol Imaging Biol* 8: 262-277

Panousis C, Rayzman VM, Johns TG, Renner C, Liu Z, Cartwright G, Lee FT, Wang D, Gan H, Cao D, Kypridis A, Smyth FE, Brechbiel MW, Burgess AW, Old LJ & Scott AM (2005) Engineering and characterisation of chimeric monoclonal antibody 806 (ch806) for targeted immunotherapy of tumours expressing de2-7 EGFR or amplified EGFR. *Br J Cancer* 92: 1069-1077

Pantaleo MA, Nannini M, Fanti S, Boschi S, Lollini PL & Biasco G (2009) Molecular imaging of EGFR: it's time to go beyond receptor expression. *J Nucl Med* 50: 1195-1196; author reply 1196, 1197

Pantaleo MA, Nannini M, Maleddu A, Fanti S, Nanni C, Boschi S, Lodi F, Nicoletti G, Landuzzi L, Lollini PL & Biasco G (2009) Experimental results and related clinical implications of PET detection of epidermal growth factor receptor (EGFr) in cancer. *Ann Oncol* 20: 213-226

Pectasides D, Gaglia A, Arapantoni-Dadioti P, Bobota A, Valavanis C, Kostopoulou V, Mylonakis N, Karabelis A, Pectasides M & Economopoulos T (2006) HER-2/neu status of primary breast cancer and corresponding metastatic sites in patients with advanced breast cancer treated with trastuzumab-based therapy. *Anticancer Res* 26: 647-653

Persson M, Tolmachev V, Andersson K, Gedda L, Sandstrom M & Carlsson J (2005) [(177)Lu]pertuzumab: experimental studies on targeting of HER-2 positive tumour cells. *Eur J Nucl Med Mol Imaging* 32: 1457-1462

Pines G, Kostler WJ & Yarden Y (2010) Oncogenic mutant forms of EGFR: lessons in signal transduction and targets for cancer therapy. *FEBS Lett* 584: 2699-2706

Regitnig P, Schippinger W, Lindbauer M, Samonigg H & Lax SF (2004) Change of HER-2/neu status in a subset of distant metastases from breast carcinomas. *J Pathol* 203: 918-926

Reilly RM, Kiarash R, Sandhu J, Lee YW, Cameron RG, Hendler A, Vallis K & Gariepy J (2000) A comparison of EGF and MAb 528 labeled with 111In for imaging human breast cancer. *J Nucl Med* 41: 903-911

Romond EH, Perez EA, Bryant J, Suman VJ, Geyer CE, Jr., Davidson NE, Tan-Chiu E, Martino S, Paik S, Kaufman PA, Swain SM, Pisansky TM, Fehrenbacher L, Kutteh LA, Vogel VG, Visscher DW, Yothers G, Jenkins RB, Brown AM, Dakhil SR,

Mamounas EP, Lingle WL, Klein PM, Ingle JN & Wolmark N (2005) Trastuzumab plus adjuvant chemotherapy for operable HER2-positive breast cancer. *N Engl J Med* 353: 1673-1684

Rosenthal EL, Kulbersh BD, King T, Chaudhuri TR & Zinn KR (2007) Use of fluorescent labeled anti-epidermal growth factor receptor antibody to image head and neck squamous cell carcinoma xenografts. *Mol Cancer Ther* 6: 1230-1238

Sampath L, Kwon S, Hall MA, Price RE & Sevick-Muraca EM (2010) Detection of Cancer Metastases with a Dual-labeled Near-Infrared/Positron Emission Tomography Imaging Agent. *Transl Oncol* 3: 307-317

Sampath L, Kwon S, Ke S, Wang W, Schiff R, Mawad ME & Sevick-Muraca EM (2007) Dual-labeled trastuzumab-based imaging agent for the detection of human epidermal growth factor receptor 2 overexpression in breast cancer. *J Nucl Med* 48: 1501-1510

Schechter NR, Wendt RE, 3rd, Yang DJ, Azhdarinia A, Erwin WD, Stachowiak AM, Broemeling LD, Kim EE, Cox JD, Podoloff DA & Ang KK (2004) Radiation dosimetry of 99mTc-labeled C225 in patients with squamous cell carcinoma of the head and neck. *J Nucl Med* 45: 1683-1687

Schechter NR, Yang DJ, Azhdarinia A, Kohanim S, Wendt R, 3rd, Oh CS, Hu M, Yu DF, Bryant J, Ang KK, Forster KM, Kim EE & Podoloff DA (2003) Assessment of epidermal growth factor receptor with 99mTc-ethylenedicysteine-C225 monoclonal antibody. *Anticancer Drugs* 14: 49-56

Schier R, McCall A, Adams GP, Marshall KW, Merritt H, Yim M, Crawford RS, Weiner LM, Marks C & Marks JD (1996) Isolation of picomolar affinity anti-c-erbB-2 single-chain Fv by molecular evolution of the complementarity determining regions in the center of the antibody binding site. *J Mol Biol* 263: 551-567

Simmons C, Miller N, Geddie W, Gianfelice D, Oldfield M, Dranitsaris G & Clemons MJ (2009) Does confirmatory tumor biopsy alter the management of breast cancer patients with distant metastases? *Ann Oncol* 20: 1499-1504

Simon R, Nocito A, Hubscher T, Bucher C, Torhorst J, Schraml P, Bubendorf L, Mihatsch MM, Moch H, Wilber K, Schotzau A, Kononen J & Sauter G (2001) Patterns of her-2/neu amplification and overexpression in primary and metastatic breast cancer. *J Natl Cancer Inst* 93: 1141-1146

Slamon DJ, Godolphin W, Jones LA, Holt JA, Wong SG, Keith DE, Levin WJ, Stuart SG, Udove J, Ullrich A & Press MF (1989) Studies of the HER-2/neu proto-oncogene in human breast and ovarian cancer. *Science* 244: 707-712

Smith-Jones PM, Solit DB, Akhurst T, Afroze F, Rosen N & Larson SM (2004) Imaging the pharmacodynamics of HER2 degradation in response to Hsp90 inhibitors. *Nat Biotechnol* 22: 701-706

Speake G, Holloway B & Costello G (2005) Recent developments related to the EGFR as a target for cancer chemotherapy. *Curr Opin Pharmacol* 5: 343-349

Steffen AC, Orlova A, Wikman M, Nilsson FY, Stahl S, Adams GP, Tolmachev V & Carlsson J (2006) Affibody-mediated tumour targeting of HER-2 expressing xenografts in mice. *Eur J Nucl Med Mol Imaging* 33: 631-638

Steffen AC, Wikman M, Tolmachev V, Adams GP, Nilsson FY, Stahl S & Carlsson J (2005) *In vitro* characterization of a bivalent anti-HER-2 affibody with potential for radionuclide-based diagnostics. *Cancer Biother Radiopharm* 20: 239-248

Stoscheck CM & King LE, Jr. (1986) Role of epidermal growth factor in carcinogenesis. *Cancer Res* 46: 1030-1037

Su H, Seimbille Y, Ferl GZ, Bodenstein C, Fueger B, Kim KJ, Hsu YT, Dubinett SM, Phelps ME, Czernin J & Weber WA (2008) Evaluation of [(18)F]gefitinib as a molecular imaging probe for the assessment of the epidermal growth factor receptor status in malignant tumors. *Eur J Nucl Med Mol Imaging* 35: 1089-1099

Tada H, Higuchi H, Wanatabe TM & Ohuchi N (2007) *In vivo* real-time tracking of single quantum dots conjugated with monoclonal anti-HER2 antibody in tumors of mice. *Cancer Res* 67: 1138-1144

Tang Y, Scollard D, Chen P, Wang J, Holloway C & Reilly RM (2005) Imaging of HER2/neu expression in BT-474 human breast cancer xenografts in athymic mice using [(99m)Tc]-HYNIC-trastuzumab (Herceptin) Fab fragments. *Nucl Med Commun* 26: 427-432

Tang Y, Wang J, Scollard DA, Mondal H, Holloway C, Kahn HJ & Reilly RM (2005) Imaging of HER2/neu-positive BT-474 human breast cancer xenografts in athymic mice using (111)In-trastuzumab (Herceptin) Fab fragments. *Nucl Med Biol* 32: 51-58

Tapia C, Savic S, Wagner U, Schonegg R, Novotny H, Grilli B, Herzog M, Barascud AD, Zlobec I, Cathomas G, Terracciano L, Feichter G & Bubendorf L (2007) HER2 gene status in primary breast cancers and matched distant metastases. *Breast Cancer Res* 9: R31

Tolmachev V, Friedman M, Sandstrom M, Eriksson TL, Rosik D, Hodik M, Stahl S, Frejd FY & Orlova A (2009) Affibody molecules for epidermal growth factor receptor targeting *in vivo*: aspects of dimerization and labeling chemistry. *J Nucl Med* 50: 274-283

Tolmachev V, Mume E, Sjoberg S, Frejd FY & Orlova A (2009) Influence of valency and labelling chemistry on *in vivo* targeting using radioiodinated HER2-binding Affibody molecules. *Eur J Nucl Med Mol Imaging* 36: 692-701

Tolmachev V, Nilsson FY, Widstrom C, Andersson K, Rosik D, Gedda L, Wennborg A & Orlova A (2006) 111In-benzyl-DTPA-ZHER2:342, an affibody-based conjugate for *in vivo* imaging of HER2 expression in malignant tumors. *J Nucl Med* 47: 846-853

Tolmachev V, Rosik D, Wallberg H, Sjoberg A, Sandstrom M, Hansson M, Wennborg A & Orlova A (2010) Imaging of EGFR expression in murine xenografts using site-specifically labelled anti-EGFR 111In-DOTA-Z EGFR:2377 Affibody molecule: aspect of the injected tracer amount. *Eur J Nucl Med Mol Imaging* 37: 613-622

Tran T, Engfeldt T, Orlova A, Widstrom C, Bruskin A, Tolmachev V & Karlstrom AE (2007) *In vivo* evaluation of cysteine-based chelators for attachment of 99mTc to tumor-targeting Affibody molecules. *Bioconjug Chem* 18: 549-558

Tran T, Orlova A, Sivaev I, Sandstrom M & Tolmachev V (2007) Comparison of benzoate- and dodecaborate-based linkers for attachment of radioiodine to HER2-targeting Affibody ligand. *Int J Mol Med* 19: 485-493

Tran TA, Ekblad T, Orlova A, Sandstrom M, Feldwisch J, Wennborg A, Abrahmsen L, Tolmachev V & Eriksson Karlstrom A (2008) Effects of lysine-containing mercaptoacetyl-based chelators on the biodistribution of 99mTc-labeled anti-HER2 Affibody molecules. *Bioconjug Chem* 19: 2568-2576

Tzahar E, Waterman H, Chen X, Levkowitz G, Karunagaran D, Lavi S, Ratzkin BJ & Yarden Y (1996) A hierarchical network of interreceptor interactions determines signal transduction by Neu differentiation factor/neuregulin and epidermal growth factor. *Mol Cell Biol* 16: 5276-5287

Urano Y, Asanuma D, Hama Y, Koyama Y, Barrett T, Kamiya M, Nagano T, Watanabe T, Hasegawa A, Choyke PL & Kobayashi H (2009) Selective molecular imaging of viable cancer cells with pH-activatable fluorescence probes. *Nat Med* 15: 104-109

Velikyan I, Sundberg AL, Lindhe O, Hoglund AU, Eriksson O, Werner E, Carlsson J, Bergstrom M, Langstrom B & Tolmachev V (2005) Preparation and evaluation of (68)Ga-DOTA-hEGF for visualization of EGFR expression in malignant tumors. *J Nucl Med* 46: 1881-1888

Vincent-Salomon A, Pierga JY, Couturier J, d'Enghien CD, Nos C, Sigal-Zafrani B, Lae M, Freneaux P, Dieras V, Thiery JP & Sastre-Garau X (2007) HER2 status of bone marrow micrometastasis and their corresponding primary tumours in a pilot study of 27 cases: a possible tool for anti-HER2 therapy management? *Br J Cancer* 96: 654-659

Weissleder R (2001) A clearer vision for *in vivo* imaging. *Nat Biotechnol* 19: 316-317

Weissleder R & Pittet MJ (2008) Imaging in the era of molecular oncology. *Nature* 452: 580-589

Wikman M, Steffen AC, Gunneriusson E, Tolmachev V, Adams GP, Carlsson J & Stahl S (2004) Selection and characterization of HER2/neu-binding affibody ligands. *Protein Eng Des Sel* 17: 455-462

Wikstrand CJ, Reist CJ, Archer GE, Zalutsky MR & Bigner DD (1998) The class III variant of the epidermal growth factor receptor (EGFRvIII): characterization and utilization as an immunotherapeutic target. *J Neurovirol* 4: 148-158

Willmann JK, van Bruggen N, Dinkelborg LM & Gambhir SS (2008) Molecular imaging in drug development. *Nat Rev Drug Discov* 7: 591-607

Xu N, Cai G, Ye W, Wang X, Li Y, Zhao P, Zhang A, Zhang R & Cao B (2009) Molecular imaging application of radioiodinated anti-EGFR human Fab to EGFR-overexpressing tumor xenografts. *Anticancer Res* 29: 4005-4011

Yang L, Mao H, Wang YA, Cao Z, Peng X, Wang X, Duan H, Ni C, Yuan Q, Adams G, Smith MQ, Wood WC, Gao X & Nie S (2009) Single chain epidermal growth factor receptor antibody conjugated nanoparticles for *in vivo* tumor targeting and imaging. *Small* 5: 235-243

Yarden Y & Sliwkowski MX (2001) Untangling the ErbB signalling network. *Nat Rev Mol Cell Biol* 2: 127-137

Yeh HH, Ogawa K, Balatoni J, Mukhapadhyay U, Pal A, Gonzalez-Lepera C, Shavrin A, Soghomonyan S, Flores L, 2nd, Young D, Volgin AY, Najjar AM, Krasnykh V, Tong W, Alauddin MM & Gelovani JG (2011) Molecular imaging of active mutant L858R EGF receptor (EGFR) kinase-expressing nonsmall cell lung carcinomas using PET/CT. *Proc Natl Acad Sci U S A* 108: 1603-1608

Zhang X, Silva E, Gershenson D & Hung MC (1989) Amplification and rearrangement of c-erb B proto-oncogenes in cancer of human female genital tract. *Oncogene* 4: 985-989

Part 3

Recent Developments and Trends

17

Recent Development and Trends in Molecular Imaging Probes for Prostate Cancer

Wenbin Zeng[1,2], Zhiguo Liu[1,2] and Wei Wang[2,3]
[1] *School of Pharmaceutical Sciences, Central South University, Tongzipo Road, Changsha,*
[2] *Molecular Imaging Research Center, Central South University, Changsha,*
[3] *Cell Transplantation & Gene Therapy Institute,*
The Third Xiangya Hospital of Central South University, Changsha,
China

1. Introduction

In 1853, a surgeon at the London Hospital, Adams J, discovered the first case of prostate cancer by histological examination [1]. In the report, he noted that the condition was "a very rare disease". Remarkably, 150 years later, prostate cancer has become a significant health problem and disease. Prostate cancer continues to have the highest incidence rate of any other type of cancer in male, and it is the second leading cause of cancer deaths in male (in the United States), with about 220k new cases diagnosed each year only in US [2-4]. Detection rates of prostate cancers vary widely across through the world, with less frequently detecting in East and South Asia than in Europe, and especially in the United States. Prostate cancer tends to develop in men over the age of fifty, and although it is one of the most prevalent types of cancer in men. However, many of those patients never have symptoms, while undergo no therapy, and eventually die of other causes. The increased incidence of prostate cancer patients has led to remarkable changes in diagnosis and treatment over the past decades. Fifty years ago the typical patient was a man in his early seventies who was diagnosed with metastases to the bone and/or soft tissues [5]. Characteristically, these lesions were bulky and histologically poorly differentiated. Diagnosis at such an advanced disease status was a death sentence, with patients dying within less than two years. Prostate cancer is currently diagnosed by sector biopsy in men presenting with an elevated serum prostate-specific antigen level. As for all biopsies, sector biopsy for prostate cancer is invasive and limited by sampling error [6]. Now there is a genetic and biochemical framework for understanding the process of both sporadic and inherited forms of prostate cancer, especially with the development of the new discipline, molecular imaging, a valuable tool for the diagnosis for prostate cancer [7]. At present, owing to the use of molecular imaging modality, together with the traditional serum PSA screening and improved biopsy techniques, most patients could be diagnosed with prostate cancer at a stage when it is potentially curable by surgical and/or radiological approaches . As a result, the good news is that the diagnosis of prostate cancer is no longer automatically a death sentence [8].

Molecular imaging is a newly emerging field, but has became an indispensable tool in cancer research, medical practice and clinical trials, with aims at noninvasive, real-time, quantitative visualization of in vivo molecular processes occurring at cellular and subcellular levels. Molecular imaging allows physicians and clinicians not only to see where a tumor is located in the body, but also to visualize the expression and activity of specific molecules (small molecular, or large molecular such as protein, antibody, and etc) and biological processes (e.g., apoptosis, metastasis, and angiogenesis) which influence tumor behavior and/or its response to therapy. At present, advancement in the molecular imaging field is promoted by the development of improved imaging hardware for use in preclinical and clinical settings, the identification and validation of new, biologically relevant imaging targets, and the development of improved imaging probes derived from novel chemicals. Of these three essential factors, which comprise the majority of current molecular imaging research, hardware developments and novel target discoveries significantly outpace the development and clinical advancement of new molecular imaging probes, particularly with respect to cancer imaging [9-12]. Hence, molecular imaging, or diagnostic imaging, could provide a full prospect of prostate tumor burden by uncovering recurrent and metastatic lesions.

Hererin, we will focus on the discovery of molecular imaging probes that exist for the use of molecular imaging as a platform for prostate cancer, rather than specific details of hardware and instrumentation. Since molecular imaging probes may also help to guide oncologists, physicians and clinicians to identify those patients that could best benefit from a given therapeutic regimen, dose, or duration of drug, we will also outline the existing molecular imaging probes and modalities that are currently undergoing preclinical and clinical tests and those, which have been described based on the different receiptor of prostate cancer, that could be rapidly translated into humans. Meanwhile, we will also discuss possible future directions and specific application of these and other potential new imaging strategies designed to both diagnosis and treatment for prostate cancer.

2. Imaging probes for prostate cancer based on androgen receptor (AR)

Androgens are fundamental for the growth, development and maintenance of the prostate. Its effects are exerted via the nuclear androgen receptor (AR) which is a ligand-dependent transcription activator involved in cellular proliferation and differentiation and is founded in all histologic types of prostate tumors. Pathologic and molecular analyses of AR would afford the evidence of the gene expression and increased protein mutation, which contributes to a change of function, and ligand-independent activation [13, 14]. Since it is particularly imperative to find approaches for assessing prostate cancer comprehensively, molecular imaging of AR might provide an unprecedented opportunity for deciphering the molecular mechanisms involved in the development and natural progression of prostate cancer from a localized process to the hormone-refractory metastatic disease. Such understanding will be the key for targeted imaging and therapy, as well as for predicting and evaluating treatment response and prognosis [15]. An alternative approach to radiolabeled antibodies, such as 111In-labeled prostate-specific membrane antigen (PSMA) monoclonal antibody (also named as ProstaScint) was reported, with a focus on the development of AR radioligands for positron emission tomography (PET), single photon emission computerized tomography (SPECT), and magnatic resonance imaging (MRI)-based imaging of the prostate. Generally speaking, AR radiolabeled ligands can be divided into two main structural classes, steroidal (such as 18F-FDHT) and nonsteroidal (such as flutamide and bicalutamide), or into two different functional classes, androgenic and antiandrogenic [16, 17].

2.1 Steroidal AR radioligands for imaging prostate cancer

Zanzonico P and co-workers discovered a steroidal AR radioligand, 18F-FDHT (16β-[18F]fluoro-5R-dihydrotestosterone), and carried out some basic research to evaluate it [18, 19]. FDHT is of a structural analog of 5R-di-hydrotestosterone, a principal intraprostatic form of androgen. A study of progressive androgen-independent prostate cancer on seven patients indicated that 18F-FDHT may be a promising new radiotracer compare with 18F-FDG. In the relevant study of fluorinated androgen analogs in baboon, performed by Welch group, the uptake of FDHT in the prostate was blocked by coadministration of cold tesosterone (reduced about 10-fold) [20]. To date, FDHT appears to bind specifically to androgen receptors in vivo and to be of the most favorable targeting properties for noninvasive imaging among all receptor-binding radiotracers studied before. In other researches, 18F-FDHT present some advantages such as fast tumor uptake and prolonged retention of radioactivity observed in human studies. However, limitations such as metabolic rate of this labeled compound rapid have been observed [21-23].

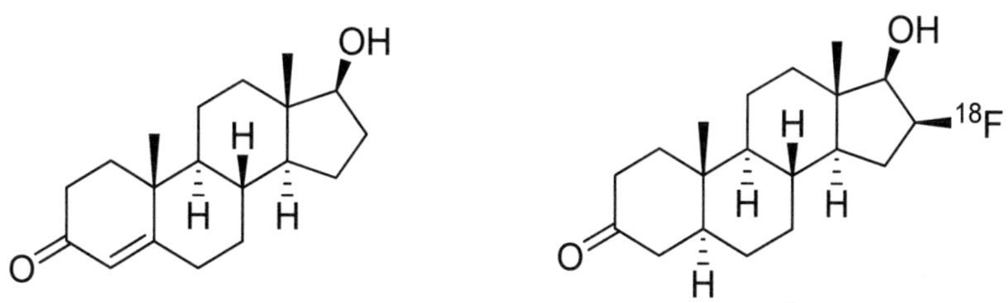

1

Testosterone 18F-FDHT

Scheme 1. The chemical structure of Testosterone and 18F-FDHT.

2.2 Nonsteroidal AR radioligands for imaging prostate cancer

Nonsteroidal AR radioligands, (R)-[11C]-dimethylaminehydroxy-flutamide derivatives (Scheme 2, probe **2**, **3**, and **4**), were designed, synthesized and radiosynthesised by Jacobson O et al in 2006 [24]. The preliminary biological evaluations of three novel nonsteroidal flutamide derivative androgen ligands demonstrated some significant benefits compared with the currently used commercial drugs. These compounds have higher or similar affinities to the AR when compared with 3-bromo-hydroxyflutamide and hydroxyflutamide. However, unlike other reported nonsteroidal radiolabeled AR ligands, these compounds have an electron-rich group (dimethylamine) located on the methyl moiety, which may confer a better stability to the molecule. Additionally, they serve as an anchor for carbon-11 labeling in a more straightforward approach than labeling with fluorine-18 or bromine-76. Furthermore, some other nonsteroidal agents are being evaluated for prostate cancer imaging, based on hydroxyflutamide and bicalutamide pharmacophores, for example, as shown in Scheme 2, (R)-[18F]-hydroxyflutamide (**5**), 3-[76Br]-bromo-hydroxyflutamide (**6**), [18F]- bicalutamide (**7**),

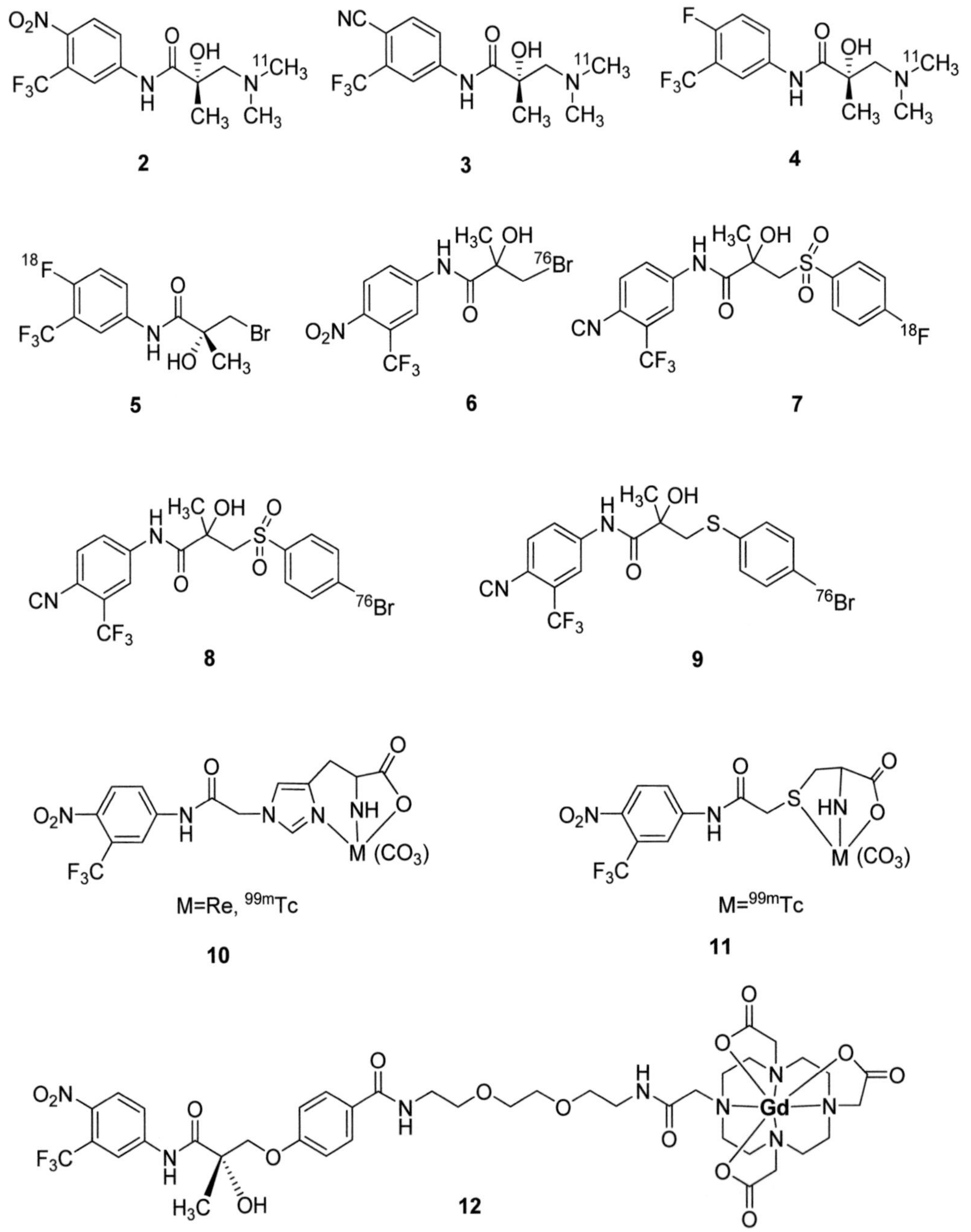

Scheme 2. Chemical structures of some nonsteroidal AR radioligands for imaging prostate cancer.

[76Br]-bromo-bicalutamide (**8**), and [76Br]-bromo-thiobicalutamide (**9**) [25, 26]. Additionally, [76Br]-bromo-bicalutamide compound has been found to have an order of magnitude higher affinity for AR than that of bicalutamide (Kd of 0.113 μM for [76Br]-bromobicalutamide versus to Kd of 1.276 μM for bicalutamide). Also, a series of novel prospective SPECT imaging agents has been reported very recently. These 99mTc-containing flutamide derivatives (**10**, **11**) were synthesized, characterized, and evaluated, with a significant selective uptake by a prostate [27]. Furthermore, Marom H et al reported a new nonsteroidal antiandrogen-lanthanoid metal complexes (**12**) as a potential MRI contrast agent for prostate cancer diagnostics [28]. These interesting results demonstrate that AR provides a more sensitive imaging-based biologic target for imaging and early assessment of treatment response.

3. Imaging probes for prostate cancer based on PSMA

Serum prostate-specific antigen (PSA) has long been used as an organ-specific biomarker and is currently the most commonly used one for prostate cancer. PSA is a 33 kDa androgen-regulated serine protease produced by the prostate gland. However, PSA and other related parameters have limited sensitivity and limited specificity to prostate cancer. Therefore, it may be affected by a manner unrelated to the effect of the therapy on tumor, and is the cause of the patients' great anxiety or overstated diagnostic expectations [29, 30]. The prostate-specific membrane antigen (PSMA) is expressed in both the benign and the neoplastic prostatic epithelial cells and in other tissues, such as kidney, liver, and brain [31]. It is upregulated in hormone-resistant states and in metastatic disease. It is a transmembrane, 750 amino acid, type II glycoprotein primarily expressed in normal human prostate epithelium but overexpressed in prostate cancer, including metastatic disease. Because PSMA is expressed by virtually all prostate cancers and its expression is further increased in poorly differentiated, metastatic and hormone-refractory carcinomas, it is a very attractive target for prostate cancer imaging and therapy [32, 33]. Recently, researchers from Johns Hopkins University presented the preparation of radiolabeled small-molecule ligands for PSMA ([125I]DCIT, [11C]DCMC, [18F]DCFBC], as well as seven technetium 99m- or rhenium-labeled chelating agents attached to an amino-functionalized PSMA inhibitor with or without a variable length linker moiety [34-36]. These probes were based on potential capitalization on PSMA as a relevant biologic target for imaging and therapy of prostate cancer. Other works indicated that biotinylated anti-PSMA antibody conjugated to streptavidin-labeled iron oxide nanoparticles could be used as the MRI probe for detection of prostate cancer cells [37]. T1-weighted signal was greater for cells with magnetic particles bound to cell surface than for cells that internalized the particles, whereas no such effect was noted with T2-weighted images. Besides, a low molecular weight PSMA-based fluorescent imaging agent have been relatively extensively studied in prostate cancer. 2-(3-(5-[7-(5-amino-1-carboxy-pentyl-carbamoyl)-heptanoy-amino]-1-carboxy-pentyl)-ureido) entanedioic acid was conjugated with a commercially available near-infrared light-emitting dye (IRDye 800CW) to afford **16** in good yield. It has a PSMA inhibitory activity of 0.37 nM, which is capable of generating target-to-nontarget ratios of at least 10 fold in PSMA-expressing PC3-PIP vs PSMA-negative PC3-flu tumors in vivo. It is useful for the study of PSMA-expressing tissue in preclinical models or for intraoperative guidance [38].

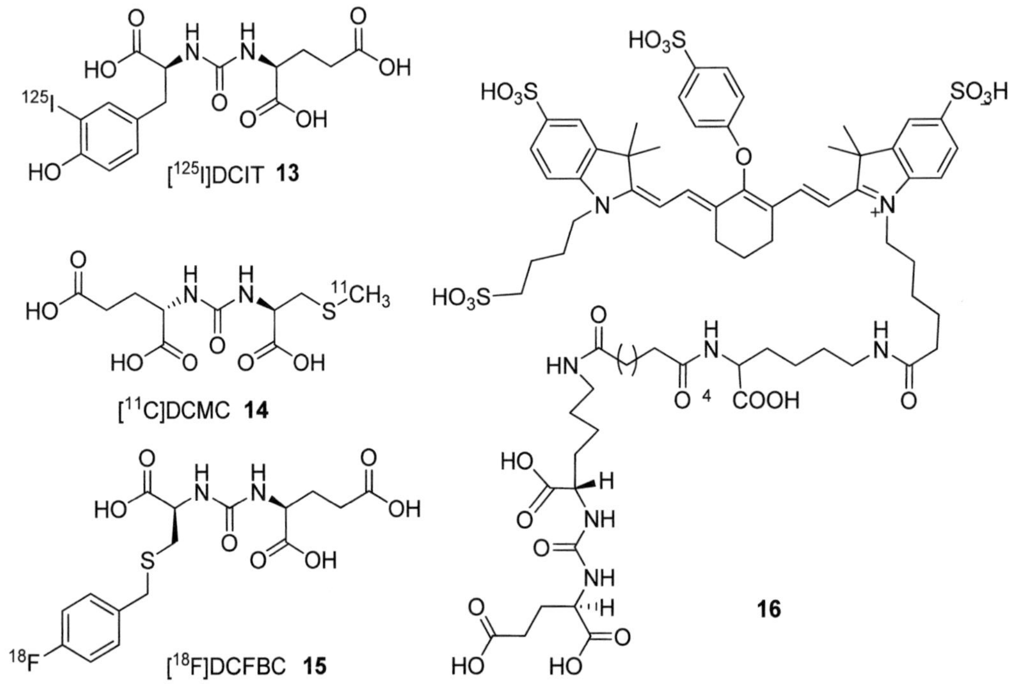

Scheme 3. Probes for imaging prostate cancer based on PSMA.

4. Other probes for imaging prostate cancer based on EGF receptor, GRP receptor, and integrin αvβ3

[18F]-fluorodeoxyglucose (FDG) (**17**) is a well known molecular imaging probe for monitoring tissue glucose metabolism in clinical trial [39, 40]. Because of the advantages of the known mechanism that most tumors are hypermetabolic with increased glucose metabolism (Warburg effect), this probe is more suitable for assessing the glucose metabolism for prostate cancer. The upregulation of glucose transporter (GLUT) proteins (such as GLUT1 and/or GLUT3) and/or increased enzymatic level of hexokinase (HK) and activity (primarily HK-II) have been observed in many cancers. GLUT, which affects the rate-limiting step, is very important for glucose metabolism. The whole procedure needs energy-independent glucose transport across the cell membrane down the concentration gradient. Then, glucose is phosphorylated to glucose-6-phosphate by efficiently using HK-II. FDG, with a similar structure to glucose, is phosphorylated to FDG-6-phosphate, but when compared with glucose-6-phosphate, it cannot be further metabolized in the glycolytic pathway and finally trapped and accumulated in the cell owing to its negative charge [41, 42]. The GLUT1 mRNA expression was observed by Northern blot analysis in both androgen-independent cell lines and the androgen-sensitive prostate cancer cell line [43]. A related study from Australia demonstrated that the expression of GLUT12 in human prostate cancer cell lines potentially enhanced glucose metabolism in prostate tumor [44]. These findings may explain the phenomenon of higher FDG accumulation in prostate cancer, especially in malignancy grade. However, there are some limitations: the role of 18F-FDG PET in prostate cancer is controversial, and the results are heavily influenced by the patient selection; The uptake of 18F-FDG is low in tumour tissue. The 60%-70% sensitivity of 18F-FDG PET for prostate cancer is not high enough to justify its routine clinical use for staging or restaging of this disease [45]. The poor performance of 18F-FDG PET is likely related to the low glucose metabolic rate that results from the relatively slow growth of most prostate cancers as well as to other factors.

Another PET tracers, such as 11C- or 18F-labeled acetate (**18, 19**) and choline (**20, 21**), have been extensively studied in prostate cancer [46, 47]. However, 11C acetate is primarily retained in prostate cancer cell lines, due to incorporation of the radiocarbon into phosphatidylcholine and neutral lipids of the cells [48]. Meanwhile, because of the alteration in several enzymes involved in the metabolism of fatty acids and enhanced beta-oxidation pathway, it has been observed that fatty acid metabolism rather than glycolysis may be dominant in prostate cancer [49]. Recent studies also confirmed that the involvement of the fatty acid synthesis pathway in 11C acetate uptake in prostate tumors is an imaging marker for fatty acid synthesis expression [50]. Previous clinical studies with 11C- labeled acetate (11C-ACE) have reported improved sensitivity, up to 100%, for detection of primary tumors in patients with untreated prostate cancer [51, 52]. However, the potential for widespread use of 11C-ACE is limited by the short radioactive half-life (20.4 min) of 11C. Accordingly, there is considerable interest in identifying positron-emitting radiopharmaceuticals labeled with isotopes with longer half-lives that are suitable for imaging of prostate cancer. One such radiopharmaceutical that has been studied is 18F-fluoroethylcholine, which also appears to be a cell membrane precursor compound [53, 54]. Another potential agent is the acetate analog 18F-fluoroacetate (18F-FAC). Fatty acid synthesis is an important pathway in cancer cell, which requires major enzyme for converting carbohydrates to fatty acids, and the upregulation of the relevant enzyme plays a key role in tumorigenesis of the prostate in the transgenic adenocarcinoma of mouse prostate (TRAMP) model [55]. Recently, [11C]acetoacetate (22) has also been evaluated as a potential PET probe of ketone body use by prostate tumors [56]. It was found that PC-3 androgen-independent prostate tumors display moderated uptake of [11C] acetoacetate with rapidly decreasing background activity. Further research would be needed to determine the exact biologic relevance of imaging ketone body use to the natural history of prostate cancer and how it may be useful in a specific clinical setting.

The epidermal growth factor receptor (EGFR) is over-expressed in a variety of human cancers, including in hormone-refractory prostate carcinomas, in which the EGFR has been associated with advanced disease stage, resistance to standard treatment and poor prognosis. Therefore, the EGFR is considered to be a promising molecular target for molecular imaging and therapy for hormone-refractory prostate cancer. Fozing T reported a synthesis an EGF receptor tyrosine kinase (EGFR-TK) inhibitor, 123I-PD153035 (**23**) as potential imaging probes. In vitro studies of 123I-PD153035 was found that it accumulats highly in human PC-3 and DU-145 prostate cancer cells cooperating with 123I-mAb425, the 123I radiolabelled IgG2a antibody [57]. In vivo studies of the human prostate cancer xenografts in mouse was accurately visualized after i.v. administration of 123I-PD153035 by a gamma camera. These data suggest that 123I-PD153035 are promising candidates as an imaging probe for EGFR- positive prostate cancer and warrant further in vivo validations to ascertain their potential as imaging agents for clinical used. Another radiolabeled bombesin (a target molecular with high affinity for GRP receptors) analogues was synthesized and assessed for SPECT (111In label) and PET (64Cu or 18F label) visualization of prostate cancer [58, 59]. However, imaging of the GRP receptor is being under the further investigation to determine whether it is useful or not in clinical trial for prostate cancer.

In relation to tumor angiogenesis, the vascular endothelial growth factor (VEGF) signaling pathway and the integrin αvβ3 (a cell adhesion molecule) have been identified to play key roles. Molecular imaging of these targets in the tumor vasculature may help tailor targeted antiangiogenic therapy [60]. Some of PET probes suitable for integrin receptor imaging have been reported, and have shown high specificity in various types of tumors, including prostate cancer models [61]. Active research continues in identifying more specific biologic markers for interrogating the tumor vessels. These investigations will not only shed more light on the biologic basis of the complex signals involved in malignancy-induced angiogenesis, but may also help facilitate the design and image-based testing of drugs targeted to tumor-specific angiogenesis.

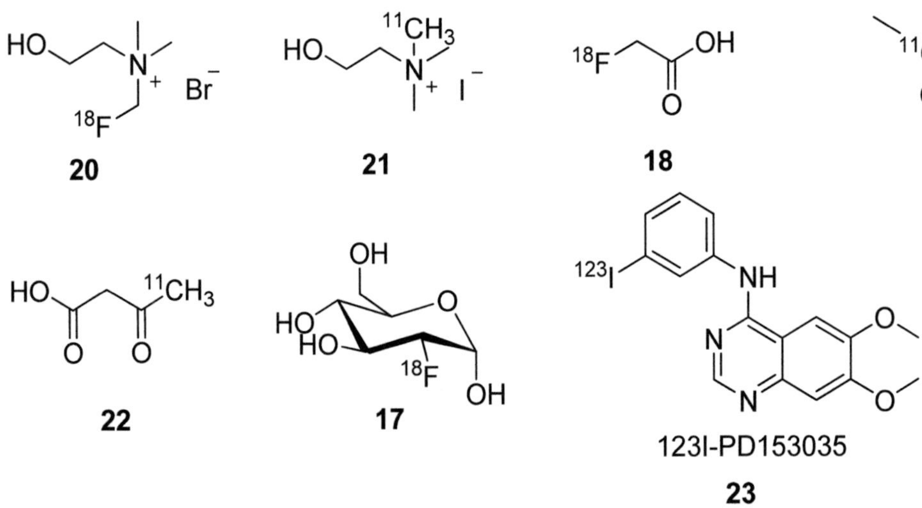

Scheme 4. Other small molecular imaging probes for prostate cancer.

5. Conclusion

Molecular imaging probes represent an important, growing class of chemical compounds for biology, pharmaceutical sciences, preclinic and clinic studies and further application. In conjunction with the imaging modality (such as PET, SPECT, MRI and etc), the identification of molecular imaging targets and the development of new labeled molecular probes for those targets are crucial for expanding the capability of in vivo molecular imaging for biological research, molecular diagnostics and drug discovery. In the post genomics era, there is the opportunity to advance probes to the point where they can target specific biochemical signatures associated with disease, including prostate cancer. Because changes in biochemistry occur before diseases reach an advanced stage, molecular imaging probes will foster earlier and more personalized diagnosis of disease. Herein, the abilities of various probes to assess different functional and molecular characteristics for prostate cancer are being explored and reviewed. The advantages and limitations of imaging agents for prostate cancer were outlined in Table 1.

Table 1.Advantages and limitations of probes used in clinical and preclinical trials for prostate cancer.

Probes for prostate cancer	Advantages	Limitations	Reference
1	fast tumor uptake, prolonged retention of radioactivity	rapid metabolic rate, not sensitive enough	21, 22, 23
2, 3, 4	stablity, easy for 11C label, high affinity	instability of the 11C labeled precursor, low radiolabeled yield	24
13, 14, 15	easy for synthesization, specificity, muti-labeled methods	not specific enough (mouse kidneys, also express PSMA)	31, 33, 34, 35, 36,
17	clinical use, safety	not sensitive enough, low cellular uptake	39, 40, 41
18, 19	clinical use, high uptake	short physical half-life of positron-emitting radionuclide (19)	51, 52
20, 21	clinical use, high sensitivity and specificity, suitable for PET (20)	short physical half-life of positron-emitting radionuclide (21)	53, 54

6. Perspective

Currently, imaging probes for prostate cancer are focused on the construction that yield an increased selectivity and sensitiveness of measurements per examination, thus higher resolution and quantification accuracy is required. Due to the complication of case difference and personalized conditions, more accurate and more efficient forward and inversion problems for improving the quantification accuracy will be speed up. The design, synthesis and application of dual- and multi-modality probe will be a hot research area, which may be the next generation of probe. The combination of different fuctional modality undoubtly will improve the accuracy of diagnosis and analysis to prostate cancer. On the other hand, a targeted gene-therapy approach is also being developed to activate the immune system to recognize prostate cancer cells. To discovery probes based on labeled gene and related macromelecule and these types of approaches might provide a new direction of prostate cancer therapies. We believe that such imaging probes will play a vital role in our further understanding of prostate cancer, in early detection and in the design of effective treatments.

7. Acknowledgement

We thank the financial supports from National Natural Foundation Science of China (30900377), Program of New Century Excellent Talents in University (NCET-09-0800), and the Fundamental Research Funds for the Central Universities.

8. References

[1] Adams J. The case of scirrhous of the prostate gland with corresponding affliction of the lymphatic glands in the lumbar region and in the pelvis. Lancet, 1853, 1, 393.

[2] Greenlee RT, Hill-Harmon MB, Murray T, and Thun M. Cancer statistics, 2001. CA Cancer J. Clin., 2001, 51, 15-36.

[3] Denmeade SR, and Isaacs JT. A history of prostate cancer treatment. Nat. Rev. Cancer, 2002, 2, 389-396.

[4] Leach F. Targeting prostate-specific membrane antigen in cancer therapy: can molecular medicine be brought to the surface? Cancer Biol. Ther., 2004, 3, 559-560.

[5] Jemal A, Bray F, Center MM, Ferlay J, Ward E, and Forman D. Global cancer statistics. CA Cancer J. Clin., 2011, 61, 69–90.

[6] Djulbegovic M, Beyth RJ, Neuberger MM, Stoffs TL, Vieweg J, Djulbegovic B, and Dahm P. Screening for prostate cancer: systematic review and meta-analysis of randomised controlled trials. Bri. Med. J., 2010, 341, c4543.

[7] Isaacs WB, Xu J, and Walsh PC. Prostate cancer: biology, genetics and the new therapeutics (eds Chung L, Isaacs W, and Simons J), Humana,Totowa, New Jersey, 2001, 13–28.

[8] Denmeade SR, and Isaacs JT. Development of prostate cancer treatment: the good news. The Prostate, 2004, 58, 211-224.

[9] Weissleder R. Molecular imaging in cancer. Science, 2006, 312, 1168-1171.

[10] Herschman HR. Molecular imaging: looking at problems seeing solutions. Science, 2003, 302, 605-608.

[11] Zeng W, and Miao W. Development of small molecular probes for the molecular imaging of apoptosis. Anti-Cancer Agents in Med. Chem., 2009, 9, 986-995.

[12] Huang J, Zeng W, Zhou M, and Gao F. Progress of the dual-modality probes for molecular imaging. Acta Biophy. Sinica, 2011, 27, 301-311.

[13] Fenton MA, Shuster TD, Fertig AM, Taplin ME, Kolvenbag G, Bubley GJ, and Balk SP. Functional characterization of mutant androgen receptors from androgen-independent prostate cancer. Clin. Cancer Res., 1997, 3, 1383–1388.

[14] Craft N, and Sawyers CL. Mechanistic concepts in androgen-dependence of prostate cancer. Cancer Met. Rev., 1998, 17, 421–427.

[15] Jadvar H. Molecular imaging of prostate cancer: a concise synopsis. Mol. Imaging, 2009, 8, 56–64.

[16] He Y, Yin DG, Perera MA, Kirkovsky L, Stourman N, and Li W. Novel ligands with high binding affinity and potent functional activity for the androgen receptor. Eur. J. Med. Chem., 2002, 37, 619–634.

[17] Dalton JT, Mukherjee A, Zhu Z, Kirkovsky L, and Miller DD. Discovery of nonsteroidal androgens. Biochem. Biophys. Res. Commun., 1998, 244, 1–4.

[18] Zanzonico P, Finn R, Pentlow KS, Erdi Y, Beattie B, Akhurst T, Squire O, Morris M, Scher H, McCarthy T, Welch M, Larson SM, and Humm JL. PET-based radiation dosimetry in man of 18F-fluorodihydrotestosterone, a new radiotracer for imaging prostate cancer. J. Nucl. Med., 2004, 45, 1966-1971.
[19] Zanzonico P. Prostate cancer: 16β-[18F] fluoro-5α-dihydrotesterone (FDHT) whole-body positron emission tomography. Methods of Cancer Diagnosis, Therapy and Prognosis, 2008, Volume 2, III, 521-530.
[20] Bonasera TA, O'Neil JP, Xu M, Dobkin JA, Cutler PD, Lich LL, Choe YS, Katzenellenbogen JA, and Welch MJ. Preclinical evaluation of fluorine-18-labeled androgen receptor ligands in baboons. J. Nucl. Med., 1996, 37, 1009 -1015.
[21] Larson SM, Morris M, Gunther I, Beattie B, Humm JL, and Akhurst TA. Tumor localization of 16h-18F-fluoro-5a-dihydrotestosterone versus 18F-FDG in patients with progressive, metastatic prostate cancer. J. Nucl. Med., 2004, 45, 366–373.
[22] Zanzonico PB, Finn R, Pentlow KS, Erdi Y, Beattie B, and Akhurst T. PET-based radiation dosimetry in man of 18F-fluorodihydrotestosterone, a new radiotracer for imaging prostate cancer. J. Nucl. Med., 2004, 45,1966- 1971.
[23] Dehdashti F, Joel P, Michalski JM, Dence CS, Siegel BA, and Katzenellenbogen JA. Positron tomographic assessment of androgen receptors in prostatic carcinoma. Eur. J. Nucl. Med. Mol. Imag., 2005, 32, 344–350.
[24] Jacobson O, Laky D, Carlson KE, Elgavish S, Gozin M, Even-Sapir E, Leibovitc I, Gutman M, Chisin R, Katzenellenbogen JA, and Mishani E. Chiral dimethylamine flutamide derivatives--modeling, synthesis, androgen receptor affinities and carbon-11 labeling. Nucl. Med. Biol., 2006, 33, 695–704.
[25] Jacobson O, Bechor Y, Icar A, Novak N, Birman A, Marom H, Fadeeva L, Golan E, Leibovitch I, Gutman M, Even-Sapir E, Chisin R, Gozin M, and Mishani E. Prostate cancer PET bioprobes: synthesis of [18F]-radiolabeled hydroxyflutamide derivatives. Bioorg. Med. Chem., 2005, 13, 6195–6205.
[26] Parent EE, Dence CS, Jenks C, Sharp TL, Welch M, and Katzenellenbogen JA. Synthesis and biological evaluation of [18F]bicalutamide, 4-[76Br]bromobicalutamide, and 4-[76Br]-bromo-thiobicalutamide as nonsteroidal androgens for prostate cancer imaging. J. Med. Chem., 2007, 50, 1028–1040.
[27] He H, Morely JE, Silva-Lopez E, Bottenus B, Montajano M, Fugate GA, Twamley B, and Benny PD. Synthesis and characterization of nonsteroidal-linked M(CO)3+ (M = 99mTc, Re) compounds based on the androgen receptor targeting molecule flutamide. Bioconjugate Chem., 2009, 20, 78–86.
[28] Marom H, Miller K, Bechor-Bar Y, Tsarfaty G, Satchi-Fainaro R, and Gozin M. Toward development of targeted nonsteroidal antiandrogen-1,4,7,10-tetraazacyclododecane-1,4,7,10-tetraacetic acid-gadolinium complex for prostate cancer diagnostics. J. Med. Chem., 2010, 53, 6316–6325.
[29] Lofters A, Juffs HG, Pond GR, and Tannock IF. "PSA-itis": knowledge of serum prostate specific antigen and other causes of anxiety in men with metastatic prostate cancer. J. Urol., 2002, 168, 2516–2520.
[30] Dreicer R. Metastatic prostate cancer: assessment of response to systemic therapy. Semin. Urol. Oncol., 1997, 15, 28–32.

[31] Gregor PD, Wolchok JD, Turaga V. Induction of autoantibodies to syngeneic prostate-specific membrane antigen by xenogeneic vaccination. Int. J. Cancer., 2005, 116, 415–421.

[32] O'Keefe DS, Bacich DJ, and Heston WD. Comparative analysis of prostate-specific membrane antigen (PSMA) versus a prostate-specific membrane antigen-like gene. The Prostate, 2004, 58, 200–210.

[33] Fair WR, Israeli RS, and Heston WD. Prostate-specific membrane antigen. The Prostate, 1997, 32,140–148.

[34] Foss CA, Mease RC, Fan H, Wang Y, Ravert HT, Dannals RF, Olszewski RT, Heston WD, Kozikowski AP, and Pomper MG. Radiolabeled small-molecule ligands for prostate-specific membrane antigen: in vivo imaging in experimental models of prostate cancer. Clin. Cancer Res., 2005, 11, 4022–4028.

[35] Banerjee SR, Foss CA, Castanares M, Mease RC, Byun Y, Fox JJ, Hilton J, Lupold SE, Kozikowski AP, and Pomper MG. Synthesis and evaluation of technetium-99m- and rhenium-labeled inhibitors of the prostate-specific membrane antigen (PSMA). J. Med. Chem., 2008, 51, 4504–4517.

[36] Mease RC, Dusich CL, Foss CA, Ravert HT, Dannals RF, Seidel J, Prideaux A, Fox JJ, Sgouros G, Kozikowski AP, and Pomper MG. N-[N-[(S)-1,3-Dicarboxypropyl]carbamoyl]-4-[18F]fluorobenzyl-L-cysteine, [18F]DCFBC: a new imaging probe for prostate cancer. Clin. Cancer Res., 2008, 14, 3036–3043.

[37] Serda RE, Adolphi NL, Bisoffi M, and Sillerud LO. Targeting and cellular trafficking of magnetic nanoparticles for prostate cancer imaging. Mol. Imaging, 2007, 6, 277–288.

[38] Chen Y, Dhara S, Banerjee SR, Byun Y, Pullambhatla M, Mease RC, and Pomper MG. A low molecular weight PSMA-based fluorescent imaging agent for cancer. Biochem. Biophys. Res. Commun., 2009, 390, 624–629.

[39] Effert PJ, Bares R. Handt S, Wolff JM, Bull D, and Jakes G. Metabolic imaging of untreated prostate cancer by positron emission tomography with 18-fluorinelabeled deoxyglucose. J. Urol., 1996, 155, 994–998.

[40] Oyama N, Akino H, Suzuki Y, Kanamaru H, Ishida H, Tanase K, Sadato N, Yonekura Y, and Okada K. FDG PET for evaluating the change of glucose metabolism in prostate cancer after androgen ablation. Nucl. Med. Commun., 2001, 22, 963–969.

[41] Shreve PD, Grossmann HB, Gross MD, and Wahl RL. Metastatic prostate cancer: initial findings of PET with 2-deoxy-2-[F-18]-fluoro-D-glucose. Radiology, 1996, 199, 751–756.

[42] Mathupala SP, Ko YH, and Pederson PL. Hexokinase II: cancer's double-edged sword acting as both facilitator and gatekeeper of malignancy when bound to mitochondria. Oncogene, 2006, 25, 4777–4786.

[43] Smith TA. Mammalian hexokinases and their abnormal expression in cancer. Br. J. Biomed. Sci., 2000, 57, 170–178.

[44] Effert P, Beniers AJ, Tamimi Y, Handt S, and Jakse G. Expression of glucose transporter 1 (GLUT-1) in cell lines and clinical specimen from human prostate adenocarcinoma. Anticancer Res., 2004, 24, 3057–3063.

[45] Chandler JD, Williams ED, Slavin JL, Best JD, and Rogers S. Expression and localization of GLUT1 and GLUT12 in prostate carcinoma. Cancer, 2003, 97, 2035–2042.

[46] Ponde DE, Dence CS, Oyama N, Kim J, Tai YC, Laforest R, Siegel BA, and Welch MJ. 18F-Fluoroacetate: a potential acetate analog for prostate tumors imaging-in vivo evaluation of 18F-fluoroacetate versus 11C-acetate. J. Nucl. Med., 2007, 48, 420–428.

[47] DeGrado TR, Coleman RE, Wang S, Baldwin SW, Orr MD, Robertson CN, Polascik TJ, and Price DT. Synthesis and evaluation of 18F-labeled choline as an oncologic tracer for positron emission tomography: initial findings in prostate cancer. Cancer Res., 2001, 61, 110–117.

[48] Shreve PD, Lannone P, and Weinhold P. Cellular metabolism of [1-C14]-acetate in prostate cancer cells in vitro. J. Nucl. Med., 2002, 43, S272.

[49] Liu Y. Fatty acid oxidation is a dominant bioenergetic pathway in prostate cancer. Prostate Cancer Prostatic Dis., 2006, 9, 230–234.

[50] Vavere AL, Kridel SJ, Wheeler FB, and Lewis JS. 1-11C-Acetate as a PET radiopharmaceutical for imaging fatty acid synthase expression in prostate cancer. J. Nucl. Med., 2008, 49, 327–334.

[51] Oyama N, Akino H, and Kanamaru H. 11C-Acetate PET imaging of prostate cancer. J. Nucl. Med., 2002, 43, 181–186.

[52] Kotzerke J, Volkmer BG, Neumaier B, Gschwend JE, Hautmann RE, and Reske SN. Carbon-11 acetate positron emission tomography can detect local recurrence of prostate cancer. Eur. J. Nucl. Med. Mol. Imaging., 2002, 29, 1380–1384.

[53] DeGrado TR, Baldwin SW, Wang S, Orr MD, Liao RP, Friedman HS, Reiman R, Price DT, and Coleman RE.. Synthesis and evaluation of 18F-labeled ncholine analogs as oncologic PET tracers. J. Nucl. Med., 2001, 42, 1805–1814.

[54] Hara T, Kosaka N, and Kishi H. PET imaging of prostate cancer using carbon-11-choline. J. Nucl. Med., 1998, 39, 990–995.

[55] Pflug BR, Pecher SM, Brink AW, Nelson JB, and Foster BA. Increased fatty acid synthase expression and activity during progression of prostate cancer in the TRAMP model. The Prostate, 2003, 57, 245–254.

[56] Authier S, Tremblay S, Dumulon V, et al Authier S, Tremblay S, Dumulon V, Dubuc C, Ouellet R, Lecomte R, Cunnane SC, and Benard F. [11C]Acetoacetate utilization by breast and prostate tumors: a PET and biodistribution study in mice. Mol. Imaging Biol., 2008, 10, 217–223.

[57] Fozing T, Scheuer C, and Samnick S. Synthesis and initial tumor affinity testing of iodine-123 labelled EGFR-affine agents as potential imaging probes for hormone-refractory prostate cancer. Eur. J. Med. Chem., 2010, 45, 3780-3786.

[58] De Visser M, Bernard HF, Erion JL, Schmidt MA, Srinivasan A, Waser B, Reubi JC, Krenning EP, and de Jong M. Novel 111In-labeled bombesin analogues for molecular imaging of prostate tumors. Eur. J. Nucl. Med. Mol. Imaging, 2007, 34, 1228–1238.

[59] Zhang X, Cai W, Cao F, Schreibmann E, Wu Y, Wu JC, Xing L, and Chen X. 18F-Labeled bombesin analogs for targeting GRP receptorexpressing prostate cancer. J. Nucl. Med., 2006, 47, 492–501.

[60] Cai W, and Chen X. Multimodality molecular imaging of tumor angiogenesis. J. Nucl. Med., 2008, 49, 113S–128S.

[61] Zhang X, Xiong Z, Wu Y, Cai W, Tseng JR, Gambhir SS, and Chen X. Quantitative PET imaging of tumor integrin alphavbeta 3 expression with 18F-FRGD2. J. Nucl. Med., 2006, 47, 113–121.